Hormonal Control of the Hypothalamo-Pituitary-Gonadal Axis

BIOCHEMICAL ENDOCRINOLOGY

Series Editor: Kenneth W. McKerns

STRUCTURE AND FUNCTION OF THE GONADOTROPINS
Edited by Kenneth W. McKerns

SYNTHESIS AND RELEASE OF ADENOHYPOPHYSEAL HORMONES
Edited by Marian Jutisz and Kenneth W. McKerns

REPRODUCTIVE PROCESSES AND CONTRACEPTION
Edited by KennethW. McKerns

HORMONALLY ACTIVE BRAIN PEPTIDES: Structure and Function
Edited by Kenneth W. McKerns and Vladimir Pantić

REGULATION OF GENE EXPRESSION BY HORMONES
Edited by Kenneth W. McKerns

REGULATION OF TARGET CELL RESPONSIVENESS, Volumes 1 and 2
Edited by Kenneth W. McKerns, Asbjørn Aakvaag, and Vidar Hansson

HORMONAL CONTROL OF THE HYPOTHALAMO-PITUITARY-GONADAL AXIS
edited by Kenneth W. McKerns and Zvi Naor

Hormonal Control of the Hypothalamo-Pituitary-Gonadal Axis

Edited by

Kenneth W. McKerns

International Foundation for Biochemical Endocrinology
Blue Hill Falls, Maine

and

Zvi Naor

Weizmann Institute of Science
Rehovot, Israel

Springer Science+Business Media, LLC

Library of Congress Cataloging in Publication Data

Main entry under title:

Hormonal control of the hypothalamo-pituitary-gonadal axis.
(Biochemical endocrinology)
"Proceedings of the eleventh annual meeting of the International Foundation for Biochemical Endocrinology, held October 2–7, 1983, at the Weizmann Institute of Science, Rehovot, Israel"—T.p. verso.
Includes bibliographical references and index.
1. Hyptothalamo-hypophyseal system—Congresses. 2. Hypothalamic hormones—Congresses. 3. Gonadotropin—Congresses. I. McKerns, Kenneth W. II. Naor, Zvi. III. International Foundation for Biochemical Endocrinology. IV. Series. [DNLM: 1. Hypothalamo-Hypophyseal System—physiology—congresses. 2. Pituitary Hormone Releasing Hormones—physiology—congresses. IN696 11th 1983h / WK 515 I588 1983h]
QP188.H9H67 1984 599′.01′42 84-13415
ISBN 978-1-4684-9962-9 ISBN 978-1-4684-9960-5 (eBook)
DOI 10.1007/978-1-4684-9960-5

Proceedings of the Eleventh Annual meeting of the International Foundation for Biochemical Endocrinology, held October 2–7, 1983, at the Weizmann Institute of Science, Rehovot, Israel

Originally published by Plenum Press, New York and London in 1984
Softcover reprint of the hardcover 1st edition 1984
A Division of Plenum Publishing Corporation
233 Spring Street, New York, N.Y. 10013

PREFACE

The eleventh monograph and meeting of the Foundation on "Hormonal Control of the Hypothalamo-Pituitary-Gonadal Axis" was held in October 1983 at the Weizmann Institute of Science. This monograph honors the memory of Professor Hans R. Lindner, a productive and innovative scientist greatly respected and admired by his colleagues.

When addressing the opening session I remarked that my impression of the Weizmann Institute was one or two large buildings housing the various departments. This was my first visit to Israel and I was overwhelmed by the beautiful semi-tropical gardens of the institute, in a setting of shrubs and trees, orange groves and flowers. Sited among this seventy-five acres are over fifty buildings and residential areas for the staff and visiting scientists. I saw pictures of this area when Dr. Chaim Weizmann founded in 1934, the Daniel Sieff Research Institute, the forerunner of the Weizmann Institute. The site was sand dunes without a blade of grass. That the desert shall bloom is illustrative of the progress made in Israel.

The topics of the monograph are grouped into twelve sections. They are: "Neuroendocrine Control of Gonadotropin Secretion," "Molecular Aspects of GnRH Biosynthesis, Release and Degradation," "GnRH Receptors and Action in the Pituitary," "Secretory Processes in the Pituitary," "Gonadotropin Antagonists," "Endocrine Regulation of Ovarian Functions," "Prolactin," "Hormones and Gene Expression," "Regulation of Testicular Function," "Extrapituitary Effects of GnRH," "Interaction of Opiates and Gonadotropins," "GnRH Analogs: Clinical Uses in the Management of Fertility and Cancer."

The chairpersons for the sessions were B. Kerdelhue, A. Beloff-Chain, S.M. McCann, D. Kanazir, M. Fridkin, M. Aubert, Z. Naor, J. de Konig, M. Dufau, Y. Orly, G. Ross, B. Eckstein, B. Lunenfeld, R. Shalgi, A. Tixier-Vidal, M. Ben-David, A.M. Kaye, I. Gozes, K. Catt, E. Bedrak, B. Cooke, Z. Laron, R. Sharpe, D. Ayalon, P.F. Kraicer, J. Sandow, H. Zakut, S. Segal and G. Leyendecker.

This monograph represents an interdisciplinary approach to the problem of regulation of gonadotropin secretion and action. Morphological, physiological, clinical and biochemical aspects are reviewed, with emphasis on recent findings.

This volume reviews the state of the art in the field of hypothalamo-pituitary-gonadal axis and is relevant to endocrinologists, reproductive biologists, obstetricians and gynecologists.

The twelfth meeting and monograph of the Foundation will be held in September at Caxtat, near Dubrovnik, Yugoslavia. Professor Vladimir Pantić will be organizer of the local arrangements. The topic will be "Neuroendocrine Correlates of Stress."

Kenneth W. McKerns
Zvi Naor

ACKNOWLEDGMENTS

The Editors express their thanks to the Organizing Committee of the Meeting, consisting of: Nava Dekel, Fortune Kohen, Yitzhak Koch, Zvi Naor (Chairman) and Uriel Zor.

The Meeting was supported by grants from: The Israel Academy of Sciences and Humanities; the Israel National Council for Research and Development; The Israel Ministry of Health; The Maurice and Gabriela Goldschleger Conference Foundation at the Weizmann Institute of Science; The University of Tel-Aviv; The Ben-Gurion University of the Negev; The Israel Society of Endocrinology; Biotechnology General (Israel) Ltd., Rehovot; Eldan Electronic Instrument Co. Ltd., Jerusalem; Inter-Yeda Ltd., Nes-Ziona; Miles-Yeda Ltd., Rehovot; Fering Sweden; Organon International B.V., The Netherlands; and Schering Aktiengesellschaft, West Germany.

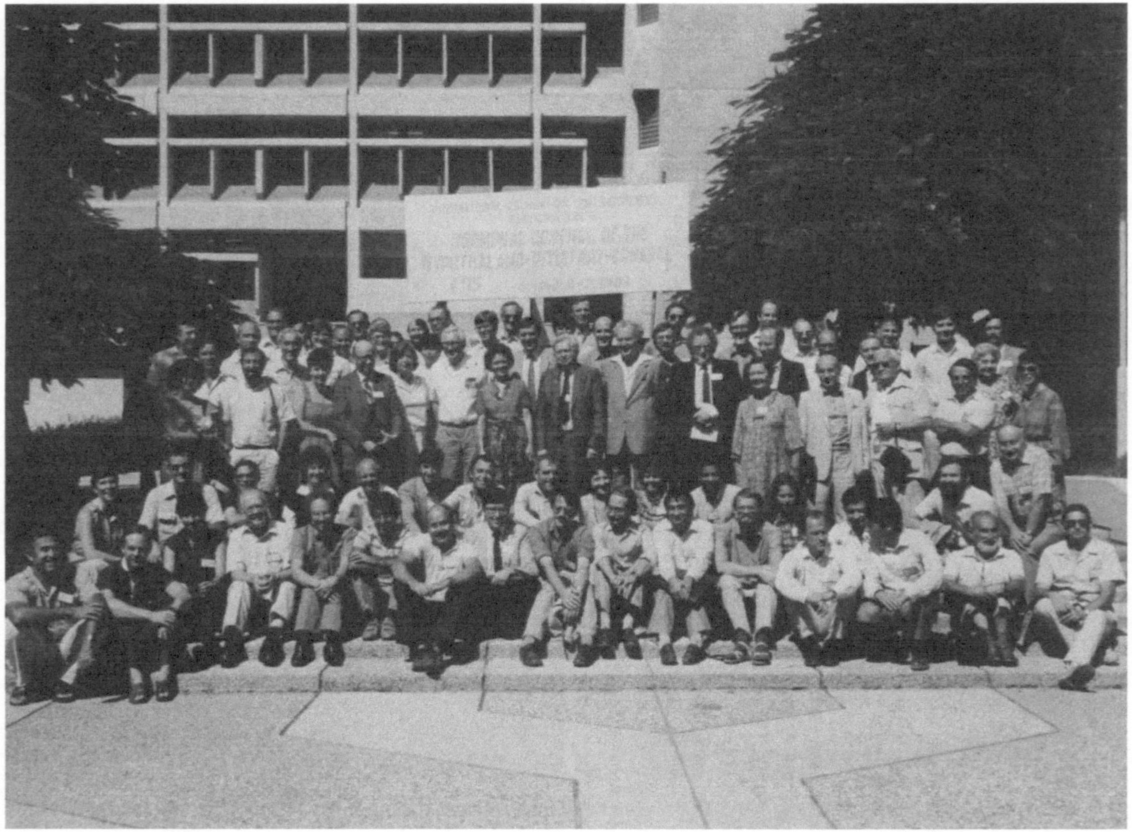

INTERNATIONAL FOUNDATION FOR BIOCHEMICAL ENDOCRINOLOGY
HORMONAL CONTROL OF THE HYPOTHALAMO-PITUITARY-GONADAL AXIS
OCTOBER 2-7, 1983

CONTENTS

GnRH RECEPTORS AND ACTION IN THE PITUITARY

SECRETORY PROCESSES IN THE PITUITARY

GONADOTROPIN ANTAGONISTS

ENDOCRINE REGULATION OF OVARIAN FUNCTIONS

PROLACTIN

HORMONES AND GENE EXPRESSION

GnRH ANALOGS: CLINICAL USES IN THE MANAGEMENT OF FERTILITY AND CANCER

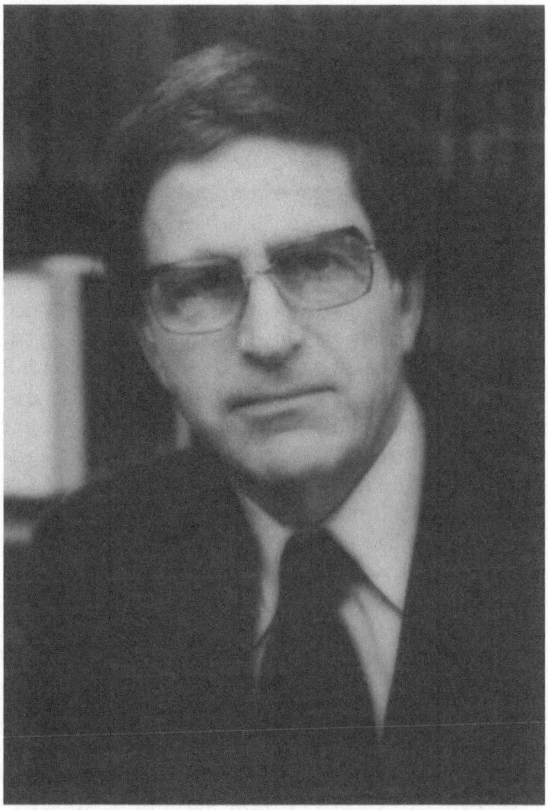

IN MEMORY OF THE LATE HANS R. LINDNER

April 21, 1922 - November 19, 1982

Hans Lindner was born in Stettin, Germany. At the rise of the Nazi regime, he and his family emigrated to the Land of Israel, then Palestine. Hans attended the Mikve-Israel Agricultural School (1938-1940) and specialized in animal husbandry. He continued to serve there as herdmaster in addition to joining the "Hagganah", the pre-state defense force. Hence, it was only at the end of the War of Independence in 1949 that he felt free to continue with his studies.

After graduating as a B.V.Sc at Sydney University, Australia (1954) he was encouraged by Dr. K.A. Ferguson to take an interest in research. This period established the continued interest of the young Hans Lindner in the functional roles of steroid hormones. In 1957, he was awarded the Commonwealth Scholarship for Advanced Studies and proceeded with his Ph.D. studies at Cambridge, under the supervision of Dr. T. Mann, F.R.S. Upon his return to Australia (1961), he established a laboratory for the endocrinology of steroid hormones at C.S.I.R.O., near Sydney.

Hans returned to Israel in 1964, joined the Weizmann Institute and in 1967 succeeded Dr. M.C. Schelesnyak as Chairman of the Department of Biodynamics, which was later renamed the Department of Hormone Research. As architect of the Department, he attracted a multi-disciplinary research group, which, within a short time, was in the forefront of current efforts to comprehend the endocrine regulation of ovarian function. These studies combined, in a unique way, approaches and methodologies of modern cell biology, biochemistry and molecular biology, with due emphasis on mechanistic and ultrastructural analysis and thus enabled in-depth understanding of complicated biological interactions and sequences. To assist these studies, as well as to serve the needs of clinical laboratories, he initiated the development of novel assay methods of high specificity and sensitivity.

Besides his activities within the Department of Hormone Research, Hans devoted much of his time to academic duties at the Weizmann Institute. He served on the advisory boards of several national and international associations. Hans Lindner's scientific contributions are widely recognized and too numerous to mention. Among the many honors bestowed on him, he was awarded the Hermann Zondek Prize for Endocrine and Metabolic Research (1972), the Israel Prize for Life Sciences (1979), the Rothschild Prize in Biology (1981) and the Axel Munthe Award in the field of Reproduction (1982). He was elected a member of the Israel Academy of Sciences and Humanities (1979), and an honorary member of the German Endocrine Society (1978). Hans was awarded honorary degrees by Cambridge University (1977) and by the University of Göteborg (1981).

In Rehovot, Hans established a warm home together with his wife, Karin, and here his son Ari and daughter Anat were born. Hans was an intellectual, possessing vast and in-depth knowledge. His interests were not limited to the biomedical sciences but also covered a variety of fields such as music and art. Hans set a fine example of modesty and trust; he possessed a warm and charming personality. Even under pressure, he always kept his composure and sense of humor. For many years he courageously fought his cruel disease and succumbed at the peak of his scientific career. Hans Lindner was ever the gentleman, whose wise counsel, professional competence, refinement and humanity will be missed by the members of the scientific community who had the privilege of being acquainted with him.

Yitzhak Koch

ROLE OF PEPTIDES IN THE CONTROL OF GONADOTROPIN SECRETION

S.M. McCANN, G.D. Snyder, S.R. Ojeda, M.D. Lumpkin, A. Ottlecz, and W.K. Samson

Department of Physiology, University of Texas Health Science Center, 5323 Harry Hines Blvd., Dallas, TX 75235

INTRODUCTION

In this chapter we will review the contributions, particularly from this laboratory, on the control of the gonadotroph by peptides acting at either the hypothalamic or pituitary level. The principal direct control is provided by LHRH which was discovered in 1960[1] and synthesized in 1971[2]. We will begin by describing the localization of LHRH in the brain, and then move to a discussion of its action on the pituitary gland. This will be followed by an examination of putative synaptic transmitters involved in control of LHRH release which include a variety of monamines and peptides. Most of these mechanisms appear to operate via the intervention of prostaglandins. Finally we will discuss recent evidence indicating the probable existance of a separate FSH- releasing factor.

Localization of LHRH in the brain. Radioimmunoassay of sections cut from the brain or of punches removed from it confirmed the early localization of LHRH by bioassay.[3] Immunocytochemical localization of the perikarya and terminals of LHRH neurons was also accomplished.[4] From all of this work it is now apparent that there is a system of LHRH neurons with cell bodies in the preoptic region and long axons which extend along the base of the brain to reach the median eminence. In most species there is also another population of LHRH neurons with cell bodies in the arcuate nucleus and short axons extending to the median eminence. It is now apparent that LHRH neurons also have axons extending down into the brain stem in the region of the central gray, a region known to be involved in sexual behavior.[5] This finding is very recent. In addition there is some evidence for projections of LHRH fibers into the amygdala and other brain regions. Very recently it has been shown that there are LHRH neurons in the olfactory system.[6] LHRH cells have even been found in gold fish retina.[7]

Actions of LHRH on the pituitary. LHRH acts on the pituitary to promote rapid release of LH and to a lesser extent FSH from the gland. Pulse injection may lead to release of only LH; however, more prolonged exposure of the gland to the peptide leads to significant FSH release.[8] The FSH-releasing potency is often of the order of 20% of the LH releasing potency; however, the FSH-releasing potency varies depending on the hormonal state of the animal and the frequency of LHRH injections. In immature rat and human the peptide tends to produce greater FSH release.[9] Frequent pulses of the peptide provoke primarily LH release, however, with more infrequent pulses a predominance of FSH release appears to occur, perhaps related in part to the longer half-time of disappearance of FSH from the circulation.[10] Responsiveness to LHRH is quite high in the castrate.[11] Following administration of estrogen to the castrate female, responsiveness declines rapidly in rat, man and other species, and this is followed by augmented responsiveness to the peptide.[12,13] In other words there is a biphasic response, first inhibition and subsequent augmentation in response, produced by estrogen. Progesterone appears to synergize with estrogen in the latter half of the cycle in rat and man to hold gonadotropin secretion in check.[14,15] Injection of progesterone in the presence of estrogen can initially augment and then suppress responsiveness to the decapeptide in both rats and humans[15,16] Testosterone has an inhibitory action suppressing responsiveness.[13]

During the menstrual cycle and rat estrous cycle, responsiveness to LHRH increases presumably because of release of estrogen from the developing follicles. Responsiveness becomes maximal just prior to the preovulatory discharge of LH.[13,15,17] This further enhancement in responsiveness is due not only to the action of estrogen but also to the so called "self-priming action" of LHRH which augments response of the pituitary to subsequent LHRH[18,19]. The estrogen secreted by the follicles brings about enhanced LHRH release by an action on the preoptic region and this then produces the self-priming action. Responsiveness to LHRH may increase 50-fold above minimal levels at the time of the preovulatory release in man and rat. In the progestational phase of the cycle, responsiveness is suppressed presumably because of inhibitory actions of both estrogen and progesterone. Responsiveness with regard to FSH release follows a similar pattern.[13,17]

There is clear evidence that there is increased LHRH release from the hypothalamus at the time of the preovulatory LH surge in rat[13] and suggestive evidence for this phenomenon in primates.[20] Recently, Knobil and his coworkers have been able to reinitiate menstrual cycles by pulsatile administration of LHRH[21] in Rhesus monkeys with arcuate nuclear lesions which suppress gonadotropin release. Spies and coworkers on the other hand have been unable to induced cyclic release of gonadotropins with pulsatile LHRH administration in Rhesus monkeys with stalk-sections and a permanent barrier placed between the cut ends of the stalk to block regeneration by portal vessels.[22] Further work is necessary to resolve this controversy.

Mechanism of action of LHRH at the pituitary. The initial event involved in the LH-releasing action of LHRH in combination with specific LHRH receptors on the surface of gonadotrophs. This has now been clearly demonstrated utilizing slowly degradable agonist analogs of LHRH.[23] The number of receptors appears to fluctuate under various conditions; noteworthy is a decline in receptors at the time of the preovulatory surge of LH. Whether this decline is due to an actual decrease in receptor numbers or to occupancy by LHRH released in increased amounts at this time of the cycle remains to be determined.

According to one theory, the receptor-hormone interaction activates adenylate cyclase leading to generation of cAMP. This cAMP is visualized to act on a protein kinase which phosphorylates proteins in the cell membrane leading to uptake of calcium. This then activates exocytosis of LH secretory granules.[24] Unfortunately, the early enthusiasm for this concept is waning. It has not been possible to demonstrate increases in cAMP following exposure to LHRH in glands taken from female rats although delayed increases in cAMP occur in males.[25] Even in populations of partially purified female gonadotrophs there was no increase in cAMP in spite of very lusty increases in LH release. On the other hand, increases cGMP in cells and in the incubation media have been demonstrated in response to LHRH under certain conditions.[26] These observations suggested that cGMP might be more important than cAMP in the release mechanism. The delayed increases in cAMP following LHRH seen in males might be involved in synthesis of LH. Recently, however, the essentiality of an increase in cGMP has been questioned since it has been possible to obtain LH release in the face of treatments which hold cGMP levels constant.[27] It is certain that increased availability of calcium is required for the release process since removal of calcium from the medium or addition of calcium-chelating agents blocks release.[28]

The most recent series of biochemical reactions to be

associated with the stimulation of the gonadotroph by LHRH are those of 1) the phosphatidylinositol cycle and 2) the metabolism of arachidonic acid. Within the last two years, it was reported that LHRH can stimulate the rate of [^{32}P]orthophosphate incorporation into phosphatidylinositol (PI)[29]. This finding is indicative that LHRH stimulates the metabolic turnover of PI (e.g., the PI cycle)[30]. This has been further substantiated by a recent report that the extent of the LHRH-stimulation of the PI cycle in the anterior pituitary varies in direct proportion with the number of LHRH receptors present in the anterior pituitary at specific stages of the estrous cycle of female rats[31].

It is now apparent, although as yet unproven, that one or more of the metabolites of the PI cycle plays an important role in the mechanism of LHRH-stimulated LH secretion. Release of arachidonic acid from phospholipids, most likely from PI, is essential for LHRH-stimulated LH secretion to occur[32]. Recent studies have also suggested that the arachidonic acid which is liberated in response to an LHRH stimulation is rapidly converted to one or more oxygenated derivatives that are essential for LHRH-stimulated LH secretion to occur[33,34]. We have recently reported that a primary epoxygenated metabolite of arachidonic acid, 5,6-eicosatrienoic acid (5,6-EET) is capable of mimicking the action of LHRH on dispersed anterior pituitary cells[33]. In vitro, the 5,6-EET stimulated the secretion of LH to equal or greater levels than does a maximal LHRH stimulation. A second observation contributes even more convincing evidence that the 5,6-EET plays an essential role in the mechanism of LHRH action. We have found that in the presence of eicosatetrayenoic acid (ETYA), a general inhibitor of AA acid metabolism, addition of the 5,6-EET to the incubation medium of a dispersed anterior pituitary cell culture circumvents the ETYA blockade and results in stimulated LH secretion[34]. Moreover, we now have evidence that the 5,6-EET also mobilizes Ca^{2+} from prelabeled cells in a manner which is parallel to that observed during an LHRH stimulation[35].

There are several other epoxygenated arachidonic acid metabolites and at least one lipoxygenated[33] arachidonic acid metabolite which are capable of stimulating secretion of LH in vitro. These compounds, however, do not appear to have nearly the biological potency of the 5,6-EET[34]. At this point in our studies we are reasonably convinced that LHRH stimulates the metabolic breakdown of phosphatidylinositol which is followed by the liberation of arachidonic acid. Our evidence also suggests that the epoxygenation of arachidonic acid is essential for LHRH-stimulated secretion to occur. Finally, we are currently of the belief that the production of the 5,6-EET or a metabolite derived directly from the 5,6-EET will be proven to be an essential participant in the cascade of events leading from LHRH-stimulation of the gonadotroph to LH secretion.

It is now apparent that continued high dose administration of LHRH, although initially stimulatory, is eventually inhibitory to gonadotropin release.[10] The mechanism of this paradoxical inhibitory effect is not known but may involve down regulation of receptors. Apparently the gland can only accept pulsatile release of LHRH or it becomes desensitized to the peptide in some manner. This phenomenon is important to keep in mind in attempting to induce ovulation with LHRH.

Putative synaptic transmitters involved in control of LHRH release. The LHRH neurons are in potential synaptic contact with a host of other transmitters, monoaminergic and peptidergic, and consequently a great deal of effort has been directed towards delineating the role of various putative synaptic transmitters in controlling LHRH release. In the median eminence there is an enormous number of terminals which contain various putative transmitters. For example, there is an overlap of the LHRH terminals in the median eminence with those containing dopamine, somatostatin and TRH. The median eminence also contains terminals which presumably contain γ-aminobutyric acid (GABA), histamine, serotonin (5-HT) and norepinephrine.[36]

Dopamine. Early incubation studies revealed that dopamine would cause the release of LHRH from the basal hypothalamus into the medium[37]. In the meantime Fuxe and coworkers on the basis of turnover of dopamine measured histofluorescently concluded that dopamine turnover was increased in the basal tuberal region at times when LH release was decreased and vice versa. They concluded that dopamine had an inhibitory role in control of LHRH release.[38] Our *in vivo* studies instead showed a stimulatory role on the basis of increased LH release following intraventricular injection of dopamine[39].

Recently we were able to show not only stimulatory effects of dopamine following its intraventricular injection, but also inhibitory effects following large doses of dopamine given peripherally.[40] This inhibitory action apparently operates via a suppression of LHRH release since the responsiveness of the pituitary to LHRH was unimpaired following administration of apomorphine, a dopamine agonist. Apomorphine was even more effective in suppressing LH than dopamine itself. Similarly others had shown that high doses of dopamine can inhibit LH release both in rats[41] and in man.[15] Our data indicate that the dose required for the inhibitory effect is quite large and we have only observed it in the ovariectomized animal. On the other hand in the ovariectomized, steroid-primed animal the stimulatory effect has always been seen.

Negro-Vilar et al.[42] have recently evaluated the action of catecholamines in an in vitro median eminence preparation and followed the release of LHRH by radioimmunoassay. Under these conditions dopamine produced a dose-related increase in LHRH release from median eminence of male rats. The effects were blocked by the dopamine receptor blocker, pimozide.

Norepinephrine. Norepinephrine was similarly active in the median eminence incubation system and the response to norepinephrine was blocked by the alpha adrenergic receptor blocker, phentolamine.[42] Similarly both norepinehprine and epinephrine will release LHRH following their injection into the third ventricle in the ovariectomized, steroid-primed rat.[43]

Further studies have characterized the role of the α and β-adrenergic receptors in the simulation of LHRH release from median eminence fragments by norepinephrine. Phentolamine, an α receptor agonist, gave a dose-related inhibition of the release of LHRH induced by norepinephrine, with a half maximal inhibitory dose of 0.9×10^{-7}M. Complete suppression of the effects of norepinephrine were observed with phentolamine at a concentration of 5×10^{-6}M. By contrast the β receptor antagonist, propranolol, was completely ineffective at this concentration. Blockade of dopamine receptors with pimozide (10^{-6}M) failed to inhibit the action of norepinephrine.[44] Further studies indicate that the effects are probably mediated by α2 rather than α1 receptors, since the α1 receptor blocker, prazosin, failed to affect either basal or clonidine-induced stimulation of LHRH release. The α2 receptor blocker, yohimbine, was effective to block the action of this α receptor-stimulating drug.[45]

Other evidence using receptor blockers and inhibitors of catecholamine synthesis favors a stimulatory role for norepinephrine in control of LHRH release.[46] LH release in the castrate is suppressed by α but not β adrenergic receptor blockers. The augmented LH release which takes place in the afternoon in the ovariectomized, steroid-primed rat or on proestrus could be blocked by inhibitors of catecholamine synthesis and specifically of norepinephrine synthesis. For example, the administration of diethyldithiocarbamate to block conversion of dopamine to norepinephrine resulted in blockade of both of these types of stimulated LH release. Reversal of the blockade by administration of dihydroxyphenylserine in most instances was capable of reinitiating LH release. The site of the presumed stimulatory synapses between noradrenergic terminals and the LHRH neurons was localized by stimulating electrochemically in the preoptic region. Electrochemical stimulation in a zone extending from preoptic region to median eminence had previously been shown to release LH. If norepinephrine synthesis was inhibited, electrochemical stimulation of the preoptic area was no longer effective, whereas if the inhibition of norepinephrine synthesis was reversed, stimulation resulted in LH release. On the other hand, LH release from stimulation in the median eminence was not blocked by blockade of norepinehprine synthesis. Presumably, in this instance the LH-RH terminals were directly activated. We postulated therefore stimulatory noradrenrgic synapses located caudal to the points of stimulation in the preoptic area.

Since the hypothalamus contains few if any cell bodies of noradrenergic neurons, we suggested that noradrenergic control was mediated by brain stem noradrenergic neurons whose axons project rostrally into the preoptic and hypothalamic regions via the ventral noradrenergic tract. This supposition was supported by the ability of injections of 6-hydroxydopamine into the ventral noradrenergic tract, which destroy catecholaminergic neurons, to block the preovulatory release of LH and that induced by progesterone in estrogen-primed animals. Control injections of 6-hydroxydopamine into other sites were ineffective as were injections of the ascorbic acid diluent into the ventral noradrenergic tract. Others have confirmed these findings, however, both our group and others have found recovery with time after these injections. In that circumstance, according to Clifton and Sawyer, the responses could not be blocked by α adrenergic blockers suggesting that another system has taken over in the chronic deafferented animals.[47] The evidence is consistent with the view that in normal animals stimulatory noradrenergic tone is associated with preovulatory LH release as well as the increased release in the castrate.

Although β receptors seemed to be uninvolved in gonadotropin control based on early studies with β receptor blockers, this position needs to be reevaluated. Recently, Caceres and Taleisnik[48] have found that the inhibitory influence on LH release produced by stimulation of the cingulate cortex can be blocked by β receptor blockers and can be mimicked by β agonists. In our recent studies[49] in conscious, ovariectomized rats third ventricle injection of isoproterenol (30 μg), a β receptor stimulator, brought about a decrease in plasma LH concentrations but propanolol, a beta receptor blocker, metapropolol, a selective β_2 antagonist, and IPS 339, a selective β_2 antagonist failed to alter plasma LH concentrations. This would suggest that β tone is not involved in the increased pulsatile LH release in castrates. In contrast, intraventricular propanolol (30 μg) increased plasma FSH in the castrates; however, there was no significant effect of the other drugs on FSH secretion. This suggests the possibility of a tonic inhibitory effect of the β system on FSH but not LH release in ovariectomized rats. In view of the dichotomy between FSH and LH release, the results also suggest the possibility of selective hypothalamic control of the two gonadotropins. Recently both β_1 and β_2 receptors have been demonstrated in the hypothalamus in nearly equal abundance[50]. Beta receptors are also found in the anterior pituitary gland[50] and a reevaluation of a possible role of these receptors in control of pituitary hormone secretion is underway.

The role of norepinephrine in stimulation of gonadotropin release is further supported by the extensive studies on turnover of catecholamines The most recent of these, carried out by Barraclough's group,[51] indicate that there is an increased turnover of norepinephrine in regions involved in control of LH release at the time of the preovulatory LH surge. This is preceded also by an increased turnover of dopamine suggesting that both dopamine and norepinehprine may be involved in the preovulatory release of LHRH.

Turnover studies also support a stimulatory role for both dopamine and norepinephrine in the increased release of gonadotropins in castrates.[52] Fig. 1 illustrates the possible interactions of norephinephrine and dopamine to alter release of LHRH.

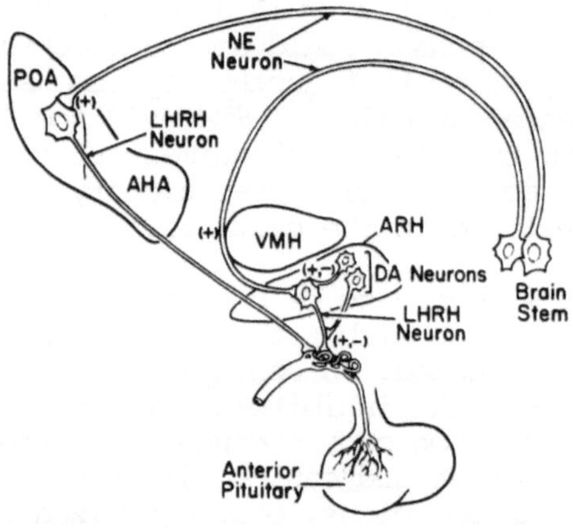

Fig. 1. Diagram showing the localization of postulated noradrenergic and dopaminergic neurons involved in the control of LHRH. Activation of noradrenergic neurons located in the brain stem stimulates LHRH neurons located at the preoptic-anterior hypothalamic area and medial basal hypothalamus-median eminence region. Activation of dopaminergic neurons can either inhibit or stimulate LHRH release depending on the steroid milieu and degree of the activation. NE=norepinephrine; DA=dopamine. (From S.R. Ojeda and S.M. McCann, In: Clinics and Obstetrics and Gynecology, Vol. 5, pp. 283-303, 1978, with permission).

Role of prostaglandins in control of LHRH release. Earlier studies indicated that intraventricular injection of prostaglandin E_2 could release LH and LHRH. Furthermore, LH release in castrates and the release provoked by steroids could be blocked by an inhibitor of prostaglandin synthetase, indomethacin. Implantation of prostaglandin E_2 in various brain loci revealed that implants in the preoptic region and in the region extending caudally and ventrally into the median eminence evoked LH release. FSH release was preferentially evoked in the dorsal anterior hypothalamic area and in the region proceeding caudally and ventrally from this to the caudal median eminence. These results suggested that the implants which provoke preferential LH release produced a release of LHRH. They also raised the possibility that those located in regions which selectively released FSH might be causing release of an FSH-RF rather than the decapeptide. Studies with receptor blockers which failed to block the response to PGE_2 suggested that the releasing action was via a direct effect on the LHRH neurons (for review, see 53).

Recently we have evaluated further the role of prostaglandins in the *in vitro* median eminence incubation system[54], and have found that prostaglandin E_2 provoked LHRH release. This effect was blocked by indomethacin. Furthermore, norepinephrine and to a lesser extent dopamine could cause release of prostaglandin E_2 into the medium. The action of norepinephrine to release LHRH was blocked by indomethacin in the face of normal responsiveness of the tissue to PGE_2-induced release of LHRH. The action of norepinephrine to release prostaglandin E_2 was blocked by the α receptor blocker, phentolamine, but not by the β receptor blocker, propranolol. These results then suggest an essential role for prostanglandin E_2 in the action of norepinephrine to release LHRH. We postulate that norepinephrine acts on the LHRH neuron to produce a release of PGE_2. This PGE_2 then either directly or via increases in cyclic AMP and/or cyclic GMP evokes release of LHRH from the terminals of the LHRH neuron. Many other prostaglandins were tested and it is clear that prostaglandin E_2 is by far the most important releaser of LHRH.[55] Figure 2 illustrates the possible mechanism of action of PGE_2 to evoke LHRH release.

LHRH SECRETING NEURON

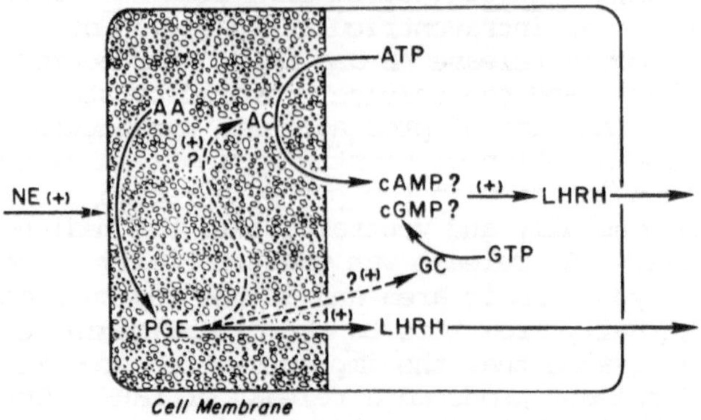

Fig. 2. Postulated series of cellular events leading to the release of LHRH by hypothalamic-secretory neurons. NE=norepinephrine; AA=arachidonic acid; AC=adenylate cyclase; GC=guanylate cyclase; ATP=adenosine triphosphate; GTP=quanosine triphosphate; cAMP=adenosine 3',5'-cyclic monophosphate; cGMP=guanosine 3',5'-cyclic monophosphate. (From S.R. Ojeda and S.M. McCann, In: Clinics in Obstetrics and Gynecology, Vol. 5, pp. 283-303, 1978, with permission).

In contrast to the stimulatory role of PGE_2 in gonadotropin secretion, prostacyclin appears to have a selective inhibitory effect on LH release. Intraventricular injection of prostacyclin suppressed LH but not FSH release in castrate females. Since there was no action of prostacyclin on LH release in vitro, it would appear that the action is exerted on the hypothalamus, perhaps to suppress selectively the release of LHRH (Ottlecz, Samson and McCann, unpublished data).

Serotonin, γ aminobutyric acid and histamine. Serotonin (5HT) may also be involved in the system. In the ovariectomized animal injection of 5HT into the third ventricle will inhibit LH release;[56] however, inhibition of 5HT biosynthesis with parachlorophenylalanine or intraventricular injection of drugs which destroy central serotoninergic neurons intereferes with the preovulatory type of LH release. Thus, serotonin may have an inhibitory action in the castrate but serotoninergic tone may be necessary for preovulatory LH release.[57]

GABA is found in the hypothalamus and there are GABA receptors in the pituitary. It is not surprising then that GABA has effects on release of most pituitary hormones.[58] In the case of

LH, intraventricular injection of GABA can stimulate LH release at relatively high doses; and these responses were blocked by bicuculline, a specific GABA antagonist. We have recently carried out additional experiments with bicuculline and have found that intravenous injection of bicuculline dissolved in alcohol can elevate plasma LH in castrates. This result is opposite to that expected following the intraventricular injection of GABA and suggests that GABA may have inhibitory as well as stimulatory effects on gonadotropin secretion and that the inhibitory effects may be tonically active in the castrate.

Intraventricular injections of histamine can also elevate plasma LH; however, since the dose required is large, it is quite possible that this may not have physiological significance.[59]

Acetylcholine. Acetylcholine was postulated many years ago to play a role in gonadotropin secretion by Everett and Sawyer and more recently intraventricular injection of acetylcholine has been shown to cause LH and FSH release in the ovariectomized animal.[60,61] The response was blocked by atropine injections into the ventricle which by themselves lowered gonadotropin levels in these animals. This suggests that acetylcholine plays a role in the normal release of LH at muscarinic type synapses. Cholinergic control may operate via the tuberoinfundibular dopaminergic tract since the response to acetylcholine was blocked by pimozide, a dopamine receptor blocker.[61]

An important mode of LH release is the increased pulsatile release which occurs in the castrate. It occurs with a certain period, characteristic of the species as a single pulse of LHRH. The effect of the LHRH then dissipates and the LH released disappears from the circulation according to its half-life, to be followed by another pulse at the appropriate interval. Recent studies in which conscious rats were cannulated and blood samples taken over a period of time, so that the pattern of pulsatile LH release could be constructed, indicate that there is a depletion of LHRH and dopamine from the median eminence on the rising limb of the LH pulse, whereas norepinephrine in the suprachiasmatic region rises just prior to the pulse.[62] This would suggest a simulatory role for dopamine in generation of the pulses and that norepinephrine is probably involved. Pulsatile LHRH release was not blocked by anterior cuts or complete hypothalamic deafferentation, a treatment which would eliminate noradrenergic input into the basal hypothalamus[63]. Furthermore this release was not blocked by lesions of the arcuate nucleus which eliminate dopaminergic input to the median eminence. However, when the lesions and cuts were combined blockade ensued. The arcuate region would be the source of the dopaminergic stimulatory drive, and the preoptic region the source of the noradrenergic drive. In animals with chronic impairments apparently pulsatile release can take place more or less in the absence of either of these drives, but if both are interrupted it ceases.

We believe that a complex interplay between noradrenergic, cholinergic and dopaminergic systems may be involved in the pulsatile release of LH in the castrate. One may speculate that the noradrenergic influence is exerted by fibers which reach the arcuate region, and stimulate cholinergic neurons there. Pulsatile release of LH may be brought about then by discharge of cholinergic neurons in the arcuate nucleus. These neurons, via synapses with the tuberoinfundibular dopaminergic neurons, stimulate the release of LHRH (Fig. 3). We also postulate that dendrites from the tuberoinfundibular dopaminergic neurons synapse with the cholinergic neurons in the arcuate nucleus. When triggered they release dopamine to inhibit the

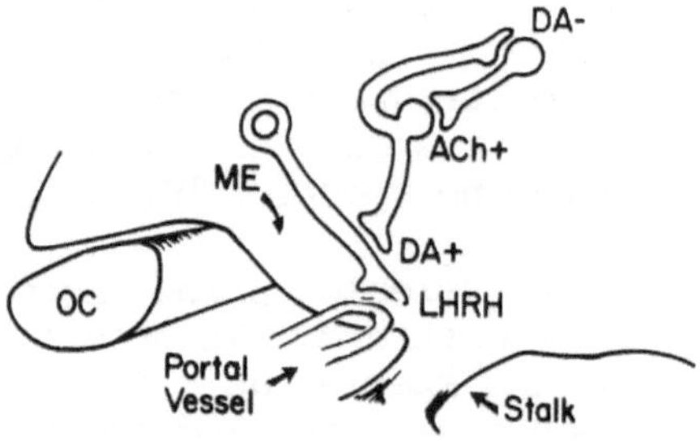

Fig. 3. Schematic diagram representing the interrelationships between dopaminergic (DA), cholinergic (ACh) and LHRH neuronal elements in the tuberoinfundibular system. ME: median eminence, OC: optic chiasm. + or - indicate stimulatory and inhibitory activity, respectively.

the cholinergic drive. This could account for the delay until the next pulse of LHRH is released and also accounts for the dual effects of dopamine to both stimulate and inhibit LH release. The failure to see inhibitory actions of dopamine with the median eminence incubation system is presumably related to the fact that these inhibitory actions occur deeper within the hypothalamus in the region of the arcuate nucleus. It is also possible that the excitatory actions of dopamine involve different dopamine receptors than the inhibitory ones.[64]

<u>Peptides</u>. In addition to these transmitters, a host of peptides has been described now in the brain and in particular in the hypothalamus. Many of them have been shown to have effects on LH release presumably mediated by altered discharge of LHRH.

Among these various peptides, it appears clear that the endogenous opioid peptides have a tonic inhibitory control over LHRH release under most circumstances.[65] We have recently examined whether or not naloxone, the opioid antagonist, operates directly on LHRH neurons or via the intervention of the muscarinic, cholinergic receptor described above. The ability of intraventricular naloxone to elevate LH was not blocked by atropine which by itself was effective in lowering LH.[66] This would indicate that the endogenous opioid peptides operate either directly on the LHRH neurons to inhibit or by the intervention of another transmitter.

In the case of the opioid peptides, convenient inhibitors of the action, such as naloxone, are available. In the case of most of the other peptides such inhibitors have yet to be discovered. This makes it difficult to assess the physiological significance of these other peptides in the control of gonadotropin secretion. A number of them are exceedingly potent to alter gonadotropin secretion. For example, vasoactive intestinal peptide (VIP) was effective to elevate LH at doses in the low nanogram range in the castrate animal and also released LHRH from hypothalamic synaptosomes.[67] Substance P was also stimulatory but required microgram doses to be effective. On the other hand cholecystokinin inhibited in low nanogram doses whereas neurotensin and gastrin required higher doses for the inhibitory effects.[65]

A number of other peptides have now been evaluated. Vasotocin is extremely potent following its intraventricular injection to inhibit LH release in ovariectomized rats, the minimal effective dose being 40 ng.[68] It may play a physiologically significant role if it can be shown to be present in the mammalian brain. Recent studies suggest that it is not.[69] None of these peptides altered gonadotropin release from hemipituitaries or dispersed pituitary cells <u>in vitro</u>.

Bradykinin did not have impressive effects on gonadotropin secretion, however, if bradykinin was injected intraventricularly along with bradykinin-potentiating factor, there was a suppression of FSH levels at 75 min after its injection in ovariectomized rats. Peculiarly, release of FSH by hemipituitaries was suppressed by the lowest dose of bradykinin tested, but not by other doses, and LH release was unaffected by any dose. Therefore, it cannot be stated that bradykinin has any clear role in gonadotropin secretion.[70]

On the other hand, angiotensin II, another peptide probably found in the median eminence, has been found active to release LH from hemipituitaries of ovariectomized female rats at a dose of 0.2 or 2μg/ml. Strangely, a high dose of 15 μg/ml had no effect. Intraventricular injection of angiotensin II was ineffective to modify LH in the ovariectomized animal.[71] However, in ovariectomized estrogen-primed animals it elevated LH dramatically.[72] That this may have physiological significance is suggested by recent experiments in which saralasin, an angiotensin antagonist, suppressed preovulatory LH release.[73] Since this was only after intraventricular and not intravenous injection of saralasin, this would suggest a central action to inhibit LHRH release.

In the meantime, angiotensin II receptors have been demonstrated in the anterior pituitary making it possible that the action of angiotensin II to release LH by pituitaries incubated <u>in vitro</u> may also have physiological significance[74]. It appears that angiotensin II is a potential candidate to have an important physiological role in control of LH release.

Calcitonin has recently also been described in brain and it has a effect to lower LH in castrate animals in intraventricular doses as low as 100 ng and no effect following intravenous injection. Also there was no effect on hemipituitary release of LH indicating a central action of calcitonin (Mangat, Samson and McCann, unpublished).

Gastric inhibitory peptide (GIP), a member of the secretin family of peptides, suppressed selectively FSH but not LH secretion following its intraventricular injection. This is another example of dissociation in factors controlling FSH and LH release. Interestingly, GIP is capable of stimulating dose-related increases in the release of both LH and FSH from dispersed pituitary cells, suggesting that the inhibitory effect of centrally administered GIP is due to an ultra-short loop feedback effect (Ottlecz, Samson and McCann, unpublished data).

Somatostatin neuronal terminals are intermingled amongst the terminals of the LHRH neurons in the median eminence. In the course of experiments evaluating the effect of intraventricular somatostatin on growth hormone release we also studied its effect on release of other pituitary hormones.[75] It produced a stimulation of growth hormone release but an inhibition of the release of LH and FSH, as well as TSH, suggesting that it inhibited LHRH and TRH release, probably in the median eminence region. It is quite likely that the various releasing factor neurons interact to augment or inhibit each other's activity in the hypothalamus, i.e. by ultrashort loop feedback.[76]

αMSH, a fragment of the proopiomelanocortin sequence, has recently been found to suppress LH release in ovariectomized females after its intraventricular injection.[77] This action appears to involve participation of dopaminergic inhibitory control since it could be blocked by the dopamine receptor antagonist, pimozide. The physiological significance of this action has not been established.

Proteins. Not only may there be interactions amongst the various releasing and inhibiting factors at the hypothalamic level to alter the release of LHRH, but also it may be affected by short-loop feedback via gonadotropins. A number of studies indicate that there is an inhibitory short-loop feedback of LH to suppress its own secretion.[76] Intraventricular injection of LH suppresses LH but not FSH secretion indicating the specificity of this feedback (Mangat and McCann, unpublished). The short-loop feedback may operate via delivery of LH to the hypothalamus by retrograde flow in portal vessels as postulated by several groups, or alternatively, it may operate via LH neurons recently described in the hypothalamus.[78]

FSH, at least in the preovulatory period, appears to act via a positive short-loop feedback which augments FSH release.[79] This may be important in the estrous elevation of FSH. It is possible that these short loop feedbacks may vary depending on the circumstances. There may be negative feedback of LH to suppress its own release in the castrate, but positive feedback to augment the preovulatory type release on proestrus. Some evidence already exists for this.[76]

Prolactin clearly operates by short-loop feedback to suppress its own secretion.[76] We have recently confirmed this and have shown that the action occurs very quickly within 5 min after intraventricular injection of prolactin in animals in which prolactin release has been augmented either by stress or by estrogen pretreatment.[80] Elevated plasma prolactin is also associated with suppression of LH secretion in certain circumstances; however, following intraventricular injection of prolactin, the suppression of LH was small and inconstant suggesting that this action of high prolactin levels may be mediated by other mechanisms. The actions of these various peptides and proteins on gonadotropin release in ovariectomized females following their injection into the third ventricle is summarized in Table 1.

TABLE 1

EFFECTS ON INTRAVENTRICULAR INJECTION OF VARIOUS PEPTIDES AND PROTEINS ON THE RELEASE OF FSH AND LH IN OVARIECTOMIZED RATS

Substance	Dosage	FSH	LH
CCK	ng	0	-
Gastrin	μg	0	-
VIP	ng	0	+
SP	μg	0	+
NT	μg	0	-
Opioids	μg	-	-
Bradykinin	μg	-	0
Angiotensin II	μg	0	0
Vasotocin	ng	0	-
Inhibin	μg	-	0
Somatostatin	μg	-	-
αMSH	μg	0	-
LH	μg	0	-
FSH	μg	0	0
Prl	μg	0	0

CCK = cholecystokinin

VIP = vasoactive intestinal peptide

SP = substance P

NT = neurotensin

0 = no effect, + = increase, - = decrease

Is there an FSH-releasing factor (FSH-RF)? A great deal of evidence obtained from stimulation and lesion experiments suggests the existence of a separate hypothalamic control of FSH, presumably mediated by an FSHRF[81]. For example, stimulations of the dorsal anterior hypothalamic area and a region extending ventrally and caudally toward the posterior median eminence can evoke selective FSH secretion. On the other hand, stimulations in the preoptic-suprachiasmatic area give selective LH release. Lesions in the dorsal anterior hypothalamic area interfere with the postcastration rise in FSH and also diminish the progesterone-induced release of FSH in the estrogen-primed spayed rat. LH release is unimpaired by these lesions. Conversely, lesions in the suprachiasmatic region lead to a suppression of the LH response in the estrogen, progesterone-treated animal while leaving the FSH response intact. Lesions of the dorsal anterior hypothalamus impair pulsatile FSH secretion in the castrate, whereas they leave the pulsatile release of LH unaltered (Lumpkin et al., Society for Neuroscience, Boston, 1983, in press). Hemi-castration of male rats is followed by a selective increase in plasma FSH which can be partially blocked by ipsilateral destruction of the dorsal anterior hypothalamic area but is unaltered by contralateral lesions.[82] Extracts of the caudal median eminence contain more FSH-releasing activity, as assayed by release of FSH from hemipituitaries incubated *in vitro*, than can be accounted for by their content of LHRH as measured by radioimmunoassay, whereas the FSH release obtained from anterior median eminence extracts can be accounted for by their content of the decapeptide[83]. In addition, assay of varying doses of extracts of the organum vasculosum lamina terminalis (OVLT), when assayed with dispersed anterior pituitary cells, revealed a steep slope for FSH release, much steeper than that produced by varying doses of decapeptide[84]. The potency of these extracts was at least 15 times greater than could be accounted for by the content of decapeptide. By contrast, there was minimal enhancement of the LH release above that accounted for by decapeptide by greater doses of these extracts.

Because of all of this evidence suggesting the existence of FSHRF, we have tried to purify such a factor from extracts of rat hypothalamus by gel filtration on a column of Sephadex G-25. The fractions eluted from the column were assayed by incubation with hemipituitaries from male rats and measurement of the FSH release by both bio- and radioimmunoassay, of the LH release by radioimmunoassay, and of the content of LHRH by radioimmunoassay. The results by bioassay confirmed our original report[85] since the bioactive FSHRF emerged in the exact tubes seen earlier. The results differed from the earlier report in that the activity persisted into the zone immediately following which contained LHRH as measured by radioimmunoassay.

When the immunoassayable FSH and LH were measured, the results differed, in that the activity could be explained by the content of LHRH present in the fractions. We further purified the bioactive FSH-releasing fractions by chromatography on carboxymethyl cellulose (CMC). Bioactive FSHRF emerged just prior to the residual decapeptide in this experiment as well and led to further purification of the bioactive FSHRF[86]. We believe the results may indicate that FSHRF alters the biological activity of FSH perhaps by further glycosylating the molecule and this leads to the detection of the bioactive FSHRF. It is possible that our use of six hours of incubation in contrast to the in vivo pulse injection previously employed enhanced the FSH-releasing activity of LHRH and that this may account for the difference between these results and those previously obtained. We are currently assaying fractions by in vivo bioassay using the ovariectomized, estrogen, progesterone-treated rat which we employed in the initial studies. It is our belief that an FSHRF will ultimately be isolated which will be quite similar chemically to LHRH. It may even be a decapeptide similar to LHRH with substitution of several of the amino acids in the molecule. The situation may be quite analogous to that of vasopressin and oxytocin which are very similar chemically, and, indeed, vasopressin has oxytocic activity.

ABSTRACT

Control of gonadotropin secretion is accomplished, at least in part, via the decapeptide, LH releasing hormone (LHRH). Within a matter of a minute of presentation LHRH acts on specific receptors on the cell membrane of the gonadotrophs to initiate LH release . The response is augmented by castration and inhibited by gonadal steroids. In the ovariectomized female, estrogen acts initially to suppress responsiveness to LHRH and this is followed by increased responsiveness. In addition, there is a self-priming action of LHRH to augment the response of the pituitary to itself which is particularly prominent in the estrogen-primed animal. These interactions, coupled to an increased release of LHRH, bring about the preovulatory surge of gonadotropins.

The mechanism of action of LHRH following its interaction with the receptor requires the presence of calcium. This may be made available via activation of phospholipase C which results in the liberation of arachidonic acid. This in turn leads to formation of metabolites by the epoxygenase pathway of arachidonic acid metabolism. These metabolites have been demonstrated to be present in the anterior pituitary and are capable of stimulating LH release in vitro. The action of LHRH can be blocked by ETYA, an inhibitor of all pathways of arachidonic acid metabolism. Even in this instance the gland is capable of responding to the epoxygenase metabolite, 5,6-EET. Interestingly, calcium is also liberated from perifused dispersed cells in response to both LHRH and the 5,6-EET.

LHRH is found in neurons within the preoptic and arcuate region which project to the median eminence and also other sites within the central nervous system. A whole host of neurotransmitters play upon the LHRH neurons. Dopamine has dual effects to either stimulate or inhibit LHRH release. Norepinephrine and epinephrine can stimulate. It is probable that dopamine and norepinephrine play roles as stimulators of LHRH release and that dopamine can also physiologically inhibit its release. There is a probable role also of serotonin and gamma aminobutyric acid and a possible role of histamine. Stimulatory muscarinic cholinergic control via acetylcholine appears very likely.

A variety of peptides now known to be in the hypothalamus influence LHRH release. The opioid peptides appear to have a physiologically significant inhibitory action. Angiotensin may act either in the brain or even directly on the pituitary to modify LH release. Several peptides, such as vasoactive intestinal peptide and substance P have a stimulatory role and a large number have inhibitory roles, such as vasotocin, neurotensin, calcitonin, and GIP. The physiological significance of these actions will ultimately be shown only by use of blocking drugs.

Releasing factors appear to interact at the hypothalamic level to modulate their own release. For example, somatostatin inhibits release of both FSH and LH while augmenting release of growth hormone. Inhibin may act at the hypothalamic as well as the pituitary level to inhibit FSH release. Lastly, an abundance of evidence now indicates that, in all probability, there is a separate FSHRF which remains to be isolated.

REFERENCES

1. McCann, S.M., Taleisnik, S. and Friedman, H.M. (1960) Proc. Soc. Exp. Biol. Med. 104: 432-434.
2. Matsuo, H., Baba, Y., Nair, R.M., Arimura, A. and Schally, A.V. (1971) Biochem. Biophys. Res. Comm. 43: 134-139.
3. Krulich, L., Quijada, M., Wheaton, J.E., Illner, P. and McCann, S.M. (1977) Fed. Proc. 36, 1953-1959.
4. Barry, J., DuBois, M.P. and Carette, B. (1974) Endocrinology 95, 1416-1423.
5. Samson, W.K., McCann, S.M., Chud, L., Dudley, C.A. and Moss,

R.L. (1980) Neuroendocrinology 31, 66-72.
6. Phillips, H.S., Hostetter, G., Kerdelhue, B. and Kozlowski, G.P. (1980) Brain Res. 193, 574-579.
7. Stell, W.K., Chohan, K.S., Lam, D.M. and Kozlowski, G.P. (1982) A.R.V.O. Abstract (in press).
8. McCann, S.M. (1974) Hand. Physiol. 4, 489-517.
9. Ojeda, S.R., Andrews, W.W., Advis, J.P. and Smith White, S. (1980) Endocrine Rev. 1, 228-257.
10. Knobil, E. (1980) Recent Prog. Horm. Res. 36, 53-88.
11. Ajika, K., Kalra, S.P., Fawcett, C.P., Krulich, L. and McCann, S.M. (1972) Endocrinology 90, 707-715.
12. Libertun, C., Orias, R. and McCann, S.M. (1974) Endocrinology 94, 1094-1100.
13. Fink, G. (1979) Ann. Rev. Physiol. 41, 571-585.
14. Goodman, R.L. (1978) Endocrinology 102, 142-150.
15. Yen, S.S.C. (1977) in Clinical Reproductive Neuroendocrinology, Hubinot, P.O., L'Hermite, M.L. and Robyn, C. ed., Karger, Basel, pp. 150-157.
16. Libertun, C. and McCann, S.M. (1974) Fed. Proc. 33, 212.
17. Zeballos, G. and McCann, S.M. (1975) Endocrinology 96, 1377-1385.
18. Castro-Vasquez, A. and McCann, S.M. (1975) Endocrinology 97, 13-19.
19. Aiyer, M.S., Chiappa, S.A. and Fink, G. (1974) J Endocrinol. 62, 573-588.
20. Neill, J.D. (1980) Front. Horm. Res. 6, 192-216.
21. Wildt, L., Hausler, R., Huchinson, J.S., Marshall, G. and Knobile, E. (1981) Endocrinology 108, 2011-2013.
22. Pavasuthitaisit, K., Hess, D.L., Norman, R.L., Adams, T.E., Baughman, W.L. and Spies, H.G. (1981) Neuroendocrinoogy 32, 42-49.
23. Marshall, J.C., Vourne, G.A., Frager, M.S. and Pieper, D.R. (1981) in Functional Correlates of Hormone Receptors in Reproduction, Mahesh, V.B., Muldoon, T.G., Saxena, B.B. and Sadler, W.A. ed., Elsevier/North-Holland, New York, 93-115. 93-115.
24. Labrie, F., Borgeat, P., Drouin, J., Beaulieu, M., Lagace, L., Ferland, L. and Raymond, V. (1979) Ann. Rev. Physiol. 41, 555-569.
25. Naor, A., Synder, G., Fawcett, C.P. and McCann, S.M. (1978) J. Cyclic Nucleotide Res. 4, 475-486.
26. Snyder, G., Naor, A., Fawcett, C.P. and McCann, S.M. (1980) Endocrinology 107, 1627-1633.
27. Naor, Z. and Catt, K.J. (1980) J. Biochem. 225, 342.
28. McCann, S.M. (1971) in Fronteirs in Neuroendocrinology, Ganong, W.F., and Martini, L., ed., Oxford Press, New York.
29. Snyder, G. and Bleasdale, J.E. (1982) Mol. Cell. Endocrinol. 28, 55-63.
30. Michell, R.H. (1975) Biochem. Biophys. Acta 415, 81-447.
31. Evans, W.S., Hellman, P.H., Uskavitch and Canonico, P.L. (1983) The Program of the 65th Annual Mtg. of the Endocine

Society. Abstract #125.
32. Naor, Z. and Catt, K.J. (1981) J. Biol Chem. 256, 2226-2229.
33. Naor, Z., Vanderhoek, J.Y., Lindner, H. R. and Catt, K. J. (1980) In: Advances in Prostaglandin, Thromboxane and Leukotriene Research, eds. Samuelsson, B., Paoleti, R., and Ramwell, P.W. (Raven, New York), pp 259-263.
34. Snyder, G., Capdevila, J., Chacos, N., Manna, S. and Falck, J.R. (1983) Proc. Natl Acad. Sci (USA) 80, 3504-3507.
35. Snyder, G., Capdevila, J., Chacos, N. and Falck, J.R. (1983) Program of the 65th Annual Mtg of the Endocrine Society. Abstract #558.
36. Elde, R. and Hokfelt, T. (1979) Ann. Rev. Physiol. 41, 587-602.
37. Schneider, H.P.G. and McCann, S.M. (1969) Endocrinology 85, 121-132.
38. Fuxe, K. and Hokfelt, T. (1969) in Frontiers in Neuroendocrinology, Ganong, W.F. and Maritni, L. ed., Oxford Press, New York, pp. 47-98.
39. Schneider, H.P.G. and McCann, S.M. (1970) Endocrinology 86, 1127-1133.
40. Vijayan, E. and McCann, S.M. (1978) Neuroendocrinology 25, 221-235.
41. Gnodde, H.P. and Schuiling, G.A. (1976) Neuroendocrinology 20, 212-223.
42. Negro-Vilar, A., Ojeda, S.R. and McCann, S.M. (1979) Endocrinology 104, 1749-1757.
43. Vijayan,E. and McCann, S.M. (1978) Neuroendocrinology 25, 150-165.
44. Ojeda, S.R., Negro-Vilar, A. and McCann, S.M. (1982) Endocrinology 110, 409-412.
45. Negro-Vilar, A. and Ojeda, S.R. (1982) 64th Ann. Mtg. Endocrine Soc. (submitted).
46. McCann, S.M., Krulich, L., Ojeda, S.R., Negro-Vilar, A. and Vijayan, E. (1979) in Central Regulation of the Endocrine System, Fuxe, K. Hokfelt, T. and Luft, R. ed., Plenum Press, New York, pp. 329-347.
47. Clifton, D.K. and Sawyer, C.H. (1980) Endocrinology 106, 1099-1102.
48. Caceres, A. and Taleisnik, S.A. (1980) J. Endocrinol. 87, 419-429.
49. Huang, X.Y. and McCann, S.M. Proc. Soc. Exp. Biol. & Med. In press.
50. Petrovic, S.L., McDonald, J.K., Snyder, G.D. and McCann, S.M. (1983) Brain Res. 261: 249-259.
51. Barraclough, C.A., Wise, P.M., (1982) Endocrine Reviews 3: 91-119.
52. Advis, J.P., McCann, S.M. and Negro-Vilar, A. (1980) Endocrinology 107, 892-901.
53. Ojeda, S.R., Negro-Vilar, A. and McCann, S.M. (1981) in Physiopathology of Endocrine Diseases and Mechanisms of

Hormone Action, Alan R. Liss, Inc., New York, pp. 229-247.
54. Ojeda, S.R., Negro-Vilar, A. and McCann, S.M. (1979) Endocrinology 104, 617-624.
55. Ojeda, S.R., Jameson, H.E. and McCann, S.M. (1976) Prostaglandins 12, 281-301.
56. Schneider, H.P.G. and McCann, S.M. (1970) Endocrinology 86, 1127-1133.
57. Hery, M., Laplant, E. and Kordon, C. (1976) Endocrinology 99, 496-503.
58. McCann, S.M., Vijayan, E. and Negro-Vilar, A. (1981) in GABA and Benzodiazepine Receptors, Costa, E., Dichiara, G. and Gessa, G.L. ed., Raven Press, New York, pp. 237-246.
59. Libertun, C. and McCann, S.M. (1976) Neuroendocrinology 20, 110-120.
60. Fiorindo, R., Justo, G., Motta, M., Simonovic, I. and Martini, L. (1974) in Hypothalamic Hormones, Motta, M., Crosignani, P. and Martini, L. ed., Academic Press, New York, pp. 195-204.
61. Vijayan, E. and McCann, S.M. (1980) Brain Res. Bull. 5, 23-29.
62. Negro-Vilar, A., Advis, J.P., Ojeda, S.R. and McCann, S.M. (1982) Endocrinology 111: 932-938.
63. Soper, B.D. and Weick, R.F. (1980) Endocrinology 106, 348-355.
64. Sarkar, D.K. and Fink, G. (1981) Endocrinology 108, 862-867.
65. McCann, S.M., In Neuroendocrine Perspectives, Vol. 1, Muller, E.E. and MacLeod, eds., Elsevier Biomedical Press, Amsterdam, pp. 1-22.
66. Huang, X.Y. and McCann, S.M., Am. J. Physiol, In Press.
67. Samson, W.K., Burton, K., Reeves, J.P. and McCann, S.M., (1981) Regulatory Peptides 2: 253-264.
68. Vijayan, E., Samson, W.K. and McCann, S.M. (1983) Proc. Soc. Exp. Biol. Med. 173: 153-158.
69. Negro-Vilar, A., Samson, W.K. and Sanchez-Franco, F. (1981) Ann. N.Y. Acad. Sci. (submitted)
70. Steele, M.K., Negro-Vilar, A., and McCann, S.M. (1980) Peptides 1, 201-205.
71. Steele, M.K., Negro-Vilar, A. and McCann, S.M. (1981) Endocrinology 109, 893-899.
72. Steele, M.K., Negro-Vilar, A. and McCann, S.M. (1982) Endocrinology 111: 722-729.
73. Steele, M.K., Brownfield, M.S., Reid, I.A. and Ganong, W.F. (1982) 64th Ann. Mtg. Endocrine Soc. pg. 1232.
74. Mukherjee, A., Kulkarni, P., McCann, S.M. and Negro-Vilar, A. (1982) Endocrinology 110, 665-667.
75. Lumpkin, M.D., Negro-Vilar, A., and McCann, S.M. (1981) Science 211, 1072-1074.
76. Piva, F., Motta, M. and Martini, L. (1979) in Endocrinology, Vol. 1, Degroot, L.J., Cahill, G.F., Martini, L., Nelson, D.H., Odell, W.D., Potts, J.T., Steinberger, E. and

Winegrad, A.I. ed., Grune & Stratton, New York, pp. 21-33.
77. Khorram, O. and McCann, S.M. Endocrinology, In Press.
78. Hostetter, G., Gallo, R.V. and Brownfield, M.S. (1981) Neuroendocrinology 33, 241-245.
79. Coutifaris, C. and Chappel, C. (1982) Endocrinology 110, 105-113.
80. Mangat, H.K. and McCann, S.M. (1983) Am. J. Physiol. 244: E3]-E36.
81. McCann, S.M., Mizunuma, H., Samson, W.K. and Lumpkin, M.D. Psychoneuroendocrinology (In press).
82. Mizunuma, H., L.R. DePalatis and S.M. McCann. Neuroendocrinology (in press)
83. Mizunuma, H., W.K. Samson, M.D. Lumpkin and S.M. McCann. Life Sci., In Press
84. Samson, W.K., S.I. Said, G. Snyder and S.M. McCann. (1980) Peptides 1: 97-102.
85. Dhariwal, A.P.S., L. Krulich, S. Katz and S.M. McCann. (1965) Endocrinology 76, 290-294.
86. Mizunuma, H., W.K. Samson, M.D. Lumpkin, J.H. Moltz, C.P. Fawcett and S.M. McCann (1983) Brain Res. Bull. 10:623-629.

MOLECULAR ASPECTS OF THE RELEASE OF LUTEINIZING HORMONE RELEASING HORMONE (LHRH) FROM HYPOTHALAMIC NEURONS

Ayalla Barnea

Department of Obstetrics and Gynecology and Physiology, Cecil H. and Ida Green Center for Reproductive Biology Sciences, The University of Texas Health Science Center at Dallas, 5323 Harry Hines Blvd., Dallas, Texas 75235

LHRH, which is stored in granule-like particles within hypothalamic neurons (Goldsmith and Ganong, 1975; Barnea et al., 1978a,b), is released into the hypophysial portal blood under various physiological conditions. Since LHRH is a peptide, and since it has been established that peptides and polypeptides are released from secretory cells by exocytosis, it is conceivable that release of LHRH also occurs by exocytosis. In spite of the large body of information collected, thus far, regarding the identity of some substances which may regulate the secretion of LHRH from the hypothalamic neurons, little is known of the intracellular processes which underlie this release mechanism.

A simplistic description of exocytosis is that a secretory granule approaches the exterior of the cell, the membrane of the secretory granule and the plasma membrane fuse and following changes in structure and permeability of the fused membranes, the interior content of the granule is expelled to the exterior of the cell. It is widely accepted that this secretory process is initiated by an extracellular stimulus acting at the level of the plasma membrane and that Ca^{2+} is an essential component of the process. Nevertheless, there are many questions that have yet to be resolved. What are the intracellular biochemical processes that underlie the interaction between the secretory granule and the plasma membrane? Are these biochemical processes specific to each type of secretory cell or are they common to all secretory cells? Is the responsiveness of the secretory granule to a stimulus that initiates exocytosis under regulatory control? Douglas (1978) has hypothesized that the essential ingredients for the fusion-fission event in exocytosis are present in the secretory granules themselves. In accordance with this postulate, several groups of investigators have shown that some of the molecular events involved in exocytosis can be studied in a cell-free system consisting of isolated granules (Taugner, 1972; Pazoles and Pollard, 1978; Russell and Thorn, 1978; Overgaard et al., 1979). Using such in vitro systems, several enzyme-mediated events, which require MgATP, have been implicated in the release of peptides and biogenic amines, for example, hydrolysis of ATP by a granule MgATPase and phosphorylation of specific granule proteins (DeLorenzo and Freedman, 1977). Therefore, we wished to ascertain if MgATP is involved in the release of LHRH from hypothalamic granules and if so, what is the characteristics of this release process.

THE ROLE OF MgATP IN LHRH RELEASE

We have developed an in vitro system for the study of the molecular events involved in LHRH release from its storage granules (Burrows et al., 1981; Rice and Barnea, 1983). In this system (Fig 1), granules containing LHRH are isolated from homogenates of rat hypothalami by hypo-osmotic shock followed by differential and Percoll-gradient centrifugations. The isolated granules are incubated in a defined medium and incubation is terminated by a rapid separation of LHRH released into the medium from that remaining in the granules (by LHRH affinity chromatography or gel filtration chromatography on Sephadex G-50). LHRH remaining in the granules after incubation is quantified by radioimmunoassay.

We found that ATP stimulates LHRH release from isolated hypothalamic granules in a Mg^{2+}-dependent manner (Burrows and Barnea, 1982a,b). In addition, we noted that some of the physico-chemical requirements for this MgATP-stimulated release of LHRH are similar to those reported by others for MgATP-stimulated release of catecholamines from chromaffin granules (Taugner, 1972; Pazoles and Pollard, 1978) and vasopressin from neurohypophysial granules (Overgaard et al., 1979): stimulation requires elevated temperature of incubation and the presence of monovalent ions (KCl) in the incubation mixture. These initial findings led us to think that the mechanism by which MgATP stimulates the release of LHRH may be similar to that of vasopressin and catecholamines. However, a close analysis of the monovalent-ion requirement for the stimulation of LHRH release by MgATP revealed that the mechanism leading to LHRH release differs markedly from that leading to the release of vasopressin and catecholamines. In the case of vasopressin and catecholamines, the MgATP-stimulated release has a selective requirement for monovalent anions but not for monovalent cations. Moreover, it appears that a functional anion-transport system is essential for this release process. In contrast, the MgATP-stimulated release of LHRH has a selective requirement for monovalent cations but not for monovalent anions nor for the activity of an anion-transport system. Thus, it became apparent

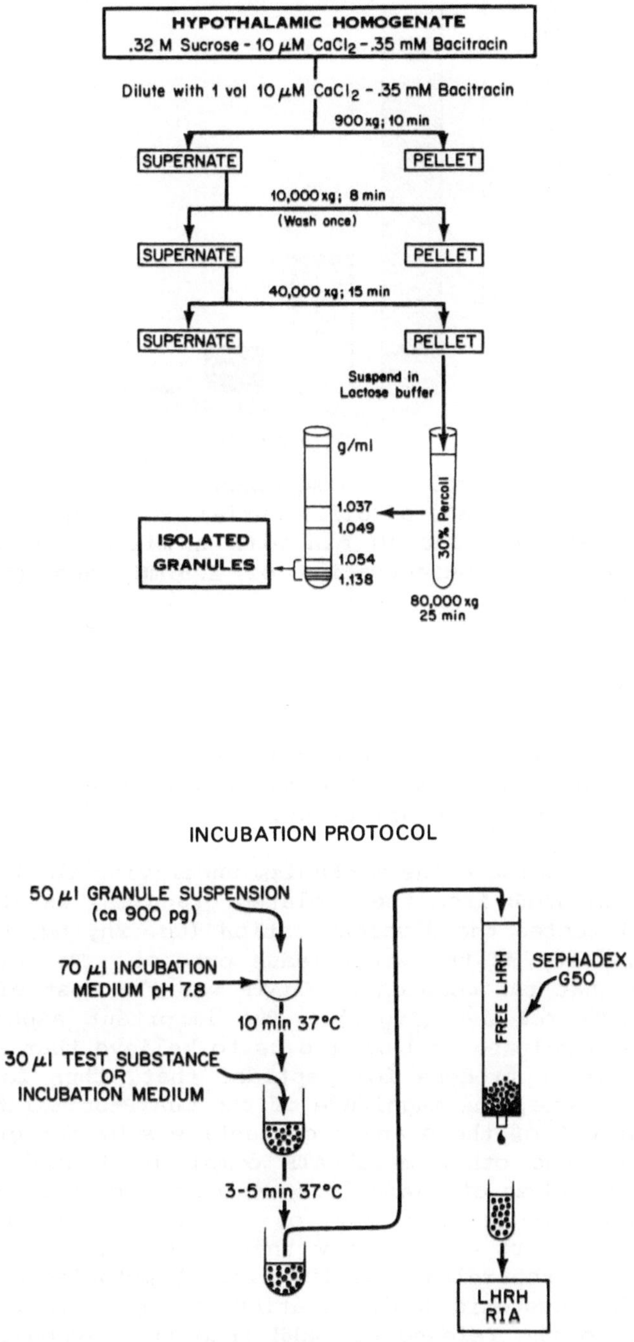

Figure 1. Scheme of isolation and incubation of LHRH granules.

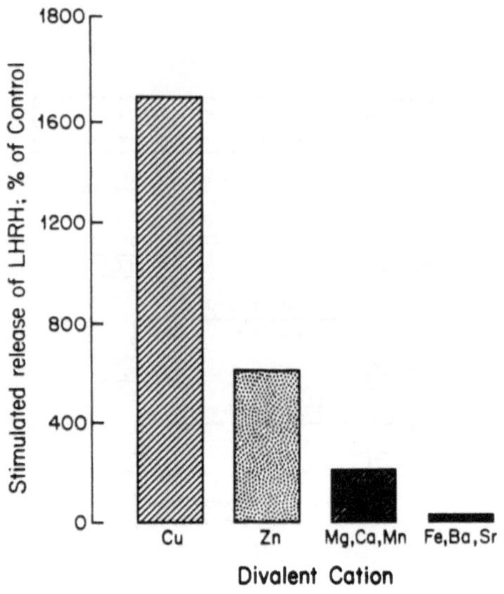

Figure 2. Effect of metal-ATP complexes on LHRH release. LHRH granules, isolated by means of differential centrifugation (Fig 1), were incubated at 37°C for 10 min with a mixture of a divalent cation and ATP at a concentration of 2.5 mM each (Burrows and Barnea, 1982c).

that although MgATP may be involved in the release process of numerous secretory substances, the molecular mechanism underlying each release process may be different.

To further elucidate the mechanism underlying the MgATP-stimulated release of LHRH from the isolated granules, we (Burrows and Barnea, 1982c) tested the divalent cation (Cu, Zn, Mg, Ca, Fe, Ba, Sr, Mn) specificity of the ATP-release process. To our surprise, we discovered that the complex of CuATP was the most effective in stimulating LHRH release (Fig 2). Two important aspects of the CuATP-stimulated release of LHRH led us to believe that we may have unraveled a release process for peptides that, thus far, has not been described. One, the magnitude of the CuATP-stimulated release of LHRH (about 65% of the granule content) was by far greater than that of any of the other metal-ATP complexes tested. Two, the minimal effective dose of CuATP (0.2 mM) required to stimulate LHRH release was much lower than that of any of the other metal-ATP complexes. In support of our view that copper may be involved in the regulation of the release of LHRH from hypothalamic neurons is the finding that systemic administration of copper salts to female rabbits leads to the release of LHRH into the hypophysial portal blood (Tsou et al., 1977) and to ovulation (Suzuki and Takahashi,

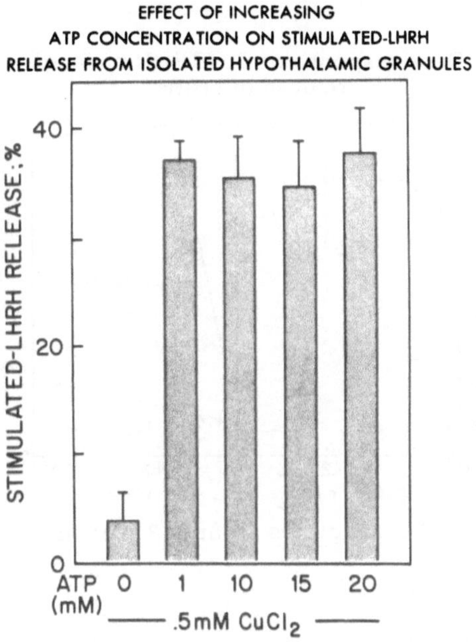

Figure 3. LHRH granules, isolated by means of differential centrifugation (Fig 1), were incubated at 37°C for 5 min with $CuCl_2$ and Na_2ATP. From Rice and Barnea (1983), reproduced with permission from Journal of Neurochemistry.

1974). Thus, it appears that blood-borne copper can stimulate LHRH release from hypothalamic neurons and that one site of action of copper is the secretory granule.

THE MECHANISM OF COPPER-STIMULATED RELEASE OF LHRH

First, we (Rice and Barnea, 1983) attempted to establish the form in which copper stimulates LHRH release: Is it chelated copper or ionic copper? Granules were incubated for 5 min in incubation medium alone, $CuCl_2$ or $CuCl_2$ mixed with various concentrations of Na_2ATP. As shown in Fig 3, copper (0.5 mM $CuCl_2$) by itself did not stimulate LHRH release. In contrast, copper, in the presence of 1 mM ATP, stimulated LHRH release by 37% and increasing the concentration of ATP up to 20 mM did not affect the copper-stimulated release of LHRH. In addition, we noted that copper complexed to tartarate was as effective in stimulating LHRH release as copper complexed to ATP. These results are indicative that chelated copper rather than ionic copper is the active form of the metal and that there is no strict requirement for ATP as the chelator for copper. It is known that at low concentrations of $\leq$ 10 μM, copper catalyzes a wide range of biological oxidative processes (Cass and Hill, 1980). However, at high concentration, copper may oxidize non-selectively several membrane components and

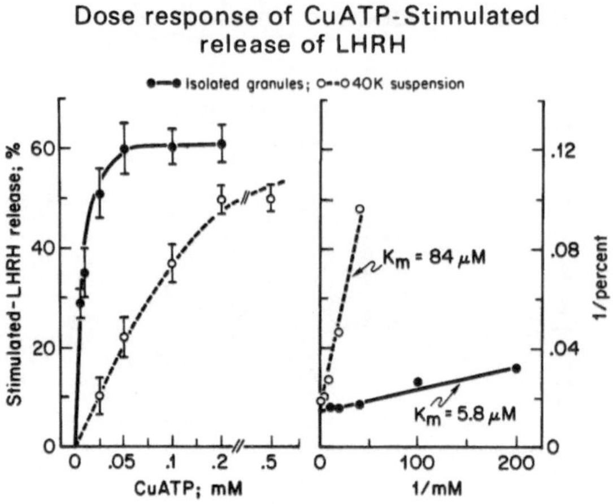

Figure 4. See figures 1 and 3 for details.

hence, lead to membrane disintegration. We were concerned with the finding that the minimal effective dose of copper stimulating LHRH release is about 200 μM (Burrows and Barnea, 1982c). In this study, granules (40K suspension) were isolated by means of differential centrifugation (Fig 1). In such a subcellular fraction, LHRH granules comprise a minor portion of the total particulate material. Therefore, we considered the possibility that the non-LHRH granule proteins compete with the LHRH granules for copper and hence, increase, artificially, the dose-requirement for the metal. This possibility was tested and, indeed, we found that when granules were further purified by means of Percoll-gradient centrifugation, the requirement for copper was drastically reduced (Fig 4). In addition, we noted that the stimulated release of LHRH was a saturable function of the concentration of copper. Using Michaelis-Menten equations for enzyme kinetics, we estimated the kinetic constant of the copper-stimulated release process and found the Vmax to be 65% of the granule content of LHRH released in 5 min and the apparent Km 6 μM copper. It should be emphasized that such a low Km for copper is well within the range of copper concentrations known to affect a number of biochemical reactions (Ting-Beall et al., 1973; Abramson et al., 1983) and of copper concentrations in blood and tissues.

It is well established that copper is present in a chelated form in biological systems and that the biological action of the chelated copper is partially determined by the nature of the

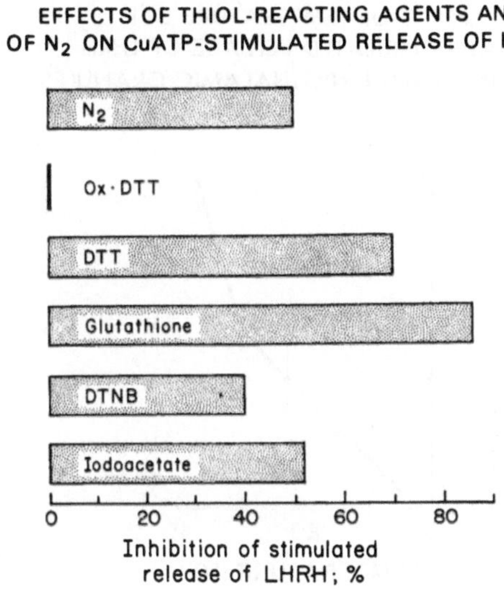

Figure 5. LHRH granules (Fig 2), were incubated with 0.5 mM CuATP as described by Rice and Barnea (1983).

chelator (Osterberg, 1974, 1980). Moreover, tissues obtain their copper supply from the circulation, where copper is chelated by proteins (ceruloplasmin, albumin), peptides (Gly-His-Lys; GHL) and amino acids (histidine, cysteine etc.). Although the mechanism(s) by which copper is transported from blood to tissues has not yet been elucidated, an important role for amino acids and albumin as transport molecules has been postulated. If indeed blood-borne copper plays a role in the release process of LHRH, then one would expect that copper, chelated by one or more of these circulating chelators, would stimulate LHRH release from the isolated hypothalamic granules. When hypothalamic granules were incubated in the presence of CuHistidine or CuCysteine (20 μM each), release of LHRH was markedly stimulated, whereas in the presence of CuGHL or CuBSA release was not stimulated (Barnea and Cho, 1983). These findings strongly support our conclusion that blood-borne copper can play a role in regulating LHRH release from hypothalamic neurons by interacting directly with the LHRH storage granules.

The involvement of granule thiol groups in the regulation of granule-membrane permeability has been proposed (Schofield, 1971; Watkins and Moore, 1974; Lorenson and Jacobs, 1982). Copper is known to catalyze a wide range of biological oxidative processes (Cass and Hill, 1980). That an oxidative reaction, most likely at the level of the granule sulfhydryl groups, is involved in the copper-stimulated release of LHRH can be implied from the following

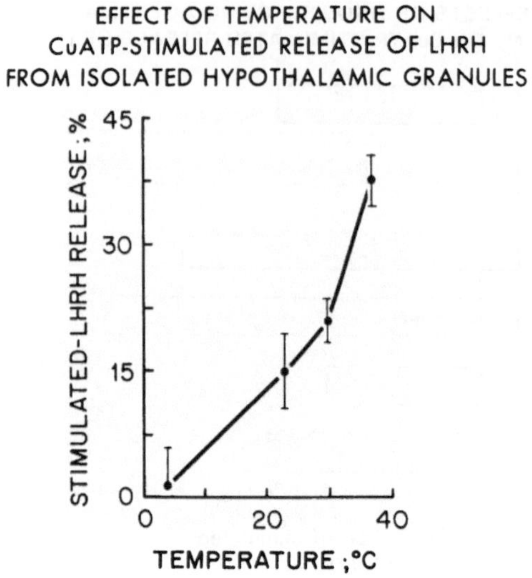

Figure 6. LHRH granules (Fig 2) were incubated for 5 min with 0.5 mM CuATP. From Rice and Barnea (1983), reproduced with permission from Journal of Neurochemistry.

observations (Rice and Barnea, 1983) (Fig 5). One, granules incubated with CuATP under an atmosphere of N_2 released half as much LHRH as those under air. Two, reduced glutathione or dithiothreitol (DTT) but not oxidized DTT inhibited the CuATP-stimulated release of LHRH. Three, incubation of granules with an alkylating agent (iodoacetate) or a disulfide-forming agent [5,5-dithiobis-(2 nitrobenzoic acid); DTNB] inhibited copper action. These observations and the fact that the apparent Km for copper is very low are suggestive that copper interacts with sulfhydryl groups of a specific granule protein.

To evaluate the energy requirement for copper action, granules were incubated with CuATP at various temperatures (Fig 6). We noted that CuATP-stimulated release of LHRH increased progressively with incubation temperature and that at 4°C, where most enzymatic and membrane transport processes are practically abolished, copper-stimulated release of LHRH did not occur (Rice and Barnea, 1983). We wished to ascertain if elevated temperature was required for the interaction between copper and the LHRH granule and/or the actual transport of LHRH from within the granule into the medium (release). First, we established the time-course of copper-stimulated LHRH release at 37°C and found that it was very rapid: maximal release was attained by 6 min of incubation. Second, DTT was added to the granules immediately after the

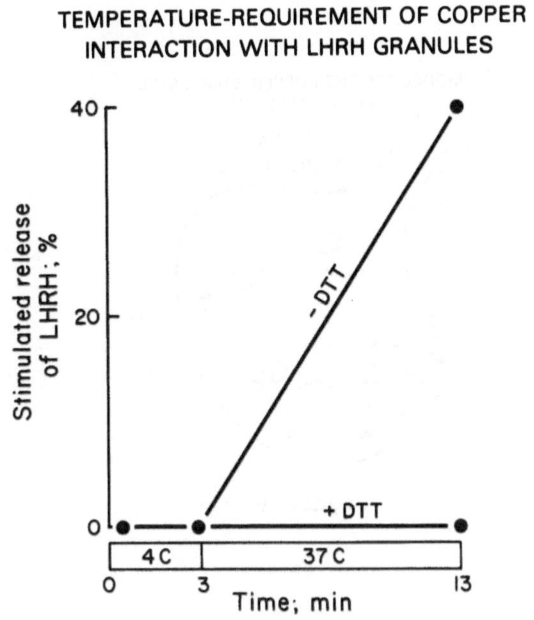

Figure 7. Isolated LHRH granules (Fig 1) were incubated with 20 µM CuHistidine for 3 min at 4°C, after which 1 mM DTT was added and the mixture was transferred to 37°C.

addition of copper and the magnitute of LHRH release was evaluated 6 min after the addition of copper. Under this condition, the stimulated release of LHRH was completely abolished. On the other hand, when DTT was added 3 min after copper, stimulated release of LHRH was not affected, indicating that DTT interferes with the interaction of copper with the granules but not with the actual release of the peptide (Barnea and Cho, 1983). Based on these findings the following experimental protocol was carried out. Granules were incubated with CuHistidine for 3 min at 4°C and then transferred to 37°C for an additional period of 10 min. Just before the transfer from 4°C to 37°C, DTT or buffer was added to the incubation mixture. If the interaction of copper with the granules does not require energy, then stimulated-LHRH release should be observed regardless whether or not DTT was added to the medium. We noted that when copper-treated granules were transferred to 37°C, without the addition of DTT, LHRH release was stimulated (40% of the granule LHRH released) (Fig 7). However, when DTT was added to the medium just before the transfer to 37°C, LHRH release was not stimulated, indicating that the interaction between copper and the LHRH granule requires energy.

It is tempting to speculate on a model which may explain the role of copper in the regulation of LHRH release from hypothalamic neurons. In this model (Fig 8), uptake of extracellular copper by

A MODEL FOR THE COPPER-STIMULATED RELEASE OF LHRH

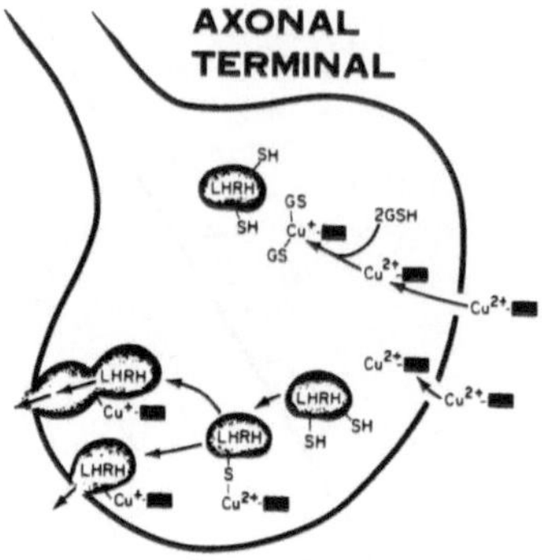

Figure 8

the LHRH neuron results in a high concentration of chelated copper in the plasma membrane and in its vicinity. Such plasma-membrane associated copper would interact with the sulfhydryl groups of LHRH granules that are in close proximity to or in the process of fusing with the plasma membrane. On the other hand, intra-neuronal copper would not interact with the LHRH granules, since it would be inactivated by reduced glutathione which occurs in high concentrations in the cytoplasm ($1 - 50 \times 10^{-4}$M, Kosower and Kosower, 1976). Such a model provides an explanation to the fact that inspite of the presence of copper in high concentrations in the brain (Osterberg, 1980), LHRH is maintained within its storage granule in the LHRH neuron. One can envision a situation in which the concentration of the plasma-membrane associated copper is too low to cause release of the peptide. Such low concentration, however, may suffice to result in a limited oxidative interaction with the sulfhydryl groups of the LHRH granule and by doing so, render the granule more susceptible to other stimuli that initiate LHRH release. Hence, copper may play a role in regulating the release process of LHRH.

ACKNOWLEDGEMENTS. The excellent technical assistance of Gloria Cho and Rashmi Doshi and the editorial assistance of Terri Zandi are highly appreciated. This work was supported by research grants AM25692 and AG00306 from the National Institutes of Health, Bethesda, Maryland.

REFERENCES

Abramson, J.J., Trimm, J.L., Weden, L., and Salama, G., 1983, Heavy metals induce rapid calcium release from sarcoplasmic reticulum vesicles isolated from skeletal muscle, Proc. Natl. Acad. Sci. 80:1526-1530.

Barnea, A., Neaves, W.B., Cho, G., and Porter J.C., 1978a, A subcellular pool of hypo-osmotically resistant particles containing thyrotropin releasing hormone, α-melanocyte stimulating hormone, and luteinizing hormone releasing hormone in the rat hypothalamus, J. Neurochem. 30:937-948.

Barnea, A., Neaves, W.B., Cho, G., and Porter, J.C., 1978b, Demonstration of a temperature-dependent association of thyrotropin releasing hormone, α-melanocyte stimulating hormone, and luteinizing hormone releasing hormone with subneuronal particles in hypothalamic synaptosomes, J. Neurochem. 31:1125-1134

Barnea, A., and Cho, G., 1983, Does blood-borne copper have a role in regulating the release of luteinizing hormone releasing hormone (LHRH) from hypothalamic neurons?, The American Society for Cell Biology, 23rd Annual Meeting, San Antonio, Texas.

Burrows, G.H., Porter, J.C., and Barnea, A., 1981, A model system for the study of the release of luteinizing hormone-releasing hormone from isolated storage granules, J. Neurochem. 36:753-758.

Burrows, G.H., and Barnea, A., 1982a, Comparison of the effects of ATP, Mg^{2+}, and MgATP on the release of luteinizing hormone-releasing hormone from isolated hypothalamic granules, J. Neurochem. 38:569-573.

Burrows, G.H., and Barnea, A., 1982b, MgATP-stimulated release of luteinizing hormone releasing hormone from isolated hypothalamic granules: Evidence for a selective requirement for monovalent cations, J. Neurochem. 39:780-787.

Burrows, G.H., and Barnea A., 1982c, Copper stimulates the release of luteinizing hormone releasing hormone from isolated hypothalamic granules, Endocrinology 110:1456-1458.

Cass, A.E.G., and Hill, H.A.O., 1980, Copper proteins and copper enzymes, Ciba Found. Symp. 79:71-91.

DeLorenzo, R.J., and Freedman, S.D., 1977, Calcium-dependent phosphorylation of synaptic vesicle proteins and its possible role in mediating neurotransmitter release and vesicle function, Biochem. Biophys. Res. Commun. 77:1036-1043.

Douglas, W.W., 1978, Stimulus-secretion coupling: variations on the theme of calcium-activated exocytosis involving cellular and extracellular sources of calcium, Ciba Found. Symp. 54:61-90.

Goldsmith, P.C., and Ganong, W.F., 1975, Ultrastructural localization of luteinizing hormone-releasing hormone in the median eminence of the rat, Brain Res. 97:181-193.

Kosower, N.S., and Kosower, E.M., 1976, The glutathione-glutathione disulfide system, in: Free Radicals in Biology (W.A. Pryor, ed.), pp. 55-84, Academic Press, Amsterdam.

Lorenson, M.Y., and Jacobs, L.S., 1982, Thiol regulation of protein, growth hormone, and prolactin release from isolated adenohypophysial secretory granules, Endocrinology 110:1164-1172.

Osterberg, R., 1974, Metal ion-protein interactions in solution, in: Metal Ions in Biological Systems, Vol. 3 (H. Sigel, ed.), pp. 45-88, Marcel Dekker Inc., New York.

Osterberg, R., 1980, Physiology and pharmacology of copper, Pharmacol. Ther. 9:121-146.

Overgaard, K., Torp-Pedersen, C., and Thorn, N.A., 1979, ATP-induced release of vasopressin from isolated bovine neurohypophyseal secretory granules. Dependency on chloride and effects of analogues of ATP, Acta Endocrinologica 90:609-615.

Pazoles, C.J., and Pollard, H.B., 1978, Evidence for stimulation of anion transport in ATP-evoked transmitter release from isolated secretory vesicles, J. Biol. Chem. 253:3962-3969.

Rice, G.E. and Barnea A., 1983, A possible role for copper-mediated oxidation of thiols in the regulation of the release of luteinizing hormone releasing hormone from isolated hypothalamic granules, J. Neurochem. In Press.

Russell, J.T., and Thorn, N.A., 1978, ATP-induced release of vasopressin associated with phosphorylation of isolated bovine neurohypophyseal secretory granule membranes, Acta Endocrinologica 87:495-506.

Schofield, J.G., 1971, Effect of sulfhydryl reagents on the release of ox growth hormone inb vitro, Biochem. Biophy. Acta. 252:516-525.

Suzuki, M., Takahashi, K., 1974, Hypothalamo-hypophyseal control of ovulation, in: Psychoneuroendocrinology (N. Hatotani, ed.), pp. 114, S. Karger, New York.

Taugner, G., 1972, The effects of univalent anions on catecholamine fluxes and adenosine triphosphatase activity in storage vesicles from the adrenal medulla, J. Biochem. 130:969-973.

Ting-Beall, H.P., Clark, D.A., Suelter, C.H., and Wells, W.W., 1973, Studies on the interaction of chick brain microsomal ($Na^+ + K^+$)-ATPase with copper, Biochem. Biophys. Acta. 291:229-236.

Tsou, R.C., Dailey, R.A., McLanahan, C.S., Parent, A.D., Tindall, G.T., and Neill, J.D., 1977, Luteinizing hormone releasing hormone (LHRH) levels in pituitary stalk plasma during the preovulatory gonadotropin surge of rabbits, Endocrinology 101:534-539.

Watkins, D.T., and Moore, M., 1974, Effect of sulfhydryl-binding reagents on insulin release from isolated secretion granules, Endocrinology 95:485-491.

ROLE OF PEPTIDES IN THE REGULATION OF GONADOTROPIN AND PROLACTIN SECRETION

M. Motta, P. Falaschi*, S. Zoppi and L. Martini

Department of Endocrinology, University of Milano and
*V Clinica Medica, Policlinico Umberto I, Roma

The discovery of different families of peptides in the brain (neurotensin, substance P, bombesin, the so-called gastrointestinal hormones, the opioids, etc.) and the fact that these principles are present in particularly high concentrations in the hypothalamus (Fernstrom et al., 1980; Frederickson, 1980; Said, 1980; Snyder, 1980) have prompted several investigations on the possible role these principles exert on the control of anterior pituitary function. Evidence is rapidly accumulating which suggests that many of these peptides may play a physiological role as modulators of the activity of the hypothalamic-pituitary system (see McCann, 1980 for references).

This paper summarizes some of the results obtained in the authors' laboratory on the effects exerted by the opioids, by neurotensin and by sauvagine in the regulation of gonadotropin and prolactin secretion.

Effects of the opioids in the control of gonadotropin secretion

Recent experimental and clinical evidence, obtained with the systemic administration of opioid agonists and antagonists, suggests that brain opioids may exert an inhibitory action on LH release (Bruni et al., 1977; Meites et al., 1979; Morley, 1981).
This concept receives support also from the data to be reported

here and obtained in the authors' laboratories while testing a new potent morphine-like peptide, dermorphin. This peptide has been recently discovered in the amphibian skin and chemically characterized as being H-Tyr-D-Ala-Phe-Gly-Tyr-Pro-Ser-NH_2 (Montecucchi et al., 1981). On the basis of the observation that this heptapeptide (a) exerts potent central and peripheral morphine-like effects (Broccardo et al., 1981; Erspamer et al., 1981), and (b) is probably present in the mammalian brain (Buffa et al., 1982; Negri et al., 1981), it was of interest to investigate whether dermorphin,

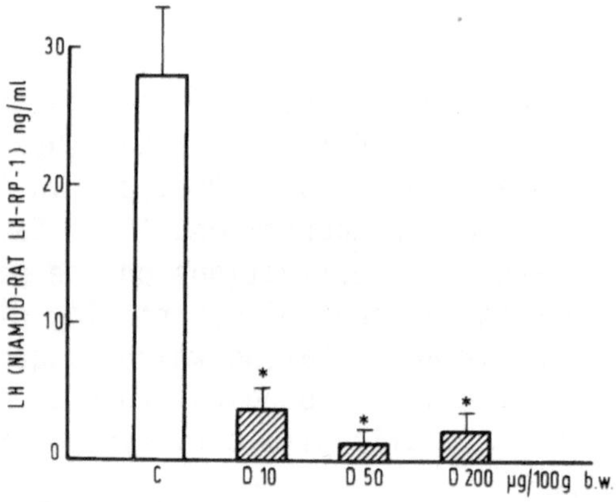

Fig. 1. Effect of subcutaneous injections of dermorphin (D) on LH release in normal male rats.

like the other opioid principles, is able to influence LH and/or FSH secretion.

The effects of systemic treatment with different doses of dermorphin on gonadotropin secretion have been evaluated in normal male rats. Dermorphin (in doses ranging from 10 to 200 μg/100 g b.w.) is able to decrease serum LH levels in normal male rats sacrificed 1 hour after injection (Fig.1).

Similar results have been obtained when dermorphin was given intraventricularly (i.v.t.) in much lower doses to long term castrated male rats. It is apparent from Fig.2 that, under the conditions of the present experiment, the i.v.t. injection of dermorphin (100 μg/100 g b.w.) significantly decreases serum LH levels in orchidectomized rats 30 minutes after treatment; an i.v.t. dose of 25 μg/100 g b.w. of this peptide is effective in decreasing serum LH levels of the orchidectomized rats at the 60 minute interval. Dermorphin proved unable to induce any significant change in serum FSH levels in either normal(systemic administration)or castrated male rats (i.v.t. injection) (data not shown).

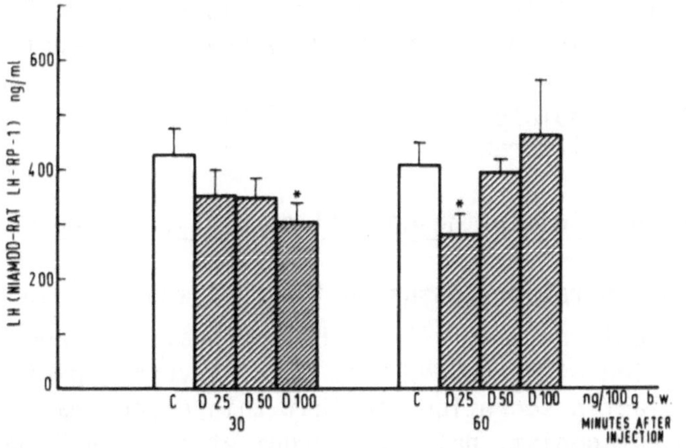

Fig. 2. Effect of i.v.t. injections of dermorphin (D) on LH release in long-term castrated male rats.

However, it must be pointed out that,in the light of the findings which will be summarized below, the partecipation of the opioids in the control of the release of LH does not seem to be as simple as it might be anticipated from the results so far described. Motta and Martini (1982) have demonstrated that the i.v.t. injection of 25 μg of either methionine-enkephalin or one of its synthetic analogs, (D-Ala^2)-methionine-enkephalinamide, induces a significant increase (rather than a decrease) of serum LH levels in long-term castrated female rats. More recently Limonta et al. (1982) have shown that the i.v.t. injection of morphine (60 or 120 μg/100 g b.w.) performed in normal adult male rats also results in a stimulation of LH release. As in the case of dermorphin, neither methio-

nine-enkephalin and its analog nor morphine proved able to modify serum levels of FSH. A stimulatory effect of the opioids on LH secretion has been reported by Takahara et al.(1978), Pang et al. (1977) and Cicero et al.(1980) following respectively the i.v.t. infusion of β-endorphin, the intraperitoneal injection of morphine and the chronic administration of morphine.
On the basis of these findings it may be postulated that the opioids may exert a dual role (inhibitory or stimulatory) in the regulation of LH secretion. These results therefore suggest the presence of at least two different opioid systems (pathways or receptors?) which exert opposite effects (inhibitory or stimulatory) on the LHRH-producing neurons. It also emerges from these data that the effect of opioids on LH secretion (indipendently on whether a stimulation or an inhibition is obtained) is rather specific, since it is not accompanied by any significant modification of FSH secretion; this further demonstrates that the control mechanisms which regulate the release of the two gonadotropins are substantially different.

Effects of the opioids in the control of prolactin secretion

There is now a general consensus on the fact that opioid peptides stimulate prolactin release. It has been repeatedly reported that the administration of these peptides or of several opioid agonists stimulates prolactin secretion and that this effect may be blocked by the opioid antagonist, naloxone (Bruni et al., 1977; Dupont et al., 1977; Johnson, 1982; Koenig et al., 1979; Meltzer et al., 1978; Mioduszewski et al., 1982; Panerai et al., 1981; Rivier et al., 1977; Van Vugt and Meites, 1980; Van Vugt et al., 1981). The following experiments, carried out in the authors' laboratories are confirmatory of this view.
The effect of dermorphin, morphine and naloxone on the release of prolactin was studied in normal male rats at different time intervals after treatment. Dermorphin, when given i.v.t. (at a dose of 100 ng/100 g b.w.) to normal male rats, causes a statistically significant increase in serum prolactin levels 10 minutes after injection (Fig.3). Serum prolactin levels return to normal at later intervals. On the contrary, the i.v.t. treatment with naloxone (10 μg/100 g b.w.) is unable to modify serum prolactin levels at any time interval considered (Fig.3). The i.v.t. administration of naloxone performed together with i.v.t. dermorphin completely

counteracts the stimulatory effect exerted by the peptide on prolactin secretion (Fig.3).

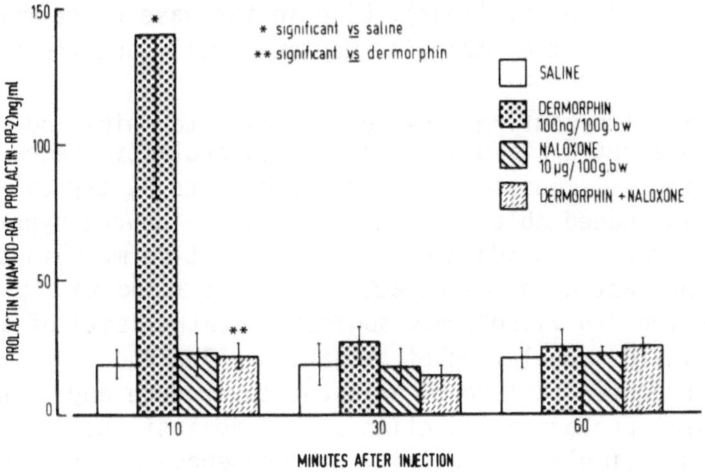

Fig. 3. Effect of i.v.t. injections of dermorphin and of naloxone on prolactin release in normal male rats.

When added "in vitro" to isolated and dispersed rat pituitary cells dermorphin does not influence the basal secretion of prolactin nor does antagonize the typical inhibitory effect exerted by dopamine (Fig.4)

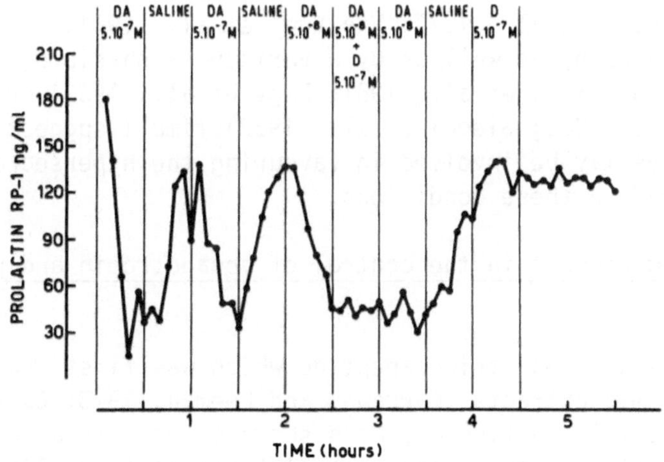

Fig. 4. Effect of dermorphin (D) on basal and dopamine (DA)-inhibited prolactin release from isolated and dispersed rat pituitary cells.

Also the i.v.t. injection of morphine (60 μg/100 g.b.w.) has been shown to induce a significant increase in serum prolactin levels 20, 40 and 60 minutes after treatment in normal male rats (Piva et al. unpublished observations). Like in the case of dermorphin, the stimulatory effect of morphine may be totally antagonized by naloxone.

The present results confirm first of all that morphine and morphine-like peptides exert a stimulatory effect on prolactin secretion and that this effect is mediated by opioid receptors; a typical opioid antagonist is indeed able to reverse the drug-induced hypersecretion of the hormone. In addition, the fact that dermorphin does not exhibit any prolactin releasing activity, when added to a pituitary cell preparation "in vitro", may suggest a central site of action of the opioids in the regulation of prolactin release.

Finally, the reported failure of naloxone to produce any significant effect on basal prolactin secretion argues against the existence of a permanent stimulating activity of endogenous opioid peptides on the release of this hormone. This has been claimed by some authors who have reported naloxone to be effective in decreasing baseline prolactin levels (Brown et al., 1978; Bruni et al., 1977; Meltzer et al., 1978; Siegel et al.,1982; Van Vugt et al., 1978). However, it must be pointed out that in these studies naloxone was injected systemically and not intraventricularly as in the present experiments. Anyway, the fact that naloxone prevents the rise of prolactin induced by the opioids (Bruni et al., 1977; Meltzer et al., 1978; Rivier et al., 1977; Van Vugt et al., 1981; and see the preceding paragraph) as well as by a variety of physiological (e. g. suckling) (Miki et al., 1981; Nagy et al., 1982) or stressful (Rossier et al., 1980; Siegel et al., 1982)stimuli suggest that opioid pathways may be involved in favouring the hypersecretion of prolactin found in these conditions.

Effects of neurotensin in the control of gonadotropin and prolactin secretion

Neurotensin is a linear tridecapeptide which was first isolated from hypothalamic extracts (Carraway and Leeman, 1973; Carraway and Leeman, 1975). This peptide has been shown to possess a large variety of biological effects on the gastrointestinal tract (Carraway and Leeman, 1973; Segawa et al., 1977)and on the cardiovascular (Carraway and Leeman, 1973) and endocrine (Brown and Vale, 1976;

Farina et al., 1978; Kaneto et al., 1978; McCann, 1980) systems. The effect of neurotensin on the release of LH, FSH and prolactin was analyzed in long-term castrated female rats. The i.v.t. injection of 30 μg/rat of neurotensin induces a significant decrease of serum LH levels (Fig.5). This decrease was not accompanied by any change in FSH or prolactin secretion (Motta and Martini, 1981).

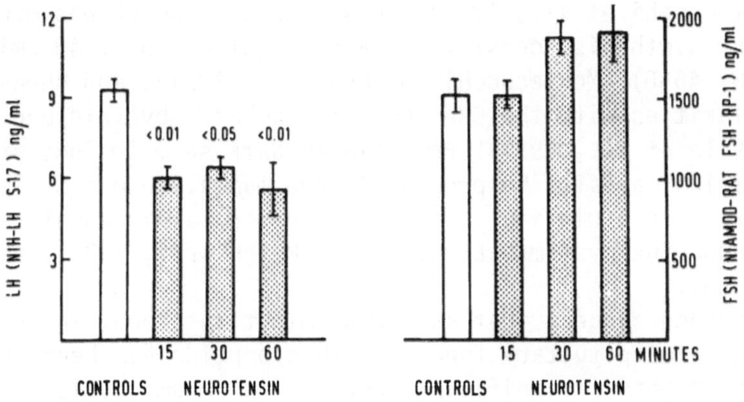

Fig. 5. Effect of i.v.t. injections of 30 μg/rat of neurotensin on serum LH and FSH levels of castrated female rats.

The present results on the effects of neurotensin on LH and FSH secretion agree with those of Vijayan and McCann (1978) obtained in ovariectomized freely moving rats, but are not consistent with those of Makino et al. (1973) who found a stimulation of the release of both gonadotropins following the intravenous injection of neurotensin into normal rats.

With regard to the effects of neurotensin on prolactin release the results of the present experiments differ from those obtained by McCann's group (Vijayan and McCann, 1978): they reported an inhibitory effect of neurotensin given i.v.t. on the release of this hormone. This discrepancy may probably be accounted for by methodological differences (doses of neurotensin used, animal preparation, way of administration, etc.).

In general the results suggest that neurotensin may partecipate in the control of LH release;as in the case of the opioids, this effect seems to be specific, since the administration of neurotensin is not associated with any modification in FSH secretion. Also the present observations provide additional data on the separate control of the release of the two gonadotropins.

Effects of sauvagine in the control of gonadotropin and prolactin secretion.

Sauvagine is a polypeptide recently isolated from the amphibian skin (Montecucchi et al., 1980). This molecule, which has now been obtained by synthesis, consists of a straight chain of 40 amino-acids (M.W. 4600) (Montecucchi and Henschen, 1981), and shows striking similarities with the CRF recently isolated by Vale and co-workers (Vale et al., 1981). Preliminary data seem to indicate that sauvagine may also be present in the mammalian brain. This peptide exhibits biological activities on the cardiovascular, renal and endocrine systems (Erspamer and Melchiorri, 1980; Erspamer et al., 1980).
Recent evidence suggest that sauvagine might intervene in the control of anterior pituitary function. This peptide has been shown to produce in rats a significant increase in serum levels of ACTH and of β-endorphin-like immunoreactivity (Falaschi et al., 1982; Falaschi et al., 1983). Sauvagine also exerts a stimulatory effect on ACTH output,when added to pituitary cells "in vitro" (Falaschi et al., 1980; Falaschi et al., 1982). These findings are not surprising due to the similarities between sauvagine and Vale's CRF. The possible effects of sauvagine on the release of LH, FSH and prolactin have been tested "in vivo" and "in vitro". It has been found that sauvagine, given i.v.t. at a dose of 0.2 μg/100 g b.w. to castrated male rats does not exert any effect on serum LH and FSH levels (Falaschi et al., 1982). Similar negative results have been obtained when this peptide was assayed in an "in vitro" system. These results may indicate that sauvagine is not involved in the control of the gonadotropic activity of the anterior pituitary gland. Subcutaneous administrations of 20 ng/100 g b.w. of sauvagine significantly decrease serum prolactin levels in normal male rats beginning 60 minutes after injection; this effect lasts for 4 hours. Moreover the subcutaneous treatment with sauvagine (0.1, 0.5 and 2μg/100 g b.w.) performed in lactating rats, is able to suppress the suckling-induced rise of prolactin (Fig.6)

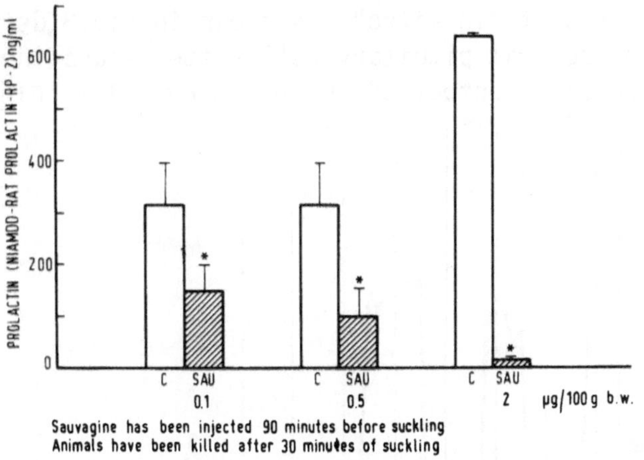

Fig. 6. Effect of subcutaneous injections of sauvagine (SAU) on prolactin release in suckling rats.

On the contrary, sauvagine, when given i.v.t. (0.2 μg/100 g b.w.) is devoid of any prolactin inhibiting effect at any time interval considered (Fig.7)

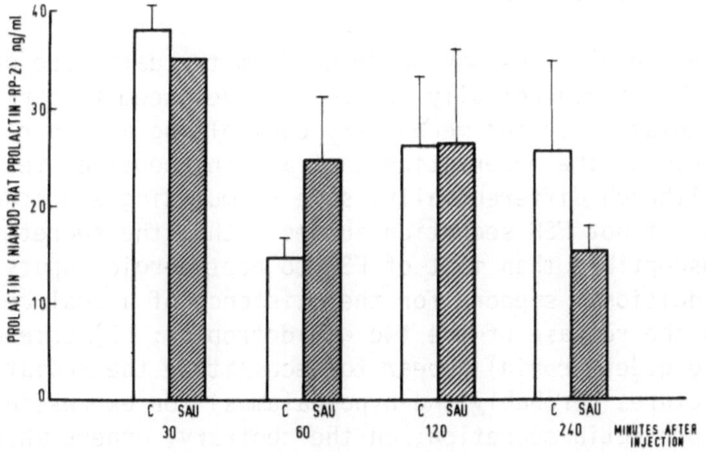

Fig. 7. Effect of i.v.t. injections of sauvagine (SAU, 200 ng/ 100 g b.w.) on prolactin release in long-term castrated male rats.

The potent and long lasting prolactin inhibitory effect of this peptide is also present "in vitro". As shown in Fig.8,using the isolated and dispersed rat pituitary cell system sauvagine remarkably reduces the prolactin output of the perfused cells (Fig. 8).

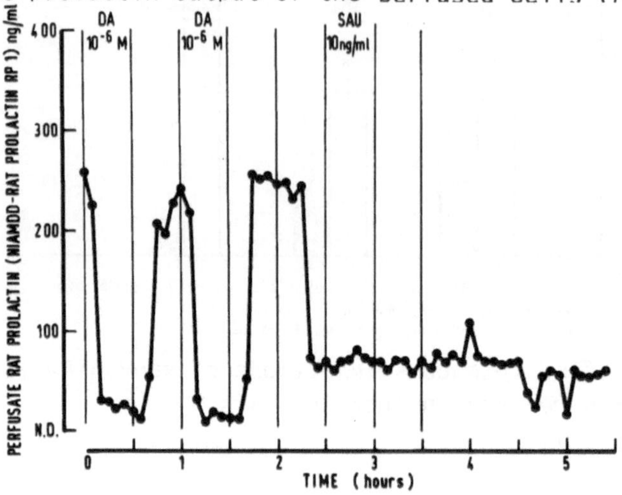

Fig. 8. Effect of sauvagine (SAU) on prolactin secretion from isolated and dispersed rat pituitary cells.

GENERAL CONCLUSIONS

Some general conclusions may be drawn from the data here presented: (1) a variety of biologically active peptides seem to participate as neuromodulators in the mechanisms controlling anterior pituitary function; (2) the observation that all the peptides tested influence (although differentially, some stimulating and others inhibiting) LH but not FSH secretion suggests that the secretion of LH is more susceptible than that of FSH to peptidergic inputs; this provides additional support for the existence of a dual central control on the release of the two gonadotropins; (3) some of the peptides (e.g.dermorphin) appear to necessitate the mediation of brain structures (probably the hypothalamus) for expressing their effect on prolactin secretion; on the contrary, others which,like sauvagine,seem to act directly at pituitary level might be included in the category of the inhibiting or releasing factors.

ACKNOWLEDGMENTS

The experiments here described were supported by a grant of the Consiglio Nazionale delle Ricerche, Rome, Italy (through the Project "Preventive and Rehabilitative Medicine"). Such support is gratefully acknowledged. Materials for LH, FSH and prolactin RIA were kindly provided by Dr. Niswender and by the Rat Pituitary Hormone Distribution Program of the NIAMDD, Bethesda, USA.

REFERENCES

- Broccardo, M., Erspamer, V., Falconieri Erspamer, G., Improta, G., Linari, G., Melchiorri, P. and Montecucchi, P.C., 1981, Pharmacological data on dermorphins, a new class of potent opioid peptides from Amphibian skin, Br.J.Pharmacol., 73: 625.
- Brown, M. and Vale, W., 1976, Effects of neurotensin and substance P on plasma insulin, glucagone and glucose levels, Endocrinology, 98: 819.
- Brown, B., Dettmar, P.W., Dobson, P R., Lym, A.G., Metcalf, G and Morgan, B.A., 1978, Opiate analgesics: the effect of agonist-antagonist character on prolactin secretion, J.Pharm.Pharmacol., 30: 644.
- Bruni, J.F., Van Vugt, D., Marshall, S. and Meites, J., 1977, Effects of naloxone, morphine and methionine enkephalin on serum prolactin, luteinizing hormone, follicle stimulating hormone, thyroid stimulating hormone and growth hormone, Life Sci., 21: 461.
- Buffa, R., Solcia, E., Magnoni, E., Rindi, G., Negri, L. and Melchiorri, P., 1982, Immunohistochemical demonstration of a dermorphin-like peptide in the rat brain, Histochemistry, 76: 273.
- Carraway, R. and Leeman, S.E., 1973, The isolation of a new hypotensive peptide, neurotensin, from bovine hypothalami, J. Biol. Chem., 248: 6854.
- Carraway, R. and Leeman, S.E., 1975, The amino acid sequence of a hypothalamic peptide, neurotensin, J. Biol. Chem., 250: 1907.
- Cicero, T.J., Meyer, E.R., Gabriel, S.M., Bell, R.D. and Wilcox, C.E., 1980, Morphine exerts testosterone-like effects in the hypothalamus of the castrated male rat, Brain Res., 202: 151.
- Dupont, A., Cusan, L., Labrie, F., Coy, D.H. and Li, C.H., 1977, Stimulation of prolactin release in the rat by intraventricular injection of beta-endorphin and methionine-enkephalin, Biochem. Biophys. Res. Commun., 75: 76.
- Erspamer, V. and Melchiorri, P., 1980, Active polypeptides: from amphibian skin to gastrointestinal tract and brain of mammals, Trends Pharmacol. Sci., 1: 391.
- Erspamer, V., Falconieri Erspamer, G., Improta, G., Negri, L. and de Castiglione, R., 1980, Sauvagine, a new polypeptide from

Phillomedusa sauvagei skin, Naunyn-Schiedeberg's Arch. Pharmacol., 312: 265.
- Erspamer, V., Melchiorri, P. and Broccardo, M., 1981, The brain-gut-skin triangle: new peptides, Peptides, 2: 7.
- Falaschi, P., Melchiorri, P., D'Urso, R., Negri, L., Rocco, A. and Erspamer, V., 1980, Sauvagine, a frog skin peptide, stimulates ACTH and beta-endorphin release from isolated and dispersed rat pituitary cells in perfusion, Hormone Metab. Res., 13: 329.
- Falaschi, P., D'Urso, R., Negri, L., Rocco, A., Montecucchi, P. C., Henschen, A., Melchiorri, P. and Erspamer, V., 1982, Potent in vivo and in vitro prolactin inhibiting activity of sauvagine, a frog skin peptide, Endocrinology, 111: 693.
- Falaschi, P., Melchiorri, P., D'Urso, R., Negri, L., Rocco, A., Messi, E., Motta, M. and Erspamer, V., 1982, Sauvagine (SAU): new perspectives in hypothalamic control of pituitary function, J. Endocrinol. Invest., (Suppl. 1) 5: 22.
- Falaschi, P., D'Urso, R., Negri, L., Proietti, A., Rocco, A., Motta, M. and Erspamer, V., 1983, Sauvagine and ovine CRF: a frog skin peptide as anticipator of a mammalian brain hormone, in: "Pituitary Hyperfunction," E. Müller, G.M. Molinatti and F. Camanni, eds., Raven Press, New York, in press.
- Farina, J.M.S., Celotti, F., Motta, M. and Martini, L., 1978, Effect of neurotensin on glucagone and insulin portal blood levels in hyperglycemic rats, J. Endocrinol. Invest., 2: 179.
- Fernstrom, M.H., Carraway, R.E. and Leeman, S.E., 1980, Neurotensin, in: "Frontiers in Neuroendocrinology, vol. 6," L. Martini and W.F. Ganong eds., Raven Press, New York, p. 103.
- Frederickson, R.C.A., 1980, Peptide receptors in the brain, in: "Comprehensive Endocrinology," M. Motta, ed., Raven Press, New York, p. 233.
- Johnson, J.H., 1982, Release of prolactin in response to injection of morphine into mesencephalic dorsal raphe nucleus, Neuroendocrinology, 35: 169.
- Kaneto, A., Kaneko, T., Kajinumana, H. and Kosaka, K., 1978, Effects of substance P and neurotensin infused intrapancreatically on glucagone and insulin secretion, Endocrinology, 102: 393.
- Koenig, J.I., Mayfield, M.A., McCann, S.M. and Krulich, L., 1979, Stimulation on prolactin secretion by morphine: role of the central serotoninergic system, Life Sci., 25: 853.
- Limonta, P., Giudici, D., Piva, F. and Martini, L., 1982, Morphine and naloxone stimulate LH secretion when given intraventricularly, Endocrinology, 110: 389A.

- Makino, R., Carraway, R., Leeman, S.E. and Greep, R.O., 1973, In vitro and in vivo effects of newly purified hypothalamic tridecapeptide on rat LH and FSH release, Program 6th Meet. Group Study Reprod., p. 26.
- McCann, S.M., 1980, Control of anterior pituitary hormone release by brain peptides, Neuroendocrinology, 31: 355.
- Meites, J., Bruni, J.F., Van Vugt, D.A. and Smith, A.F., 1979, Relation of endogenous opioid peptides and morphine to neuroendocrine functions, Life Sci., 24: 1325.
- Meltzer, H.Y., Miller, R.J., Fessler, R.G., Simonovic, M. and Fang, V.S., 1978, Effects of enkephalin analogues on prolactin release in the rat, Life Sci., 22: 1931.
- Miki, N., Sonntag, W.E., Forman, L.J. and Meites, J., 1981, Suppression by naloxone of rise in plasma growth hormone and prolactin induced by suckling, Proc.Soc.exp.Biol.Med., 168: 330.
- Mioduszewski, R., Zimmermann, E. and Critchlow, V., 1982, Effects of morphine dependence, withdrawal and tolerance on prolactin and growth hormone secretion in the rat, Life Sci., 30: 1343.
- Montecucchi, P.C., Anastasi, A., de Castiglione, R. and Erspamer, V., 1980, Isolation and amino acid composition of sauvagine an active polypeptide from methanol extracts of the skin of the South American frog Phyllomedusa sauvagei, Int. J. Peptide Protein Res., 16: 191.
- Montecucchi, P.C. and Henschen, A., 1981, Amino acid composition and sequence analysis of sauvagine, a new active peptide from the skin of the Phyllomedusa sauvagei, Int. J. Peptide Protein Res., 18: 113.
- Montecucchi, P.C., de Castiglione, R., Piani, S., Gozzini, L. and Erspamer, V., 1981, Amino acid composition and sequence of dermorphin, a novel opiate-like peptide from the skin of Phyllomedusa sauvagei, Int.J.Peptide Protein Res., 17: 275.
- Morley, J.E., 1981, The endocrinology of the opiates and opioid peptides, Metabolism, 30: 195.
- Motta, M. and Martini, L., 1981, Neurotensin inhibits LH release, Proc. Soc.exp. Biol. Med., 168: 62.
- Motta, M. and Martini, L., 1982, Effect of opioid peptides on gonadotrophin secretion, Acta Endocrinol., 99: 321.
- Nagy, G., Kacsoh, B. and Halasz, B., 1982, Effect of naloxone on the suckling induced prolactin release in rats, Endocr. Exp., 16: 239.
- Negri, L., Melchiorri, P., Falconieri Erspamer, G. and Erspamer, V., 1981, Radioimmunoassay of dermorphin-like peptides in mammalian and non mammalian tissue, Peptides, 2: 45.

- Panerai, A.E., Casanueva, F., Martini, A., Mantegazza, P. and Di Giulio, A.M., 1981, Opiates act centrally on GH and PRL release, Endocrinology, 108: 2004.
- Pang, C.N., Zimmermann, E. and Sawyer, C.H., 1977, Morphine inhibition of the preovulatory surges of plasma luteinizing hormone and follicle stimulating hormone in the rat, Endocrinology, 101: 1726.
- Rivier, C., Vale, V., Ling, N., Brown, M. and Guillemin, R., 1977, Stimulation in vivo of the secretion of prolactin and growth hormone by beta-endorphin, Endocrinology, 100: 238.
- Rossier, J., Fench, E., Rivier, C., Shibasaki, T., Guillemin, R. and Bloom, F.E., 1980, Strees-induced release of prolactin: blockade by dexamethasone and naloxone may indicate beta-endorphin mediation, Proc. Natl. Acad. Sci. U.S.A., 77: 666.
- Said, S.I., 1980, Peptides common with the nervous system and the gastrointestinal tract, in: "Frontiers in Neuroendocrinology, vol. 6," L. Martini and W.F. Ganong, eds., Raven Press, New York, p. 293.
- Segawa, T., Mosokawa, M., Fitigawa, K. and Yajima, H., 1977, Contractile activity of synthetic neurotensin and related polypeptides on guinea-pig ileum, J. Pharm. Pharmacol., 29: 57.
- Siegel, R.A., Chowers, I., Conforti, N. and Weidenfeld, J., 1982, Effects of naloxone on basal and stress-induced prolactin secretion in intact, hypothalamic deafferented adrenalectomized, and dexamethasone-pretreated male rats, Life Sci., 30: 1691.
- Snyder, H.S., 1980, Brain peptides as neurotransmitters. Science, 209: 976.
- Takahara, J., Kageyama, J., Yunoki, S., Yakushiji, W., Yamauchi, J., Kageyma, N. and Ofuji, T., 1978, Effects of 2-bromo-alpha-ergocriptine on beta-endorphin-induced growth hormone, prolactin and luteinizing hormone release in urethane anesthetized rats, Life Sci., 22: 2205.
- Vale, W., Spiess, J., Rivier, C. and Rivier, J. 1981 , Characterization of a 41-residue ovine peptide that stimulates, Science, 213: 1394.
- Van Vugt, D.A., Bruni, J.F. and Meites, J., 1978, Naloxone inhibition of stress-induced increase in prolactin secretion, Life Sci., 22: 85.
- Van Vugt, D.A. and Meites, J., 1980, Influence of endogenous opiates on anterior pituitary function, Fed. Proc., 39: 2533.
- Van Vugt, D.A., Sylvester, P.W., Aylsworth, C.F. and Meites, J., 1981, Comparison of acute effects of dynorphin and beta-endorphin on prolactin release in the rat, Endocrinology, 107: 2017.

- Vijayan, E. and McCann, S.M., 1978, Effects of intraventricular injection of substance P (SP), Neurotensin (NT), and gastrin (G) on pituitary hormone release in conscious ovariectomized (OVX) rats, Endocrinology, 102: 217A.

ESTROUS CYCLE DEPENDENT MODULATION OF MUSCARINIC CHOLINERGIC RECEPTORS IN THE HYPOTHALAMUS AND ADENOHYPOPHYSIS

Mordechai Sokolovsky, Ethy Moscona-Amir and Yaakov Egozi

Department of Biochemistry
George S. Wise Faculty of Life Sciences,
Tel Aviv University, 69978 Tel-Aviv, Israel

INTRODUCTION

Muscarinic acetylcholine receptors mediate the response of cells to the neurotransmitter acetylcholine (AcCho). The physiological significance of muscarinic receptors in the parasympathetic nervous system has been well documented.[1] Among the most marked effects of muscarinic agonists are those observed in gastric and salivary glands, smooth muscle and the cardiovascular system.[1] In the central nervous system most of the cholinergic receptors are of the muscarinic type;[2] some of them, e.g. cerebral cortex receptors, are mainly excitatory while others, particularly in the hypothalamus, are mostly inhibitory.[3]

With increasingly sensitive techniques of receptor detection, muscarinic receptors have been biochemically characterized in both the peripheral and the central nervous systems.[4,5,6] Among the tissues in which cholinergic muscarinic receptors have been biochemically characterized are the rat adenohypophysis[7,8,9] and rat hypothalamus.[8,9,10] Although their physiological role in these regions is not yet understood, a cholinergic mediation has been implicated in the modulation of release of growth hormone,[11] prolactin and luteinizing hormone[12] from the anterior pituitary. Studies have demonstrated that carbamylcholine stimulates the release of growth hormone and thyroid stimulating hormone from anterior pituitary cells;[13] it also inhibits prolactin release, an effect that can be reversed by atropine.[14] Other studies have indicated the possible involvement of cholinergic mechanisms in the regulation of gonadotropin secretion: atropine, an anticholinergic drug, was shown to block ovulation,[15] while cholinomimetic drugs were shown to depress the secretion of luteneizing hormone in ovariectomized, estrogen-primed rats.[16] These findings thus imply a multireceptor regulation of the adenohypophyseal neuroendocrine system, with hormonal release mechanisms involving not only hypothalamic releasing hormones[17] and steroid hormones acting at the hypothalamic[18] and adenohypophyseal levels,[19] but also neurotransmitters such as acetylcholine.

It has been demonstrated that properties of cell surface receptors can be regulated by hormones and neurotransmitters in endocrine and other tissues subject to hormonal control.[20] One might thus reasonably expect that muscarinic receptors in the adenohypophysis and hypothalamus, if they have a functional role to play in the hypothalamus-adenohypophysis axis, would be regulated by hormones. To examine this possibility, we studied in vitro the binding properties of muscarinic receptors in male and female rats at the various stages of the estrous cycle, in the presence and absence of steroid hormones. The experiments were carried out using homogenates from ovariectomized rats and steroid-treated homogenates from cyclic rats.

Muscarinic receptors in the rat adenohypophysis

Muscarinic receptors in various tissues have been characterized by means of binding studies using potent tritiated muscarinic antagonists such as [^{3}H]-4-N-methyl piperidyl benzilate ([^{3}H]-4NMPB), [^{3}H]-quinuclidinyl benzilate ([^{3}H]-QNB) and [^{3}H]-methyl scopolamine. In most cases these [^{3}H]-antagonists bind to a homogeneous population of sites, the number of sites being constant for a given tissue.[4,5,6] In the adenohypophysis, however, these same [^{3}H]-antagonists bind to an apparently heterogeneous population of binding sites,[7] as indicated by the curvilinear Scatchard plots of the binding data which also reflect negative cooperativity.[21] Nevertheless, the number of muscarinic binding sites occupied by any of the radiolabeled antagonists is the same (∿280 fmol/mg protein),[7] and antagonist binding is inhibited by muscarinic agonists at the physiologically relevant (μM) concentration range.[7]

The mixed cooperative-heterogeneous interaction of muscarinic antagonists with their receptors in the adenohypophysis necessitates a complex model for the evaluation of binding parameters.[21] In the absence of a quantitative measure of the contribution by each of the factors influencing the mode of antagonist binding, the simplest analysis of binding data would be based on a two-site model involving two heterogeneous, non-interacting sites.[7,9] Using this model one can evaluate the apparent characteristics of antagonist binding, which in turn reflects the properties of the receptor. Thus, male adenohypophyseal muscarinic receptors are apparently characterized by two subpopulations: [^{3}H]-4NMPB is bound by one of them (comprising 63% of the receptors) with low affinity (Kd_β=2.0 nM), and by the other (38% of receptors) with high affinity (Kd_α=0.41 nM).[7] Similar binding characteristics were observed in the adenohypophyses of female rats at the diestrous stage. However, binding differed at the proestrous and estrous stages, as manifested by an increased Kd_β and a marked decrease in the density of muscarinic receptors from 218 fmole/mg protein to 161 fmole/mg protein (Table 1). This decrease is attributable mainly to a reduction in density of the low affinity subpopulations. These results clearly indicate that changes occur in the adenohypophyseal muscarinic receptors during the estrous cycle. Such changes might be accounted for in terms of variations in endogenous cholinergic activity and/or in the levels of endogenous sex hormones.

Table 1. Binding characteristics of adenohypophyseal muscarinic receptors from male rats and female rats during the estrous cycle

	Maximal binding capacity for the antagonist [^{3}H]-4NMPB (fmole/mg protein)	Proportion of high affinity agonist binding sites (%)
Male	176	42
Female androgenized	166	40
diestrous	183	57
proestrous	218	85
estrous	161	55
ovariectomized	174	40
ovariectomized + 17β-estradiol	211	26
proestrous + in vitro incubation with 17β-estradiol	220	22

Binding capacity was calculated by Scatchard plot analysis. Proportion of high affinity agonist binding sites was calculated from competition binding data ([^{3}H]-4NMPB/oxotremorine) using a two site model[7] for agonist binding. Accordingly, binding sites X% is the proportion of high affinity and 100-X% is the proportion of low affinity binding sites.

If endogenous cholinergic activity contributes to the state of muscarinic receptors observed in vitro, then the binding characteristics of muscarinic agonists should also vary during the estrous cycle. Indeed, binding of the agonist oxotremorine undergoes changes during the estrous cycle, as shown in Fig. 1: the apparent affinity of oxotremorine towards the receptors (as measured by its inhibition

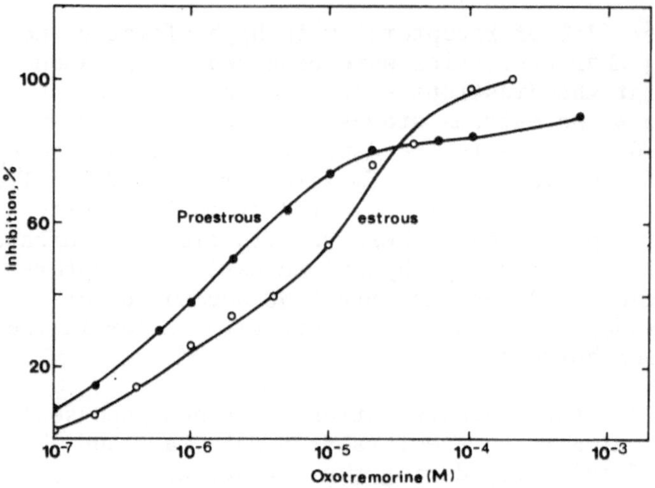

Fig. 1. Inhibition of [^{3}H]-4NMPB binding to adenohypophyseal muscarinig receptors by the agonist oxotremorine. Adenohypophysis from rat on the proestrus (•) or estrus (o) days were homogenized and used for binding studies at 25°C in Krebs buffer (containing 1.8 mM $CaCl_2$) as described before.[7] Data represent % inhibition of [^{3}H]-4NMPB binding by various concentrations of oxotremorine. [^{3}H]-4NMPB concentration was 2.0 nM.

of [^{3}H]-4NMPB binding) is lower at the estrous than at the proestrous stage. This lowered affinity stems mainly from a decrease in the proportion of high affinity agonist binding sites, which comprise ∿85% of the total during proestrus and 55% during estrus (Table 1). At the diestrous stage and in male rats only about 50% of the total are high affinity sites. Thus, adenohypophyseal muscarinic receptors typically undergo a change during the transition from the proestrous to the estrous stages: the total number of receptors is decreased, and this is accompanied by a reduction in proportion of high affinity agonist binding sites. This phenomenon is identical with that observed in cultured heart cells upon exposure to carbamylcholine,[22] viz., a reduction in both receptor density and the proportion of high affinity agonist binding sites. It therefore seems most likely that cholinergic activity is the immediate source of the observed changes in adenohypophyseal muscarinic receptors. However, the dependence of these changes on the estrous cycle suggests that the sex hormones are also involved.

The possible participation of steroid sex hormones in the regulation of muscarinic receptors was investigated in the ovariectomized rat (OVX), in which the primary source of estrogen and progesterone is eliminated.[23] The binding of [^{3}H]-4NMPB (Fig. 2) and of oxotremorine

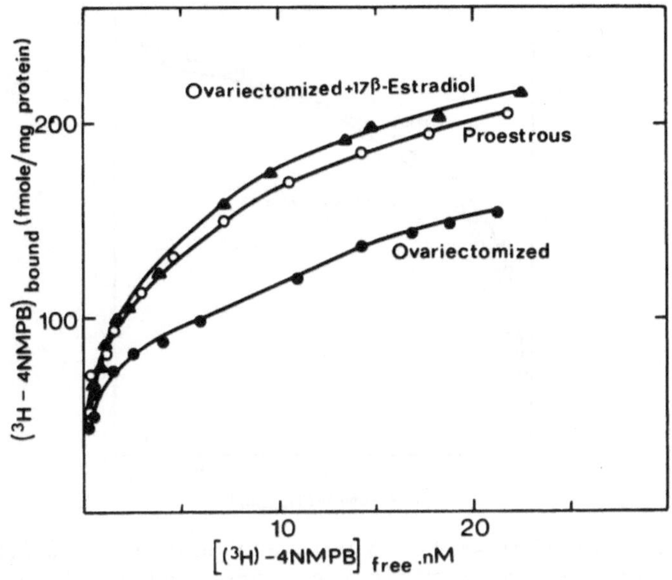

Fig. 2. Binding of [^{3}H]-4NMPB to adenohypophyseal muscarinic receptors in homogenates from rats in proestrus (o), from ovariectomized rats (•) or ovariectomized rats with 17β-estradiol implant (▲). Binding of [^{3}H]-4NMPB to the homogenates was measured at 25°C in Krebs buffer (containing 1.8 mM $CaCl_2$) by methods described before.[7]

to adenohypophyseal receptors in these animals was similar to that observed in male rats or in female rats at estrus and diestrus, but different significantly from that observed in the proestrous stage (Table 1). An alternative endocrine manipulation, namely, administration of testosterone to 1-day-old female rats, was also employed. This treatment results in the development of androgenized adults[9] in which the pattern of adenohypophyseal muscarinic receptors resembles that in normal male rats (Fig. 3). In the androgenized rat, the OVX rat, and the normal female at estrus, estradiol levels are low compared to those observed at the proestrous stage, suggesting that estrogenic activity plays a role in the regulation of levels of adenohypophyseal muscarinic receptors. Indeed, the implantation of 17β-estradiol capsule in OVX rats resulted in an increase in muscarinic receptor density to the level observed in normal females at proestrus (Fig. 2). However, unlike the situation at proestrus, elevated levels of high affinity agonist binding sites were not observed; on the contrary, following implantation the proportion of high affinity agonist binding sites was decreased from 40% (OVX) to 26% (OVX + 17β-estradiol). These data indicate that estrogen may exert a dual effect on the adenohypophyseal muscarinic system:
1) An indirect effect through which new receptors are synthesized;
2) a direct effect, manifested in the properties of pre-existing receptors.

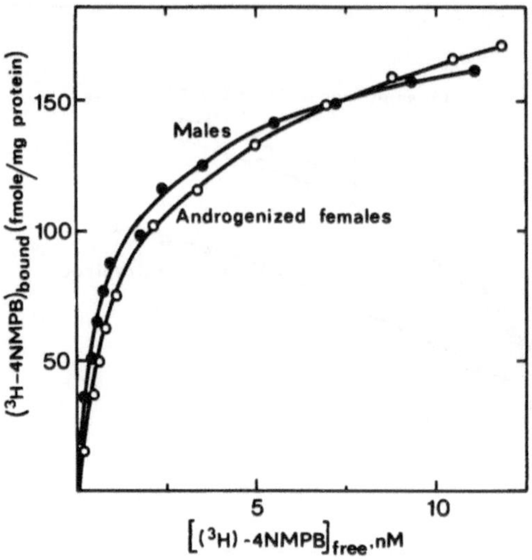

Fig. 3. Binding of [^{3}H]-4NMPB to male and androgenized female adenohypophyseal muscarinic receptors. Androgenized females were prepared by testosterone treatment of 1-day-old female rats.[9] Binding was measured as described before, at 25°C, in Krebs buffer (containing 1.8 mM $CaCl_2$).[7]

The direct effect could be demonstrated in vitro. Incubation of adenohypophyseal homogenates from proestrous rats (in which despite high estrogen levels the muscarinic receptors are present mostly in their high affinity state) with estradiol (50 ng/ml) resulted in a decrease in the proportion of high affinity agonist binding sites (Table 1). This decrease is not a consequence of reduction in receptor density (Table 1); it therefore reflects estrogen-induced conversion of high affinity to low affinity binding sites. Thus, estrogen acts in this case as an allosteric effector. Direct evidence for an allosteric effect of estrogen on muscarinic receptors also comes from studies with the antiestrogenic drug clomiphene,[24] which was shown to inhibit the binding of the antagonist [^{3}H]-4NMPB noncompetitively. Since clomiphene acts on the estrogen receptor or on a component associated with it,[25] these findings indicate that the muscarinic and the estrogen receptors can be coupled either directly or via an additional component which is itself coupled to the muscarinic receptor, thus preventing the estradiol-induced conversion of high affinity to low affinity agonist state at the proestrous stage.

We were able to demonstrate in vitro the direct coupling of a Ca^{2+}-dependent component to muscarinic receptors from the adenohypophysis. As shown, the binding of [^{3}H]-4NMPB (Fig. 4A) as well as of oxotremorine (Fig. 4B) to these receptors is strongly affected

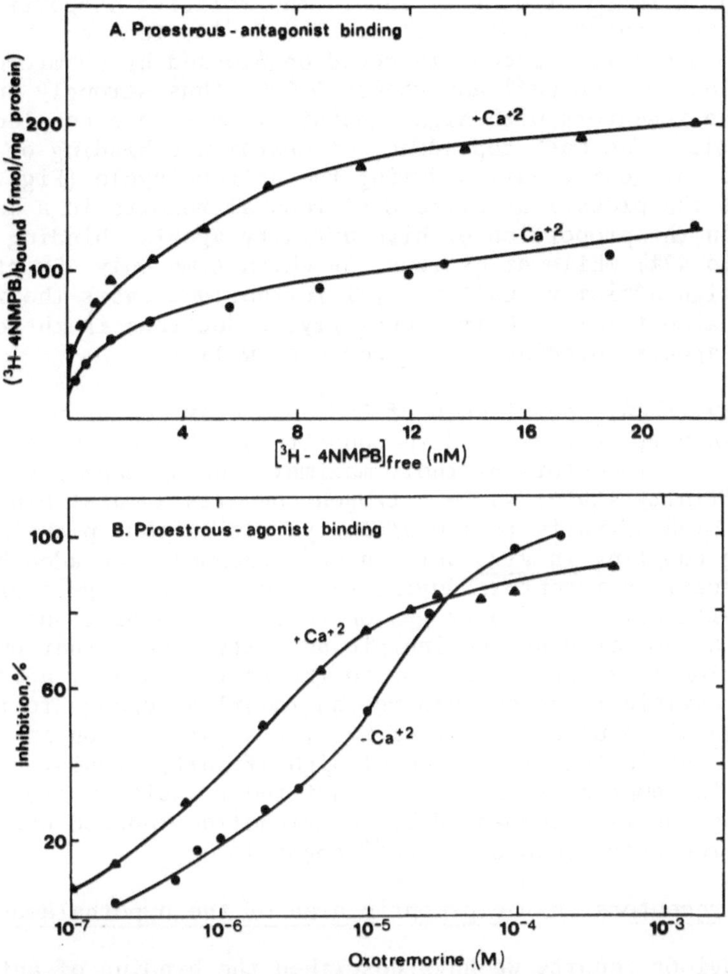

Fig. 4. Effect of Ca^{2+} on binding of [^{3}H]-4NMPB and oxotremorine to adenohypophyseal muscarinic receptors in homogenates from rats on the proestrus day. Binding was determined as described before,[7] at 25°C in Krebs buffer (containing 1.8 mM $CaCl_2$) (▲) or Krebs buffer without $CaCl_2$ containing 0.1 mM EGTA (●). A. Binding of [^{3}H]-4NMPB. B. Inhibition of [^{3}H]-4NMPB binding by oxotremorine. [^{3}H]-4NMPB concentration was 2.0 nM.

by the presence of Ca^{2+}. The maximal binding capacity and the high affinity agonist state manifested by the receptors at proestrus are both absolutely dependent on Ca^{2+}; removal of these ions results in a reduction in receptor density and in the relative proportion of high affinity agonist binding sites. The Ca^{2+} effect on the adenohypophyseal muscarinic receptors could be blocked by submicromolar concentrations of the Ca^{2+} antagonist D-600, thus strongly suggesting that the receptors with high agonist affinity are coupled to Ca^{2+} channels. The Ca^{2+}-dependency of muscarinic binding of both agonist and antagonist varies during the estrous cycle (Figs. 4 and 5): at the proestrous stage Ca^{2+} removal results in a marked reduction in the proportion of high affinity agonist binding sites (from 85% to 47%) while at estrous, by which time only 45% of the sites are high affinity, Ca^{2+} removal further decreases their proportion to almost zero. Correspondingly, reductions in the densities of antagonist binding sites occurs as well.

Clearly, then, the effects of Ca^{2+} and estrogen on muscarinic receptors in vitro are exerted in opposite directions: Ca^{2+} tends to maintain the receptors at their maximal binding capacity and in the high affinity state, while estrogen converts agonist binding sites from high affinity to low affinity. It is thus plausible that strong coupling in vivo between Ca^{2+} channels and adenohypophyseal muscarinic receptors during the proestrous stage overcomes the allosteric effects of estrogen on those receoptors. Such coupling could be achieved by cholinergic activity. Note that during the transition from the proestrous to the estrous stage, adenohypophyseal muscarinic receptors undergo an identical change to that occurring in vitro upon removal of Ca^{2+}, viz., reduction in receptor density and in the proportion of high affinity agonist binding sites. It is tempting to speculate that the transition from proestrus to estrus is accompanied by acetylcholine-induced changes in muscarinic receptors coupled to Ca^{2+} channels.

Muscarinic receptors in the preoptic area of the hypothalamus

In previous reports we have described the binding of antagonists and agonists to the muscarinic receptor in the preoptic area (POA).[10] Binding of the potent muscarinic antagonist [^{3}H]-4NMPB pointed to the existence of a homogeneous population of binding sites for the ligand in the POA of female rats at both the proestrous and estrous stages. No differences were observed either in the number of sites or in their affinity towards [^{3}H]-4NMPB at the various stages of the estrous cycle. Binding of agonists to muscarinic receptors in the POA differs from that of antagonists in two respects: (1) Agonist binding at both the proestrous and estrous stages is heterogeneous, i.e., it results in the formation of at least two agonist-receptor complexes indicating the possible existence of high and low affinity forms of agonists binding sites.

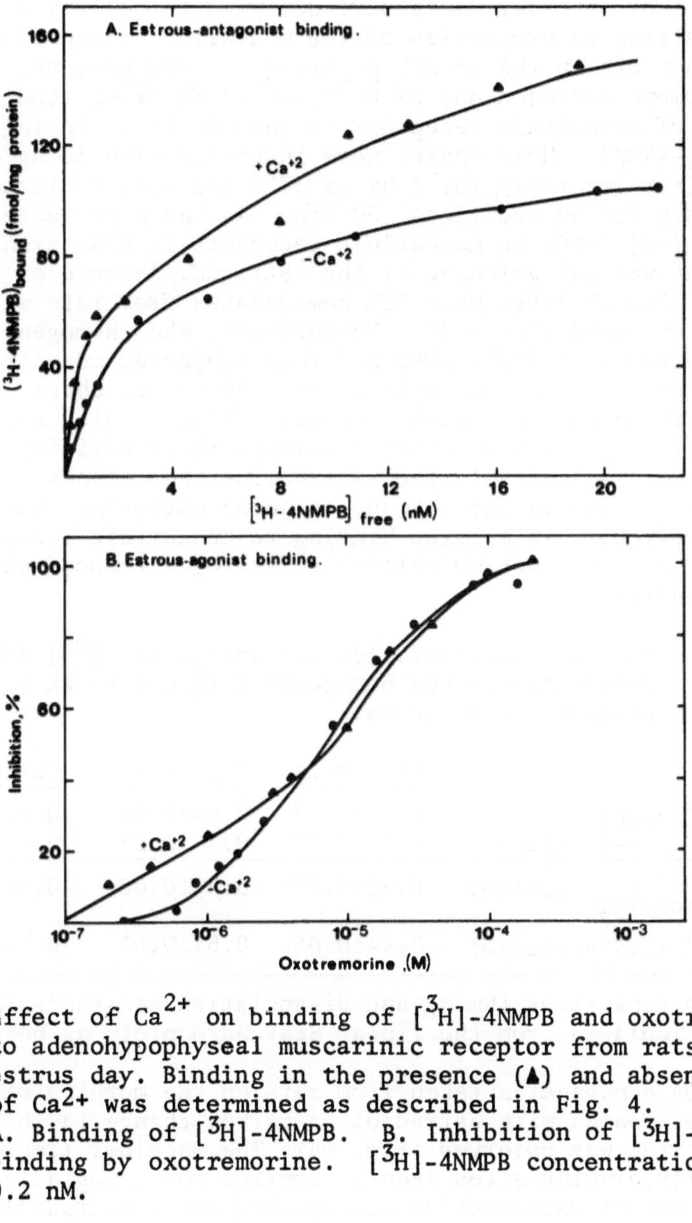

Fig. 5. Effect of Ca^{2+} on binding of $[^3H]$-4NMPB and oxotremorine to adenohypophyseal muscarinic receptor from rats on the estrus day. Binding in the presence (▲) and absence (●) of Ca^{2+} was determined as described in Fig. 4. A. Binding of $[^3H]$-4NMPB. B. Inhibition of $[^3H]$-4NMPB binding by oxotremorine. $[^3H]$-4NMPB concentration was 0.2 nM.

(2) The properties of agonist binding are changed during the estrous cycle, the proportion of high affinity binding sites varying from 66% at proestrus to 39% at estrus.[10]

The following experiments were designed to determine whether these variations in properties of the muscarinic receptor are related as they are in the adenohypophysis, to the presence of the steroid hormone estrogen and of Ca^{2+} ions. We first studied the properties of muscarinic receptors in the POA by employing the antagonist [^{3}H]-4NMPB. Homogenates were incubated with 30 ng of estradiol or buffer (control) for 1 hr at 37°C and then subjected to the binding assay for an additional 30 min. As shown in Table 2, the binding of [^{3}H]-4NMPB to muscarinic receptors in POA taken from rats at proestrus was not affected by the estrogen. Absence of estrogen effect was also observed when POA homogenates from rats at diestrus and estrus was used (Table 2). Furthermore, when homogenates were first incubated with [^{3}H]-4NMPB and then subjected to estradiol treatment, no effect on the antagonist binding was observed. These results indicate that the number of muscarinic binding sites in the POA, as well as properties which determine their affinity for antagonists, remain essentially the same during the estrous cycle, both in the presence and in the absence of added estrogen. Variations observed previously in agonist binding to muscarinic receptors in the POA[8,10] can thus not be related to estrogen-induced change in receptor density.

Table 2. Binding parameters for the antagonist [^{3}H]-4NMPB determined in POA homogenates from rats at various estrous cycle stages.

		Diestrous	Proestrous	Estrous
Kd nM	Control	0.41±0.08	0.62±0.04	0.83±0.03
	+ 17β-estradiol	0.97±0.23	0.76±0.13	0.96±0.39
Bmax pmole/mg protein	Control	0.35±0.03	0.52±0.08	0.46±0.05
	+17β-estradiol	0.44±0.03	0.51±0.01	0.44±0.07

Binding capacities (Bmax) and dissociation constants (Kd) were calculated from the linear Scatchard plots as before.

When POA homogenates taken from rats on the morning of proestrus were treated with estradiol, a marked change in the binding of oxotremorine was observed (Fig. 6A). The shoulder (representing high affinity binding sites seen in control POA homogenates at low concentrations of oxotremorine disappeared after estradiol treatment; i.e. almost all of the muscarinic receptors were now present in the low affinity state. Since this treatment did not alter the total number of muscarinic binding sites (Table 2), it is concluded that estradiol mediated in vitro their interconversion from high affinity to low affinity. Moreover, the estradiol-mediated conversion of high affinity to low affinity muscarinic receptors was restricted to a specific period of time, viz., up to 13.00 hours on the day of proestrus (Fig. 6B). Estradiol pretreatment failed to affect high affinity agonist binding sites two hours later, although most of the receptors were then in the high affinity binding state for agonist (Fig. 6C). Furthermore, estradiol did not affect either the density (Table 2) or the proportions of POA receptors taken from rats on the day of estrus (Fig. 6D).

These results indicate that during the critical period[26] a dramatic change occurs in the factors which induce interaction between muscarinic and estrogen receptors in the POA. During this period POA cells are highly active in the synthesis and trasport of luteinizing hormone releasing hormone (LHRH),[27] as a consequence of elevated levels of estradiol on the day of proestrus up to noon.[28] It is therefore clear that in the intact rat, in spite of elevated estrogen levels, muscarinic receptors maintain on the morning of proestrus their high affinity state, whereas they are extremely sensitive to the steroid in vitro. It follows that the operation of some other component, which is itself changed during the initial period, is preventing estradiol induced conversion of high affinity to low affinity muscarinic agonist binding sites. Two likely factors are acetylcholine and Ca^{2+} ions.

The experiments described above were carried out in a modified Krebs solution containing 1.8 mM Ca^{2+}. Clearly, then, the presence of Ca^{2+} does not interfere with the estrogen-induced interconversion of binding sites. In order to examine whether Ca^{2+} ions are required for this process, we omitted Ca^{2+} from the buffer and added 0.1 mM EGTA. Binding properties of the muscarinic antagonist [^{3}H]-4NMPB, as well as those of the agonist oxotremorine, were then determined at all stages of the estrous cycle, as described before. Omission of Ca^{2+} from the incubation mixtures of control POA homogenates did not change the binding properties of either [^{3}H]-4NMPB or oxotremorine. In the absence of Ca^{2+}, POA homogenates taken from rats on the morning of proestrus contained a high proportion of high affinity muscarinic agonist binding sites, even after treatment with estradiol (Fig. 6A). This finding implies that the omission of Ca^{2+} ions from the incubation medium prevented the steroid-induced conversion of high affinity to low affinity sites which occurs in the presence of Ca^{2+}. These results confirm that Ca^{2+} is an essential factor in the in vitro estrogen-induced interconversion of muscarinic agonist binding sites. However, the cooperative effects of Ca^{2+} and estrogen suggest that it is not the Ca^{2+} ion itself which prevents in vivo conversion of high to low affinity agonist binding sites in the POA. The involvement of cholinergic activation should therefore be considered as a possibility.

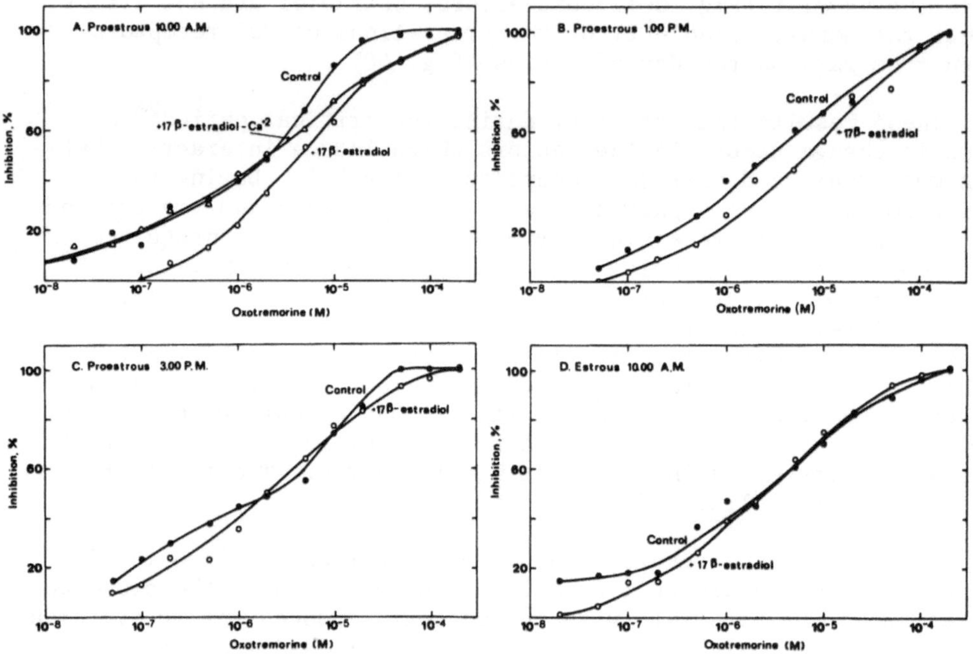

Fig. 6. Inhibition of [^{3}H]-4NMPB binding to muscarinic receptors in POA homogenates pretreated with estradiol by the agonist oxotremorine. POA's were taken from rats on the day of proestrus at the hours 10.00 (A), 13.00 (B) and 15.00 (C) and on the day of estrus (D). The tissues were homogenized and used for competition binding studies (as described in Fig. 1). After 1 hour incubation at 37°C in the presence (o) and absence (●) of 30 ng/ml 17β-estradiol. In part A are given also results of experiments in which homogenates were incubated in the absence of Ca^{2+} and in the presence of estradiol and 0.1 mM EGTA (Δ).

In order to mimic in vitro the postulated occupation of muscarinic receptor in vivo, we performed experiments in which POA homogenates were first exposed to the cholinergic ligands oxotremorine and [^{3}H]-4NMPB and then incubated in the presence of 17β-estradiol. The results are shown in Fig. 7. Under these conditions muscarinic receptors taken from the POA from rats on the morning of proestrus were not affected by the estrogen, i.e. prior occupation of the muscarinic receptors protected against the in vitro estradiol-induced interconversion of agonist binding sites. Further studies should determine whether the levels of endogenous acetylcholine are correspondingly higher on the morning of the proestrus.

SUMMARY

Properties of muscarinic acetylcholine receptors were studied in two distinct tissues which are involved in the estrous cycle, namely, the adenohypophysis and the hypothalamic preoptic area (POA). The latter contains cells synthesizing releasing hormones[27] which activate adenohypophyseal hormone release.[29] In both tissues the properties of the muscarinic receptors underwent cyclic changes

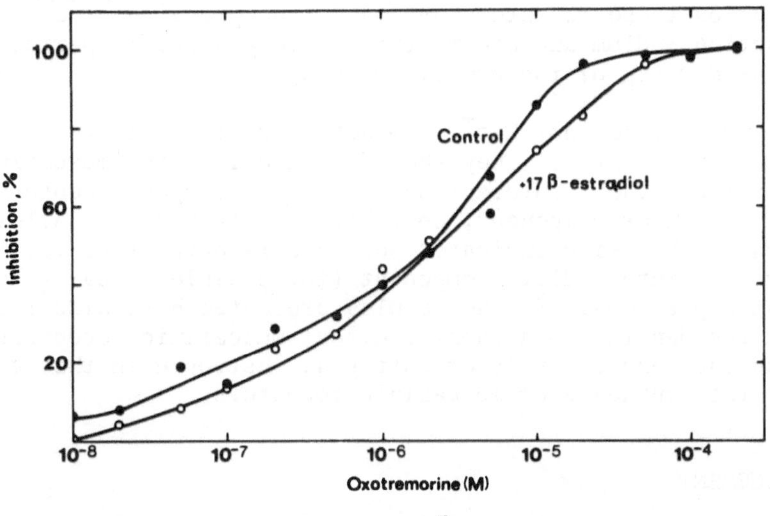

Fig. 7. Oxotremorine inhibition of [^{3}H]-4NMPB binding to muscarinic receptors in POA homogenates exposed to estradiol after incubation with the ligands. POA's from rats on the day of proestrus at 10.00 were homogenized and incubated with 2.0 nM [^{3}H]-4NMPB and various concentrations of oxotremorine at 37°C for 30 min. Then estradiol was added for additional 60 min. Results of control (•) and estradiol-treated homogenates (o) are presented.

during the estrous cycle. Factors which are crucial for a normal estrous cycle (estradiol) and for its accompanying hormonal release (Ca^{2+}) were shown to modulate muscarinic receptor properties. These findings suggest that muscarinic receptors may participate in the regulation of both hypothalamic neurosecretory cells and adenohypophyseal secretory cells. In spite of the distinct differences between these two cell types,[30] both of them require calcium ions for the hormone-releasing activities[29] and both are affected by estrogen.[30] It is therefore not surprising that Ca^{2+} and estrogen each have a distinct influence on adenohypophyseal and on POA muscarinic receptors. In the adenohypophysis, reduction in the number of muscarinic receptors during the transition from proestrus to estrus can be mimicked in vitro by the omission of Ca^{2+} from the medium; it seems that accompanying reduction in proportion of high affinity agonist binding sites is due to loss of receptors. On the other hand, the reduction in high affinity muscarinic agonist binding sites estrogen-induced in the adenohypophysis, is due to the conversion from high affinity to low affinity sites; the steroid does not affect in vitro the number of muscarinic receptors. Similarly, in the POA estrogen induced in vitro conversion of high affinity to low affinity sites with no effect on receptor density. Here, unlike in the adenohypophysis, the number of receptors does not vary during the estrous cycle, and their properties (as manifested in vitro) are not affected by Ca^{2+}. However, the in vitro effects of estrogen on these receptors depend on the presence of Ca^{2+} in the incubation medium and are restricted to a specific period, namely, the morning of the proestrous stage.

Neither estrogen nor Ca^{2+} interacts directly with the muscarinic recognition sites. They therefore modulate the muscarinic receptor through their interaction with the estrogen receptors and/or a Ca^{2+}-dependent component, possibly a Ca^{2+}-channel. Allosteric modulation of this kind indicates possible receptor-receptor interactions via an intermediate component (for example, a Ca^{2+}-channel) as suggested previously.[8] The results presented here also indicate that the density of adenohypophyseal muscarinic receptors depends on endogenous levels of estrogen. Estrogen in this case increases the synthesis of muscarinic receptors.

ACKNOWLEDGEMENT

The enlightening discussions and suggestions of Drs. Yoel Kloog and Yoav Henis are greatly appreciated. This work was supported in part by the Recanati Fund for Medical Research.

REFERENCES

1. G. Pepeu and H. Ladinsky, "Cholinergic Mechanisms," Plenum Press, New York (1981).
2. K. Krnjevic and J.W. Phillis, Inotophoretic studies of neurons in the mammalian cerebral cortex, J. Physiol. (Lond.) 165:274 (1963).
3. K. Krnjevic, Chemical nature of synaptic transmission in vertebrates, Physiol. Rev. 54:418 (1974).
4. M. Sokolovsky, D. Gurwitz, and Y. Kloog, Biochemical characterization of the muscarinic receptors, Adv. in Enzymology 55:137 (1983).
5. M. Sokolovsky, Muscarinic receptors in the central nervous system, Int'l Review of Neurobiology 25, in press (1983).
6. N.J.M. Birdsall, and E.C. Hulme, Biochemical studies on muscarinic receptors, J. Neurochem. 27:7 (1976).
7. S. Avissar, Y. Egozi, and M. Sokolovsky, Bicochemical characterization and sex dimorphism of muscarinic receptors in rat adenohypophysis, Neuroendocrinology 32:303 (1981).
8. M. Sokolovsky, Y. Egozi, and S. Avissar, Molecular regulation of receptors: Interaction of β-estradiol and progesterone with the muscarinic system, Proc. Natl. Acad. Sci. USA 78:15554 (1981).
9. Y. Egozi, S. Avissar, and M. Sokolovsky, Muscarinic mechanisms and sex hormone secretion in rat adenohypophysis and preoptic area, Neuroendocrinology 35:93 (1982).
10. S. Avissar, Y. Egozi, and M. Sokolovsky, Studies on muscarinic receptors in mouse and rat hypothalamus: A comparison of sex and cyclical differences, Neuroendocrinology 32:295 (1981).
11. P.W. Young, R.J. Bicknell, and J.G.L. Schofield, Acetylcholine stimulates growth hormone secretion, phosphatidyl inositol labeling $^{45}Ca^{++}$ efflux and cyclic GMP accumulation in bovine anterior pituitary gland, J. Endocr. 80:203 (1979).
12. C. Libertun, and S.M. McCann, Blockade of the release of gonadotropin and prolactin by subcutaneous or intraventricular injection of atropin in male and female rats, Endocrinology 92:1714 (1973).
13. W. Vale, C. Rivier, M. Brown, L. Chan, N. Ling, and J. Rivier, Application of adenohypophyseal cell cultures to neuroendocrine studies, in: "Hypothalamus and Endocrine Function," F. Labrie, J. Mietes, and G. Pelleties, eds., Plenum Press, New York (1976).
14. S.R. Vivian, and F.S. Labella, Cellular mechanisms of anterior pituitary secretion: estimation of several hormones release in vitro, Mem. Soc. Endocr. 19:203 (1971).
15. L.H. Lindstrom, and N.J. Meyerson, The effect of pilocarpin, oxotremorine and arecoline in combination with methylatropin on hormone activated oestrous behaviour in ovariectomized rats, Psychopharmacology 11:405 (1967).
16. D.K. Sarkar, and G. Fink, Luteinizing hormone releasing factor in pituitary stalk plasma from long-term ovariectomized rats: Effects of steroids, J. Endocr. 86:511 (1980).

17. G. Fink, Feedback actions of target hormones on hypothalamus and pituitary with special reference to gonadal steroids, A Rev. Physiol. 41:571 (1979).
18. R.L. Goodman, and E. Knobil, The sites of action of ovarian steroids in regulation of LH secretion, Neuroendocrinology 32:57 (1981).
19. J. Drouin, and F. Labrie, Interactions between 17β-estradiol and progesterone in the control of luteinizing hormone and follicle stimulating hormone release in rat anterior pituitary cells in culture, Endocrinology 108:52 (1981).
20. K.J. Catt, S.P. Harwood, G. Aguilera, and M.C. DuFau, Hormonal regulation of peptide receptors and target cell responses, Nature 280:109 (1979).
21. Y.I. Henis, R. Galron, S. Avissar, and M. Sokolovsky, Interactions between antagonist occupied muscarinic binding sites in rat adenohypophysis, FEBS Lett. 140:173 (1982).
22. J.B. Galper, L.C. Dziekan, D.S. O'Hara, and T.W. Smith, The biphasic response of muscarinic cholinergic receptors in cultured heart cells to agonists, J. Biol. Chem. 257:10344 (1982).
23. S.J. Legan, G.A. Coon, and F. Karsch, Role of estrogen as initiator of daily LH surges in the ovariectomized rat, Endocrinology 96:50 (1975).
24. L.C. Huppert, Induction of ovulation with clomiphene citrate, Fertil. Steril. 31:1 (1979).
25. G. Ben-Baruch, G. Schreiber, and M. Sokolovsky, Cooperativity pattern in the interaction of the antiestrogen drug clomiphene with the muscarinic receptors, Mol. Pharmac. 21:287 (1982).
26. J.W. Everett, Brain, pituitary gland and the ovarian cycle. J. Biol. Reprod. 6:3 (1972).
27. B. Flerko, Hypothalamic mediation of neuroendocrine regulation of hypophyseal gonadotrophic functions, in: "MTP International Review of Science, Physiology Section, series 1, Reproductive Physiology," R.O. Greep, ed., Butterworths, London (1972).
28. L.G. Nequin, J. Alvarez, and N.B. Schwartz, Measurement of serum steroid and gonadotropin levels and uterine and ovarian variables throughout 4 day and 5 day estrous cycles in the rat, J. Biol. Reprod. 20:659 (1979).
29. G.W. Bennett, and S.A. Whitehead, "Mammalian Neuroendocrinology," Oxford University Press, New York (1983).
30. A.M. Poisner, and J.M. Trifaro, "The Secretory Granule," Elsevier Biomedical Press, New York (1982).

HORMONES AND OTHER MESSENGER MOLECULES: AN APPROACH TO UNITY

Jesse Roth, Derek LeRoith, Joseph Shiloach[#], and
Chaim Rabinowitz [#]

Diabetes Branch and [#]Pilot Plant, Laboratory of
Nutrition and Endocrinology, NIADDK, NIH
Bethesda, Maryland 20205

Endocrinology was formulated in the late 19th and early 20th centuries. The central concept of endocrinology was that a group of specialized cells limited to one location in the body release chemical messengers which travel through the blood stream to act upon and regulate target cells throughout the body. These chemical messengers were named hormones [1].

With the recognition of endocrine systems, coordination and communication between cells were conceptually assigned to two systems, the traditional (nervous) and the novel (endocrine) system. Initially the two systems were seen as separate and independent (Fig.1). Soon, however, breaches in the boundaries between the two were detected but unappreciated. In the last decade, the breaks in the boundaries between the two systems have become more numerous (Table 1) and several attempts have been made conceptually to unite these two systems of intercellular communication into one. The major approach, taken by several groups of investigators, has been to suggest that cells of neural origin are the phylogenetic and ontogenetic precursors of the endocrine system of vertebrates [2-4].

Concommitantly, many intercellular communication systems have been discovered that do not conform to the rules established for either the endocrine or nervous systems (Fig. 1D). Among the exceptions are hormone molecules that have gone astray, i.e. molecules that are widely accepted as traditional hormones which are found in places that were unexpected (Table 2) or behave as messengers in modes other than strictly endocrine. Another larger, more important category is composed of non-hormone messengers which are very much like hormones in structure, biological function, and interactions with target cells, including receptors, which fail to meet the criteria established for hormones. For example, these messengers are manufactured by many cell types, or at multiple sites rather than at a single dominant site, or may act upon target cells without passing first through the blood stream (Table 3).

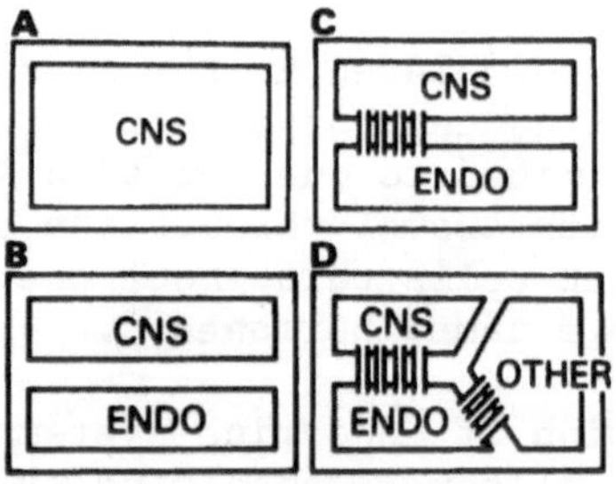

Figure 1: Evolution of concepts about intercellular communication. (A) The central nervous system (CNS) was considered to be the unique coordinator among cells of multicellular animals; (B) integration and coordination were performed by two separate but equal systems, the CNS and the endocrine system (ENDO); (C) penetrations in the boundaries that separate the two systems became apparent, especially in recent years; (D) there are a large number of examples of intercellular communication that we now recognize which do not fit either system, designated OTHER.*

In our recent studies we have attempted to provide a unified concept with a single focus with which to describe intercellular communication. By taking an evolutionary approach, we hope that

Table 1: Penetrations of the Boundaries Between Endocrine and Nervous System.

A. Classic Examples
1. Nerves signal other cells via chemical messengers (neurotransmission).
2. Neurons, like epithelial cells, can serve as a glandular source of hormone (neurosecretion).
3. Catecholamines, among the first of the neurotransmitters to be discovered, had already been recognized as bona fide hormones of the adrenal medulla.

B. Recent Examples
1. Neuropeptides are also found in non-neural tissues.
2. Gastro-entero-pancreatic hormones are also found in nervous tissue.
3. Receptor-effector mechanisms that are initiated by intercellular messenger molecules are very similar or possibly identical in brain and peripheral non-neural tissues (e.g. catecholamines bind to β-adrenergic receptors and activate adenylate cyclase-protein kinase mechanisms in both brain and liver).

Table 2: Hormone Molecules Gone Astray.

1. Many peptide hormones have been identified in brain cells and peripheral nerves of vertebrates and multicellular invertebrates.
2. Nonendocrine cancers may produce and release hormonal peptides, which can cause disabling clinical syndromes.
3. Hormonal peptides may be present in embryos before the development of the glands that we associate with that hormone.
4. Placental tissue can synthesize several hormones and neuropeptides that we associate with other glands.
5. Multiple hormonal peptides are present in exocrine secretions.
6. The glands in the skin of some amphibia can be a particularly rich source of mammalian type neuropeptides.

Table 3: Examples of Nonhormone Messengers that are Very Hormone-like in Structure or Function.

Insulin-like growth factors (IGF); nerve growth factor (NGF); epidermal growth factor (EGF)
Interferons and other endogenous antiviral substances
Interleukins and other intercellular messengers used in the immune system
Prostaglandins and other arachidonic acid derivatives
Nucleotides; amino acids

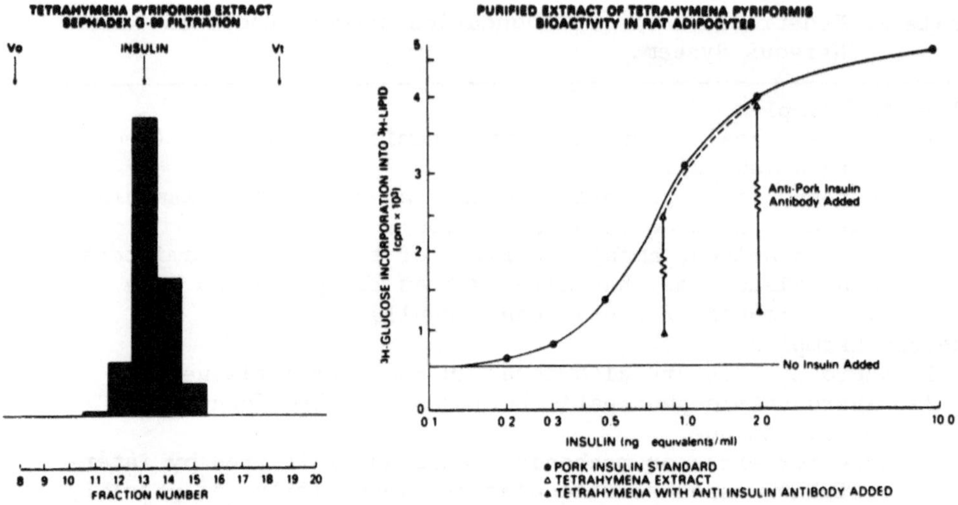

Figure 2: Insulin-related material in Tetrahymena. Tetrahymena cells were homogenized and extracted in acid ethanol. The immunoactive insulin-related material was purified by several chromatographic techniques. The figure (left panel) shows gel filtration on a column of Sephadex G-50 fine; a peak of immunoactive insulin was recovered in the region where purified mammalian insulins migrate (left panel). The peak fractions from the gel filtration were pooled and tested in a bioassay for insulin measuring ^{3}H-glucose incorporation into ^{3}H-lipids in isolated adipocytes from young rats (right panel). The immunoactivity predicted the bioactivity. In addition, most of the bioactivity was neutralized in the presence of anti-(pork) insulin antibody but not by nonimmune serum, indicating that the immunoactivity and bioactivity resided on the same molecular species. Further, the addition of anti-sera that block the receptor for insulin also blocked the bioactivity of the tetrahymena extract (data not shown) indicating that the bioactivity of the purified material was being expressed through the insulin receptor on the adipocytes.* (Adapted from references [5,6]).

we can unite not only the traditional endocrine and nervous systems (which others have done before us) but also integrate with them the growing number of other intercellular communication systems and messenger molecules.

We grew Tetrahymena pyriformis, a common laboratory protozoa, in a defined simple medium. The cells and the medium in which the cells had been grown contained material quite similar to authentic insulins. The insulin-related immunoactive material eluted from a Sephadex G-50 column close to the position typical of genuine mammalian insulins. This material stimulated adipocytes (isolated from young rats) to accelerate the metabolism of glucose. Further, this biological activity was largely (though not completely) neutralized by anti-insulin antibodies [5] (Fig. 2). The bioactivity of the microbial material was fully neutralized by antibodies that bind to and block the insulin receptor [6]. These studies indicated to us that the size of the insulin-related molecule was about that appropriate for insulin. Further its surface topography was remarkably similar to insulin since it binds to insulin receptors on mammalian cells and when bound to these receptors it initiates a program of insulin-related effects on the cell. In addition, the surface of the molecule is also recognized by antibodies against insulin.

Preliminary studies have shown that the microbial material further resembles mammalian insulins in its behavior on DEAE cellulose, DEAE Sephadex, and on reverse phase liquid chromatography [7]. Because we have not yet refined these separation systems adequately, we must limit our conclusion to stating that the microbial material is quite similar to authentic insulins without providing a more precise indication of how closely the material resembles known species of vertebrate insulins.

We have found that the insulin-related material that is native to the protozoa differs from authentic insulins in its subcellular distribution. Thus, when unlabeled or labeled mammalian insulin is added to the microbes just before or just after they are homogenized, the distribution of the endogenous insulin gives a pattern that is clearly distinct from the distribution of the added insulins [7]. While the cause for the differences in subcellular distribution is as yet unclear, the differences appear to be reproducible.

While we do not yet know what stimulates production of insulin-related material by the protozoa, its production does follow a characteristic time pattern. We found that there was a rapid rise in the insulin content of both the cells and the medium over the first 18-24 hours of culture. Beyond 24 hours, the insulin content reaches a plateau or may even show a progressive decline. It should be emphasized that fresh medium, when carried through the entire procedure, is free of detectable insulin. Moreover, when an innoculum of the microbe is introduced into the medium and extracted immediately, the amount of insulin recovered is only that predicted by the insulin content of the innoculum itself[7].

We also detected material resembling insulin in other microbes including two species of fungi and in five strains of E. coli. These studies included filtration on Sephadex G-50, radioimmunoassay, assay of biological activity with isolated fat cells and neutralization of bioactivity by anti-insulin antibodies [5,6].

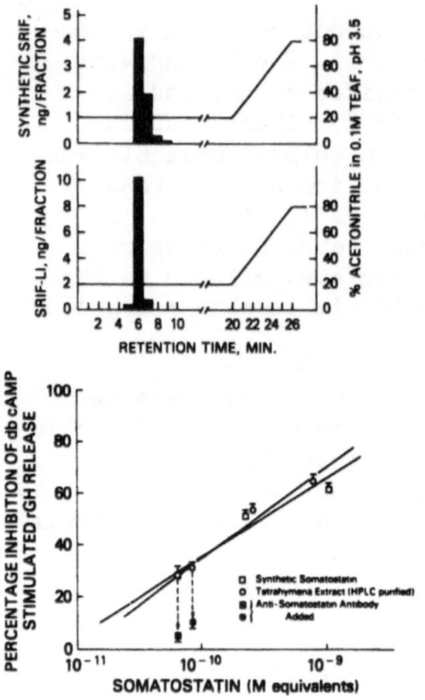

Figure 3: Somatostatin-like material in Tetrahymena pyriformis. Purification of the tetrahymena extracts for somatostatin-like material included reverse phase high performance liquid chromatography (HPLC, upper panel). The retention time of the somatostatin-like material from tetrahymena (SRIF-LI) was similar to that of synthetic somatostatin (SRIF). This HPLC purified material was tested for bioactivity (inhibition of release of growth hormone from dispersed rat pituitary cells); the bioactivity of both synthetic somatostatin as well as SRIF-LI from tetrahymena was neutralized by anti-somatostatin antibody (lower panel).* (Adapted from reference 8).

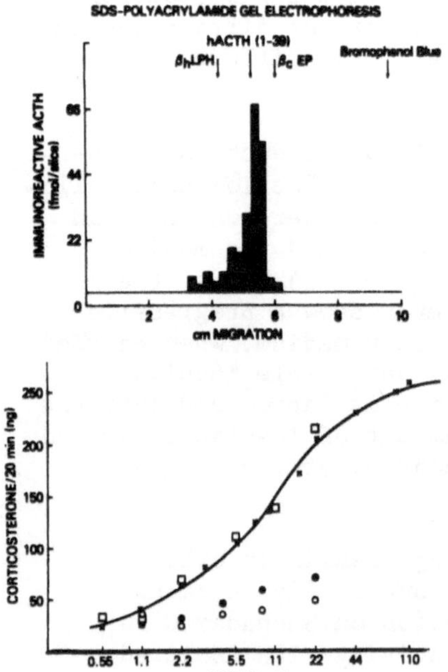

Figure 4: ACTH-like and beta-endorphin-like material in Tetrahymena pyriformis. Multiple steps were used to purify the ACTH-like and beta-endorphin-like material from extracts of tetrahymena. Following SDS-polyacrylamide gel electrophoresis most of the ACTH-like immunoactivity eluted in a single region (upper panel). Standard mammalian ACTH (solid line-lower panel) was compared with purified extract (□,X) in a bioassay that measures corticosterone release from dispersed adrenal cells of the rat. Most of the bioactivity of the purified extract was removed (●,○) by anti-ACTH antibody.* (Adapted from reference 9.)

In collaboration with colleagues at the University of Cincinnati we detected somatostatin-related material in protozoa. This material is similar to mammalian somatostatin in its immunoactivity and behavior in gel filtration, HPLC, biological assay, and neutralization of biological activity by anti-somatostatin antibodies [8] (Fig. 3).

In collaboration with colleagues at the Mount Sinai School of Medicine, we detected (Fig. 4) materials in protozoa that resembled ACTH and β-endorphin [9]. In vertebrates these two peptides are synthesized as part of a high molecular weight precursor, pro-opiomelanocortin. In the extracts from protozoa we also detected a high molecular weight component, which on gel filtration was similar in size to pro-opiomelanocortin and which had immunoactivities of both ACTH and β-endorphin, like its vertebrate counterpart; however, as yet we have not demonstrated its precursor role.

We and others [10-15] have also detected other hormone-related materials in these and other microbes (Table 4).

Proteins have been found in bacteria that can bind labeled hCG[16]. Weiss et al. have demonstrated binding sites on gram negative organisms that bind TSH and closely related hormones but not unrelated substances[17]. Interestingly, the binding of labeled TSH to the bacteria is also inhibited by human immunoglobulins that react with the receptor for TSH on human thyroids. They speculate that in patients with diffuse hyperthyroidism (Graves' disease), bacterial components may be the immunogens that stimulate the production of "autoantibodies" against TSH receptors that are characteristic of this disease [17]. Whether these hormone binding proteins function as receptors in the microbes is unknown but pharmacological evidence has been provided for a receptor in amoebae that closely resembles the opiate receptor of vertebrates [18] (Fig.5).

In summary, we and others have demonstrated that microbes produce materials that closely resemble those of peptide hormones and related messenger molecules typical of vertebrates. We have tried to demonstrate that the reactivities in the radioimmunoassays and biological assays were specific and not due to interference. We also performed extensive studies to convince ourselves that the materials were endogenous to the microbes and not introduced inadvertently from external sources (for example, see ref. 5-7).

In considering "non-specific" effects in the assays and "contamination" of the extracts, the reader should recall that the two problems and the experiments designed to rule out one or the other are mutually exclusive. It is important to emphasize that we do not as yet have any of these materials purified and

Table 4: Material Resembling Vertebrate Hormonal Peptides in Unicellular Organisms.

TSH	Clostridium (12)
hCG	Many bacteria (13,14)
Insulin	Tetrahymena, Neurospora, Aspergillus (5); E.coli (6)
Somatostatin	Tetrahymena (8)
ACTH, β-endorphin	Tetrahymena (9)
Relaxin	Tetrahymena (10)

Additional studies have shown materials resembling calcitonin in bacteria, fungi, and protozoa (I. MacIntyre et al.; L. Deftos et al.), vasotocin in protozoa (E. Collier et al.) somatostatin in E. coli (D. LeRoith et al.) and cholecystokinin in protozoa (J. Taylor et al.). Microbes also contain non-peptide molecules (e.g. steroids, acetylcholine, amines, nucleotides) that serve as intercellular and intracellular messengers in vertebrates. We have focused on the peptides because their existence implies the coexistence (and evolutionary conservation) of the appropriate DNA. For the non-peptides, it may be argued that their existence is for another purpose or solely accidental, whereas for peptides, existence alone has much stronger biological implications.

therefore do not really know their structure. Likewise, our study implies that the microbes have specific DNA and RNA that correspond to these proteins; it remains for future work to provide these data. Also, we have assumed that the vertebrate-type messenger molecules in microbes originated there evolutionarily; we have not excluded their origin in complex organisms with transfer of DNA or RNA to the microbes at a later stage. Now let us turn briefly to speculate on the possible roles of these materials in the microorganisms themselves.

We do not know whether the hormone-related molecules act as messengers in the microorganisms themselves. We speculate that they do but all of our evidence is totally circumstantial. First, the extreme conservation of the structure of each molecule suggests the presence of a biological function that is providing strong constraints against evolutionary change. In addition there are data, albeit less extensive, for binding sites or receptor sites in microbes that have similarities to vertebrate-type receptors. Finally, there are numerous examples of intercellular communication among microbes mediated by humoral messengers [19–23]; these systems show remarkable resemblances to intercellular communication among vertebrate cells.

In addition to food, the other major subject for communication between microbes is sex. In Streptococcus faecalis, the

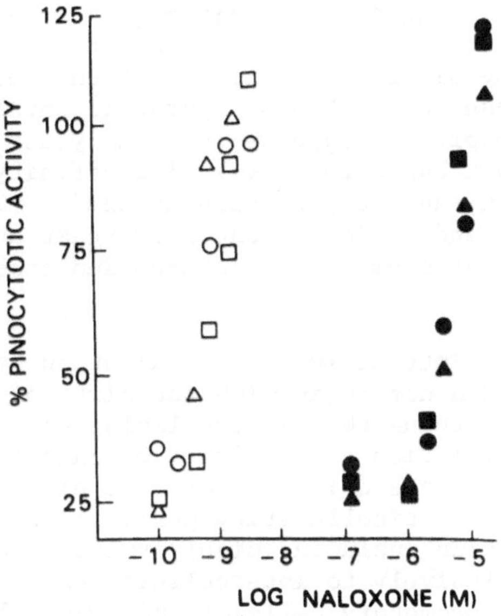

Figure 5: Vertebrate-type receptor and effector mechanism in a microbe. Pinocytotic activity in Amoeba proteus was inhibited in the presence of endorphin (□) and enkephalin (○) as well as morphine (△). The effect of these opioids was markedly reduced by the active form of naloxone, a specific blocker of opioid receptors (solid symbols) but was unaffected by the inactive isomer of the antagonist (open symbols). (Reproduced with permission of the authors[18]).*

transfer of genetic material is highly regulated by humoral factors released into the culture medium [22]. In many unicellular eukaryotes, mating is regulated by humoral messengers released by the organisms themselves. The chemical classes of these mediators include sterols, amino acids, peptides, and glycoproteins. One of the best studied examples is Saccharomyces cerevisiae, a common yeast [23]. Here the mating of two haploids of opposite sexual type to yield a diploid requires the presence of two sex factors, peptides released into the medium which promote the sexual union (Fig.6). Interestingly, one of the sexual mating factors, the alpha factor, has a structure that is similar to that of LHRH or GnRH [24](Fig.7). Yeast alpha factor at high concentrations can mimic LHRH in causing the release of

LH from pituitary glands of rats [25]. Since the natural and synthetic preparations of alpha factor are equally potent, it is likely that this activity is due to the yeast peptide rather than to some extraneous component. In addition, the yeast peptide, like LHRH, competes for binding of ^{125}I-LHRH to receptors of the rat pituitary and the biological activity of the yeast peptide, like that of LHRH, can be blocked by synthetic antagonists that block the LHRH receptor. It appears that the yeast sex factor is an analog of LHRH that has a relatively low affinity but full intrinsic activity in the rat pituitary system[25]. Thus a chemical mediator for mammals and a similar one from yeast share common functions, have similar chemical structures and cross react biologically.

We conclude that intercellular communication by soluble messenger molecules did not begin with the birth of multicellular organisms. Rather we think that intercellular communication was devised earlier in evolution at the level of unicellular organisms and that it became widespread long before the emergence of multicellularity (Fig.8). Multicellularity permitted extremes of cellular differentiation including highly specialized cells devoted largely or exclusively to intercellular communication, cells like nerves or secretory cells of endocrine glands. Moreover, the aqueous compartment that joined the secretory cell to the target cell could now be controlled and soon developed into much more special forms such as those provided by the closed circulatory systems of vertebrates. While the cell biology and gross anatomy of the components have evolved dramatically the biochemical elements by which the secretory cell and the target cell actually communicate have been highly conserved [26,27].

Vertebrate-type messenger molecules occur not only in unicellular organisms but are also found widely in multicellular invertebrate animals (metazoa). Material related to insulin has been described in many metazoan forms in many laboratories [28] but the findings have not been widely appreciated. In some, the insulin secretory cells appear among the cells lining the gastro-intestinal tract [29] while in others insulin appears to be associated with the brain and peripheral neuroendocrine systems [30,31]. Interestingly, insulin deficiency may produce a diabetes-like state in both molluscs and insects [29-31].

These findings and speculations lead us to think that the extraordinary overlap between the nervous and endocrine systems of vertebrates did not arise because the nervous system or one of its neural elements gave rise to the endocrine system. Rather we propose that both of these relatively specialized systems inherited their key molecular components including the messenger and receptor molecules from simpler unicellular ancestors. The common ancestry of the two (rather than the nervous system

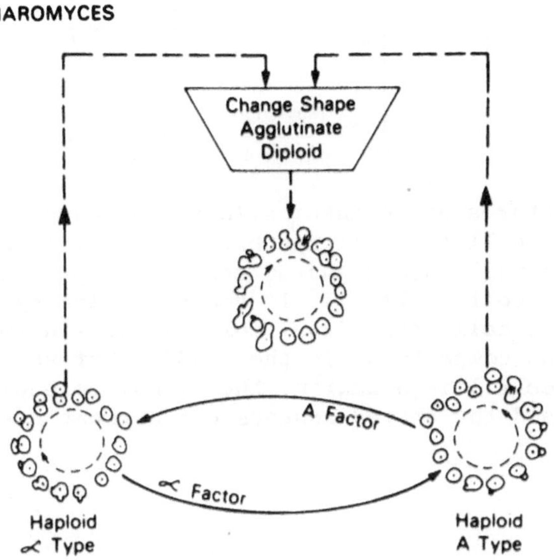

Figure 6: Saccharomyces cerevisiae, a common yeast, exists in a diploid form as well as in two haploid types, designated A and α. To initiate the union of haploids to form diploids, the alpha type organism secretes a small peptide "α mating factor" which reacts with specific receptors on the surface of A cells. The A cells respond by secreting a different peptide, "A factor", which acts on α cells. In response to the specific peptide, the cells change shape, develop new surface properties and agglutinate; opposite cell types then pair up, fuse cytoplasma and later nuclei to form diploid organisms.*

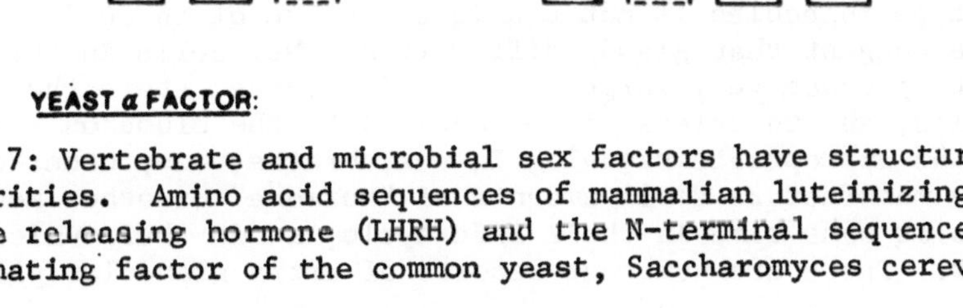

Figure 7: Vertebrate and microbial sex factors have structural similarities. Amino acid sequences of mammalian luteinizing hormone releasing hormone (LHRH) and the N-terminal sequence of alpha mating factor of the common yeast, Saccharomyces cerevisiae.*

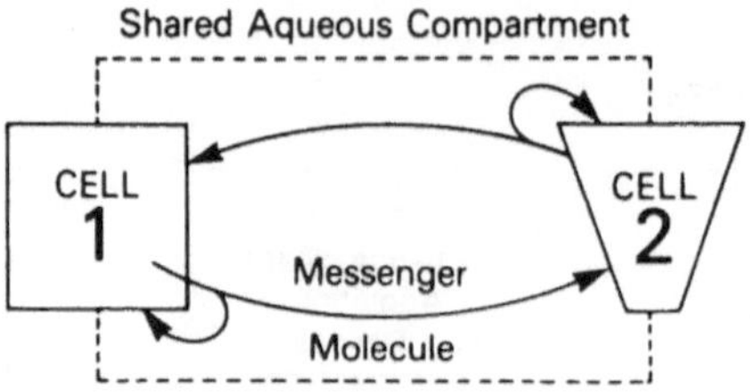

Figure 8: Features of an intercellular communication system. The secretory cell (cell 1) synthesizes and releases a soluble messenger (signal) into a shared aqueous compartment and acts on the target cell (cell 2). In the endocrine system, cell 1 is a glandular cell, the signal molecule is a hormone and the shared aqueous compartment is the blood, whereas in the nervous system cell 1 is a neuron, the signal molecule a neurotransmitter and the shared aqueous compartment a synapse.*

leading to the endocrine system) better explains to us why catecholamines act as both hormones and neurotransmitters, why epithelial cells and neural cells both can act as glandular sources of hormone, and why individual neurons can have both amino acid-derived and peptide messengers. (Likewise, we think that the similarities and overlaps between the nervous systems, GI tract, and skin are better ascribed to a primitive ancestor that is shared by the three).

Similar considerations allow us to rationalize comfortably the overlaps and similarities of tissue factors with hormones as well as the overlaps between the exocrine and endocrine systems. At the level of unicellular organisms, the intercellular communication molecules are more like tissue factors than they are like hormones.

Our present formulation suggests that the ability to produce hormone type molecules is not a unique feature of endocrine glands. Rather we suggest that glands differ from other cells in their ability to produce very large amounts of hormone, store the hormone in granules, and to release it promptly into the blood on receiving the appropriate signal. In vertebrates, many other cell types may manufacture small amounts of "hormone" or other messenger molecules at some time in their life cycle, as do their unicellular ancestors. There are numerous reports of extra-glandular produc-

Table 5: Materials in Plants Related to Messenger Molecules of Vertebrates.

Steroid & Steroid-related:	Cortisol, corticosterone, estrogen, testosterone, progesterone; sex pheromone of hogs; ecdysone.
Peptide:	LHRH-like bioactivity; TRH-like immunoactivity;interferon-related materials; opioid-related materials
Alkaloids:	Muscarine, nicotine, morphine, ephedrine, yohimbine, et al.

tion of hormones in vertebrates. Multiple laboratories have detected material very similar to chorionic gonadotropin in cells from normal non-pregnant, non-tumor bearing animals[32, 33], in contrast with the long held belief that hCG was a product limited to placenta or tumors. There is compelling evidence that ACTH in addition to being made in the pituitary is also produced in brain and in cancers, and can also be produced at other sites including normal lung and placenta[34]. There is increasing evidence to suggest the possibility that insulin may be produced in vertebrate cells other than the pancreatic beta cells; the salivary gland, pituitary gland, and peripheral nerves appear to be strong candidates [35–37].

Our hypothesis which suggests that the biochemical elements of intracellular messenger systems of vertebrates had their origins in unicellular organisms before the evolutionary division of life forms into the major kingdoms, provides a rational explanation of the finding that higher plants may contain molecules that are identical with or are very similar to messenger molecules of vertebrates (Table 5). Among the peptides are materials related to neuropeptides (TRH, LHRH, and opioid). In addition recent studies demonstrated that interferon-like substances are native to higher plants and that a mammalian interferon can produce a biological response in plants [38,39]. Our hypothesis may also suggest a basis for understanding why plants contain novel compounds like alkaloids that have such precise specificities for the binding region present on vertebrate receptors; are these receptors found in plants and did these alkaloids evolve in the presence of the receptors?

In summary, since the introduction of concepts about the nervous and endocrine systems in the late 19th and early 20th centuries data have been accumulated in vertebrates, metazoa, microbes, and higher plants that suggest that the messenger molecules associated with intercellular communication in vertebrates are very widely distributed and possibly may have originated at the level of unicellular organisms. Using this information, we have re-examined observations in vertebrates to try to provide a more unified focus for a wide range of biological and medical phenomena.

ACKNOWLEDGMENTS

Hans Lindner through his warmth, intellect, published works, family and younger colleagues has endowed us with a very precious legacy in which we all have a share.

*Figures reproduced with permission from Clinical Research 31:354-363, 1983.

REFERENCES

1. Starling, E.H. The Croonian Lectures. Lancet August 26: 579-583, (1905).
2. Pearse A.G.E. The cytochemistry and ultrastructure of polypeptide hormone-producing cells of the APUD series, and the embryologic, physiologic and pathologic implications of the concept. J. Histochem. Cytochem. 17:303-313, (1969).
3. Pearse, A.G.E., Polak, J.M., Facer, P., and Marangos, P.J. Neuron specific enolase in gastric and related endocrine cells. The facts and their significance. Hepatogastroenterology 27:78-86 (1980).
4. Fujita, T. The gastro-enteric endocrine cell and its paraneuronic nature. In:Chromafin, Enterochromafin and Related Cells, R.E. Coupland and T. Fujita, ed., Elsevier, Amsterdam, 191-208 (1976).
5. LeRoith, D., Shiloach, J., Roth, J. and Lesniak, M.A. Insulin or a closely related molecule is native to Escherichia coli. J. Biol. Chem. 256:6533-6536 (1981).
6. LeRoith, D., Shiloach, J., Roth, J. and Lesniak, M.A. Evolutionary origins of vertebrate hormones:substances similar to mammalian insulins are native to unicellular organisms. Proc. Natl. Acad. Sci. (USA) 77:6184-6188 (1980).
7. LeRoith, D., Shiloach, J., Heffron, R., Rubinovitz, C., Tanenbaum, R. and Roth, J. Insulin-related material in microbes: Similarities and differences from mammalian insulins (submitted for publication).
8. Berelowitz, M., LeRoith, D., Von Schenk, H., Newgard, C., Szabo, M., Frohman, L.A., Shiloach, J. and Roth, J. Somatostatin-like immunoactivity and biological activity is present

in T. pyriformis, a ciliated protozoan. Endocrinology 110: 1939-1944 (1982).

9. LeRoith, D., Liotta, A.S., Roth, J., Shiloach, J., Lewis, M.E., Pert, C.B., and Krieger, D.T. Corticotropin and β-endorphin-like materials are native to unicellular organisms. Proc. Natl. Acad. Sci. (USA) 79:2086-2090 (1982).
10. Schwabe, C., LeRoith, D., Thompson, R.P., Shiloach, J. and Roth, J. Relaxin extracted from protozoa (Tetrahymena pyriformis). J. Biol. Chem. 258:2778-2781 (1983).
11. Perez-Cano, R., Murphy, P.K., Girgis, S.I., Arnett, T.R., Blenkharn, L. and MacIntyre, I. Unicellular organisms contain a molecule resembling human calcitonin. Endocrinology, 110: 673A (abstract) (1982).
12. Macchia, V., Bates, R.W. and Pastan, I. Purification and properties of thyroid stimulating factor isolated from Clostridium perfringens. J. Biol. Chem. 242:3726-3730 (1967).
13. Maruo, T., Cohen, H., Segal, S.J. and Koide, S.S. Production of choriogonadotropin-like factor by a microorganism. Proc. Natl. Acad. Sci. (USA) 76:6622-6626 (1979).
14. Acevedo, H.F., Slifkin, M., Pouchet, G.R. and Pardo, M. Immunocytochemical localization of a choriogonadotropin-like protein in bacteria isolated from cancer patients. Cancer 41:1217-1219 (1978).
15. Domingue, G.J., Acevedo, H.F., Powell, F.E. and Stevens, V.C. In vivo production by bacterial vaccines of choriogonadotropin antibodies in the rabbit. Endocrinology 112:157A (1983).
16. Richert, N.D. and Ryan, R.J. Specific gonadotropin binding to Pseudomonas maltophilia. Proc. Natl. Acad. Sci. (USA) 74:878-882 (1977).
17. Weiss, M., Ingbar, S.H., Winblad, S., and Kasper, D.L. Demonstration of a saturable binding site for thyrotropin in Yersinia enterocolitica. Science 219:1331-1333 (1983).
18. Josefsson, J.O. and Johansson, P. Naloxone-reversible effects of opioids on pinocytosis in Amoeba proteus. Nature 282: 78-80 (1979).
19. Stephens, K., Hegeman, G.D. and White, D. Pheromone produced by the myxobacterium Stigmatella aurantiaca. J. Bacteriology 149:739-747 (1982).
20. Sarkar, N., Langley, D. and Paulus, H. Biological function of gramicidin: Selective inhibition of RNA polymerase. Proc. Natl. Acad. Sci. (USA) 74:1478-1482 (1979).
21. Bonner, J.T. Aggregation and differentiation in the cellular slime molds. Ann. Rev. Microbiology 25:75-92 (1971).
22. Dunny, G.M., Craig, R.A., Carron, R.L. and Clewell, D.B. Plasmid transfer in Streptococcus fecalis; production of multiple sex pheromones by recipients. Plasmid 2:454-465 (1979).
23. O'Day, D.H. Modes of cellular communication and sexual interactions in eukaryotic microbes. In: Sexual Inter-

actions in Eukaryotic Microbes, O'Day, D.H. and P.A. Horgen eds. Acad. Press, N.Y., 3-17 (1981).
24. Hunt, L.T. and Dayhoff, M.D. Structural and functional similarities among hormones and active peptides from distantly related eukaryotes. In: Peptides: Structure and Biological Function. Gross, E. and Meienhofer, J. eds. Pierce Chemical Co., Proceedings of The Sixth American Peptide Symposium, Rockford, Il. 757-760 (1979).
25. Loumaye, E., Thorner, J., and Catt, K.J. Yeast mating pheromone activates mammalian gonadotrophs: Evolutionary conservation of a reproductive hormone? Science 218:1324-1325 (1982).
26. Roth, J., LeRoith, D., Shiloach, J., Lesniak, M.A., Rosenzweig, L., and Havrankova, J. The evolutionary origins of hormones, neurotransmitters and other extracellular chemical messengers. N. Eng. J. Med. 306:523-526 (1982).
27. Roth, J., LeRoith, D., Shiloach, J. and Rubinovitz, C. Intercellular Communication: An Attempt at a Unifying Hypothesis. Clin. Res. 31:354-363 (1983).
28. Kramer, J.J. Vertebrate hormones in insects. In: Comprehensive Insect Physiology, Biochemistry and Pharmacology 7: Endocrinology, Chap. 20 (in press).
29. Plisetskaya, E., Kazakov, V.K., Solititskaya, L., and Leibson, L.G. Insulin producing cells in the gut of freshwater bivalve molluscs Anodonta cygnea and Unio pictorum and the role of insulin in the regulation of their carbohydrate metabolism. Gen. Comp. Endocrinol. 35:133-145 (1978).
30. Duve, H., Thorpe, A. Immunofluorescent localization of insulin-like material in the median neurosecretory cells of the blowfly Calliphora vomitoria. Cell Tiss. Res. 200:187-191 (1979).
31. Duve, H., Thorpe, A. and Lazarus, N.R. Isolation of material displaying insulin-like immunological and biological activity from the brain of the blowfly, Calliphora vomitoria. Biochem. J. 184:221-227 (1979).
32. Braunstein, G.D., Kandar, V., Rasor, J., Swaminathan, N. and Wade, M.E. Widespread distribution of chorionic gonadotropin-like substance in normal human tissues. J. Clin. Endocrinol. Met. 49:917-925 (1979).
33. O'dell, W.D. and Wolfsen, A.R. Hormones from tumors. Are they ubiquitous? Amer. J. Med. 68:317-318 (1980).
34. Liotta, A.S., Osathanondh, R., Ryan, K.J., and Krieger, D.T. Presence of corticotropin in human placenta: Demonstration of in vitro synthesis. Endocrinology 101:1552-1558 (1977).
35. Murakami, K., Taniguchi, H. and Baba, S. Presence of insulin-like immunoreactivity and biosynthesis in rat and human parotid gland. Diabetologia 22:358-361 (1982).
36. Budd, G.C., Pansky, B. and Cordell, B. Insulin or insulin-like peptides in the pituitary gland. J. Cell. Biol. 163:

404A (abstract) (1983).

37. Uvnas-Möberg, K., Uvnas, B., Posloncec, B. Castensson, S., Hagerman, M. and Rubio, C. Occurrence of an insulin-like peptide in extracts of peripheral nerves of the cat and in extracts of human vagal nerves. Acta Physiol. Scand. 115: 471 (1982).
38. Sela, I. Plant-virus interactions related to resistance and localization of viral infections. Advances Virus Res. 26:201-237 (1981).
39. Orchansky, P., Rubenstein, M., Sela, I. Human interferons protect plants from virus infection. Proc. Natl. Acad. Sci. 79: 2278-2280 (1982).

REGULATION OF THE SYNTHESIS, RELEASE AND ACTION OF HYPOTHALAMIC LUTEINIZING HORMONE RELEASING HORMONE

George Fink, Ann Curtis and Val Lyons

MRC Brain Metabolism Unit
Department of Pharmacology
1 George Square
Edinburgh EH8 9JZ, Scotland

INTRODUCTION

Hans Lindner like Geoffrey Harris was an adherent of the law of parsimony. Although the application of this law ('Occam's razor') to physiology has been challenged by a number of recent discoveries, the law appears to be upheld in the case of luteinizing hormone releasing hormone (LHRH) the decapeptide that mediates the neural control of gonadotropin secretion. This peptide not only stimulates the release of luteinizing hormone (LH) and follicle stimulating hormone (FSH) but also stimulates the synthesis of the gonadotropins, maintains the structure of the gonadotrophs and has the apparently unique property (for neuropeptides studied so far) of sensitizing the pituitary gland to itself (the priming effect of LHRH). Furthermore, as discussed in other chapters of this book, LHRH may exert a direct effect on the gonads, and may serve as a neurotransmitter in parts of the nervous system remote from the hypothalamus.

The physiology and pharmacology of LHRH has been the subject of many reviews in the past decade (1,2,3,4,5,6,7) and here attention will be focussed on recent studies related to the synthesis, release and some aspects of the mechanism of action of hypothalamic LHRH.

REGULATION OF THE SYNTHESIS OF LHRH

Synthesis of LHRH is under genetic control: direct evidence from the hypogonadal mouse

It has generally been assumed that the synthesis of LHRH is regulated genomically, and direct evidence for this was provided by the discovery of the hypogonadal (*hpg*) mouse (8). The hypogonadism is found in both sexes of the mutant, is transmitted as an autosomal recessive trait, and is due to the total absence in the hypothalamus of any immunoreactive (8) or bioactive LHRH (A. Speight, H.M. Charlton and G. Fink, unpublished). In addition to providing direct evidence for the genomic control of LHRH synthesis, the hpg mouse has proved important for studies of the mechanisms of synthesis and action of LHRH and these aspects are discussed below.

The nature of the precursor for LHRH

There is considerable evidence that most if not all biologically active peptides are synthesized as components of larger precursors which are subsequently cleaved by enzymes to yield the active principle. Gel filtration studies of extracts of hypothalamus showed the presence of LHRH-immunoreactive forms that are larger than the decapeptide (9,10), and we have recently demonstrated that the translation products of Poly A^+ mRNA from extracts of human, rat and normal mouse hypothalamus contained a single 28,000 MW polypeptide which immunoprecipitated with a specific anti-LHRH serum (11,12). Total RNA was extracted from rat, mouse and human (3-12 h post-mortem) hypothalamus by the guanidinium thiocyanate procedure. The Poly A^+ mRNA enriched fractions, isolated by oligo (dT)-cellulose chromatography, were translated in an amino-acid depleted rabbit reticulocyte lysate system supplemented with 1 µCi/µl of a ^{3}H-amino acid mix. The incorporation of labelled amino acids into protein was monitored by trichloroacetic acid precipitation of a small aliquot of the translation mix after incubation for 60 min. Approximately 70,000 acid precipitable counts of each sample were loaded (generally 5-10 µl) in SDS-β-mercaptoethanol sample buffer. Electrophoresis was carried out at 15 mA constant current for 15 hours on 12% SDS polyacrylamide slab gels with a 4.75% stacking gel according to the method of Laemmli (13). The gels were fluorographed and exposed to film (Kodak X-omat R) for 10 days. Aliquots of the translation mixes containing a minimum of 10^6 acid precipitable counts (typically 80-150 µl) were taken for treatment with the specific LHRH antiserum. This antiserum (HC6), which was raised in rabbits against a LHRH-haemocyanin conjugate, did not cross react with either nine different analogues of LHRH modified at either the N or C terminus, or pituitary hormones, but did cross react 100% with the free acid of LHRH. The translation products from all four sources were immunoprecipitated using either the second antibody (anti-rabbit IgG) or the staphylococcal protein A method. The precipitate was washed four times with 1.5 ml of immunoprecipitation buffer by gentle homogenisation and centrifugation. The final precipitate was boiled for 5 min in SDS-β-mercaptoethanol sample buffer and the supernatant was electrophoresed on a 12% slab gel and fluorographed.

The translation products of human hypothalamus spanned a similar molecular weight range to those of the rat and mouse and were of comparable specific activity despite the delay between death and RNA extraction (Fig. 1) confirming (14) that the *in vitro* translation of

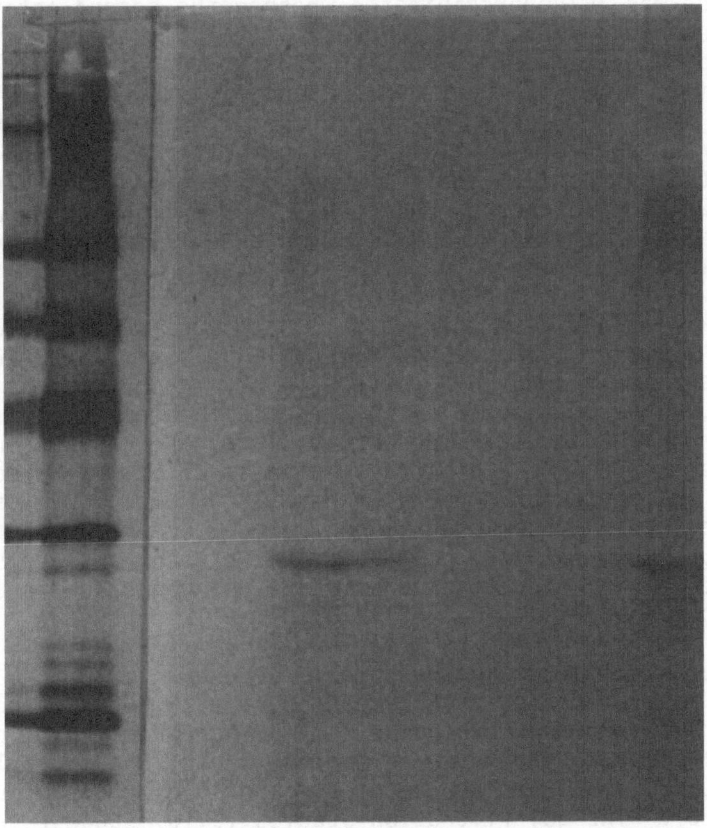

Fig. 1. PAGE and autoradiography of ^{3}H-labelled translation products of hypothalamic mRNA samples of human (lane B), normal mouse (lane D), <u>hpg</u> mouse (lane E) and rat (lane F). Lane C - translation mix with no added mRNA. Lane A - ^{14}C-labelled molecular weight standards: phosphorylase b, 92500; bovine serum albumin, 69000; ovalbumin, 46000; carbonic anhydrase, 30000; and lysozyme, 14300. Reproduced from ref. 12 with the permission of Academic Press.

mRNA occurs with similar efficiency irrespective of whether the original tissue is fresh or is stored at 4°C for several hours. Immunoprecipitation of the translation products of the human and normal mouse and rat hypothalamic mRNA showed a single major band with an apparent molecular weight of 28,000 (Figs. 2 and 3). This same polypeptide was immunoprecipitated whether the second antibody or protein A techniques were used (Fig. 2). The polypeptide could not be detected, however, when an excess (10 μg) of cold LHRH was added before immunoprecipitation (Figs. 2 and 3), showing that the decapeptide is able to compete for the antiserum and block its binding with the precursor completely. The 28,000 molecular weight band was also not detected by the identical immunoprecipitation of a translation mix to which no exogenous mRNA was added or in which normal rabbit serum replaced the anti-LHRH serum or when ^{35}S methionine was the only radiolabelled amino acid in the translation mix (11).

Similar experiments were carried out on Poly A^{+} mRNA extracted from the hypothalami of 60 adult hpg mice of both sexes. The translation products contained no polypeptides that immunoprecipitated with the anti-LHRH serum (Fig. 3). The precise mechanism of the inherited defect in the hpg mouse is not known, but these results suggest that it is unrelated to the processing mechanism of a large precursor molecule since the precursor appears to be either completely absent, or present in a mutated form which is not recognised by the anti-LHRH serum. It is unlikely that the polypeptide is present at levels below our limits of detection since the genetics of the hpg condition clearly show that the primary defect is either all or none.

These results show that in the human, rat and normal mouse hypothalamus, LHRH is synthesized as a component of a 28,000 MW precursor which contains little or no methionine. Allowing for cleavage of a putative signal sequence, the size of the precursor is comparable to the 26,000 MW LHRH immunoreactive peptide found in extracts of rat hypothalamus (10). The gel filtration studies (9,10) suggest that the 28,000 precursor may be processed by way of several intermediate forms to finally yield LHRH. Nucleic acid probes will be required to determine the precise nature of the primary defect in the hpg mouse. However, unless the hpg condition is due to a point mutation, the fact that the hpg mouse appears to be free of any other obvious abnormalities suggests that active components of the precursor, other than LHRH, are unlikely to be crucial for the normal function of the animal.

REGULATION OF THE RELEASE OF LHRH

Characteristics of LHRH release into hypophysial portal blood

The regulation of LHRH release into hypophysial portal blood has been reviewed in detail recently (4,6,7) and so here only a summary will be given. Measurements of LHRH in the rat (6), rabbit (15),

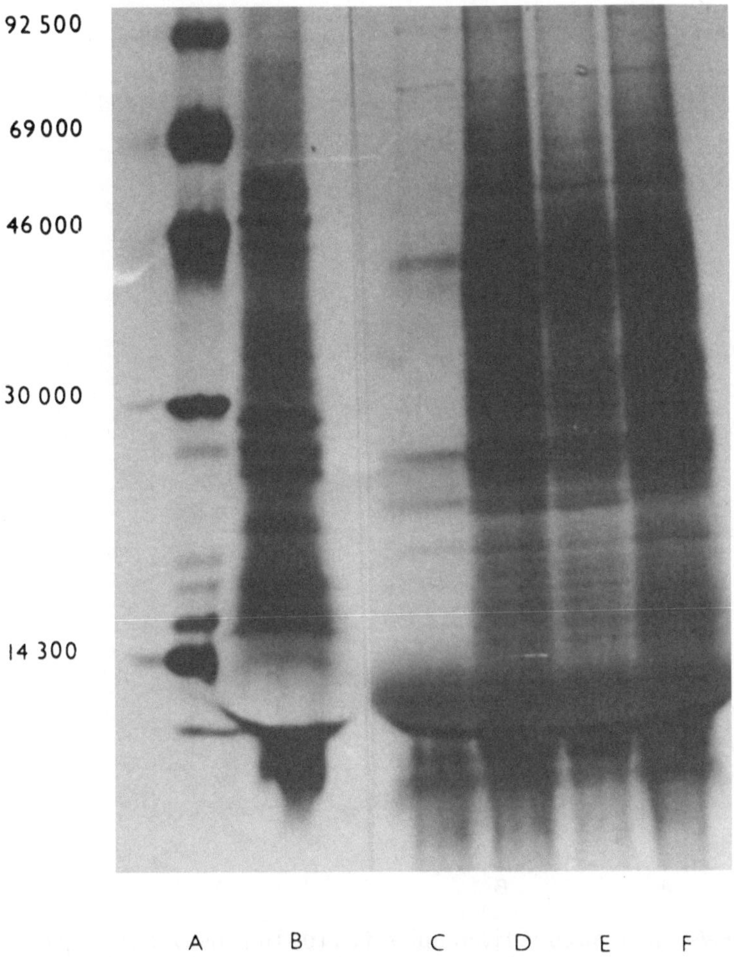

Fig. 2. PAGE and autoradiography following immunoprecipitation of rat and human hypothalamic mRNA translation products with an anti-LHRH serum. Lanes B, C and D show the rat hypothalamic translation products immunoprecipitated in the presence of excess cold LHRH (lane B), or using either the second antibody (lane C) or the Staphylococcal protein A immunoprecipitation technique (lane D). Lane E - translation mix without exogenous mRNA. Lane G - immunoprecipitation product in an human translation mix was a 28,000 MW polypeptide; no immunoprecipitation was seen in the presence of excess cold LHRH (lane F). Lane A: MW standards as in Fig. 1. Reproduced from ref. 12 with the permission of Academic Press.

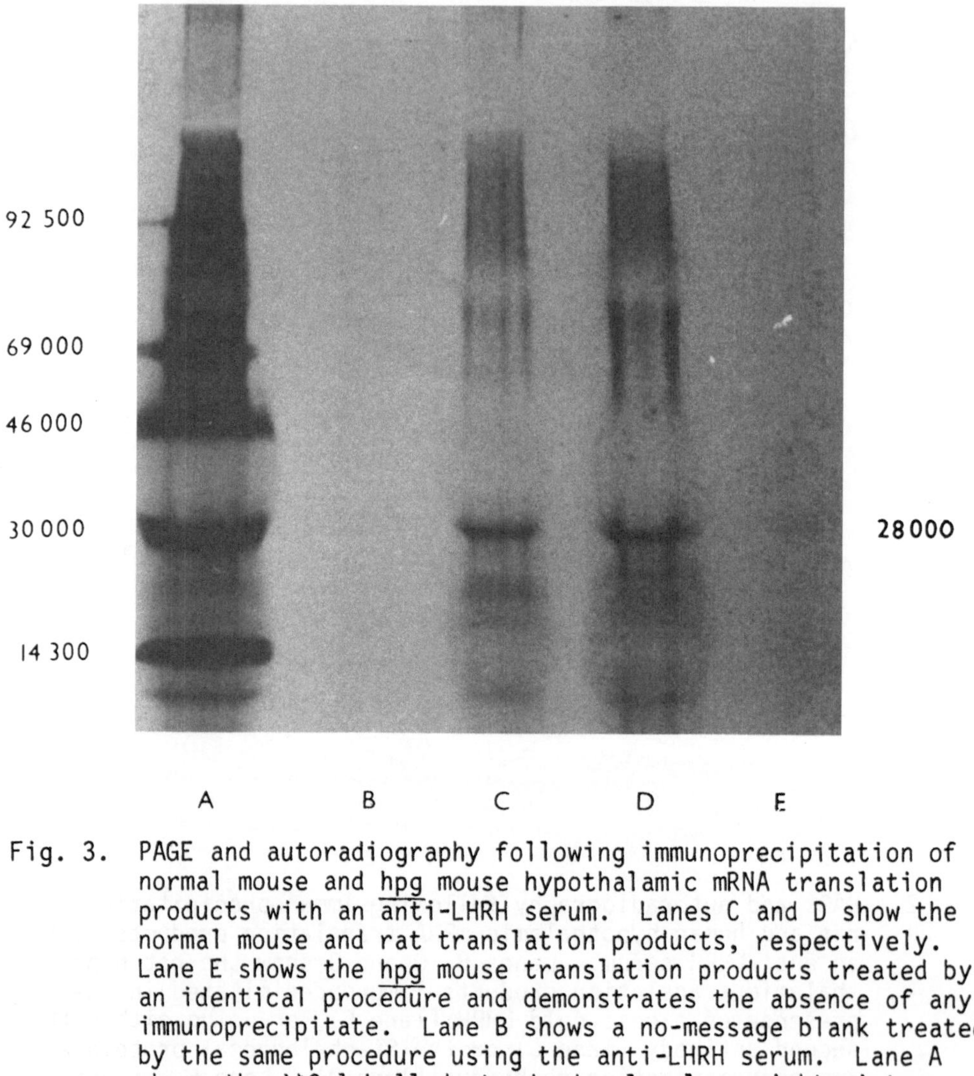

Fig. 3. PAGE and autoradiography following immunoprecipitation of normal mouse and hpg mouse hypothalamic mRNA translation products with an anti-LHRH serum. Lanes C and D show the normal mouse and rat translation products, respectively. Lane E shows the hpg mouse translation products treated by an identical procedure and demonstrates the absence of any immunoprecipitate. Lane B shows a no-message blank treated by the same procedure using the anti-LHRH serum. Lane A shows the ^{14}C-labelled standard molecular weight mixture as detailed in Fig. 1. Reproduced from ref. 12 with the permission of Academic Press.

sheep (16) and rhesus monkey (17,18,19) have shown that the amount of LHRH in hypophysial portal blood is considerably greater than in peripheral blood, and in most situations is related to LH release. Electrical stimulation of the hypothalamus significantly increases LHRH output into portal blood (20,21). The output of LHRH is dependent upon the pulse amplitude (20) and, as assessed by studies of LH release (22), the pulse frequency of the stimulus. The stimulus-evoked release of LHRH is site-specific being greatest when the stimulus is applied to the median eminence (ME) (23). The amount of LHRH released (above basal) by stimulation of either the medial preoptic area, suprachiasmatic nuclei and anterior hypothalamic area was, respectively, 52%, 35% and 9% relative to the amount released by ME stimulation (23). Stimulation of the hippocampus or amygdala had no effect on the amount of LHRH released into portal blood, but stimulation of the ventral hippocampus did reduce the amount of LHRH released by stimulation of the medial preoptic area (23). The responsiveness of the preoptic LHRH system to electrical stimulation could be enhanced by estradiol benzoate (EB) and testosterone, but not by 5α dihydrotestosterone (24).

More important than the release evoked by hypothalamic stimulation is the spontaneous release of LHRH. Advances in this area occurred when it was found that the steroid anaesthetic, alphadalone (Althesin) does not block completely, although it does reduce the magnitude of, the spontaneous ovulatory surge of LH (25). Measurement of LHRH in hypophysial portal blood collected from female rats anaesthetized with Althesin showed that in fact a surge of LHRH did occur and that this coincided with the spontaneous ovulatory surge of LH (25,26,27,28). A spontaneous surge of LHRH was also found to coincide with the first, pubertal, surge of LH (29). Experimental studies showed that the spontaneous surge of LHRH depended upon the increase in the plasma concentration of estradiol-17β (E_2) that begins on diestrus and reaches a peak at or about midday of proestrus (30). Surprisingly, depending upon dose, progesterone had either no effect or inhibited the stimulation of LHRH release by EB. However, in female rats exposed to continuous illumination, progesterone stimulated LHRH release and this explains in part how progesterone stimulates a surge of LH in these rats.

In long-term ovariectomized rats the release of LHRH was found to be pulsatile (31). The amplitude of the pulses increased with time after ovariectomy (31) and this coincided with the changes in the pattern of LH release seen after ovariectomy (31,32). Intravenous injection of E_2 caused a rapid reduction in the release of LHRH into portal blood, and long-term exposure to high plasma concentrations of E_2 (produced by s.c. implants of silicone elastomer capsules containing E_2) resulted, after 3 d, in a daily increase in LHRH release during the afternoon which corresponded with the afternoon increase in the plasma concentration of LH in this preparation (31). However, in spite of several different studies and approaches it was not possible to demonstrate a surge of LHRH in long-term ovariectomized rats injected with EB followed 72 h later by progesterone or a second injection of EB (31). In this preparation a massive surge of LH occurs with a peak about 5 h after the second steroid injection. Preliminary studies showed that Althesin did not block the LH surge induced by EB followed by progesterone. The responsiveness of the anterior pituitary gland to LHRH in long-term ovariectomized rats treated with EB followed by progesterone is about 2-3 times that at the peak of responsiveness at proestrus. Thus, while a blocking effect of Althesin on LHRH release in this particular preparation cannot be excluded, it is plausible that the massive surge of LH is due primarily to the massive increase in pituitary responsiveness to LHRH which occurs after the injection of progesterone.

The mechanisms by which E_2 and progesterone exert their different effects on LHRH release are not clear; however, it would appear that the effects are not necessarily direct on LHRH neurons but may be mediated or influenced by the activity of monoaminergic (6,33,34,35, 36,37,38) and opioid neurons (39,40,41,42,43).

The nature of LHRH in hypophysial portal blood

Although, as outlined above, a number of groups have studied the release of immunoreactive LHRH in hypophysial portal blood it is not known whether the peptide is released as only one or more forms. Conceivably, like somatostatin (44) larger peptides (derived from the LHRH precursor) containing the LHRH sequence could be released into portal blood. However, so far studies of extracts of portal blood with reverse phase HPLC (using the method in ref. 45) have shown only one peak of LHRH which coincides precisely with the authentic decapeptide (W.J. Sheward, A.J. Harmar and G. Fink, unpublished). However, the variable 'exclusion limit' of the HPLC system may have prevented detection of large molecules, and so further studies are in progress to determine whether in fact no large forms of the decapeptide are released *in vivo*.

EFFECT OF LHRH ON GONADOTROPIN SYNTHESIS: STUDIES ON THE HYPOGONADAL MOUSE

The way in which the gonadotropin-releasing action of LHRH is modified dramatically by steroids, E_2 and progesterone in particular, has been reviewed in detail as has the priming effect of the peptide (4,5,6,46). Studies of pituitary grafts (47,48,49,50) and development (51,52) provided strong indirect evidence that LHRH is also necessary for the synthesis of the gonadotropins. Direct evidence for this was provided by experimental studies on the rat (53,54,55) and our studies on the *hpg* mouse (8,56,57). Recently, Charlton et al (58) carried out a detailed study on the effect of different modes (frequency and dose) of LHRH administration on the pituitary gonadotropin content and the weights of the gonads and secondary sex organs in male and female hpg mice. In male hpg mice, single daily injections of LHRH at doses from 50 ng to 20 μg for 20 days increased the pituitary FSH content to values similar or greater than that in normal mice (∼ 36 to 60-fold increase in content), but only increased slightly the pituitary content of LH. The weights of the tests was increased to about a third of those in normal adult mice and, by 60 days of injection, all stages of spermatogenesis were present. However, in none of the animals was there any growth of the seminal vesicles. However, when LHRH was administered as 12 injections each day (at 2 h intervals) for 15 days, there was an increase in pituitary LH (although not to normal adult levels) as well as pituitary FSH content, and a significant increase in the weights of the seminal vesicles as well as the testes. Injection of 60 ng LHRH 12 times daily for 15 days produced increases in pituitary LH content, plasma FSH concentration, and seminal vesicle weights which were much greater than those produced by the much larger total dose of 1 μg LHRH administered once daily; pituitary FSH contents were similar in the 2 groups of animals. Castration alone or castration with either adrenalectomy or the implantation of silicone elastomer capsules containing testosterone propionate did not inhibit the increase in the LHRH-stimulated increase in pituitary FSH content.

In female hpg mice single daily s.c. injections of LHRH for 10-15 days increased pituitary FSH content to a level 4 times that in normal adult female mice, but there was no increase in uterine weight. Injections of LHRH, given either 4 or 12 each day for 10-15 days, increased pituitary FSH content to the level in normal adult female mice and also increased significantly the weights of the uteri. Pituitary LH content was increased to nearly normal values by 12 injections of 60 ng LHRH/day but remained low in animals given single daily injections of LHRH even at doses as high as 1 μg. Treatment with EB significantly reduced, whereas ovariectomy significantly enhanced, the increase in pituitary FSH content produced by multiple LHRH injections.

These data showed that 1) multiple daily injections of LHRH produce a more normal function of the pituitary-gonadal-accessory sex organ system in hpg mice of either sex compared with the effect of single daily injections of the peptide, 2) in the female hpg mouse, E_2 exerts its inhibitory effect at the level of the anterior pituitary gland, whereas in the male testosterone appears to exert its inhibitory effect at the hypothalamus or above, and 3) with every injection regimen used, LHRH is considerably more potent at stimulating FSH compared with LH synthesis in the hpg mouse. These data are consistent with those reviewed in other chapters of this book which show that pulsatile LHRH release is likely to be the most common physiological mode of the secretion of this peptide. These data also show that in spite of the fact that the possibility of a separate FSH-RH cannot be excluded (see Chapter by McCann) at least in the mouse, LHRH is a potent stimulant of FSH synthesis and release.

The *hpg* mouse should prove to be a valuable model for more sophisticated studies on the trophic and synthesis-stimulating actions of LHRH. In addition, this mutant may provide a useful model for studies of the interactions, if any, between the several other pituitary hormone systems and the gonadotropin control system. Thus, for example, studies of PRL in the *hpg* mouse (59) showed that the stimulatory effect of E_2 of PRL synthesis by the pituitary was not impaired in *hpg* compared with normal mice of both sexes. However, for reasons that have yet to be established E_2 could significantly increase plasma PRL concentrations in normal but not *hpg* mice.

SUMMARY

As assessed by the immunoprecipitation of Poly A^+ mRNA extracted from human, rat or mouse hypothalamus, LHRH is synthesized as a component of a 28,000 MW precursor. The decapeptide is released into hypophysial portal blood in amounts that are consistent with one of its main actions, the stimulation of LH release. The release of LHRH is modulated by steroids, predominently E_2, the action of which may be mediated and/or modified by central neurotransmitters such as the monoamines and the opioids. In addition to its action as a gonadotropin releasing hormone, LHRH sensitizes the pituitary to itself (priming effect) and plays a crucial role, as shown clearly in the *hpg* mouse, in maintaining the integrity of the gonadotrophs and stimulating the synthesis of FSH and LH.

ACKNOWLEDGEMENTS

We are grateful to Miss Jo Donnelly for the careful preparation of the typescript.

REFERENCES

1. A.V. Schally, A. Arimura and A.J. Kastin, *Science* 179:341 (1973).
2. W. Vale, C. Rivier and M. Brown, *Ann. Rev. Physiol.* 39:473 (1977).
3. G. Fink, in: Recent Advances in *Obstetrics and Gynaecology*, J. Stallworthy and G. Bourne, eds., pp. 4-54, Churchill Livingstone, Edinburgh (1977).
4. G. Fink, *Brit. Med. Bull.* 35:155 (1979).
5. G. Fink and A. Pickering, *in*: Synthesis and Release of Adenohypophyseal Hormones, M. Jutisz and K. McKerns, eds., pp. 617-638, Plenum Press, New York (1980).
6. G. Fink, M. Aiyer, S. Chiappa, S. Henderson, M. Jamieson, V. Levy-Perez, A. Pickering, D. Sarkar, N. Sherwood, A. Speight and A. Watts, *in*: Hormonally Active Brain Peptides, K. McKerns and V. Pantic, eds., pp. 397-426, Plenum Press, New York (1982).
7. G. Fink, H.F. Stanley and A.G. Watts, *in*: Brain Peptides, D. Krieger, M. Brownstein and J. Martin, eds., pp. 413-435, John Wiley & Sons Inc., New York (1983).

8. B.M. Cattanach, C.A. Iddon, H.M. Charlton, S.A. Chiappa and G. Fink, Nature 269:338 (1977).
9. R.P. Millar, C. Ashnelt, G. Rossier, Biochem. Biophys. Res. Commun. 74:720 (1977).
10. J.P. Gautron, E. Pattou and C. Kordon, Mol. Cell Endocrinol. 24:1 (1981).
11. A. Curtis and G. Fink, Endocrinology 112:390 (1983).
12. A. Curtis, V. Lyons and G. Fink, Biochem. Biophys. Res. Commun. 117:872 (1983).
13. U. Laemmli, Nature 222:680 (1970).
14. M.R. Morrison and W.S.T. Griffin, Anal. Biochem. 113:318 (1981).
15. R.C. Tsou, R.A. Dailey, C.S. McLanahan, A.D. Parent, G.T. Tindall and J.D. Neill, Endocrinology 101:534 (1977).
16. I.J. Clarke and J.T. Cummins, Endocrinology 111:1737 (1982).
17. P.W. Carmel, S. Araki and M. Ferin, Endocrinology 99:243 (1976).
18. J.D. Neill, R.A. Dailey, R.C. Tsou, J. Patton and G. Tindall, in: Ovulation in the Human, P.G. Crosignani and D.R. Mishell, eds., pp. 115-125, Academic Press, New York (1976).
19. J.D. Neill, J.M. Patton, R.A. Dailey, R.C. Tsou and G.T. Tindall, Endocrinology 101:430 (1977).
20. G. Fink and M.G. Jamieson, J. Endocrinol. 68:71 (1976).
21. R.L. Eskay, R.S. Mical and J.C. Porter, Endocrinology 100:263 (1977).
22. M.G. Jamieson and G. Fink, J. Endocrinol. 68:57 (1976).
23. S.A. Chiappa, G. Fink and N.M. Sherwood, J. Physiol. 267:625 (1977).
24. N.M. Sherwood, S.A. Chiappa and G. Fink, Endocrinology 70:501 (1976).
25. D.K. Sarkar, S.A. Chiappa, G. Fink and N.M. Sherwood, Nature 264:461 (1976).
26. N.M. Sherwood and G. Fink, Endocrinology 106:363 (1980).
27. N.M. Sherwood, S.A. Chiappa, D.K. Sarkar and G. Fink, Endocrinology 107:1410 (1980).
28. M. Ching, Neuroendocrinology 34:279 (1982).
29. D.K. Sarkar and G. Fink, J. Endocrinol. 83:339 (1979).
30. D.K. Sarkar and G. Fink, J. Endocrinol. 80:303 (1979).
31. D.K. Sarkar and G. Fink, J. Endocrinol. 86:511 (1980).
32. R.E. Leipheimen and R.V. Gallo, Neuroendocrinology 37:421 (1983).
33. C.H. Sawyer, Neuroendocrinology 17:97 (1975).
34. G. Fink and L.B. Geffen, in: International Review of Physiology, vol. 17, Neurophysiology III, R. Porter, ed., pp. 1-48, University Park Press, Baltimore (1978).
35. R.I. Weiner and W.F. Ganong, Physiol. Rev. 58:905 (1978).
36. D.K. Sarkar and G. Fink, Endocrinology 108:862 (1981).
37. C.A. Barraclough and P.M. Wise, Endocrinol. Rev. 1:91 (1982).
38. D.K. Sarkar, G.C. Smith and G. Fink, Brain Res. 213:335 (1981).
39. T.J. Cicero, T.M. Badger, C.E. Wilcox, R.D. Bell and E.R. Meyer, J. Pharmacol. 203:548 (1977).
40. T.J. Cicero, B.A. Schainker and E.R. Meyer, Endocrinology 104:1286 (1979).

41. D.A. Van Vugt, P.W. Sylvester, C.F. Aylsworth and J. Meites, Neuroendocrinology 34:274 (1982).
42. R. Bhanot and M. Wilkinson, Endocrinology 113:596 (1983).
43. R. Bhanot and M. Wilkinson, Endocrinology 112:399 (1983).
44. R.P. Millar, W.J. Sheward, I. Wegener and G. Fink, Brain Res. 260:334 (1983).
45. W.J. Sheward, A.J. Harmar, H.M. Fraser and G. Fink, Endocrinology 113:1865 (1983).
46. G. Fink, Ann. Rev. Physiol. 41:571 (1979).
47. G.W. Harris and D. Jacobsohn, Proc. R. Soc. B. 139:263 (1952).
48. M. Nikitovitch-Winer and J.W. Everett, Endocrinology 63:916 (1958).
49. M. Nikitovitch-Winer and J.W. Everett, Endocrinology 65:357 (1959).
50. P.E. Smith, Endocrinology 68:130 (1961).
51. G. Fink and G.C. Smith, Z. Zellforsch. 119:208 (1971).
52. S.A. Chiappa and G. Fink, J. Endocrinol. 71:211 (1977).
53. T.-C. Liu and G.L. Jackson, Endocrinology 103:1253 (1978).
54. T.-C. Liu and G.L. Jackson, Endocrinology 104:962 (1979).
55. S. Azhar, J.R. Reel, C.A. Pastushok and K.M.J. Menon, Biochem. Biophys. Res. Commun. 80:659 (1978).
56. C.A. Iddon, H.M. Charlton and G. Fink, J. Endocrinol. 85:105 (1980).
57. I.F.W. McDowell, J.F. Morris, H.M. Charlton and G. Fink, J. Endocrinol. 95:331 (1982).
58. H.M. Charlton, D.M.G. Halpin, C. Iddon, R. Rosie, G. Levy, I.F.W. McDowell, A. Megson, J.F. Morris, A. Bramwell, A. Speight, B.J. Ward, J. Broadhead, G. Davey-Smith and G. Fink, Endocrinology 113:535 (1983).
59. H.M. Charlton, A. Speight, D.M.G. Halpin, A. Bramwell, W.J. Sheward and G. Fink, Endocrinology 113:545 (1983).

DEGRADATION OF LH-RH

Karl Bauer and Bernhard Horsthemke

Institut für Biochemie
Technische Universität Berlin
Berlin (West)

INTRODUCTION

The neuropeptide Luteinizing Hormone - Releasing Hormone (LH-RH, pyroGlu-His-Trp-Ser-Tyr-Gly-Leu-Arg-Pro-Gly-NH_2) participates in synaptic events and the hypothalamic control of adenohypophyseal hormone secretion. Since the peptide is rapidly hydrolyzed by various tissue homogenates, it has been postulated that the biological inactivation of LH-RH at the target site is catalyzed by a peptidase, which might possibly be specific for this neuropeptide. Furthermore, it has been suggested that the feedback-controlled alterations of such an enzymatic activity might be involved in the regulation of the LH-RH metabolism and thus in the control of the biological activity of this peptide (Griffiths et al., 1975; Fridkin et al., 1977; Kuhl et al., 1978; Advis et al., 1982). Alternatively, it is conceivable that LH-RH is degraded by general proteolytic enzymes, which might fulfill a scavenger function at the site of target interaction (if located in the vicinity of the receptors) or a more general metabolic clearance function at other sites. It is clear that such enzymes cannot serve a regulatory function. For answering these questions it is a prerequisite to delineate the pathway of LH-RH fragmentation and to evaluate the biochemical properties of the enzymes capable of hydrolyzing this neuropeptide.

EXPERIMENTAL RESULTS

Degradation of LH-RH by Adenohypophyseal and Hypothalamic Tissue Homogenates

Enzymatic hydrolysis of the strongly basic decapeptide amide LH-RH generates N-terminal fragments which contain a free carboxy group and thus are less basic than LH-RH. They can be separated from LH-RH by ion-exchange chromatography on cellulose phosphate paper using 25 mM ammonium acetate as eluant. Under these conditions, LH-RH remains at the origin. Basic N-terminal fragments containing an arginine residue (e.g. deamido-LH-RH) exhibit a R_f-value of 0.15 and are separated from the slightly acidic fragments such as LH-RH (1-6) hexapeptide, LH-RH (1-5) pentapeptide and LH-RH (1-3) tripeptide ($R_f = 0.5$) and also from the strongly acidic pyroglutamic acid, which migrates with the solvent front (see Fig.1).

On this basis a highly sensitive, accurate and convenient test using commerially available [pyroglutamyl-^{3}H]LH-RH could be developed. After incubation of this substrate with rat adenohypophyseal or hypothalamic tissue homogenates, the reaction mixtures could be resolved as described above. Scanning for radioactivity revealed three zones of radioactive material separated from LH-RH (zone I). For both incubates, qualitatively the same fragmentation pattern could be observed. However, LH-RH is degraded more rapidly by adenohypophyseal tissue homogenates than by homogenates from hypothalamic tissues. As identified later, zone II contains LH-RH (1-9) nonapeptide, zone III mainly LH-RH (1-5) pentapeptide and trace amounts of LH-RH (1-4) tetrapeptide and LH-RH (1-3) tripeptide and zone IV pyroglutamic acid.

The kinetical analysis (Fig.2) shows that these fragments are formed without any lag phase and therefore most likely represent primary cleavage products. Zone II is the most rapidly formed fragment (compare the initial rates of product formation), but after 5 minutes its concentration reaches a steady state. At this time the rate of formation of zone III increases, and this zone becomes the major product. This indicates that the fragments of zone III, besides being generated by primary cleavage of LH-RH, are also formed by rapid degradation of the fragment of zone II. The fragment of zone IV (pyroGlu) is slowly released and may be generated from LH-RH and the N-terminal fragments of zone II and III.

The formation of several primary cleavage products strongly indicates that LH-RH is not degraded by only one enzyme (Koch et al., 1974; Kuhl et al., 1978), but by several peptidases. Therefore, the degradation of LH-RH can ultimately be analyzed only after purification of the individual LH-RH degrading enzymes.

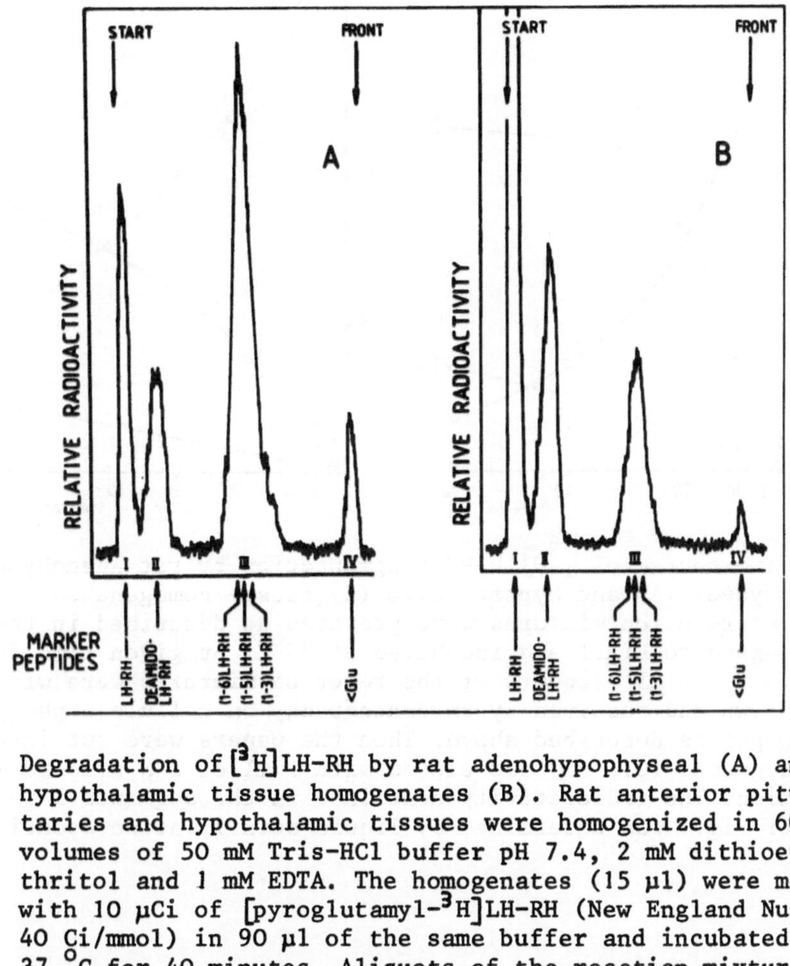

Fig.1. Degradation of [^{3}H]LH-RH by rat adenohypophyseal (A) and hypothalamic tissue homogenates (B). Rat anterior pituitaries and hypothalamic tissues were homogenized in 60 volumes of 50 mM Tris-HCl buffer pH 7.4, 2 mM dithioerythritol and 1 mM EDTA. The homogenates (15 µl) were mixed with 10 µCi of [pyroglutamyl-^{3}H]LH-RH (New England Nuclear, 40 Ci/mmol) in 90 µl of the same buffer and incubated at 37 °C for 40 minutes. Aliquots of the reaction mixtures (10 µl) were added to a solution of marker peptides and resolved by chromatography on P81 cellulose phosphate paper using 25 mM ammonium acetate as eluant. After scanning the chromatogram for radioactivity, the marker peptides were visualized by spraying with Pauly's reagent. [^{14}C]pyroGlu was chromatographed at the edge of the paper and localized by scanning for radioactivity.

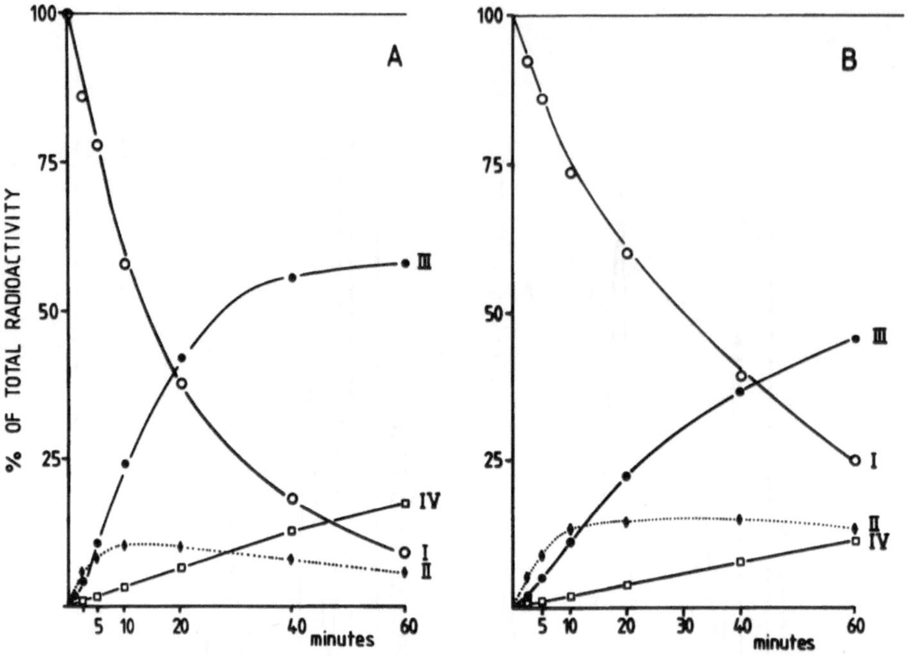

Fig.2. Time course of [^{3}H]LH-RH fragmentation by rat adenohypophyseal (A) and hypothalamic (B) tissue homogenates. The reaction mixtures were prepared as described in the legend to Fig.1 and incubated at 37°C. At given time intervals, 10 µl aliquots of the reaction mixtures were withdrawn and resolved by chromatography on cellulose phosphate paper as described above. Then the papers were cut into segments (0.5 cm) and eluted with 1 ml of 2 N ammonia solution. The radioactivity contained in the segments I to IV of Fig.1 was determined by liquid scintillation counting.

Purification and Characterization of LH-RH Degrading Tissue Enzymes

The degradation of LH-RH by pituitary and brain homogenates is mainly due to soluble enzymes, which could be separated from each other as well as from amino- and carboxypeptidases by ion-exchange chromatography, gel filtration, hydroxylapatite chromatography and hydrophobic interaction chromatography of tissue extracts. Recently, a particle bound LH-RH degrading activity was also partially purified. After incubation of these enzyme preparations with LH-RH and [pyroGlu-^{3}H]LH-RH as radioactive tracer, the N-terminal fragments were isolated by ion-exchange chromatography on Aminex-resin and thin-layer chromatography on silica gel (Fig.3). A negative reaction with ninhydrin indicated that the peptides were not contaminated by internal or C-terminal fragments and that they contained intact pyroglutamic acid. Amino acid analysis then allowed the identification of the fragments and hence the cleavage sites of LH-RH (see upper part of Tab.1). After intensive characterization these enzymes were found to be general proteolytic enzymes capable of hydrolyzing several substrates (Knisatschek and Bauer, 1979; Bauer and Kleinkauf, 1980; Horsthemke and Bauer, 1980; Horsthemke and Bauer, 1981; Horsthemke and Bauer, 1982; Hersh and McKelvy, 1979; Orlowski et al., 1979; Wilk and Orlowski, 1980; Leblanc et al., 1980) Their physical, chemical and biochemical properties are summarized in Tab.1.

The primary specificity of these enzymes is not directed towards the whole substrate but only towards certain structural elements. This fact, however, does not exclude the possibility that the rate of hydrolysis is influenced by neighbouring groups or even the total conformation of the substrate. This effect is especially obvious when the degradation of LH-RH and LH-RH (1-9) nonapeptide by the nonchymotrypsin-like endopeptidase are compared (see Fig.4). In contrast to the cation-sensitive endopeptidase, which also cleaves the Tyr-Gly peptide bond, this enzyme hydrolyzes the nonapeptide 50 times more rapidly than LH-RH. Similar observations were reported for the endo-oligopeptidase A from rabbit brain, which seems to be identical to the nonchymotrypsin-like enzyme (Horsthemke and Bauer, 1980; Camargo et al., 1982). The rapid degradation of LH-RH (1-9) nonapeptide by this enzyme explains the finding mentioned above, that this fragment (zone II in Fig.1 and 2) does not accumulate during the incubation of LH-RH with tissue homogenates, although it is most rapidly formed.

Evaluation of the Biochemical Studies

The characterization of the LH-RH degrading enzymes clearly demonstrates that this neuropeptide is not degraded by a LH-RH specific peptidase but by general proteolytic enzymes. Therefore, these studies do not provide any direct information about the biological functions of these enzymes but are the basis for developping enzyme-specific tests and inhibitors suitable for further investigations. The activity of an individual enzyme, for example, can selectively be determined by including appropriate inhibitors for the other enzymes (see Tab.1) in the [^{3}H LH-RH] degradation assay. Alternatively, enzyme-specific substrates can be employed in rapid and highly sensitive tests for these enzymes. PyroGlu-ß-naphthylamide, for example, serves as an excellent substrate for the pyroglutamate aminopeptidase (Szewczuk and Mulczyk, 1979).

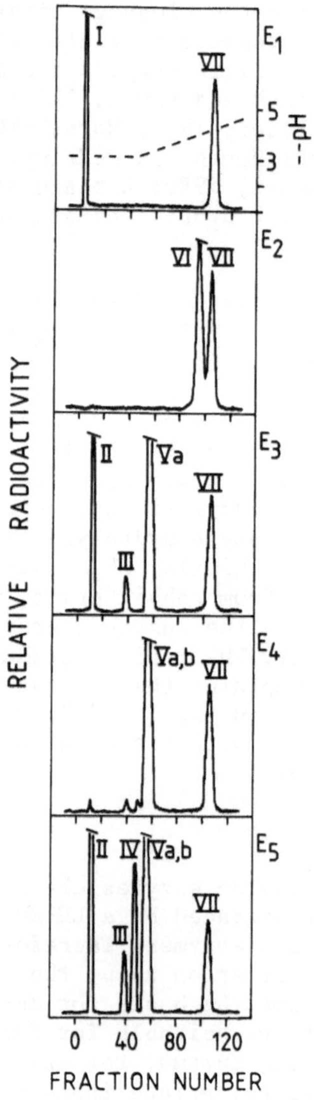

Fig.3. Isolation of LH-RH fragments. LH-RH and [^{3}H]LH-RH were incubated with the enzyme preparations at 37 °C. The reaction mixtures were then resolved by ion-exchange chromatography on Aminex-resin using pyridine/acetate buffers as described (Horsthemke and Bauer, 1981). For continuous scintillation counting, about 25% of the effluent was separated by stream splitting with the aid of a sampling valve and mixed with 9 volumes of scintillation cocktail. The radioactive compounds were further purified by thin-layer chromatography on silica gel using the following solvent system: 2-butanon/1-propanol/pyridine/water/acetic acid (40:40:40:40:20 v/v/v/v/v). By this technique the material of peak V formed by enzyme E_4 and E_5 was resolved into two compounds (Va,b), whereas the other peaks were homogeneous (not shown). After amino acid analysis the fragments could be identified as follows:

I: pyroGlu,
II: (1-2) LH-RH,
III: (1-4) LH-RH,
IV: (1-6) LH-RH,
Va: (1-5) LH-RH,
Vb: (1-3) LH-RH,
VI: (1-9) LH-RH,
VII: LH-RH.

E_n denotes the enzymes as given in Tab.1.

Tab.1. Physical, chemical and biochemical properties of the LH-RH degrading enzymes

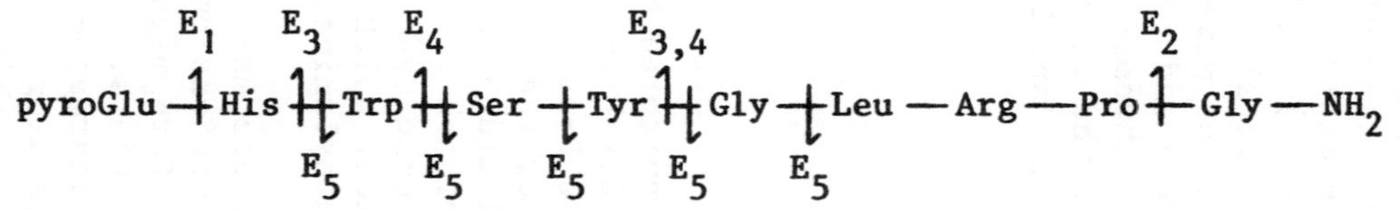

E_n	enzyme	molecular weight [d]	inhibitors	primary specificity	peptides known to be substrates	K_M for LH-RH [µM]
E_1	pyroglutamate aminopeptidase	28,000	Hg^{2+}, NEM, J-Ac-NH_2	carboxy-side of pyroGlu	LH-RH, TRH, neurotensin, etc.	76
E_2	post-proline-cleaving enzyme	77,000	DFP, Hg^{2+}, NEM, J-Ac-NH_2	carboxy-side of Pro	LH-RH, TRH, neurotensin, substance P, bradykinin, etc.	2
E_3	nonchymotrypsin-like endopeptidase	83,000	Hg^{2+}, NEM	carboxy-side of hydrophobic and basic amino acids	LH-RH, bradykinin	190
E_4	cation-sensitive endopeptidase	700,000	Na^+, K^+, Hg^{2+}	carboxy-side of hydrophobic amino acids, Arg and Glu	LH-RH, bradykinin, substance P, etc.	not determined
E_5	particle-bound metallopeptidase	100,000	Hg^{2+}, NEM, EDTA	amino- and carboxy-side of hydrophobic amino acids	LH-RH	20

NEM, N-ethyl-maleimide; J-Ac-NH_2, 2-iodoacetamide; DFP, diisopropylfluorophosphate

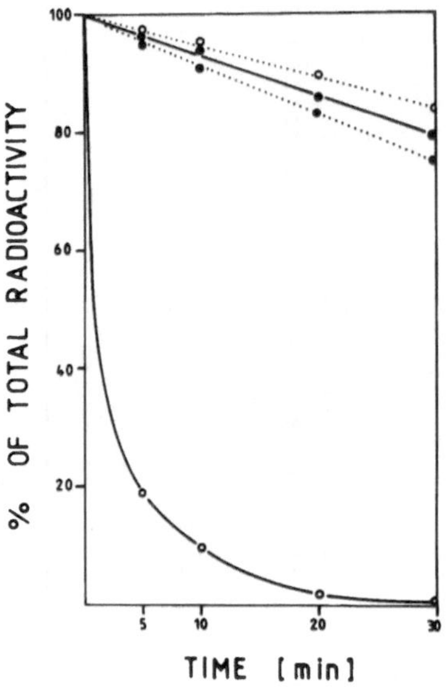

Fig.4. Degradation of [^{3}H]LH-RH and [^{3}H]LH-RH (1-9) nonapeptide by the nonchymotrypsin-like endopeptidase and the cation-sensitive endopeptidase. [^{3}H]LH-RH (•) and [^{3}H]LH-RH (1-9) nonapeptide (o) were incubated with the nonchymotrypsin-like endopeptidase (———) and the cation-sensitive endopeptidase (·····). At given time intervals aliquots of the reaction mixtures were resolved and analyzed by paper chromatography as described in the legends to Fig.1 and 2.

The enzymatic release of ß-naphthylamine can easily be monitored by the highly sensitive fluorometric detection method. Cbz-Gly-Pro-ß-naphthylamide (Knisatschek et al., 1980) or Cbz-Gly-Pro-ß-naphthylamide (Yoshimoto et al., 1979) are specific substrates for the post-proline-cleaving enzyme. Succinyl-Phe-Gly-Leu-ß-naphthylamide can be used in a coupled enzyme assay with leucine aminopeptidase for determing the nonchymotrypsin-like endopeptidase (Horsthemke and Bauer, 1980). The enzyme generates Gly-Leu-ß-naphthylamide, which is successively degraded by the aminopeptidase to ß-naphthylamine.

The biochemical studies also allow the synthesis of enzyme-specific inhibitors, which might be suitable for investigations on intact animals or cell cultures. For example, such inhibitors might induce conditions comparable to certain pathological disorders. Although some care has to be taken in interpreting such pharmacological data, these studies may contribute to an understanding of the biological functions of these enzymes. Ideally, such inhibitors should be specific for a given peptidase, capable of penetrating the plasma membrane (when intracellular enzymes are concerned) and of low toxicity for the cells. In the case of the post-proline-cleaving enzyme, Cbz-Gly-Pro-diazomethylketone might possibly fulfill these requirements (Knisatschek and Bauer, unpublished). Biological studies with this inhibitor are in progress.

Degradation of LH-RH Analogues

It has been suggested that the prolonged and increased LH/FSH releasing activity of some analogues directly reflects their resistance against enzymatic degradation (Koch et al., 1977). Using purified enzyme preparations and a fluorescamine-based assay, which detects C-terminal fragments containing a free amino-group, we have determined the relative rates of hydrolysis of various LH-RH analogues by the individual enzymes (Horsthemke et al., 1981). It is true that superactive agonists modified at position 6 and 10 (such as [D-Ser(tBu)^6]LH-RH(1-9)ethylamide, which is 150 times more active than LH-RH) are degraded more slowly than LH-RH itself, and some of them are resistant to the hydrolysis by the nonchymotrypsin-like endopeptidase or the post-proline-cleaving enzyme, but there is no strict colinearity between the resistance to degradation and the biological activity of the analogues. This indicates that resistance to degradation (if at all) is not the only factor in rendering these analogues superactive, but that increased receptor binding or stimulation must be considered also. Studies about the receptor binding activities performed with tissue homogenates or crude membrane preparations, however, are hampered by ligand degradation. The characterization of the LH-RH degrading enzymes may help to design new superactive agonists and enzyme-specific inhibitors to overcome these difficulties.

Regulation of Enzyme Activities

It has been postulated that the enzymatic degradation of LH-RH might be involved in the metabolic regulation of the decapeptide-amide and thus in the regulation of the neuroendocrine or behavioral effects of LH-RH (Griffiths et al., 1975; Fridkin et al., 1977; Kuhl et al., 1978; Advis et al., 1982). To test this hypothesis, we have determined the activity of the individual LH-RH degrading enzymes after physiological manipulations of experimental animals (Bauer et al., 1981). Confirmatory to the findings of Loudes et al. (1978) we did not observe any significant change in the total LH-RH degrading activities of hypothalamic homogenates from gonadectomized or estradiol benzoate treated rats. Using hypophyseal tissue homogenates from such animals, some fluctuations in the specific activities of the total peptidasic pool as well as of the individual LH-RH degrading enzymes could be detected. Treatment of ovariectomized rats with estradiol benzoate, for example, increases the specific activity of the post-proline-cleaving enzyme and decreases the activity of the pyroglutamate aminopeptidase, the nonchymotrypsin-like endopeptidase and the cation-sensitive endopeptidase. Minor changes in specific activities comparable to those of the LH-RH degrading enzymes could also be observed for other peptidases such as the cystinyl arylamidase, which has been assumed to fulfill a regulatory function for the LH-RH metabolism (Kuhl et al., 1978). This enzyme, however, does not degrade LH-RH (Horsthemke and Bauer, 1981).

As a typical aminopeptidase it can only act on fragments of LH-RH containing a free amino-group. In contrast to the proteolytic enzymes, however, there are very pronounced changes in the specific activities of enzymes involved in the glycolysis and pentose phosphate pathway, which provide energy for the cell. Therefore, these results do not support the hypothesis that LH-RH degrading enzymes fulfill a regulatory function. Moreover, the changes in the specific activities of these enzymes do not correlate in time with changes in neuroendocrine or behavioral events. There is only a very slight increase (less than 5%) in the LH-RH degrading activities within the 24-36 hour period necessary for induction of ovulation or lordosis. Therefore, the observed fluctuations most likely reflect changes within homeostatic adaption processes rather than specific changes within feedback regulatory mechanisms.

Subcellular Distribution of LH-RH Degrading Enzymes

Since the main effects of LH-RH are exerted via receptors on the cell surface, only extracellular or plasma-membrane bound enzymes can directly affect the concentration of LH-RH after its release. Intracellular enzymes may be involved in the degradation of LH-RH in the synthesizing cell before secretion or in the target cell after internalization. Therefore the subcellular localization of the peptidases is of great importance for determining their biological function. This was investigated in collaboration with Drs. P. Leblanc, C. Kordon (Paris), S. Wattiaux-De Coninck and R. Wattiaux (Namur, Belgium) using rat anterior pituitaries. The pyroglutamate aminopeptidase, the post-proline-cleaving enzyme, the nonchymotrypsin-like endopeptidase and the cation-sensitive endopeptidase are mainly present in the cytosol. The particle-bound metallopeptidase was found to be an innermitochondrial enzyme and therefore seems to be excluded from the degradation of LH-RH (Leblanc et al., 1983). Despite other reports (Clayton et al., 1977; Elkabes et al., 1981) no evidence for a plasma-membrane bound enzyme capable of hydrolyzing LH-RH could be obtained (Horsthemke et al., 1983). This was confirmed by studies with intact pituitary and brain cells in culture (performed in collaboration with Drs. B. Hamprecht, Würzburg, FRG and C. Denef, Leuven, Belgium). Concerning pituitary cells, these results have recently been verified by Nikolics et al. (1983). Since TRH, Leu-enkephalin and substance P degrading enzymes have been detected in analoguous studies, these results do not seem to represent experimental artefacts, but strongly suggest the existence of other mechanisms for the removal of LH-RH from its target sites in the pituitary.

Degradation of LH-RH by Serum

Since LH-RH is secreted into the hypothalamic-hypophyseal portal blood vessels and transported to the target cells by the blood, the effective peptide concentration at the receptor might be influenced by serum peptidases. This is apparently not the case, because LH-RH is degraded only very slowly by serum, and this degradation is due to low levels of circulating post-proline-cleaving enzyme.

CONCLUSIONS

So far, there is no experimental evidence supporting the hypothesis that LH-RH degrading enzymes are directly involved in the mechanisms regulating the metabolism of this neuropeptide. The biochemical studies clearly demonstrate that LH-RH is not degraded by a specific enzyme but by several general proteolytic enzymes. These enzymes are capable of degrading a variety of peptides and do not provide the specificity and selectivity required for an regulatory function. This interpretation is supported by the experimental findings:

a) The LH-RH degrading enzymes are neither tissue nor cell specific, but are widely distributed throughout all tissues.
b) They do not exhibit a high affinity towards LH-RH as substrate.
c) Their activity is apparently not a limiting factor within a regulatory system.
d) There is no experimental evidence that these peptidasic activities are controlled by feedback-regulatory mechanisms.
e) Changes in enzymatic activities do not correlate in time with neuroendocrine or behavioral events.
f) The LH-RH degrading enzymes are intracellularly located and therefore can not directly control the extracellular concentration of LH-RH.

Due to the lack of enzymes capable of degrading extracellular LH-RH, other mechanisms must exist for the removal of this peptide from the target sites. For example, the peptide may be diluted to ineffective concentrations after its dissociation from the receptor and finally be degraded in the liver or the kidneys. Alternatively, the peptide may be internalized by receptor-mediated endocytosis and subsequently degraded by lysosomal or cytosolic enzymes of the gonadotrophic cells. Since the frequency of LH-RH release is in the hour range, slow processes like diffusion and internalization may be adequate for the clearance of LH-RH in the pituitary.

For the LH-RH synthesizing cell we should also expect that the site of degradation is necessarily separated from the site of synthesis, storage and release. Therefore, the LH-RH degrading enzymes can also not directly act on the neuropeptide and thus do not fulfill a specific function for the regulation of intracellular LH-RH concentrations.

In both situations, the mechanisms regulating the availability of the substrate to the enzymes (such as receptors, carriers, the mechanism of the crinophagic disposal of secretion granules etc.) represent the decisive factors which govern the enzymatic event. The physiological importance of the LH-RH degrading enzymes is restricted to the destruction of peptides at secondary sites.

SUMMARY

For LH-RH, as for other highly active substances, efficient inactivation mechanisms are likely to exist. Since the peptide is rapidly degraded by various tissue homogenates, it has been suggested that LH-RH is inactivated by a specific peptidase which might even serve a regulatory function. After fractionation of brain and pituitary homogenates, however, only general proteolytic enzymes capable of degrading LH-RH and other peptides have been identified. A pyroglutamate aminopeptidase and a post-proline-cleaving enzyme liberate pyroGlu and glycineamide, respectively. Internal peptide bonds (preferentially Tyr-Gly) are hydrolyzed by a nonchymotrypsin-like endopeptidase and a cation-sensitive endopeptidase. These enzymes are mainly present in the cytosol. A mitochondrial metalloendopeptidase cleaves the decapeptideamide at the amino and carboxy side of hydrophobic amino acids. Studies with subcellular fractions and intact cells did not reveal any evidence for a plasma-membrane bound LH-RH degrading enzyme. These results suggest that LH-RH is not removed from the target site by hydrolysis, but that it is degraded only after internalization by the target cells or after diffusion into the peripheral circulation.

ACKNOWLEDGEMENT

This work was supported by the Deutsche Forschungsgemeinschaft.

REFERENCES

Advis, J.P., Krause, J.E., and McKelvy, J.F., 1982, Luteinizing Hormone - Releasing Hormone peptidase activities in discrete hypothalamic regions and anterior pituitary of the rat: apparent regulation during the prepubertal period and first estrous cycle at puberty, Endocrinolgy 110:1238

Bauer, K., and Kleinkauf, H., 1980, Catabolism of thyroliberin by rat adenohypophyseal tissue extract, Eur. J. Biochem. 106:107

Bauer, K., Beier, S., Horsthemke, B., Knisatschek, H., and Sievers, J., 1980, Estrogen effects on LH-RH degrading brain and pituitary enzymes, Exptl. Brain Res. Suppl. 3:93

Camargo,A.C.M.D., Fonseca,M.J.V.D., Caldo,H., and Carvalho,K.D.M., 1982, Influence of the carboxyl terminus of Luteinizing Hormone-Releasing Hormone and bradykinin on hydrolysis by brain endo-oligopeptidases, J. Biol. Chem. 257:9265

Clayton,R.N., Shakespear,R.A., and Marshall,J.C.,1977, LH-RH degrading activity associated with a purified pituitary plasma membrane fraction, J. Endocrinol. 73:34

Elkabes,S., Fridkin,M., and Koch, Y., 1981, Studies on the enzymic degradation of Luteinizing Hormone - Releasing Hormone by rat pituitary plasma membranes, Biochem. Biophys. Res. Commun. 103:240

Fridkin,M., Hazum,E., Baram,T., Lindner,H.R., and Koch,Y., 1977, Hypothalamic and pituitary LRF-degrading enzymes: characterization, purification and physiological role, in: Proceedings of the Vth American Peptide Symposium, Goodman,M., and Meienhofer,J., eds., Halsted Press, New York, p.193

Griffiths,E.C., Hooper,K.C., Jeffcoate,S.L., and Holland,D.T., 1975, The effects of gonadectomy and gonadal steroids on the activity of hypothalamic peptidases inactivating Luteinizing Hormone - Releasing Hormone (LH-RH), Brain Res. 88:384

Hersh,L.B., and McKelvy,J.F., 1979, Enzymes involved in the degradation of Thyrotropin - Releasing Hormone (TRH) and Luteinizing Hormone - Releasing Hormone (LH-RH) in bovine brain, Brain Res. 168:553

Horsthemke,B., and Bauer,K., 1980, Characterization of a nonchymotrypsin-like endopeptidase from anterior pituitary that hydrolyzes Luteinizing Hormone - Releasing Hormone at the tyrosylglycine and histidyl-tryptophane bonds, Biochemistry 19:2867

Horsthemke,B., and Bauer,K., 1981, Chymotryptic-like hydrolysis of luliberin (LH-RF) by an adenohypophyseal enzyme of high molecular weight, Biochem. Biophys. Res. Commun. 103:1322

Horsthemke,B., Knisatschek,H., Rivier,J., Sandow,J., and Bauer,K., 1981, Degradation of Luteinizing Hormone - Releasing Hormone and analogs by adenohypophyseal peptidases, Biochem. Biophys. Res. Commun. 100:753

Horsthemke,B., and Bauer,K., 1982, Substrate specificity of an adenohypophyseal andopeptidase capable of hydrolyzing Luteinizing Hormone - Releasing Hormone: Preferential cleavage of peptide bonds involving the carboxyl terminus of hydrophobic and basic amino acids, Biochemistry 21:1033

Horsthemke,B., Leblanc,P., Kordon,C., Wattiaux-De Coninck,S., Wattiaux,R., and Bauer,K., 1983, Subcellular distribution of particle-bound neutral peptidases capable of hydrolyzing gonadoliberin, thyroliberin, enkephalin and substance P, submitted

Knisatschek,H., and Bauer,K., 1979, Characterization of "Thyroliberin deamidating enzyme" as a post-proline-cleaving enzyme, J. Biol. Chem. 254:10936

Knisatschek,H., Kleinkauf,H., and Bauer,K., 1980, Specific fluorogenic substrates for the TRF-deamidating post-proline-cleaving enzyme, *FEBS Lett.* 111:157

Koch,Y., Baram,T., Chobsieng,P., and Fridkin,M., 1974, Enzymic degradation of Luteinizing Hormone - Releasing Hormone (LH-RH) by hypothalamic tissue, *Biochem. Biophys. Res. Commun.* 61:95

Koch,Y., Baram,T., Hazum,E., and Fridkin,M., 1977, Resistance to enzymic degradation of LH-RH analogues possessing increased biological activity, *Biochem. Biophys. Res. Commun.* 74:488

Kuhl,H., Rosniatowski,C., and Taubert,H.D., 1978, The activity of an LH-RH-degrading enzyme in the anterior pituitary during the rat oestrus cycle and its alteration by injections of sex hormones, *Acta endocr. (Kbh.)* 87:476

Leblanc,P., Pattou,E., L'Heritier,A., and Kordon,C., 1980, Some properties of peptidasic activity bound to the anterior pituitary membranes, *Biochem. Biophys. Res. Commun.* 96:1457

Leblanc,P., L'Heritier,A., Kordon,C., Horsthemke,B., Bauer,K., Wattiaux-De Coninck,S., Dubois,F., and Wattiaux,R., 1983, Characterization of a neutral metalloendopeptidase localized in the mitochondrial matrix of rat anterior pituitary tissue with GnRH as a substrate, submitted

Loudes,C., Josepho-Bravo,P., Leblanc,P., and Kordon,C., 1978, Specific activity of LH-RH and TRH degrading enzymes in various tissues of normal and castrated male rats, *Biochem. Biophys. Res. Commun.* 83:921

Nikolics,K., Szöke,B., Kéri,G., and Teplán,I., 1983, Gonadotropin-Releasing Hormone (GnRH) is not degraded by intact pituitary tissue in vitro, *Biochem. Biophys. Res. Commun.* 114:1028

Orlowski,M., Wilk,E., Pearce,S., and Wilk,S., 1979, Purification and properties of a prolyl endopeptidase from rabbit brain, *J. Neurochem.* 33:461

Szewczuk,A., and Mulczyk,M., 1969, Pyrrolidonyl peptidase in bacteria, *Eur. J. Biochem.* 8:63

Wilk,S., and Orlowski,M., 1980, Cation-sensitive neutral endopeptidase: Isolation and specificity of the bovine pituitary enzyme, *J. Neurochem.* 35:1172

Yoshimoto,T., Ogita,K., Walter,R., Koida,M., and Tsuru,D., 1979, Post-proline-cleaving enzyme, synthesis of a new fluorogenic substrate and distribution of the endopeptidase in rat tissues and body fluids of man, *Biochim. Biophys. Acta* 569:184

DEGRADATION OF LUTEINIZING HORMONE-RELEASING HORMONE BY RAT PITUITARY PLASMA MEMBRANE ASSOCIATED ENZYMES

Yitzhak Koch, Stella Elkabes and *Mati Fridkin

Departments of Hormone Research and *Organic Chemistry
The Weizmann Institute of Science
Rehovot, 76100, Israel

INTRODUCTION

The hypothalamic decapeptide luteinizing hormone-releasing hormone (LHRH) is known to be inactivated by peptidases present at its site of synthesis and release, the hypothalamus (1-8), at its target organ, the pituitary (3,9-16), as well as in other locations such as in brain (3,17,18), kidney and liver (19,20,21), in serum and plasma (22,23). Little is known about the mechanism of action of these enzymes and their physiological significance is still uncertain. Since the stimulation of gonadotropin secretion from the pituitary gland is initiated by specific binding of LHRH to plasma membrane receptors (11,24), the presence of membrane-bound, LHRH degrading enzymes (11,14) may be of potential significance. These peptidases may be involved in the mechanism of action of LHRH, by regulating the amount and duration of action of the decapeptide at its receptor site. The elucidation of the degradation products of LHRH, the design of analogs modified at the site of cleavage and determination of their resistance to enzymatic degradation can provide a better insight into the mode of action of these peptidases. Investigation of a possible relation between LHRH at the receptor site and the enzymatic activity may provide evidence for the involvement of these enzymes in the regulation of LHRH action.

Plasma membranes of rat anterior pituitaries were purified by a modification of the procedure employed by Fleisher and Kervina (25) for the preparation of rat liver plasma membranes. This procedure is described in Fig. 1.

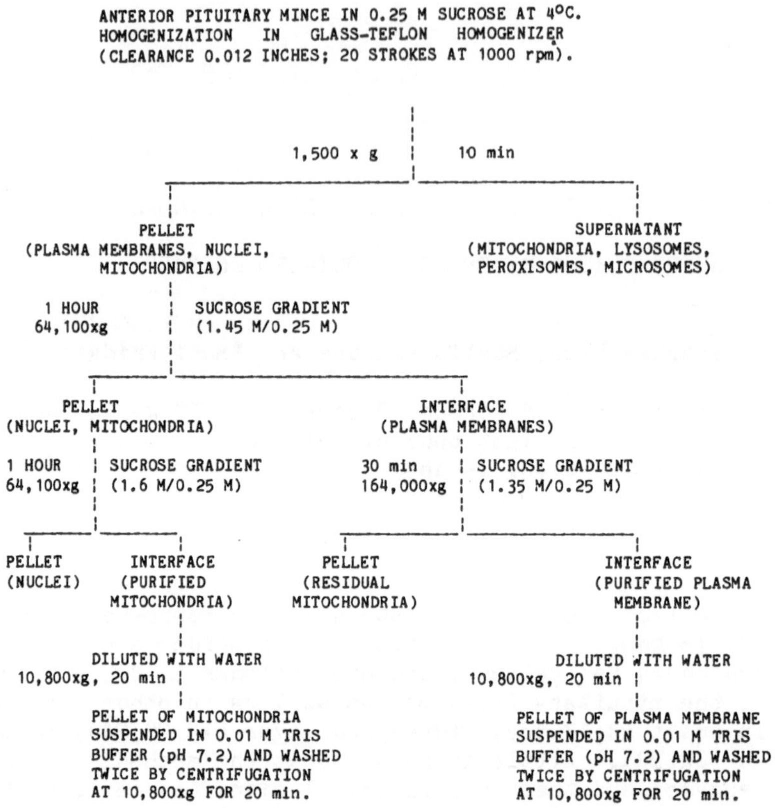

Fig. 1. Preparation of subcellular fractions of rat pituitaries.

The fraction containing the membranes showed (Table 1) a several fold enrichment (4-8 folds in different experiments) in 5'-nucleotidase activity as compared to the homogenate, while the activity of the mitochondrial marker enzyme Succinate-Cytochrome C reductase was low, indicating that there was not a significant contamination of this fraction by mitochondria. Moreover, the specific binding of the LHRH analog was 30 fold higher in the plasma membrane enriched fraction, than in the starting homogenate, and 54 fold higher than in the mitochondrial fraction.

Incubation of aliquots of plasma membranes (100 ug protein) with synthetic LHRH (10 nmoles) at neutral pH (10 mM Tris buffer pH 7.2) for 20 min at 37°C, resulted in the partial degradation of LHRH (14). The main products observed were the N-terminal tripeptide (pGlu-His-Trp) and the N-terminal hexapeptide (pGlu-His-Trp-Ser-

Table 1. Specific binding of LHRH analog [D-Ser(t-Bu)^6, des Gly^{10} ethylamide]LHRH and specific activity of marker enzymes in pituitary whole homogenate and its subcellular fractions. The 5'-nucleotidase activity is expressed as umole phosphate hydrolysed/mg protein/hour. Specific activity of Succinate-Cytochrome C reductase is expressed in umole Cytochrome C reduced/mg protein/min. Specific binding of LHRH analog is expressed as bound over total/ ug tissue protein.

	5'nucleotidase	Succinate-Cytochrome C reductase	Specific binding
Homogenate	0.82±0.01	0.120±0.020	0.023±0.005
Plasma membrane	3.91±0.52	0.007±0.002	0.703±0.040
Mitochondria	0.24±0.04	0.440±0.040	0.013±0.004

Tyr-Gly) although the N-terminal tetrapeptide (pGlu-His-Trp-Ser) and N-terminal pentapeptide (pGlu-His-Trp-Ser-Tyr) were also present, but in a smaller ratio (Fig. 2). When the incubation reaction was carried out at a more basic pH (8.7), an increase in the production of the N-terminal pentapeptide and N-terminal hexapeptide was observed while there was no change in the amount of the N-terminal tripeptide (Table 2). These findings suggest that several enzymes are involved in the production of the different LHRH fragments. This notion is further supported by additional studies on the effect of the chelating agents EDTA and EGTA on the activity of the enzymes. As shown in Fig. 3, when the degradation reaction was performed at neutral pH in the presence of 1 mM EDTA or EGTA, there was a decrease in the production of (1-3)LHRH whereas the production of the other degradation products was increased.

The increase in the amount of (1-5)LHRH and (1-6)LHRH fragments (collected together) concomitantly with a decrease in the concentration of the (1-3)LHRH fragment (Fig. 3) raises the question whether the N-terminal tripeptide fragment of LHRH is a primary or secondary degradation product. Whether it is produced by the cleavage of the intact neurohormone or by a further cleavage of larger LHRH fragments (N-terminal hexapeptide or pentapeptide). In order to elucidate these two possibilities, synthetic (1-6)LHRH or (1-5)LHRH were incubated with plasma membrane preparations under the same conditions as LHRH. Fig. 4 shows that (1-6)LHRH was indeed further processed to produce the (1-3)LHRH, as well as some of

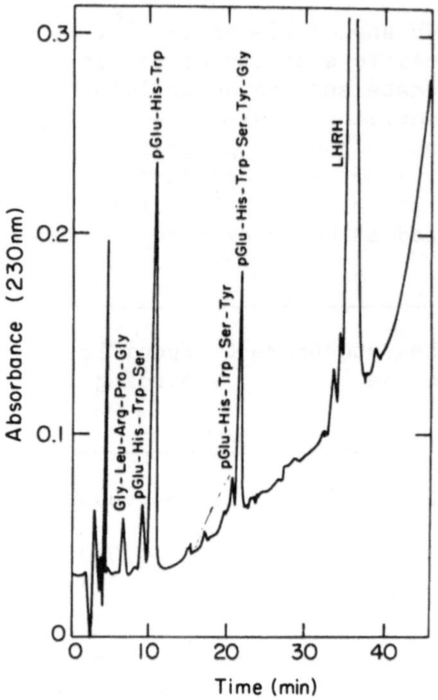

Fig. 2. High pressure liquid chromatography of the degradation products of LHRH. The LHRH degradation mixture was injected to a reversed-phase Lichrosorb RP-18 column (Merck, Darmstadt, Germany 0.4x2.5 cm, particle size 10 u). The column was eluted with a linear gradient of isopropanol in 0.05 M Ammonium acetate pH 5.5 starting with 5% isopropanol and ending with 20% isopropanol. The flow rate was 1 ml/min and the gradient lasted for 50 min. Elution was followed continuously by monitoring UV absorbance at 230 nm.

Table 2. Effect of pH on the degradation of LHRH by pituitary plasma membrane bound enzymes. Aliquots of plasma membranes (100 ug protein) were incubated with LHRH (10 nmoles) and ^{3}H-LHRH in Tris buffer, for 20 min at 37°C. Incubation was terminated by boiling the samples.

pH	Degradation Product (uM)		
	(1-3)LHRH	(1-5)LHRH	(1-6)LHRH
7.2	2.50±0.60	0.53±0.02	1.16±0.31
8.7	2.60±0.80	1.60±0.02	2.70±0.10

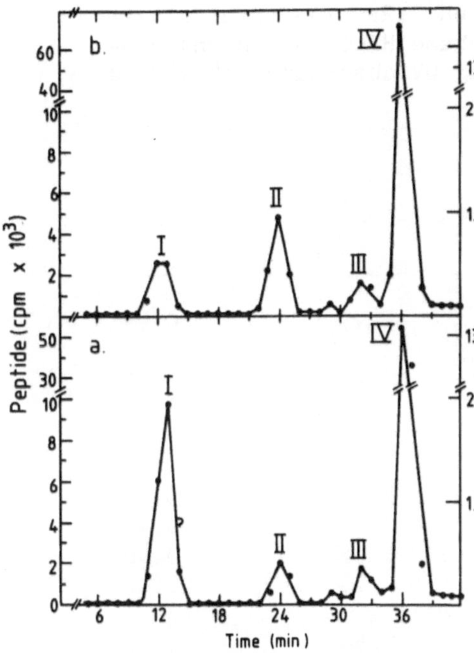

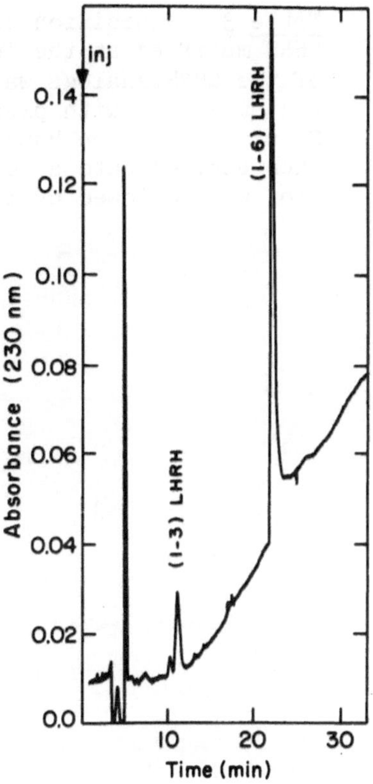

Fig. 3. High pressure liquid chromatography of the degradation products of LHRH. (A) in the absence, and (B) in the presence, of 1 mM EDTA at pH 7.2. I, (1-3)LHRH; II, (1-5)LHRH and (1-6)LHRH; III, modified LHRH; IV, intact LHRH.

Fig. 4. High pressure liquid chromatography of the synthetic N-terminal hexapeptide sequence of LHRH and its degradation products (conditions are as described in Fig. 2).

the (1-4)LHRH fragment (compare with Fig. 2). The (1-5)LHRH was also further processed (results not shown) but produced only the N-terminal tripeptide. These results would suggest that (1-3)LHRH is a secondary degradation product. However, since the decrease in the total production of (1-3)LHRH in the presence of EDTA is greater than the increase observed in the total (1-6)LHRH and (1-5)LHRH production, it can be concluded that (1-3)LHRH is probably produced by two mechanisms: further processing of large LHRH fragments as well as by cleavage of intact LHRH. Time course studies (data not shown) also support this notion demonstrating that a significant amount of (1-3)LHRH is detected even after two minutes of reaction.

Table 3. Inhibition of LHRH degradation by analogs of LHRH modified at the Trp^3 or Gly^6 positions. Degradation of the LHRH analogs was studied by incubating 10 ug of the substrate with plasma membranes (100 ug protein) for 20 minutes or one hour (*) at pH 7.2. The samples were then applied onto a reversed phase HPLC column and elution was followed by monitoring UV absorbance at 230 nm.

Analog	LHRH:Analog ratio	(1-3)LHRH (uM)	(1-6)LHRH (uM)
LHRH	1:0	4.90	0.99
$[Phe(Me)_5]^3$LHRH	0:1*	0.00	0.00
	1:1	1.30	0.25
	1:2	0.00	0.00
$[(N^{\varepsilon}$-Indolyl)-Lys$]^3$-LHRH	0:1*	0.00	0.00
	1:1	2.90	0.48
	1:2	1.96	0.40
	1:10	0.00	0.00
$[D\text{-}Phe]^6$LHRH	0:1	0.64	0.00
	0:1*	1.30	0.00
	1:1	3.14	0.29
$[D\text{-}Lys]^6$LHRH	0:1*	0.00	0.00
	1:1	1.72	0.17

Studies with the LHRH analogs modified at the Gly^6 position, ($[D\text{-}Phe]^6$LHRH and $[D\text{-}Lys]^6$LHRH) also indicated that the (1-3)LHRH fragment is produced by the cleavage of the intact neurohormone. Incubation of $[D\text{-}Phe]^6$LHRH with plasma membranes for 20 min resulted in limited degradation of the analog. The only degradation product observed was the (1-3)LHRH fragment which was doubled when the reaction was continued for one hour. $[D\text{-}Lys]^6$LHRH, and the LHRH analogs with modification at the Trp^3 position, $[Phe(Me)_5]^3$LHRH and $[(N^{\varepsilon}$-indolyl-Lys$]^3$LHRH, were found to be completely resistant to enzymic action even when the degradation reaction was continued for one hour (Table 3).

Although these findings suggest that modifications at the Trp^3 or Gly^6 positions increase the resistance of the analogs to both enzymes, the identification of the (1-3)LHRH as the only degradation product of [D-Phe]^{6}LHRH, suggest that alterations at the Gly^{6} position may result in analogs which are resistant to the Gly^{6}-Leu^{7} bond cleavage, while degradation at the Trp^{3}-Ser^{4} bond can still occur but at a slower rate. This implies that (1-3)LHRH is produced by an enzyme that cleaves the Trp^{3}-Ser^{4} bond of LHRH. Further, [Gln]^{8}LHRH, an analog which is modified at a position which is remote from the site of cleavage was susceptible to enzymic attack. Its degradation produced both the (1-3)LHRH and the (1-6)LHRH fragments, although at a slower rate as compared with LHRH (45% and 27% of that produced by LHRH). These findings suggest that resistance to enzymic degradation is mainly observed in analogs with alterations at the site of cleavage. However, modifications at the vicinity of these sites may still affect the rate of degradation. In the case of [Gln]^{8}LHRH, the decrease in the cleavage of the Gly^{6}-Leu^{7} bond was greater than the decrease in the Trp^{3}-Ser^{4} bond, indicating that the activities of the two enzymes were affected to a different extent. Nevertheless, modifications of the Trp^{3} residue of LHRH protected also the degradation at the mid-portion of the neurohormone.

When LHRH was incubated with plasma membranes in the presence of different concentrations of the analogs mentioned above, the degradation of LHRH was inhibited (Table 3). Although all analogs affected the cleavage at the Trp^{3}-Ser^{4} and Gly^{6}-Leu^{7} bonds, analogs with modifications at the Gly^{6} position were more effective in inhibiting cleavage at the Gly^{6}-Leu^{7} bond, suggesting a higher affinity of these analogs for the enzyme cleaving at this bond. The [Gln]^{8}LHRH did not affect the enzymic degradation of LHRH indicating that it had lower affinity for both enzymes.

In an attempt to further characterize these enzymes and to study their properties, the effects of different inhibitors on the degradation of LHRH was studied. Table 4 shows that the most potent inhibitors were pepstatin and bacitracin. Although the thiol blocking agent iodoacetamide did not inhibit the enzymic activity, NEM, another thiol agent, was effective. The discrepancy between the mode of action of these two thiol blocking agents may perhaps be explained on the basis of their different polarity. The serine protease inhibitor diisopropylfluorophosphate, benzamidine, the trypsin inhibitor TLCK and chymotrypsin inhibitor TPCK did not affect significantly the degradation of LHRH. This indicates that the LHRH degrading enzymes are not chymotrypsin- or trypsin-like enzymes.

The presence of high affinity binding sites for LHRH as well as degrading enzymes on plasma membranes suggest that these enzymes may be involved in the regulation of LHRH action at the receptor site. To investigate this possibility a photoactive analog of LHRH ([(p-azidobenzoyl glycyl)D-Lys]^{6}LHRH) was incubated with plasma membranes at 4°C for 90 min. The samples were then photolysed

Table 4. Effect of various inhibitors on the degradation of LHRH by pituitary membrane-bound enzymes. Inhibitors were preincubated with plasma membranes for 10 min at 37°C at pH 7.2. 10 ug LHRH and ^{3}H-LHRH were then added and incubation was continued for 20 min. DFP = Diisopropyl fluoro phosphate; TPCK = L-1-Tosylamide-2-phenylethylchloromethyl ketone; TLCK = N-α-p-Tosyl-L-Lysine chloromethyl ketone HCl; NEM = N-Ethylmaleimide.

Inhibitors	mM	N-terminal fragments tripeptide (uM)	Penta and hexapeptides (uM)
None		4.90	0.99
Pepstatin	0.1	4.90	0.99
	0.3	1.22	0.63
	0.7	0.00	0.00
Bacitracin	1	0.00	0.00
DFP	1	3.90	0.76
TPCK	1	4.90	0.99
TLCK	1	4.60	0.77
Benzamidine	1	4.60	0.99
Iodoacetamide	1	4.30	0.70
NEM	1	0.80	0.24

through a $CuSO_4$ filter and excess of ligand was removed by extensive washings. The iodinated analog [D-Ser^6(t-Bu)-des Gly^{10} ethylamide]LHRH did not bind significantly to the membranes treated as described above, indicating that the receptors were labelled covalently by the photoactive LHRH analog. Enzymatic activity of the labelled membranes was also studied. As shown in Table 5, covalent binding of the photoreactive LHRH analog to the receptors decreased the activity of the membrane-bound enzymes. These findings may indicate that the enzymes are located at the vicinity of the receptors and that alterations at these sites affect the enzymatic activity. However, the possibility of certain direct interaction between the enzymes and the photoactive analog of LHRH cannot be excluded. This would imply that the inhibition of the enzymatic activity observed in the presence of the [(p-azidobenzoyl glycyl)D-Lys]^{6}LHRH is due to its binding to the enzyme and is not mediated through the receptor. However, studies with kidney plasma membranes do not support this possibility. Rat kidney plasma membrane-bound enzymes cleave LHRH to produce mainly the (1-3)LHRH fragment but do not have any high affinity binding sites for LHRH.

Table 5. Degradation of LHRH by pituitary or kidney plasma membrane-bound enzymes after photolysis of the membranes in the presence of a photoreactive analog of LHRH ([(p-azidobenzoyl glycyl)D-Lys]^{6}LHRH = PAL). Exp. 1, 2 and 3 are the results of three different experiments with pituitary plasma membranes; in Exp. 4, the results with kidney plasma membranes are reported.

	Degradation products (uM)			
	(1-3)LHRH	(1-5)LHRH	(1-6)LHRH	LHRH
Exp. 1				
Control	4.41	2.85	5.85	11.67
PAL	0.60	0.27	0.33	26.20
Exp. 2				
Control	4.41	2.16	3.99	15.23
PAL	1.38	0.84	1.26	23.79
Exp. 3				
Control	1.68	0.75	0.93	24.54
PAL	0.90	0.48	0.48	26.70
Exp. 4				
Control	22.60	-	-	6.00
PAL	22.70	-	-	5.70

As shown in Table 5 (experiment 4), the photoactive analog of LHRH does not inhibit this enzymatic activity. Although there is some similarity in the degradation pattern of LHRH by pituitary and kidney plasma membrane associated enzymes, the identity of the two enzymes has not yet been demonstrated. Therefore, the finding that the photoreactive analog of LHRH does not inhibit the enzymic activity in the kidney provides only suggestive evidence for an interaction between the LHRH receptor and the degrading enzyme in the pituitary plasma membrane.

GENERAL DISCUSSION

Studies on the localization of LHRH-degrading enzymes have indicated their existence in various subcellular fractions such as the cytosol (8,9), mitochondria (8,26) and plasma membrane (11,12,14). The pattern of LHRH degradation by these enzymes is still contraversial (8,9,13,14,27,28) and this may stem from the different methods that were used for tissue fractionation, conditions of reaction and methods for elucidation of the degradation products. Recently it has been demonstrated (26) that LHRH-degrading enzymes reside in the mitochondrial fraction. We have also observed previously (29) an interaction between LHRH and mitochondria. Recent studies in our laboratory (data not shown) indicated that the pattern of degradation of LHRH by pituitary mitochondrial fraction is similar to that exhibited by purified pituitary plasma membrane preparations. It seems, however, that the LHRH degrading enzymes present in these two subcellular fractions are not due to contamination of either of the fractions by the other since the specific activity of the enzymes is similar in the mitochondrial and the plasma membrane fractions (data not shown). This notion is further supported by assay of marker enzymes in the purified subcellular fractions as well as by demonstration that the LHRH-receptor binding activity was enriched only in the pituitary plasma membrane fraction (Table 1). In addition, we have recently observed that the activity of the mitochondrial enzymes, unlike that of the plasma membrane enzymes (Table 2), was not modified by alteration of the pH of the reaction.

The results presented here clearly demonstrate LHRH degrading enzymes which are associated with the pituitary plasma membrane. The major sites of cleavage are the Trp^3-Ser^4, Gly^6-Leu^7, and Trp^5-Gly^6 bonds of the neurohormone. Studies on the degrading activities at different pH values, in the presence of chelating agents and with analogs of LHRH, suggest that more than one enzyme is involved in the degradation of the neurohormone. Analogs of the decapeptide with modifications at the sites of cleavage are more resistant than LHRH to enzymic degradation. Preliminary results utilizing a photoaffinity derivative of LHRH suggest that the enzymes are located in close proximity to the receptor.

The bioactivity of LHRH can be terminated by different mechanisms such as: dissociation of the hormone-receptor complex followed by escape and dilution of the neurohormone in the general circulation; degradation of the neurohormone at its binding site by plasma membrane associated enzymes, or by internalization of the hormone-receptor complex (30-32), followed by degradation of the hormone by lysosomal and cytosolic enzymes. It is possible that plasma membrane associated enzymes are important also for the degradation of the internalized hormone since it has been demonstrated by autoradiographic techniques that only part of the internalized complexes are found in lysosomes whereas a significant portion of the radioactive material is localized on secretory vesicles (33). This may indicate a mechanism for rapid recycling of the receptor which may occur upon fusion of the secretory granules with the plasma membrane. It is possible that degrading enzymes in the internalized plasma membrane vesicle are involved in the process of the dissociation of the hormone-receptor complex.

ACKNOWLEDGMENT

This work was supported by a grant from the Rockefeller Foundation, N.Y. We thank Mrs. M. Kopelowitz for expert text processing of the manuscript. Y.K. is the Adlai E. Stevenson III Professor of Endocrinology and Reproductive Biology.

REFERENCES

1. E.C. Griffiths, K.C. Hooper, S.L. Jeffcoate and D.I. Holland, Acta Endocr. 77:435 (1974).
2. Y. Koch, T. Baram and P. Chobsieng, Biochem. Biophys. Res.Commun. 61:95 (1974).
3. K. Kochman, B. Kerdelhue, U. Zor and M. Jutisz, FEBS Lett. 50:190 (1975).
4. E.C. Griffiths, Hormone Res. 7:179 (1976).
5. D.K. Sundberg and K.M. Knigge, Brain Res. 139:89 (1978).
6. P. Joseph-Bravo, C. Loudes, J.L. Charli and C. Kordon, Brain Res. 166:321 (1979).
7. C.A. Powers and D.C. Johnson, J. Neurochem. 36:670 (1981).
8. J.R. McDermott, A.I. Smith, J.A. Biggins, J.A. Edwardson and E.C. Griffiths, Regul. Peptides 3:257 (1982).
9. M. Fridkin, E. Hazum, T. Baram, H.R. Lindner and Y. Koch, in: "Peptides" Proceedings of the Fifth American Peptide Symposium, 193, J. Wiley and Sons, Inc., New York (1977).
10. H. Kuhl, C. Rosniatowski and H.D. Taubert, Acta Endocr. 87:476 (1978).
11. R.N. Clayton, R.A. Shakespear, J.A. Duncan and J.C. Marshall, Endocrinology, 104:1484 (1979).
12. P. Leblanc, E. Pattou, A. L'Heritier and C. Kordon, Biochem. Biophys. Res. Commun. 96:1457 (1980).
13. B. Horsthemke and K. Bauer, Biochem. 19:2867 (1980).
14. S. Elkabes, M. Fridkin and Y. Koch, Biochem. Biophys. Res. Commun. 103:240 (1981).
15. E. Hazum, H. Fridkin, T. Baram and Y. Koch, FEBS Lett. 127:273 (1981).
16. B. Horsthemke, H. Knisatschek, J. Rivier, J. Sandow and K. Bauer, Biochem. Biophys. Res. Commun. 100:753 (1981).
17. E.C. Griffiths, K.C. Hooper, S.L. Jeffcoate and D.T. Holland, Brain Res. 85:161 (1975).
18. S. Wilk, M. Benuck, M. Orlowski and N. Marks, Neurosci. Lett. 14:275 (1979).
19. T.W. Redding and A.V. Schally, Life Sci. 12:23 (1973).
20. A. Duport, F. Labrie, G. Pelletier, R. Puviani, D.H. Coy, E.J. Coy and A.V. Schally, Neuroendocrinology 16:65 (1974).
21. M.A. Stetler-Stevenson, G. Flouret, S. Nakamura, B. Gulcrynski and F.A. Corone, Am. J. Physiol. 244:F628 (1983).
22. A.D. Swift and D.B. Crighton, J. Endocr. 80:141 (1979).

23. J.R. McDermott, A.I. Smith, J.A. Biggins, J.A. Hardy, P.R. Dodd and J.A. Edwardson, Regul. Peptides 2:69 (1981).
24. R. Meidan and Y. Koch, Life Sci. 28:1961 (1981).
25. S. Fleisher and M. Kervina, in: "Methods in Enzymology" vol. 31, 6, Academic Press, New York (1974).
26. K. Bauer and B. Horsthemke. In this book.
27. T.N. Akopyan, A.A. Arutunyan, A.I. Oganisyan, A. Lajtha and A.A. Galoyan, J. Neurochem. 32:629 (1979).
28. T. Towatari and N. Katunuma, J. Biochem. 93:1119 (1983).
29. M. Liscovitch and Y. Koch, Peptides, 3:55 (1982).
30. E. Hazum, P. Cautrecasas, J. Marian and P.M. Conn, Proc. Natl. Acad. Sci. USA, 77:6692 (1980).
31. Z. Naor, D. Atlas, R.N. Clayton, D.S. Forman, A. Amsterdam and K.J. Catt, J. Biol. Chem. 256, 3049 (1981).
32. E. Hazum, R. Meidan, M. Liscovitch, D. Keinan, H.R. Lindner and Y. Koch, Molec. Cell. Endocr. 30:291 (1983).
33. E. Hazum, R. Meidan, D. Keinan, E. Okon, Y. Koch, H.R. Lindner and A. Amsterdam, Endocrinology, 111:2135 (1982).

GnRH RECEPTORS: IDENTIFICATION, LOCALIZATION AND IMPLICATIONS FOR BIOLOGICAL FUNCTION

Eli Hazum

Department of Hormone Research
The Weizmann Institute of Science
Rehovot, 76100, Israel

INTRODUCTION

Gonadotropin-releasing hormone (GnRH) is a hypothalamic decapeptide, which stimulates gonadotropin release from the anterior pituitary. The first step in GnRH action (Conn et al., 1981b) is its recognition by specific binding sites (receptors) at the surface of gonadotrope cells. The interaction of GnRH with pituitary membrane preparations or cultured pituitary cells has been studied in detail by using radioiodinated, metabolically stable GnRH analogs (Clayton et al., 1978; Conne et al., 1979; Clayton and Catt, 1980, 1981; Marian and Conn, 1980; Naor et al., 1980; Hazum, 1981a; Marian et al., 1981; Meidan and Koch, 1981a). These studies have indicated the presence of a single class of high-affinity binding sites for both agonists and antagonists of GnRH in the pituitary. Recently, the presence of similar high affinity binding sites have been shown in the ovary and testis (reviewed by Clayton and Catt, 1981; Hsueh and Jones, 1981; Hazum, 1983). Characterization of the GnRH-receptor in the pituitary have indicated that the receptor is a glycoprotein which contains sialic acid residues (Hazum, 1982a) and that membrane phospholipids are involved in the interaction between the hormone and the receptor (Hazum et al., 1982a).

IDENTIFICATION OF THE GnRH RECEPTOR AND CRITERIA FOR SPECIFICITY

Characterization of Photoaffinity Derivative of GnRH

In order to identify directly the postulated GnRH receptors by biochemical techniques, a photoaffinity derivative of GnRH, [azidobenzoyl-D-Lys^{6}]GnRH (Fig. 1), was prepared by chemical modipGlu - His - Trp - Ser - Tyr - Gly ↕ Leu - Arg - Pro - Gly - NH_2

pGlu - His - Trp - Ser - Tyr - D-Lys - Leu - Arg - Pro - Gly - NH_2

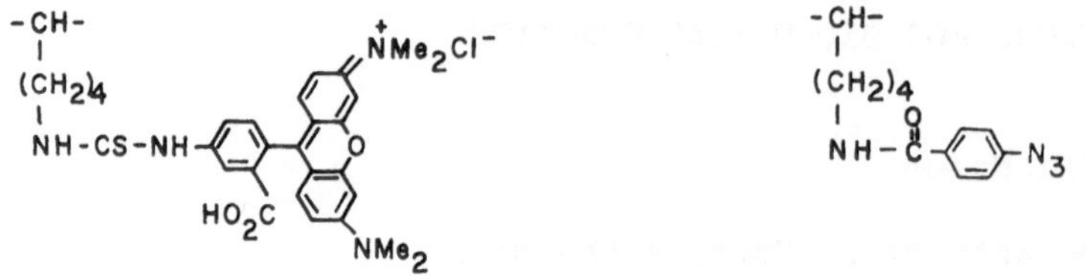

Fig. 1. The structures of GnRH, [D-Lys^6]GnRH and the analogs modified at the epsilon amino group of [D-Lys^6]GnRH: [azidobenzoyl-D-Lys^6]GnRH and [Rhod-D-Lys^6]GnRH. Top of figure, cleavage of native GnRH at the Gly^6-Leu^7 bond.

fication of the epsilon amino group in position 6 of [D-Lys^6]GnRH with N-hydroxysuccinimide ester of 4-azidobenzoic acid (Hazum, 1981b). [D-Lys^6]GnRH was selected as the starting material for derivatization since:

i) Pituitary enzymes cleave GnRH at the Gly^6-Leu^7 bond (Fig. 1) and substitution of D-amino acids in position 6 of GnRH results in more potent and metabolically stable derivatives (Koch et al., 1977; Hazum et al., 1981).

ii) The epsilon amino group of lysine serves as a spacer for substitution reactions and thus the GnRH conformation is less likely to be disturbed.

The photoreactivity of this analog was established by its spectral changes when irradiated with ultraviolet light and by its ability to bind covalently to pituitary membrane preparations after photoactivation (Hazum, 1981b, c). The photoaffinity derivative binds to the GnRH receptor with higher apparent affinity than GnRH and [D-Lys^6]GnRH and it is 3 to 4 times more active than GnRH in LH release in pituitary cell cultures (Hazum and Keinan, 1983a).

Table 1. Identification of Pituitary and Gonadal GnRH Receptors Using ^{125}I-labeled [azidobenzoyl-D-Lys^6]GnRH

Tissue	Identification of receptors	References
Pituitary	Specific labeling of a 60K dalton band	Hazum 1981c; Hazum and Keinan 1982, 1983b
Ovary: granulosa cells	Specific labeling of 2 proteins (Mr=60K and 54K)	Hazum and Nimrod, 1982
Testis: Leydig cells	Specific labeling of 2 proteins (Mr=60K and 54K)	Hazum and Keinan (unpublished)

Photoaffinity Labeling of Pituitary and Gonadal GnRH Receptors

Photoaffinity labeling of pituitary GnRH receptors after preincubation with the iodinated photoaffinity derivative (90 min at 4°C, in the dark) results in the identification of a single specific band with an apparent molecular weight of 60,000 daltons (Table 1). Our findings suggest that some differences exist between the GnRH binding sites of the pituitary and that of the gonads, as the latter have an additional specific component of 54,000 daltons (Table 1). This additional band may represent a degradation product of the receptor by peptidases that are specifically present in the gonads but not in the pituitary. Alternatively, the 54,000 dalton component may be related to the different functional effects of the hormone at the two locations (pituitary and gonads). The common 60,000 dalton band probably accounts for the similarity in binding and recognition properties of these three tissues towards the hormone.

Criteria for the Specificity of Pituitary GnRH Receptor

To evaluate the specificity of photolabeling of the 60K dalton band by [^{125}I][azidobenzoyl-D-Lys^6]GnRH, the ability of various concentrations of Buserelin or TRH to inhibit photolabeling of this band is determined as shown in Table 2. These results of inhibiting the labeling of the 60K dalton band are similar to the potency in inhibiting the binding of the ^{125}I-labeled analog to pituitary

Table 2. Specificity of Photolabeling of the 60K Dalton Band.

Concentration of peptides (M)	% of specific cpm incorporated
None	100
Buserelin, 10^{-10}	68
10^{-9}	43
10^{-8}	4
10^{-7}	0
TRH, 10^{-7}	100

Pituitary membranes are photolabeled in the presence of various concentrations of Buserelin during the incubation of the membranes with ^{125}I-labeled [azidobenzoyl-D-Lys^6]GnRH. The membranes are then subjected to SDS-polyacrylamide gel electrophoresis and the amount of radioactivity incorporated into the 60K dalton band determined. Modified from Hazum (1981c).

membranes. In addition, the labeling of the 60K dalton band is not affected by TRH, thus indicating specificity (Hazum, 1981c).

To further evaluate the specificity of photolabeling of the 60K dalton band, Hazum and Keinan (1982) have examined whether physiological alterations in pituitary GnRH receptor content during the rat estrous cycle are accompanied by similar changes in the radioactivity incorporated into this band. Photoactivation of the ^{125}I-labeled [azidobenzoyl-D-Lys^6]GnRH after preincubation (90 min at 4°C) with pituitary membrane preparations derived from various stages of the rat estrous cycle results in the identification of a single specific band with an apparent molecular weight of 60,000 daltons. The amount of radioactivity incorporated into the 60K dalton band throughout the rat estrous cycle is shown in Table 3. In diestrus and proestrus female rats there is a 2.3 to 2.4 fold increase in the amount of radioactivity incorporated into the 60K dalton band, as compared to that of metestrus and estrus female rats. The differences in radioactivity incorporated into the 60K dalton band is due to changes in receptors content, since all previous binding studies during the estrous cycle (Clayton et al., 1980; Savoy-Moore et al., 1980; Adams and Spies, 1981; Marian et al., 1981; Meidan and Koch, 1981b) have shown a single population of binding sites without any alteration in binding affinity. Similar patterns of receptor changes throughout the rat estrous cycle

Table 3. Radioactivity Incorporated into the 60K Dalton Band During the Rat Estrous Cycle.

Animal status	% of specific cpm incorporated
Metestrus	100
Diestrus	240
Proestrus	230
Estrus	110

Pituitary membranes have been photolabeled with ^{125}I-labeled photoaffinity derivative of GnRH and then subjected to SDS-polyacrylamide gel electrophoresis. The amount of specific radioactivity (cpm in the absence of Buserelin minus cpm in the presence of 10^{-6} M Buserelin) incorporated into the 60K dalton band determined. Modified from Hazum and Keinan (1982).

have been reported by other investigators using binding assays (Clayton et al., 1980; Savoy-Moore et al., 1980; Marian et al., 1981; Meidan and Koch, 1981b), thus providing additional evidence for the specificity of labeling of the 60K dalton band.

Finally, another approach for determining that the GnRH binding sites have physiological significance is that covalent linking of photoreactive GnRH to gonadotropes should result in persistent activation of LH release. The results in Fig. 2 show that irradiation of pituitary cells has no effect on the basal LH release. Pituitary cells preincubated with high concentrations (10^{-7} M) of GnRH or [D-Lys^6]GnRH, 100% receptor occupancy, and subsequently photolyzed and washed extensively gave similar values of LH release as non-photolyzed cells. Incubation of pituitary cells with 10^{-7} M [azidobenzoyl-D-Lys^6]GnRH in the dark (no covalent attachment of the peptide) and subsequent washing results in a low stimulation of LH release (150 ng/5 x 10^5 cells). When the pituitary cells are photolyzed in the presence of 10^{-7} M [azidobenzoyl-D-Lys^6]GnRH and washed, the LH release became maximal (550 ng/5 x 10^5 cells), indicating that covalent linking of photoreactive GnRH to gonadotropes produces a prolonged signal. The persistent activation of LH release by the photoreactive GnRH analog is time dependent and concentration dependent (Hazum and Keinan, 1983a).

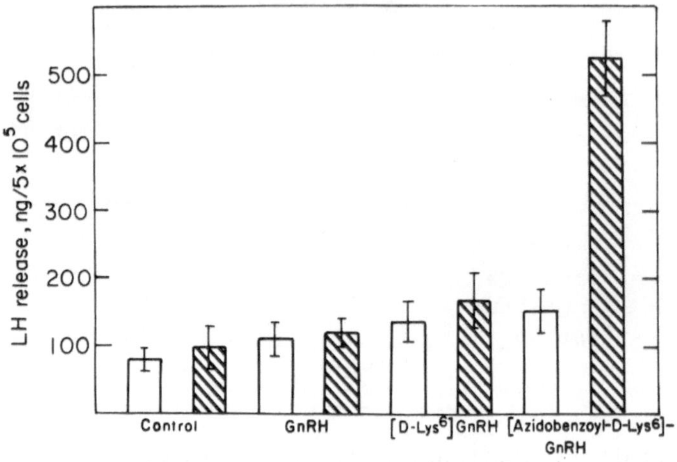

Fig. 2. Persistent activation of LH release by photolysis. Pituitary cells in monolayer culture are incubated with the indicated compounds. After a 90 min pre-incubation in the dark, experiments are carried out with a 5 min irradiation period (▧) or without irradiation (□). The cells are then washed extensively (4 times over a period of 1 hr) to remove non-covalently bound hormone and re-incubated in medium 199-0.1% BSA for 6 hrs at 37°C. LH contents are measured by radioimmunoassay. Each bar represents mean ± S.E. of 12 determinations in two separate experiments. Data from Hazum and Keinan (1983a).

LOCALIZATION OF GnRH RECEPTORS IN THE PITUITARY

GnRH receptors in the pituitary have been localized by various methods (Sternberger and Petrali, 1975; Hopkins and Gregory, 1977; Duello and Nett, 1980; Hazum et al., 1980, 1982b; Dacheux, 1981; Naor et al., 1981; Duello et al., 1983).

The distribution of GnRH receptors in pituitary cells was first reported after electron microscopic studies (Hopkins and Gregory, 1977) using a bioactive GnRH analog coupled to ferritin. Short incubations with this ferritin analog show an even distribution of ferritin particles over the cell surface of gonadotropes. Longer incubations result in aggregates of the bound conjugate, followed by internalization into lysosome-like structures in the Golgi area. Immunocytochemical staining of pituitary sections (Sternberger and

Petrali, 1975; Dacheux, 1981) with antisera to GnRH shows that GnRH receptors are found in plasma membranes of rat pituitaries but are mainly concentrated on the membranes of large secretory granules of rat and porcine gonadotropes. In vivo uptake studies (Duello and Nett, 1980) with ^{125}I-labeled GnRH and its agonists also indicate an intracellular locus of radioactivity after the initial binding at the membrane.

Recently, image-intensified fluorescence microscopy has proved useful in visualizing the cellular distribution of receptors for GnRH (Hazum et al., 1980; Naor et al., 1981). Incubation of cultured rat pituitary cells (120 min, 4°C) with a bioactive rhodamine derivative of GnRH, Rhod-GnRH ([D-Lys^{6}-N$^{\epsilon}$-rhodamine]GnRH; Fig. 1) results in a uniform distribution of the fluorescent hormone over the surface of gonadotropes. The uniform distribution observed is specific because the fluorescence is much reduced in the presence of 10^{-5}M [D-Ala^{6}]GnRH or 10^{-5}M native GnRH. If the cells that have bound Rhod-GnRH at 4°C are warmed to 37°C, aggregation and subsequent internalization of the fluorescent peptide by the gonadotropes can be observed.

More recently, the photoaffinity derivative of GnRH, [azidobenzoyl-D-Lys^{6}]GnRH, was used for localization studies (Hazum et al., 1982b, 1983a), which circumvent some of the problems described in previous studies, such as rapid dissociation of the hormone from its receptor. Dispersed rat pituitary cells are incubated with the photoaffinity analog for 90 min at 4°C or for various time periods at 37°C and subsequently photolized. The distribution of the labeled hormone by light and electron microscopic autoradiography indicates that after exposure of pituitary cells to the ^{125}I-labeled hormone at 4°C (90 min), most of the labeled hormone is associated with the cell surface membrane. At 37°C (15 min) about 25% of the cell-bound labeled hormone is internalized. After 45 min at 37°C, only half of the label is associated with the plasma membrane, while the rest is found in lysosome like structures (21%), in secretory granules (20%)and in the Golgi complex. The incidence of clustered grains over the cell membrane is high both after 15 min and 45 min incubation at 37°C, and a significant fraction of the grain is associated with coated pits of the cell membrane. Similar distribution has been observed after electron microscopic autoradiography, using ^{125}I-labeled [D-Ala^{6}-des-Gly^{10}-ethylamide]GnRH taken up by rat pituitary gonadotropes in vivo (Duello et al., 1983).

GnRH RECEPTOR REDISTRIBUTION: IMPLICATIONS FOR BIOLOGICAL FUNCTION

Receptors for polypeptide hormones appear to have a common topological redistribution. The occupied receptors are initially evenly distributed over the cell surface and quickly form clusters that are subsequently internalized. However, there are two possibilities in the subsequent events that could mediate hormone action. In the first, the binding of ligand to receptors leads to cross-linking of receptors (or receptor-effector) at the cell surface, which is by itself sufficient to trigger the subsequent biochemical events of hormone action. Although ligand internalization and degradation may occur, it is not a prerequisite for ligand function. In the second, however, internalization and degradation of hormone-receptor complexes are important for biological activity. Thus, internalization may serve as a selective transport mechanism, or processing of the hormone-receptor complexes may produce a "second messenger" in the action of the hormone (for review see Hazum, 1982b).

In the pituitary, it has been shown that an immobilized GnRH analog ([D-Lys^6]GnRH coupled by its epsilon amino group, through a 10-Å spacer, to agarose matrix) can stimulate luteinizing hormone (LH) release from pituitary cells (Conn et al., 1981a). This immobilized analog is stable under various conditions, including exposure to cell cultures, thus excluding the possibility of leakage from the matrix. The apparent potency of the immobilized analog (which cannot be internalized) is one-quarter that of the free hormone. Nevertheless, it is still capable of evoking a full LH secretory response (Conn et al., 1981a). These studies indicate that internalization of GnRH is not required for stimulation of gonadotropin release from pituitary cells.

Three different approaches have also been described that indicate that GnRH-receptor internalization as well as cluster formation are not required for GnRH-stimulated LH release from pituitary cells (Conn and Hazum, 1981). The first approach utilized again the immobilization technique. A more potent GnRH agonist, [D-Lys^6-des-Gly^{10}-ethylamide]GnRH, immobilized at a higher hormone/bead ratio (providing additional evidence for the stability of the immobilized agonist) also induced LH release with full efficacy. In these highly derivatized beads, the quantity of LH release is restricted by the number of beads added as a result of the fact that the hormone is exposed to only a small number of cells. In the second approach, it has been shown that the removal of external GnRH from the cells at different times throughout the GnRH stimulation results in a prompt return of LH release to basal levels. Thus, under conditions in which internalization takes place, continuous release of LH can only occur when external GnRH is present. These results again indicate that LH release with full efficacy does not require internalization of the hormone-receptor complex. Finally, comparative studies on receptor distribution and LH release have been undertaken. Cluster formation and internalization of Rhod-GnRH are not observed in the presence of 0.1 mM vinblastine, and the fluorescence is evenly distributed over the cell surface of gonadotropes. Under these conditions, gonadotropin secretion by GnRH or its agonist is not affected. This result suggests that internalization, as well as large-scale clusters of GnRH receptors, are not important in eliciting the biological effects of GnRH.

Recently, the conversion of a GnRH antagonist to an agonist and the potency enhancement of a GnRH agonist by bridging two molecules within a critical distance d ($15\ \text{Å} < d < 150\ \text{Å}$) suggest that receptor cross-linking as such is sufficient to activate the effector system in pituitary cells to evoke release (Conn et al., 1982a,b; Gregory et al., 1982). On the basis of these experimental data a mathematical model of hormone action that quantitatively accounts for the release of LH has recently been proposed (Blum and Conn, 1982).

Another important question regarding receptor redistribution is what is the function of an antagonist of a hormone. An antagonist of GnRH is capable of binding to the receptor but it is unable to induce biological activity and refractoriness. Therefore, it is of interest to examine whether an antagonist of GnRH will induce a similar or different pattern of receptor distribution to that observed with a GnRH agonist. Recent studies (Hazum et al., 1983b) have indicated that GnRH antagonist can also induce receptor clustering and internalization in pituitary cells using a fluorescently labeled antagonist and the image intensification technique. In addition, the internalization of both GnRH agonists and antagonists was established by biochemical methods. These results suggest that the GnRH antagonists can by-pass receptor cross-linking and directly induce clustering and internalization. Alternatively, the mechanisms in inducing clustering and internalization by GnRH agonists and antagonists may be different. The internalization of GnRH (and presumably its receptor) may have some other intracellular action or may simply be degraded or recycled.

SUMMARY

Identification of the GnRH receptors by biochemical techniques has been achieved by using a bioactive photoaffinity derivative of GnRH [azidobenzoyl-D-Lys^{6}]GnRH. Photoaffinity labeling of pituitary GnRH receptors led to the identification of a single specific band of 60K daltons. In contrast, photoaffinity labeling of gonadal GnRH receptors resulted in the identification of two specific components with apparent molecular weights of 60K and 54K daltons. These findings suggest that some differences exist between the GnRH binding sites of the pituitary and the gonads. The specificity and the physiological role of the photoaffinity labeled components was established.

The distribution of GnRH receptors, after binding to gonadotropes, was followed by light and electron microscopic autoradiography using ^{125}I-labeled GnRH analogs, as well as by image-intensified fluorescence microscopy utilizing rhodamine-labeled hormone. These studies indicated that, after exposure of gonadotropes to the hormone at 4°C, the receptors are evenly distributed, while at 37°C aggregation and subsequent internalization of the hormone-receptor complex into subcellular organelles can be observed. Similar pattern of receptor redistribution was observed with a GnRH antagonist.

Three different approaches indicated that GnRH-receptor internalization, as well as cluster formation, are not required for GnRH-stimulated LH release from pituitary cells. In addition, recent studies have indicated that receptor cross-linking per se is sufficient to activate the effector system in pituitary cells to evoke LH release.

ACKNOWLEDGEMENTS

This work was supported by the Ford Foundation and the Rockefeller Foundation, New York, and by the fund for basic research administered by the Israel Academy of Sciences and Humanities. I am grateful to Mrs. M. Kopelowitz for typing the manuscript.

REFERENCES

Adams, T.E., and Spies, H.G., 1981, Binding characteristics of gonadotropin-releasing hormone receptors throughout the estrous cycle of the hamster, Endocrinology, 108:2245.

Blum, J.J., and Conn, P.M., 1982, Gonadotropin-releasing hormone stimulation of luteinizing hormone release: A ligand-receptor-effector model, Proc. Natl. Acad. Sci. U.S.A., 79:7307.

Clayton, R.N., and Catt, K.J., 1980, Receptor-binding affinity of gonadotropin-releasing hormone analogs: Analysis by radioligand receptor assay, Endocrinology, 106:1154.

Clayton, R.N., and Catt, K.J., 1981, Gonadotropin-releasing hormone receptors: Characterization, physiological regulation, and relationship to reproductive function, Endocrine Rev., 2:186.

Clayton, R.N., Shakespear, R.A., and Marshall, J.C., 1978, LHRH binding to purified plasma membranes: Absence of adenylate cyclase activation., Mol. Cell. Endocrinol., 11:63.

Clayton, R.N., Solano, A.R., Gracia-Vela, A., Dufau, M.I., and Catt, K.J., 1980, Regulation of pituitary receptors for gonadotropin-releasing hormone during the rat estrous cycle , Endocrinology, 107:699.

Conn, P.M., and Hazum, E., 1981, LH release and GnRH-receptor internalization: Independent actions of GnRH, Endocrinology, 109:2040.

Conn, P.M., Smith, R., and Rogers, D.C., 1981a, Stimulation of pituitary gonadotropin release does not require internalization of gonadotropin-releasing hormone, J. Biol. Chem., 256:1098.

Conn, P.M., Marian, J., McMillian, M., Stern, J., Rogers, D., Hamby, M., Penna, A., and Grant, E., 1981b, Gonadotropin-releasing hormone action in the pituitary: A three step mechanism, Endocrine Rev., 2:174.

Conn, P.M., Rogers, D.C., Stewart, J.M., Niedel, J., and Sheffield, T., 1982a, Conversion of gonadotropin-releasing hormone antagonist to an agonist, Nature, 296:653.

Conn, P.M., Rogers, D.C., and McNeil, R., 1982b, Potency enhancement of a GnRH agonist: GnRH-receptor microaggregation stimulates gonadotropin release, Endocrinology, 111:335.

Conne, B.S., Aubert, M.L., and Sizoneko, P.C., 1979, Quantification of pituitary receptor sites for LHRH: Use of superactive analog as a tracer, Biochem. Biophys. Res. Commun., 90:1249.

Dacheux, F., 1981, Ultrastructural localization of gonadotropin-releasing hormone in porcine gonadotrophic cells, Cell Tissue Res., 216:143.

Duello, T.M., and Nett, T.M., 1980, Uptake, localization, and retention of gonadotropin-releasing hormone and gonadotropin-releasing hormone analogs in rat gonadotrophs, Mol. Cell. Endocrinol., 19:101.

Duello, T.M., Nett, T.M., and Farquhar, M.G., 1983, Fate of a gonadotropin-releasing hormone agonist internalized by rat pituitary gonadotrophs, Endocrinology, 112:1.

Gregory, H., Taylor, C.L., and Hopkins, C.R., 1982, Luteinizing hormone release from dissociated pituitary cells by dimerization of occupied LHRH receptors, Nature, 300:269.

Hazum, E., 1981a, Some characteristics of GnRH-receptors in rat pituitary membranes: Differences between an agonist and an antagonist, Mol. Cell. Endocrinol., 23:275.

Hazum, E., 1981b, Photo-affinity inactivation of gonadotropin-releasing hormone receptors, FEBS Lett., 128:111.

Hazum, E., 1981c, Photoaffinity labeling of luteinizing hormone releasing hormone receptors of rat pituitary membrane preparations, Endocrinology, 109:1281.

Hazum, E., 1982a, GnRH-receptor of rat pituitary is a glycoprotein: Differential effect of neuraminidase and lectins on agonists and antagonists binding, Mol. Cell. Endocrinol., 26:217.

Hazum, E., 1982b, Receptor regulation by hormones: Relevance to secretion and other biological functions, in: "Cellular Regulation of Secretion and Release", P.M. Conn, ed., Academic Press, New-York.

Hazum, E., 1983, Nature of the GnRH receptors in the ovary, in: "Regulation of Target Cell Responsiveness" K.W. McKerns, ed., Plenum Press, New-York.

Hazum, E., and Keinan, D., 1982, Photoaffinity labeling of pituitary gonadotropin releasing hormone receptors during the rat estrous cycle, Biochem. Biophys. Res. Commun., 107:695.

Hazum, E., and Keinan, D., 1983a, Covalent linking of photoreactive gonadotropin-releasing hormone to gonadotropes produces a prolonged signal, Proc. Natl. Acad. Sci. U.S.A., 80:1902.
Hazum, E., and Keinan, D., 1983b, Gonadotropin releasing hormone receptors: photoaffinity labeling with an antagonist, Biochem. Biophys. Res. Commun., 110:116.
Hazum, E., and Nimrod, A., 1982, Photoaffinity labeling and fluorescence distribution studies of gonadotropin-releasing hormone receptors in ovarian granulosa cells, Proc. Natl. Acad. Sci. U.S.A., 79:1747.
Hazum, E., Cuatrecasas, P., Marian, J., and Conn, P.M., 1980, Receptor-mediated internalization of gonadotropin-releasing hormone by pituitary gonadotropes, Proc. Natl. Acad. Sci. U.S.A., 77:6692.
Hazum, E., Fridkin, M., Baram, T., and Koch, Y., 1981, Degradation of gonadotropin-releasing hormone by anterior pituitary enzymes, FEBS Lett., 127:273.
Hazum, E., Garritsen, A., and Keinan, D., 1982a, Role of lipids in gonadotropin releasing hormone agonist and antagonist binding to rat pituitary, Biochem. Biophys. Res. Commun., 105:8.
Hazum, E., Meidan, R., Keinan, D., Okon, E., Koch, Y., Lindner, H.R., and Amsterdam, A., 1982b, A novel method for localization of gonadotropin releasing hormone receptors, Endocrinology, 111:2135.
Hazum, E., Liscovitch, M., Koch, Y., and Amsterdam, A., 1983a, Distribution of gonadotropin releasing hormone (GnRH) receptors in pituitary cells, 65th Ann. Meet. Endocrine Soc., San Antonio, Abs. 386.
Hazum, E., Meidan, R., Liscovitch, M., Keinan, D., Lindner, H.R., and Koch, Y., 1983b, Receptor-mediated internalization of LHRH antagonists by pituitary cells, Mol. Cell. Endocrinol., 30:291.
Hopkins, C.R., and Gregory, H., 1977, Topographical localization of the receptors for luteinizing hormone-releasing hormone on the surface of dissociated pituitary cells, J. Cell Biol., 75:528.
Hsueh, A.J.W., and Jones, P.B.C., 1981, Extrapituitary actions of gonadotropin-releasing hormone, Endocrine Rev., 2:437.
Koch, Y., Baram, T., Hazum, E., and Fridkin, M., 1977, Resistance to enzymic degradation of LHRH analogues possessing increased biological activity, Biochem. Biophys. Res. Commun., 74:488.
Marian, J., and Conn, P.M., 1980, The calcium requirement in GnRH-stimulated LH release is not mediated through a specific action on receptor binding, Life Sci., 27:87.
Marian, J., Cooper, R.L., and Conn, P.M., 1981, Regulation of the rat pituitary gonadotropin-releasing hormone receptor, Mol. Pharmacol., 19:399.
Meidan, R., and Koch, Y., 1981a, Binding of luteinizing-hormone releasing hormone analogues to dispersed pituitary cells, Life Sci., 28:1961.

Meidan, R., and Koch, Y., 1981b, Variations in luteinizing hormone-releasing hormone receptors in pituitary cells from immature and mature cycling female rats, FEBS Lett., 132:114.

Naor, Z., Clayton, R.N., and Catt, K.J., 1980, Characterization of GnRH receptors in cultured rat pituitary cells, Endocrinology, 107:1144.

Naor, Z., Atlas, A., Clayton, R.N., Forman, D.S., Amsterdam, A., and Catt, K.J., 1981, Interaction of fluorescent gonadotropin-releasing hormone with receptors in cultured pituitary cells, J. Biol. Chem., 256:3049.

Savoy-Moore, B.T., Schwartz, N.B., Duncan, J.A., and Marshall, J.C., 1980, Pituitary gonadotropin-releasing hormone receptors during the rat estrous cycle, Science, 209:942.

Sternberger, L.A., and Petrali, J.P., 1975, Quantitative immunocytochemistry of pituitary receptors for luteinizing hormone-releasing hormone, Cell Tissue Res., 162:141.

PHYSIOLOGICAL REGULATION OF PITUITARY GnRH RECEPTORS

R.N. Clayton, S.I. Naik, L.S. Young, H.M. Charlton*

Dept. of Medicine, University of Birmingham, *and
Dept. of Human Anatomy, University of Oxford, U.K.

INTRODUCTION

In common with other oligo- and poly-peptide hormones, gonadotrophin releasing hormone (GnRH) initiates the processes leading to release and synthesis of LH and FSH following interaction with specific receptors in gonadotroph cell membranes. Initial attempts at measurement of pituitary GnRH-R employed (^{125}I)-GnRH as the radioligand in receptor assays (RRA) and were unsuccessful. However the availability of iodinated non-degradable agonist analogs of GnRH (GnRH-A) resolved the major problem viz: ^{125}I-GnRH binding was largely to low-affinity sites. Thus, a reliable GnRH receptor assay was validated, which measured only high-affinity GnRH binding sites, is highly specific for a whole series of GnRH agonist and antagonist analogs, and ligand binding is restricted to gonadotrophs (for review see 1). Assays based upon ^{125}I-GnRH-A ligands are now widely accepted as the method of choice for receptor quantitation. By analogy with other ligand cell surface membrane receptor systems, it seemed likely that changes at the first site of cellular interaction could be a site for regulation of the target cell's responses. Thus, with a reliable RRA it was possible to directly measure the GnRH-R content of individual rat pituitaries in different physiological circumstances to establish the relationship, if any, between GnRH-R, pituitary gonadotrophin content, and serum LH and FSH concentrations. The present review is concerned largely with these relationships *in vivo* in laboratory animals, although some more recent *in vitro* studies will also be briefly discussed.

Physiological regulation of GnRH receptor in rats

Initial studies in rats examined the effect of gonadectomy. In both males and females there was a 2-3 fold rise in GnRH-R detectable at the time of the plasma gonadotrophin increase[2-4], which could be prevented by appropriate sex steroid replacement. During the rat estrous cycle GnRH-R increase on the evening of diestrous and are maintained at the higher level until the time of the proestrous gonadotrophin surge when a small decline is observed[5]. By the morning of estrous GnRH-R levels return to those found before the increase on diestrous[5,6]. Therefore in both these situations an increase in GnRH receptors can contribute to the enhanced gonadotrophin secretion observed under these circumstances. Conversely, when gonadotrophin secretion is reduced during lactation, and in hyperprolactinaemic states, GnRH receptors are also lower by about 50%[6-8]. The detailed changes of GnRH-R in rats can be found in recent reviews[1,9], and will not be further elaborated here.

Mechanism for the GnRH receptor regulation in rats

It was apparent from these early studies that pituitary GnRH-R content could be positively correlated with the level of endogenous GnRH secretion (Table 1).

Table 1. Correlation between pituitary GnRH receptors and endogenous GnRH secretion.

Physiological state	GnRH secretion	GnRH receptors
GONADECTOMY	direct measurement of GnRH in pituitary stalk blood indicates an increase	increased 2-3 fold
LACTATION	reduced/absence of LH pulsatility, low basal serum LH, diminished response to exogenous GnRH suggest decreased GnRH secretion.	reduced by 50%

Thus, the hypothesis was formulated that GnRH-R levels could be induced by their own ligand (receptor up-regulation) in a manner analogous to angiotensin II receptors in adrenal glomerulosa[10], and prolactin receptors in the liver[11]. Experiments were performed to test the hypothesis that GnRH regulates its own receptors *in vivo*. The principle was to determine whether removal of endogenous GnRH would prevent the post-castration increase in GnRH-R in male rats. The experimental approaches and results, summarised in Table 2, provided good support for this hypothesis. Furthermore, *in vitro*

Table 2. Evidence that endogenous GnRH is essential for the post-castration increase in pituitary GnRH-R

Rationale and Experimental design (ref)	Result
1) Removal of GnRH at source by mechanical destruction of the median eminence. (17)	a) Placed before orchidectomy-prevents GnRH-R and serum LH increase. GnRH-R values 30% below intact controls. b) Reduced GnRH-R values when chronically castrated animals are lesioned. Lesion effect completely reversed by exogenous GnRH.
2) Abolition of endogenous GnRH by passive immunoneutralisation with GnRH antiserum (18)	a) Post-orchidectomy GnRH-R and serum LH increase prevented. GnRH-R values 30% below intact controls. b) Decrease in GnRH-R partly prevented by exogenous GnRH agonist analogue which does not cross-react with antiserum.
3) Blockade of GnRH action at pituitary receptor sites by continuous infusion of a GnRH antagonist analogue (17)	Prevents the post-orchidectomy GnRH-R and serum LH increase. GnRH-R reduced to 75% below control largely due to receptor occupancy.

studies have clearly indicated that GnRH and its agonist analogs induce GnRH-R in cultured pituitary cells in a dose- and time-dependent manner[12-14]. Receptor induction in vitro is prevented by a GnRH antagonist, indicating its mediation through GnRH receptors, and protein synthesis inhibitors. In addition, GnRH rapidly increases GnRH-R in pituitaries that have never previously been exposed to GnRH in vivo, in the hypogonadotrophic hypogonadal (hpg) mouse (vide infra). The hypothesis of GnRH receptor up-regulation, therefore, has considerable support. This does not necessarily presuppose that all in vivo changes in GnRH-R are secondary to alterations in endogenous GnRH secretion. Influences of factors, particularly sex-steroids, acting directly on the pituitary are not precluded. Indeed, Loumaye et al have clearly demonstrated induction of pituitary GnRH-R by oestrogens in vitro[15], and reduction of GnRH-R by androgens in vitro has also been reported[16].

Desensitisation of pituitary gonadotrophin secretion and GnRH receptor down-regulation

Numerous studies in primates[19], rodents[20], and *in vitro*[13,21], have shown that when high-doses of GnRH or more dramatically its long-acting analogs are administered chronically gonadotrophin secretion rather than being stimulated, falls. This refractoriness to the ligand, or desensitisation, is reminiscent of insulin resistant states and treatment with high doses of hCG (see 22 for review). In these latter cases a large component of the desensitisation is net loss of ligand receptors (down-regulation). To determine whether a similar mechanism operates with GnRH and the pituitary we infused graded doses of GnRH, or a potent agonist analog (GnRH-A), for 1 week into both intact and orchidectomised male rats[23]. Surprisingly, with the lowest doses of GnRH or GnRH-A, which resulted in 'physiological' serum levels of the peptides (30-100 pg/ml), GnRH receptor levels were actually increased by 30-50% in intact rats. This increase was accompanied by a 2-fold rise in serum LH in the analog-infused, but not the GnRH-infused, animals. Increasing the infusion dose to produce serum GnRH and GnRH-A levels of around 1 ng/ml markedly depleted free GnRH-R though serum LH was still increased 2-3 fold in intact rats. However, in castrated rats there was never any further increase in GnRH-R or serum LH with the lowest doses of GnRH, while higher doses decreased free GnRH-R, serum LH, and pituitary LH in parallel. The GnRH-R content was measured in individual pituitary homogenates without any attempt to remove GnRH bound to the receptors. If pituitary membranes from glands exposed to 1 ng/ml GnRH-A *in vivo* were extensively washed to allow dissociation of occupied receptors[23], then the proportional fall in GnRH-A relative to control was much reduced. This provided good evidence of considerable receptor occupancy. Thus, true net receptor loss accounted for only about 25-30% of the fall in measurable GnRH-R. However, in castrates, despite a marked degree (about 75%) of receptor occupancy serum and pituitary LH values fall considerably which indicates that disruption of post-receptor events plays a considerable role in the desensitisation phenomenon. A similar conclusion was reached by Smith and Vale when examining responses of desensitised pituitary cells *in vitro*[13]. Thus, the process of desensitisation to GnRH is caused by disruption of a combination of cellular biochemical mechanisms which remain to be fully defined.

GnRH receptor regulation in normal mice

It seems clear from the evidence summarised above that GnRH is an important *in vivo* receptor regulator in rats. However, whether this function is widely applicable has not been investigated in any detail. We, therefore, decided to test the hypothesis that GnRH positively regulates its own receptors in another rodent species - that is laboratory mice. The strategy was essentially similar to that employed for rats - namely to examine GnRH-R regulation *in vivo* after manipulation of the sex steroid hormone environment.

a) Gonadectomy

As in rats there is a brisk rise in serum levels of both gonadotrophins after castration. However, when GnRH-R are measured, contrary to rats, there is a 30-50% decrease in pituitary GnRH-R in both male and female mice[24,25]. In both sexes there is a very early (between 3-12 hours post-castration) receptor fall with a subsequent return to near-intact receptor values at 24 hours, which is then followed by a second fall in GnRH-R to values which remain about 50% below those of intact controls for up to three months. We have never observed any increase in GnRH-R at any time following castration of either male or female mice, despite a persistent elevation in serum LH and FSH. Furthermore, this result has been observed in two different strains of mice and in neither can changes in receptor affinity be responsible, since this was the same ($Ka = 2.0 \times 10^9 M^{-1}$) in intact and castrated mouse pituitaries. This unexpected result is the opposite to that seen in rats following castration.

The post-castration GnRH-R fall can be prevented by testosterone treatment of males and estrogen plus progesterone treatment of females. As regards pituitary hormone content, this falls and remains reduced (again by about 50%) for up to 3 months post-orchidectomy, but after ovariectomy the fall is only transient, with an elevation above intact control values occurring about one week post-ovariectomy. The explanation for this sex difference in pituitary hormone content response to gonadectomy is unclear. No information is available concerning GnRH levels in pituitary stalk blood after gonadectomy of mice. If, as in rats, this is increased then the persistent fall in GnRH-R could be the result of receptor occupancy or down-regulation - both of which could be attributed to greater pituitary exposure to endogenous GnRH. We have attempted to determine the contribution of occupancy by measurement of GnRH-R in pituitary membrane preparations rather than unprocessed homogenates. The membrane preparation protocol, which involves dilution and washing of receptors prior to centrifugation, would be expected to remove the majority of endogenously bound GnRH, which dissociates very rapidly from its receptors under these conditions[1,23]. In such membrane preparations from gonadectomised mouse pituitaries a fall in GnRH-R is still observed, although by only about 30% as opposed to 50% in homogenates. This suggests that occupancy may contribute, albeit in a minor way, to the receptor decrease. The possibility of true ligand-dependent GnRH receptor down-regulation remains to be explored. Alternatively, the post-castration receptor fall may be entirely independent of endogenous GnRH and result from an as yet undetermined mechanism.

We have also measured GnRH receptors in genotypic male mice with the syndrome of testicular feminisation (Tfm). These animals are phenotypic females owing to complete androgen insensitivity because of a genetic absence of androgen receptors. These animals may therefore be considered to represent life-long castrates. They too have reduced GnRH-R, elevated serum gonadotrophins, and reduced pituitary LH and FSH contents, very similar to long-term orchidectomised normal mice[24].

b) Lactation

Pituitary GnRH receptors in female mice suckling 4-8 pups are reduced by 40-50%, as are serum LH and FSH levels. This is entirely analogous to the data obtained in lactating rats[6]. We have not yet examined the effect of induced hyperprolactinaemia on GnRH-R regulation in mice.

c) Effects of GnRH antiserum treatment

In orchidectomised rats the GnRH-R increase can be prevented by concurrent administration of a GnRH antiserum, implicating a role for endogenous GnRH in the receptor increase (Table 2). If the GnRH decrease post-gonadectomy of mice is a consequence of altered endogenous GnRH secretion we would expect the administration of the GnRH antiserum to prevent the receptor fall. In fact, this does not occur, the post-castration GnRH-R fall is accentuated rather than prevented, despite the complete suppression of the post-gonadectomy increase in serum gonadotrophins. Furthermore, like in rats, GnRH antiserum treatment reduces GnRH-R and serum gonadotrophins in both intact normal male and female mice[26]. These data indicate that GnRH is required to maintain a 'normal' complement of GnRH-R in intact mice, as in rats. Furthermore the data suggest that GnRH is not the mediator of the post-gonadectomy GnRH-R fall.

GnRH receptor regulation in hypogonadotrophic hypogonadal mice (hpg)

The hypogonadal hypogonadotrophic mouse (hpg) appeared as a spontaneous mutation at the Atomic Energy Research Establishment, Harwell, Oxford, U.K. It is characterised by a genetic absence of hypothalamic GnRH[27]. Consequently, pituitary and serum levels of gonadotrophic hormones are extremely low, with all other pituitary trophic hormones being normal. These animals are phenotypically normal males and females but fail to undergo sexual maturation at puberty. Electrical stimulation of the hypothalamus does not elicit any rise in serum gonadotrophins, whereas a single injection of exogenous GnRH will produce a small increment in serum LH, though only about 1/10th that found in normal littermates. If endogenous GnRH is essential for gonadotroph differentiation and acquisition of GnRH receptors, then hpg animals should have undetectable levels of receptors. In fact, GnRH-R are easily measurable in pituitaries from hpg mice of both sexes and the values are about 30% of those of their normal male littermates. The receptor affinity is identical with that of normal mice[28]. As previously reported[27], we confirmed the very much reduced content of LH and FSH in the pituitaries of hpg mice and undetectable serum gonadotrophin levels. Thus, it would seem that GnRH-R can be expressed in the apparent absence of any endogenous GnRH. The failure of the most sensitive RIA (using the Nett-Niswender R42 antiserum which requires intact unmodified N- and C-temini of the GnRH molecule for recognition) to detect immunoreactivity in hypothalamic extracts does not categorically exclude the possibility that the pituitary is exposed to a minute amount of the decapeptide, or some similar 'trophic' material. Immunocytochemistry reveals that the gonadotroph population is not much reduced in hpg mice, being 70% of normal. However, gonadotroph size, surface area and granule content are dramatically reduced[29,30]. The morphological data are therefore consistent with the GnRH-receptor data and imply that hypothalamic GnRH is not essential for gonadotroph differentiation, though as suggested earlier this is necessary for maintenance of 'normal' gonadotroph function. The possibility that gonadotroph differentiation, which begins at about day 11-12 of foetal life, is stimulated by placental GnRH is supported by findings that the placenta appears to synthesise GnRH de novo[31].

Using this hpg mouse model we have been able to examine, in some detail, the role of exogenous GnRH on gonadotroph function. Repetitive subcutaneous injections of 60 ng GnRH, given in a physiological regime (i.e. once every 2 hours) for 15 days reproduces the serum hormonal profiles akin to those of animals undergoing spontaneous puberty, i.e. FSH rises before LH. GnRH receptors are already increased to about 50% of normal values after one day of treatment, while by day 3 values are indistinguishable from normal[28]. The receptor increase precedes the rise in pituitary and serum FSH implying that the former is a prerequisite for normal gonadotrophin synthesis. The stimulation of pituitary function is followed by testicular and ovarian development. As yet, longer studies (>15D) have not been performed. In parallel with the biochemical changes induced by GnRH treatment are morphological changes in the gonadotrophs, which include increases in size, surface area, and the secretory elements of the cells as evidenced by electron microscopy[30]. Further details of the effects of single and multiple GnRH injections on pituitary/gonadal function in hpg mice can be found in Charlton et al[32]. These data indicate the central role of GnRH in regulation of gonadotroph function. This hpg mouse model is ideal for investigation of sites of gonadal steroid hormone feedback regulation of GnRH-R, gonadotrophin release and synthesis since this animal model is not complicated by changes in hypothalamic GnRH secretion. The interaction of known exposure to GnRH and sex steroids on the pituitary can be examined and represents an ideal in vivo parallel to studies with pituitary cells in vitro.

Hypothalamic implants into hpg mice

The concept that transplantation of foetal brain tissue from a normal healthy donor to an animal with selected neurotransmitter deficiency could improve the functional deficiencies has been shown for dopamine[33], and vasopressin[34]. This same principle has been applied to adult hpg mice whose hypogonadism can be partly reversed by implantation of normal foetal hypothalamus into the IIIrd ventricle of the recipient[35]. We have extended this study to look in more detail at pituitary gonadal function in both male and female hpg mice. The foetal hypothalamic transplants were performed in Oxford (by HMC) and their localisation and viability verified by histological staining of brain sections at the time of sacrifice. Judged by the increases in testicular and ovarian weights, only those grafts that visibly communicated with the median eminence were successful. When pituitary GnRH receptors were analysed a gradual increase to near 'normal' littermate values was observed by 40 days post-implantation in 9/10 male hpg mice. In these same animals pituitary and serum gonadotrophin levels increased dramatically[36]. Testicular and seminal vesicle weights increased and testicular LH receptors, expressed/testis, attained near-normal values. In the one animal that failed to respond none of the variables measured showed any change from cerebral-cortex grafted controls, which were not different from unimplanted hpg animals. The 'sex' of the donor foetal hypothalamus did not appear to influence the response of the recipient.

Foetal hypothalamic implants into hpg females increased pituitary GnRH-R in 10/13 recipients, though only to about 60% of normal control values. Ovarian and uterine weights increased as did ovarian LH receptors. In contrast to the males, pituitary and serum gonadotrophins were increased to normal female values. Again absence of response correlated well with either absence or poor position of the implants in the IIIrd ventricle. Vaginal opening in females occurs anything from 13-41 days post-implantation, and the animals remain in constant oestrous for up to 256 days post-transplantation. No evidence of ovarian cyclicity has been observed to date. Whether longer periods of time will see mating behaviour and ovarian cyclicity remains to be seen, although currently available data suggest that the grafts do not form the functional neural connections with host neurones required for cyclic ovarian function. This technique is of enormous theoretical interest since it may provide another model for analysis of the effects of hormonal feedback signals both on the function of the implant and at the pituitary level. However, it is probable that in the absence of appropriate 'wiring' into the host hypothalamic neuronal circuits, GnRH secretion will be a continuous trickle rather than being released in the 'physiological' pulsatile mode. This remains to be determined but does present a potential theoretical disadvantage of the model, compared to administration of exogenous GnRH, for physiological studies. Nevertheless, whatever the mode of GnRH release from the implant, it is clearly effective in stimulating GnRH receptors, gonadotroph, and gonadal function.

CONCLUSIONS

With the exception of gonadectomy, currently available data on mice (both normal and hpg) indicate an important role for GnRH in the regulation of its own pituitary receptors in this species. The data obtained from the mouse studies clearly support the general applicability of the GnRH receptor auto-regulation hypothesis. The failure of gonadectomy to elicit a GnRH-R increase may be unrelated to endogenous GnRH levels, or if it is so related then the mouse pituitary clearly responds differently from that of the rat in respect of the GnRH receptor response. There are certainly some minor species differences in other areas, e.g. the pituitary gonadotrophin content response to orchidectomy differs in mice and rats. We are currently attempting to determine what factor(s) are responsible for the post-gonadectomy receptor fall in mice and performing prolonged pulsatile GnRH injection studies in hpg female mice in attempts to induce cyclical ovarian function and even pregnancy. Our in vivo receptor regulation data, particularly in the hpg mouse, is qualitatively very similar to that which we and others have observed in cultured pituitary cells. This lends 'physiological' validity to the in vitro systems designed to investigate the molecular mechanism of GnRH receptor regulation and its precise relationship to secretion and synthesis of gonadotrophic hormones.

REFERENCES

1. R.N. Clayton and K.J. Catt. Gonadotrophin-releasing hormone receptors: characterisation, physiological regulation, and relationship to reproductive function. Endocrine Reviews 2: 186 (1981).
2. M.S. Frager, D.R. Pieper, S. Tonetta, J.A. Duncan and J.C. Marshall, Pituitary gonadotrophin releasing hormone (GnRH) receptors: effects of castration, steroid replacement, and the role of GnRH in modulating receptors in the rat. J.Clin. Invest. 67:615 (1981).
3. R.N. Clayton and K.J. Catt. Regulation of pituitary gonadotrophin releasing hormone receptors by gonadal hormones. Endocrinol. 108:887 (1981).
4. B.S. Conne, S. Scaglioni, U. Lang, P.C. Sizonenko, and M.L. Aubert. Pituitary receptor sites for GnRH: effect of castration and substitutive therapy with sex steroids in the male rat. Endocrinol. 110:70 (1982).
5. R. Savoy-Moore, N.B. Schwartz, J.A. Duncan and J.C. Marshall. Pituitary gonadotrophin releasing hormone receptors during the rat estrous cycle. Science 209: 942 (1980).

Endocrinology 107: 699 (1980).

7. R.N. Clayton and L.C. Bailey. Hyperprolactinaemia attenuates the gonadotrophin releasing hormone receptor response to gonadectomy in rats. J. Endocrinol 95: 267 (1982).

8. H.M. Fraser,, R.M. Popkin, A.S. McNeilly and R.M. Sharpe. Changes in pituitary LHRH receptor levels in situations of increased or decreased gonadotrophin secretion in the male rat. Mol. Cell. Endocrinol. 28: 321 (1982).

9. R.N. Clayton. The role of pituitary gonadotrophin-releasing hormone receptors in the physiological regulation of gonadotrophin secretion. Clinical Science 64: 1 (1983).

10. R.L. Hauger, G. Aguilera, and K.J. Catt. Angiotensin II regulates its receptor sites in the adrenal glomerulosa zone. Nature 271: 176 (1978).

11. B.I. Posner, P.A. Kelly, and H.G. Friesen. Prolactin receptors in rat liver: possible induction by prolactin. Science 188: 57 (1975).

12. E. Loumaye and K.J. Catt. Homologous regulation of gonadotrophin releasing hormone receptors in cultured pituitary cells. Science 215: 983 (1982).

13. M.A. Smith, M.H. Perrin, and W.W. Vale. Desensitisation of cultured pituitary cells to gonadotrophin releasing hormone: evidence for a post-receptor mechanism. Mol. Cell. Endocrinol. 30: 85 (1983).

14. L.S. Young, S.I. Naik and R.N. Clayton. Adenosine 3'5' monophosphate derivatives induce GnRH receptors in cultured pituitary cells - Endocrinol Submitted.

15. E. Loumaye and L. Forni. Regulatory actions of 17β-estradiol and progesterone upon pituitary GnRH receptors in vitro. Abst No. 825 Programme of the 64th Mtg of the American Endocrine Society. San Francisco. June 1982.

16. V. Giguere, F-A. Lefebvre and F. Labrie. Androgens decrease LHRH binding sites in rat anterior pituitary cells in culture. Endocrinology 108: 350 (1981).

17. R.N. Clayton, K. Channabasavaiah, J.M. Stewart and K.J. Catt. Hypothalamic regulation of pituitary gonadotrophin releasing hormone receptors: effects of hypothalamic lesions and a gonadotrophin releasing hormone antagonist. Endocrinol 110: 1108 (1982).

18. R.N. Clayton, R.M. Popkin and H.M. Fraser. Hypothalamic regulation of pituitary gonadotrophin releasing hormone receptors: Effects of gonadotrophin releasing hormone immunoneutralisation. Endocrinol. 110: 1116 (1982).

19. E. Knobil. The neuroendocrine control of the menstrual cycle. Recent Prog. Horm. Res. 36:53 (1980).

20. J. Sandow. Gonadotrophic and antigonadotrophic actions of LHRH analogues. in Neuroendocrine Perspectives I, Ed. Muller E.E. and MacLeod R.M. Elsevier, North Holland. p.339 (1982).

21. M.A. Smith and W.W. Vale. Desensitisation to gonadotrophin releasing hormone observed in superfused pituitary cells on

cytodex beads. Endocrinol. 108: 752 (1981).
22. K.J. Catt, J.P. Harwood, G. Aguilera and M.L. Dufau. Hormonal regulation of peptide receptors and target cell responses. Nature 280: 109 (1979).
23. R.N. Clayton. Gonadotrophin-releasing hormone modulation of its own pituitary receptors: evidence for biphasic regulation. Endocrinol. 111: 152 (1982).
24. S.I. Naik, L.S. Young, H.M. Charlton, and R.N. Clayton. Pituitary gonadotrophin-releasing hormone receptor regulation in mice I: males. Endocrinology - Submitted.
25. S.I. Naik, L.S. Young, H.M. Charlton, and R.N. Clayton. Pituitary gonadotrophin-releasing hormone receptor regulation in mice II: females. Endocrinology - Submitted.
26. S.I. Naik, L.S. Young, H.M. Charlton and R.N. Clayton - unpublished observations.
27. B.M. Cattanach, C.A. Iddon, H.M. Charlton, S.A. Chiappa and G. Fink. Gonadotrophin-releasing hormone deficiency in a mutant mouse with hypogonadism. Nature 269: 338 (1977).
28. L.S. Young, A. Speight, H.M. Charlton and R.N. Clayton Pituitary gonadotrophin-releasing hormone receptor regulation in the hypogonadotrophic hypogonadal (hpg) mouse. Endocrinology 113: 55 (1983).
29. I.F.W. McDowell, J.F. Morris, and H.M. Charlton. Characterisation of the pituitary gonadotroph cells of hypogonadal (hpg) male mice: comparison with normal mice. J. Endocrinol. 95: 321 (1982)
30. I.F.W. McDowell, J.F. Morris, H.M. Charlton and G. Fink. Effects of luteinising hormone releasing hormone on the gonadotrophs of hypogonadal (hpg) mice. J. Endocrinol. 95: 331 (1982).
31. G.S. Khodr and T.M. Siler-Khodr. Placental luteinising hormone-releasing factor and its synthesis. Science 207: 31 (1980).
32. H.M. Charlton, D.M.E. Halpin, C. Iddon, R. Rosie, G. Levy, I.F.W. McDowell, A. Megson, J.F. Morris, A. Bramwell, A. Speight, B.J. Ward, J. Broadhead, G. Davey-Smith and G. Fink. The effects of daily administration of single and multiple injections of gonadotrophin-releasing hormone on pituitary and gonadal function in the hypogonadal (hpg) mouse. Endocrinology. 113: 535 (1983).
33. M.J. Perlow, W.J. Freed, B.J. Hoffer, A. Seiger, L. Olson and R.J. Wyatt. Brain grafts reduce motor abnormalities produced by destruction of nigrostriatal dopamine system. Science 204: 643 (1979).
34. D. Gash, J.R. Sladek, C.D. Sladek. Functional development of grafted vasopressin neurons. Science 210: 367 (1980).
35. D.T. Kreiger, M.J. Perlow, M.J. Gibson, T.F. Davies, E.A. Zimmerman, M. Ferin, H.M. Charlton. Brain grafts reverse hypogonadism of gonadotrophin releasing hormone deficiency. Nature 298: 468 (1982).
36. L.S. Young, A. Detta, H.M. Charlton, and R.N. Clayton - Unpublished observations.

GnRH RECEPTOR MICROAGGREGATION: REGULATION OF GONADOTROPIN RELEASE, GnRH RECEPTORS, AND GONADOTROPE RESPONSIVENESS

P. Michael Conn, Deloris C. Rogers, Sallie G. Seay,
Lothar Jennes, Hyder Jinnah, Michael Bates,
David Clapper and Diana Luscher

Department of Pharmacology
Duke University Medical Center
Durham, N.C.

INTRODUCTION

Gonadotropin releasing hormone (GnRH) stimulates luteinizing hormone (LH) and follicle stimulating hormone (FSH) release from pituitary gonadotropes. Additional receptor-mediated actions of the releasing hormone include regulation of both the GnRH receptor and of cell responsiveness. While it is apparent that the release mechanism is Ca^{2+} mediated, it remains unclear how this receptor-mediated action is integrated with regulation of the receptor and of cell responsiveness. It is the purpose of this presentation to describe the requirements of gonadotropin release as well as receptor and response regulation in order to prepare an integrated model for these actions of the releasing hormone.

BINDING OF GnRH AND ITS ANALOGS BY THE RECEPTOR

Biochemistry

The binding step has been studied in great detail owing to the availability of a wide variety of useful analogs. Highly satisfactory radioligands can be prepared by using high affinity, metabolically stable agonists (1,2). Such synthetic compounds have in common the presence of a D-amino acid^{6} (inhibiting degradation) and the substitution des-Gly^{10}-Pro^{9} ethylamide (enhancing receptor binding affinity). Detailed studies employing these analogs (which can be radioiodinated to high specific activity) have shown changes in GnRH receptor number (but not binding affinity) during the rat estrus cycle (3,4,5), lactation, castration and aging (3) and other endocrine states. In a general way the frequency of the receptors is predictive of the responsiveness of the gonadotrope cell to GnRH.

Occupancy of the plasma membrane GnRH receptor (6) mobilizes extracellular Ca^{2+} via a plasma membrane Ca^{2+} ion channel. The channel appears to be similar to that found in nervous and muscle tissue. Interestingly, however, structure-activity relationships with Ca^{2+} ion channel antagonists reveal that the channel is not identical to that observed in these other tissues (7).

Patching, Capping and Internalization

Observations of the cell biology of the receptor can be made by preparation of fluorescent GnRH analogs which can be monitored on living cells by image intensified microscopy (8,9). As has been observed for many polypeptide hormones, the fluorescently labeled GnRH (presumably occupying the receptor, since the process is saturable and specific for gonadotropes) can be seen to undergo patching, capping, and internalization at 37°C.

Recently (10) a metabolically stable gonadotropin releasing hormone agonist (D-Lys^6-GnRH) was coupled to electron opaque markers (colloidal gold and ferritin) in order to characterize the intracellular pathway of the releasing hormone bound by pituitary gonadotropes. This approach has the advantage of increasing the resolution of localization to a "circle of uncertainty" about 10-20 fold smaller than that which can be obtained by autoradiography. After an initial uniform distribution on the cell surface, the derivatives were taken up individually as well as in small clusters in coated and uncoated membrane invaginations and moved to the lysosomal compartment either directly or after passage through the Golgi apparatus. The results suggest that labeled GnRH or GnRH-receptor complex may be routed to two distinct intracellular compartments: the lysosome and the Golgi cisternae. Examples of images obtained in this fashion are presented in a timed order in Figures 1-19.

An early question therefore was: Is patching, capping and internalization necessary for the molecular events which ensue? In order to answer this question, D-Lys^6-GnRH (which has a reactive amino group) was covalently attached to an immobile support (11,12); LH release could then be measured when GnRH was prevented from entering the cell. The derivative provoked LH release at full efficacy and therefore suggested that internalization is not necessary for GnRH to exert its affect.

It was apparent that vinblastin could inhibit receptor patching, capping and internalization in response to the releasing hormone but could not inhibit LH release (11). This also suggested that the process of patching, capping, and internalization could be uncoupled

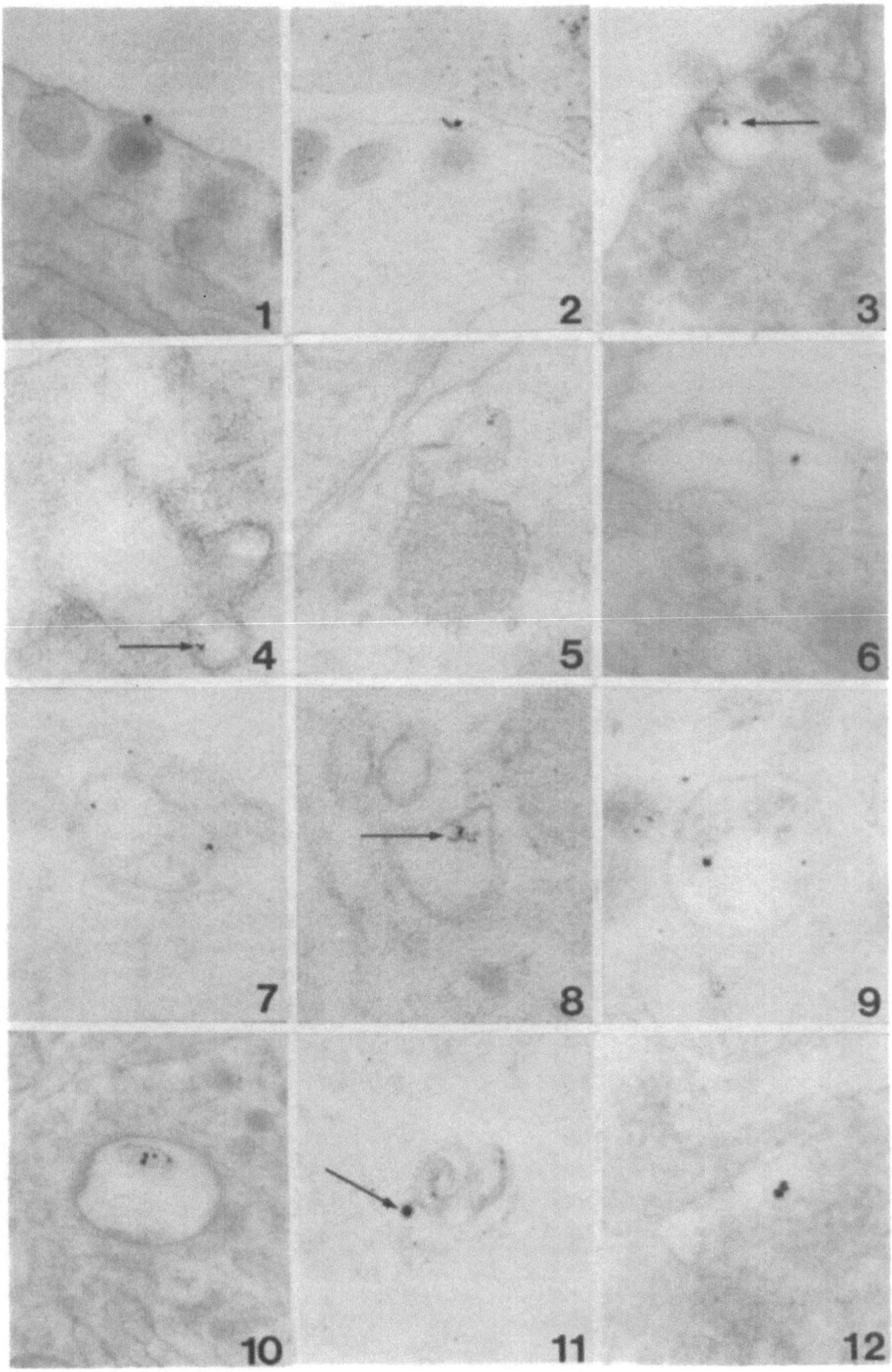
1
2
3
4
5
6
7
8
9
10
11
12

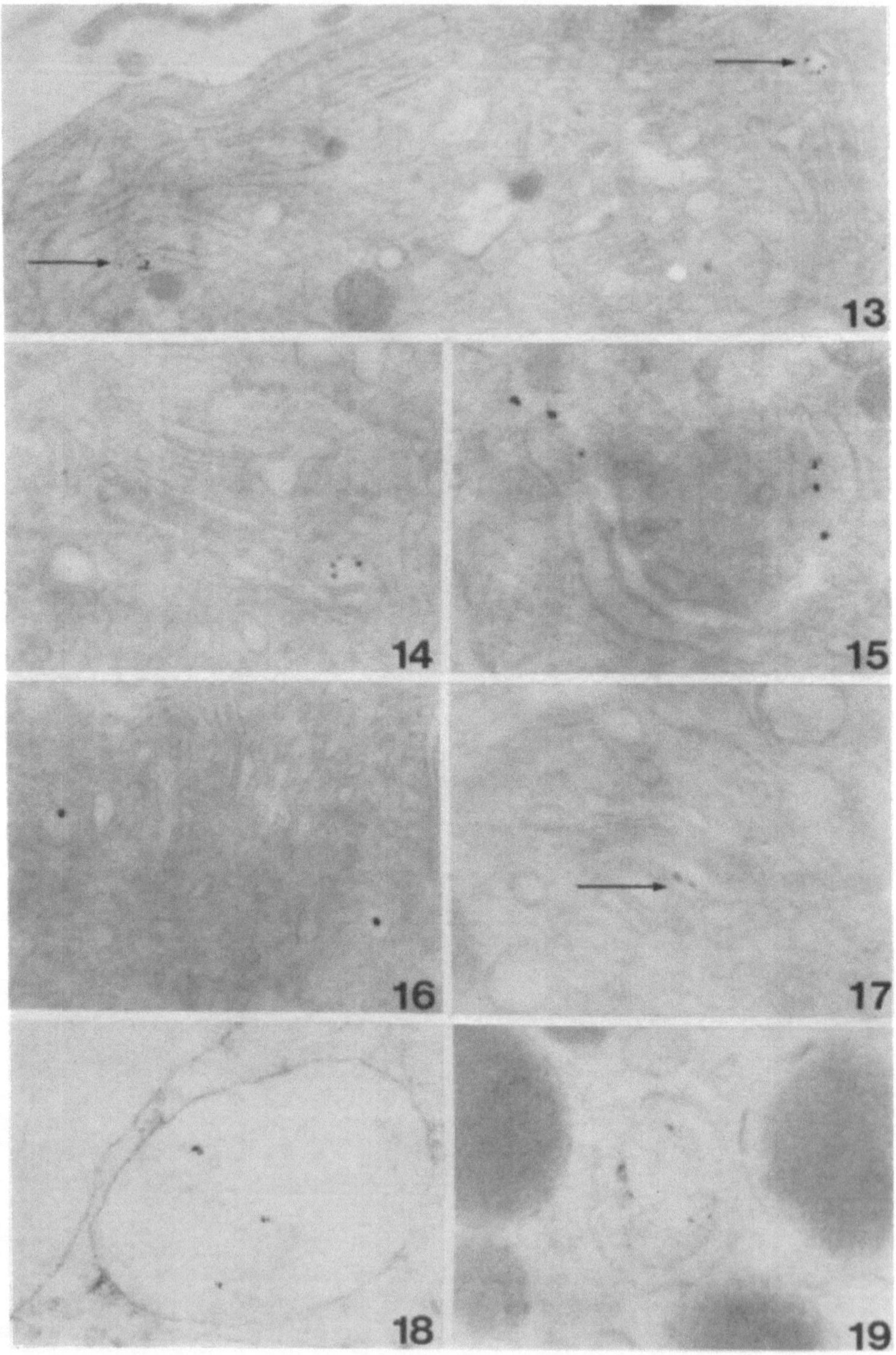
13
14
15
16
17
18
19

from release. Patching and capping refers to events that can be seen by image intensified microscopy. The resolution of such a technique is only about a hundred molecules. Therefore events which occur as the result of receptor dimerization or multimerization (that is receptor microaggregation, which is described below) would not be seen by this technique.

An additional approach has been a two-incubation experiment (11). In these studies, cells were first incubated in various concentrations of GnRH for various times. After about 15 min at ED_{50} or higher concentrations, considerable internalization of the releasing hormone occurs. If the releasing hormone is then removed from outside the media, one of two things will happen. If the internalized GnRH is sufficient to support continued gonadotropin release, this event should continue. If, in contrast, a continuously applied extracellular source of GnRH is required, then the response system should undergo extinction--the latter appears to be the case.

After washing GnRH from outside the cells, the cells rapidly stop releasing gonadotropin. Extinction occurs. Consequently, an externally applied, continuous source of GnRH is necessary for the response system to continue. It then appeared that patching, capping and internalization were not necessary for the releasing hormone to exert its effect.

Receptor-Receptor Interactions: Microaggregation

In order to examine the significance of receptor-receptor interaction at levels below that which can be measured by image intensification, additional use can be made of the GnRH analogs. Because of the interest of drug companies in this compound and support from the Contraceptive Development Branch of the NIH, a large number of GnRH antagonists are available. Many of these antagonists appear to work by the classic pharmacologic means; that is, they occupy the receptor but do not produce efficacy (i.e. gonadotropin release). A particular GnRH antagonist was used: D-p-Glu^1-D-Phe^2-D-Trp^3-D-Lys^6 (13). The substitution of D-amino acids in the first three positions leads to considerable antagonism intrinsic in this molecule. The substitution with a D-Lys^6 at the sixth position provides protection against biologic degradation and, in addition, introduces the only amino group in this molecule (the N-terminus is blocked, pyro-Glu^1). It was then a simple matter to prepare a GnRH dimer with a very short bridge length (about 12 Å) between the antagonist molecules (Fig. 20). This could then be used almost like a male-male plumbing fitting to change the specificity of a antibody initially directed against the antagonist. It is possible then to prepare a molecule which is a derivatized antibody having a GnRH antagonist dimer at either F_{ab} arm. This compound when applied to cells, has considerable efficacy as an agonist. This strange event, i.e. the conversion of a GnRH antagonist to an

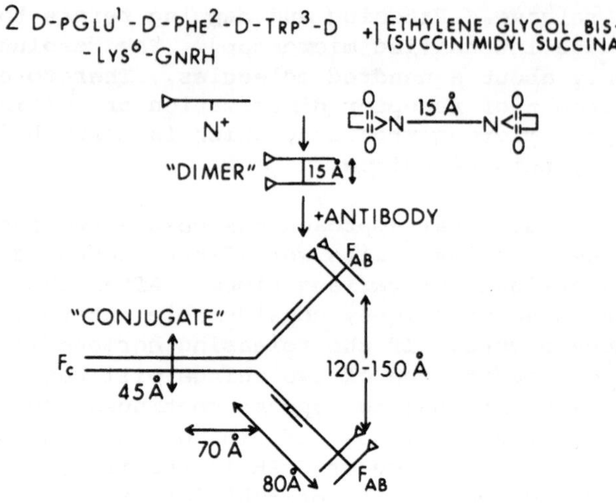

Figure 20. Synthesis of antibody conjugate. Two GnRH antagonist molecules are crosslinked by (lysyl) epsilon aminos. Further incubation with a cross-reactive antibody results in antagonists being separated by 120-150 Å.

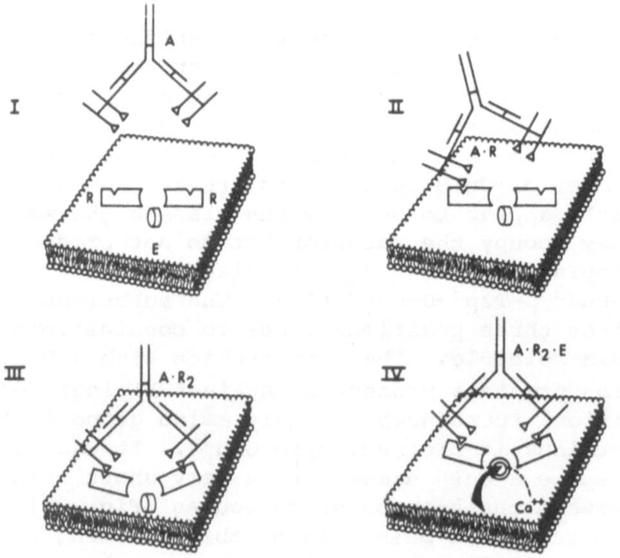

Figure 21. Model showing crosslinking (microaggregation) of GnRH receptors by antibody conjugate described in Figure 20 and text.

agonist as a result of its dimerization, was a confusing result. In a number of human disease states antibodies have been identified which crosslink receptors and consequently provide agonist efficacy. Because of these observations, receptor-receptor interactions were considered in the present situation.

Indeed, when a papain or reduced-pepsin cleavage product of the antibody (i.e. univalent "antibody") is coupled with the dimer, we now have a pure antagonist. The antibody alone has no agonist efficacy and consequently the inescapable conclusion appeared to be that receptor-receptor interactions, that is, the dimerization of receptors, could stimulate the response system. A model for what might be occurring is presented in Fig. 21. An antagonist then might be a compound which could occupy the receptor, but, because of its inability to promote receptor-receptor dimerization, would then behave antagonistically. When one takes an antagonist and confers upon it the ability to cross-link receptors, we are now able to see agonist efficacy. It was also possible to demonstrate that the efficacy of the agonist in this system shared much in common with the authentic native molecule of GnRH. Both, for example, are inhibited by calmodulin antagonists. Both, additionally, require extracellular calcium. It was therefore presumed that the mechanism by which the receptor dimerization event was able to provide agonist efficacy was very much similar to that which was provided by the native molecule (that is, GnRH). It was also possible to use this technique to potentiate the action of a GnRH agonist (D-Lys^6-GnRH). This compound is a biologically stable compound because of the D-amino acid^6 substitution, and, additionally, has the amino group for substitution to prepare dimers. Following preparation of the agonist dimer, it was possible to show that when it was administered to cells at a ED_{10} dose, its efficacy could be super-potentiated by addition of antibody, suggesting, then, that the agonist was able to occupy receptors and then at the appropriate concentrations was able to be cross-linked by antibodies to that molecule.

Recently, computer simulations (15) were prepared for this model. If we assume that two receptors are able to come together about a previously closed calcium ion channel and if these two receptors are able to stimulate opening of the ion channel, an equilibrium model can be built. Such a model, interestingly enough, fits the data within approximately 5% over 5 dose logs.

RECEPTOR MEDIATED ACTIONS OF THE RELEASING HORMONE

Gonadotropin Release

Ca^{2+} while clearly fulfills the requirements of a second messenger (dealt with previously: 16,17), the steps which follow its mobilization remain unclear. A likely candidate for the intracellular receptor is calmodulin, which redistributes inside pituitary cells following treatment with GnRH. GnRH provokes calmodulin disappearance in the cytosolic fraction and appearance in the plasma membrane fraction (18). The constitutive expression of calmodulin in these cells suggests that the redistribution may actually reflect translocation within the cells.

A related observation is that calmodulin inhibitors (19), some of which are highly specific (20), block GnRH stimulated LH release in the same potency order as they bind calmodulin. Thus, a role for calmodulin in this system appears reasonable. Although we are uncertain of the action of calmodulin once occupied with calcium, a number of possibilities have been described previously (18).

Desensitization

In addition to LH release, receptor occupancy (by an agonist) leads to desensitization (that is, refractoriness of the cells as a result of prior administration of GnRH, 21). This process has some fundamental differences with the release process. It can be shown, for example, that desensitization, unlike the gonadotropin releasing process, is not calcium dependent. Advantage was taken of a technique for growing pituitary cells on beads (22). This provides a good model system for kinetic studies. It was possible to demonstrate conditions which led to desensitization following a physiological dose of GnRH. The question remained, then, whether this reduced efficacy was a result of LH depletion from the cells or whether it was a true receptor-mediated sort of desensitization (i.e. receptor depleted population). In order to answer this question in a very direct manner, responsiveness of the cells following administration of ionophore A23187 was measured. As mentioned above, calcium behaves as a second messenger in this system; therefore, ionophore A23187, which allows calcium to freely enter the cell, behaves as a secretagogue (22). It was possible to show then that if A23187 was first given to cells, then washed out and GnRH given in the second administration, that the cells did have the potential to respond fully to this challenge, suggesting that LH depletion was not the explanation for this reduced sensitivity. This also suggested that secretion and desensitization may be mediated by fundamentally different processes in this system.

In order to probe this question further, advantage was taken of the fact that extracellular calcium is an absolute requisite for GnRH stimulated LH response from these cells (23). In these studies, calcium was first removed from outside the cells, GnRH was then added and the receptor was occupied under a condition (diminished extracellular calcium) which did not lead to gonadotropin release. Here we have a condition in which the receptor is occupied but gonadotropin is not released from the cells because of the low extracellular calcium. GnRH was then removed and calcium added back. Surprisingly, we found cells so treated to be desensitized. Thus, a result of occupancy is desensitization whether or not release of LH occurs. This suggests, in addition, that the release system and the desensitization system are mediated by chemically fundamentally different means. It further could be seen that, while LH release has an absolute requirement for calcium, desensitization appears not to be a calcium-mediated event. It could also be seen that GnRH antagonist alone did not lead to desensitization. Thus, simple receptor occupancy did not result in desensitization. Occupancy had to be by an agonist in order for desensitization to occur. Therefore, in comparing desensitization with the release process we find that the release process has an absolute requirement for calcium while desensitization does not. We find that both systems require occupancy by an agonist; an antagonist is not satisfactory. It was, at this point, desirable to see if the dimerized antagonist could provide desensitization. Indeed, it was able to do so (24); suggesting then that there is a slightly more complicated and branched mechanism of response of this system, which will be described below.

<u>Biphasic Regulation of the Receptor</u>

Pituitary cell cultures were used to examine the effect of GnRH and other treatments on the GnRH receptor (25). GnRH occupancy of its receptor promotes an initial decrease, then increase in receptor numbers but not affinity ($=3.0 \pm 0.6 \times 10^9$ M^{-1}). Occupancy of the receptor by an antagonist is not in itself sufficient to evoke down- or up-regulation and blocks these actions of GnRH. Up-regulation, but not down-regulation, can be blocked by depletion of extracellular Ca^{2+} or by the presence of the Ca^{2+} ion channel blocker D600 (methoxyverapamil).

Additional evidence that up-regulation is a Ca^{2+}-mediated process comes from the observation that ionophore A23187 and veratridine, which mobilize extracellular Ca^{2+} by acting at loci other than the GnRH receptor, both stimulate LH release and provoke increases in GnRH receptor number without the initial drop in receptor numbers seen in response to the releasing hormone. Indeed, the enhancement of receptor number appears to be independent of LH release since this action persists (unlike release, 22) when releasing hormone is washed out. Moreover, low concentrations of both A23187 and veratridine were capable of stimulating up-regulation while LH release was not evoked (25,26). At higher concentrations of ionophore a smaller increase in receptors was noted, suggesting a biphasic action of Ca^{2+}. A regulatory role for Ca^{2+} in gene expression is consistent with another report (27) implicating such an action at low concentrations (ED_{50} about 100 μM).

The observation that up-regulation is uncoupled from LH release makes unlikely the possibility up-regulation is mediated by receptors which may be on secretion granules. Additionally, unlike desensitization, up-regulation appears to be dependent on both protein and RNA synthesis, as low concentrations of cycloheximide and actinomycin D block the latter process.

Both down- and up-regulation are provoked by receptor microaggregation since a GnRH antagonist, which alone provokes neither process, becomes active when the ability to dimerize receptors is conferred upon it. It appears likely that such actions are mediated by the ability of this conjugate to crosslink GnRH receptors and mimic GnRH actions. The requirement of gonadotropin release, receptor regulation and regulation of cell responsiveness is shown below in Table 1.

While it is attractive to consider that a relationship exists between receptor number and cell responsiveness the precise relationships remains to be established, some workers arguing for such a relation (29-31) and others arguing against one (32,33). The present study suggest that during the period of receptor recovery (5-10 h), when the cells are clearly refractory to GnRH (33), receptor number and cell responses are clearly uncoupled. Following short term exposure, when the effect of LH depletion is minimized, down-regulation and desensitization clearly appear to have some components in common.

Domains Associated with the GnRH Receptor

While it has not yet been shown that GnRH itself stimulates receptor microaggregation as a component of its mechanism of action, the observation that a GnRH antagonist can be converted to an agonist (as described above) suggests that it may be convenient to consider that there are two functional domains associated with the GnRH molecule. One of these is required for recognition of the molecule by the active site of the receptor ("R" site), and the other is necessary for activation of microaggregation ("M" site). An agonist possesses both sites. An antagonist in this scheme possesses an R site, (thus binding somewhat similarly to an agonist, which appears to be the case, 34) but not an M site. It becomes an agonist when it is (artifically) conferred with the ability to crosslink receptors. While a compound lacking both sites would not be either a receptor agonist or an antagonist, one could imagine that compounds with M sites but no R sites could be biologically significant. Such compounds might lack specificity but could activate the system by provoking microaggregation. Compounds which restrict the movement of the GnRH receptor to a small domain (and thus might enhance the chances of random microaggregation) are an example of a compound of this type. A related type of compound might have a specificity component conferred upon it by recognition of a site other than the active site (i.e. that which recognizes the GnRH molecule). An example of this type of molecule would be an antibody

Table 1. Requirements of gonadotropin release, receptor regulation, and regulation of gonadotrope responses. While desensitization and down-regulation share much in common, this table should not be taken to suggest that they are conclusively manifestations of the same process.

	LH Release	Desensitization and Down-Regulation	Up-Regulation
Evoked By:			
Antagonist	No	No	No
Agonist	Yes	Yes	Yes
Microaggregation	Yes	Yes	Yes
↑Intracellular Ca^{2+}	Yes	No	Yes
Requires:			
Time	0-3 h	0-3 h	5-10 h
Protein Synthesis	No	No	Yes
↑Intracellular Ca^{2+}	Yes	No	Yes

developed against the GnRH receptor. Such specific anti-receptor antibodies clearly stimulate other hormone receptors.

Considerable evidence exists which suggests that the R and M sites correspond to definite physical domains of the GnRH molecule: pGlu^1-His^2-Trp^3-Ser^4-Tyr^5-Gly^6-Leu^7-Arg^8-Pro^9-Gly^{10}-NH_2. It was initially observed that deletion of the His^2 (i.e. des-His^2-GnRH) resulted in a molecule which bound to the GnRH receptor (albeit with lower affinity) but which had no LH releasing activity. This molecule first demonstrated the potential of synthesizing GnRH analogs which behaved as antagonists.

Further studies (35) identified the His^2 and, later, Trp^3 as sites which could be substituted without total loss of receptor binding activity but with loss of the ability to evoke LH release (receptor level competitive antagonists). Substitutions in this position (His^2-Trp^3) then allow the molecule to be recognized by the receptor (R site) but not activate the effector (likely M site). Thus the His^2-Trp^3 region likely corresponds to the M site.

Conformational analysis of the GnRH molecule suggests that the least energy state favors close association of the N- and C-termini (perhaps something like the letter C). Deletion of p-Glu^1 or even opening the pyro-Glu ring results in dramatic loss of binding affinity. Substitutions at the Gly^{10} position such as replacement with an ethylamide group results, when coupled with a D-amino acid in the sixth position, in considerably enhanced receptor binding affinity. Interestingly, except for this "substituted 10" derivative, peptides with less than 10 amino acids have not been identified which bind with appreciable affinity. This observation may emphasize the importance of the 1-10 amino acids in receptor recognition; this site is likely the R site.

CONCLUSION

The available data support a model shown in Figure 22 in which GnRH-receptor microaggregation is the last step in common to a branched pathway. This event evokes at least four physiological actions attributed to the releasing hormone: LH release, receptor down-regulation, desensitization, and receptor up-regulation. Down-regulation and desensitization, on one hand, appear to be Ca^{2+} independent while gonadotropin release and GnRH receptor up-regulation are Ca^{2+}-mediated actions. (This work was supported by HD13220, RCDA HD00337 and the Mellon Foundation.)

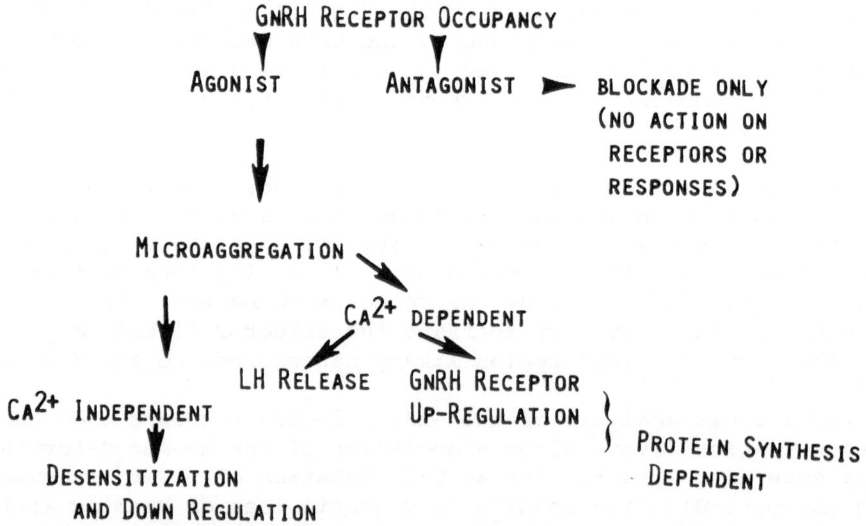

Figure 22. Integrated model showing roles of receptor occupancy and microaggregation, Ca^{2+}, and synthetic events in regulation of receptors, LH release, and cell responsiveness.

REFERENCES

1. R.N. Clayton, R.A. Shakespear, J.A. Duncan, and J.C. Marshall, Radioiodinated nondegradable GnRH analogs: new probes for the investigation of pituitary GnRH receptors. Endocrinol. 105: 1369, (1979).
2. R.N. Clayton, Preparation of radiolabeled neuroendocrine peptides. in: "Methods in Enzymology: Neuroendocrine Peptides," P.M. Conn, ed., Academic Press, in press (1983).
3. J. Marian, R. Cooper, and P.M. Conn, Regulation of the rat pituitary GnRH-receptor. Mol. Pharmacol. 19:399, (1981).
4. R.T. Savoy-Moore, N.B. Schwartz, J.A. Duncan, and J.C. Marshall, Pituitary gonadotropin-releasing hormone receptors during the rat estrous cycle. Science 209:942, (1980).
5. R.N. Clayton, A.R. Solano, M. Garcia-Vela, M.L. Dufau, and K.J. Catt, Regulation of pituitary receptors for GnRH during the rat estrous cycle. Endocrinol. 106:699, (1980).
6. J. Marian, and P.M. Conn, Subcellular localization of the receptor for gonadotropin-releasing hormone in pituitary and ovarian tissue. Endocrinol. 112:104 (1983).
7. P.M. Conn, D.C. Rogers, and S.G. Seay, Structure-function relationships of calcium ion channel antagonists at the pituitary gonadotrope, Endocrinol. in press, (1983).
8. E. Hazum, P. Cuatrecasas, J. Marian, and P.M. Conn, Receptor-mediated internalization of fluorescent gonadotropin releasing hormone by pituitary gonadotropes. Proc. Natl. Acad. Sci. 77: 6692, (1980).
9. Z. Naor, A. Atlas, R.N. Clayton, D.S. Forman, A. Amsterdam, and K.J. Catt, Interaction of fluorescent GnRH with receptors in pituitary cells. J. Biol. Chem. 256:3049, (1981).
10. L. Jennes, W.E. Stumpf, and P.M. Conn, Intracellular pathways of electron opaque GnRH-derivatives bound by cultured gonadotropes. Endocrinol. in press, (1983).
11. P.M. Conn, R.G. Smith, and D.C. Rogers, Stimulation of pituitary release does not require internalization of gonadotropin releasing hormone. J. Biol. Chem. 256:1098, (1981).
12. P.M. Conn, and E. Hazum, LH release and GnRH-receptor internalization: independent actions of GnRH. Endocrinol. 109:2040, (1981).
13. P.M. Conn, D.C. Rogers, J.M. Stewart, J. Neidel, and T. Sheffield, Conversion of a gonadotropin releasing hormone antagonist to an agonist: Implication for a receptor microaggregate as the functional unit for signal transduction. Nature 296:653, (1982).
14. P.M. Conn, D.C. Rogers, and R. McNeil, Potency enhancement of a GnRH agonist: GnRH-receptor microaggregation stimulates gonadotropin release. Endocrinol. 111:335, (1982).
15. J.J. Blum, and P.M. Conn, Gonadotropin releasing hormone stimulation of luteinizing hormone: A ligand-receptor-effect model for receptor mediated responses. Proc. Natl. Acad. Sci. USA,

79:7307, (1982).

16. P.M. Conn, J. Marian, M. McMillian, J.E. Stern, D.C. Rogers, M. Hamby, A. Penna, and E. Grant, Gonadotropin releasing hormone action in the pituitary: A three step mechanism. Endo. Rev. 2:174 (1981).
17. P.M. Conn, Molecular mechanism of gonadotropin releasing hormone action. in: "Biochemical Actions of the Hormones," vol. 11, G. Litwack, ed., Academic Press, in press (1983).
18. P.M. Conn, J. Chafouleas, D. Rogers, and A.R. Means, Gonadotropin releasing hormone stimulates calmodulin redistribution in the rat pituitary. Nature 292:264, (1981).
19. P.M. Conn, D.C. Rogers, and T. Sheffield, Inhibition of gonadotropin releasing hormone stimulated luteinizing hormone release by pimozide: evidence for a site of action after calcium mobilization. Endocrinology 109:1122, (1981).
20. P.M. Conn, M.D. Bates, D.C. Rogers, S.G. Seay, and W.A. Smith, GnRH-receptor-effector-response coupling in the pituitary gonadotrope: A Ca^{2+} mediated system. in: "Role of Drugs and Electrolytes in Hormonogenesis," K. Fotherby, S.B. Pal, eds., Walter de Gruyter and Company, New York, in press, (1983).
21. W.A. Smith, and P.M. Conn, GnRH-mediated desensitization of the pituitary gonadotrope is not calcium dependent, Endocrinol. 112:408, (1983).
22. P.M. Conn, D.C. Rogers, and F.S. Sandhu, Alteration of intracellular calcium level stimulates gonadotropin release from cultured rat pituitary cells. Endocrinol. 105:1122, (1979).
23. J. Marian, and P.M. Conn, GnRH stimulation of cultured pituitary cells requires calcium. Mol. Pharmacol. 16:196 (1979).
24. W.A. Smith, and P.M. Conn, Microaggregation of the GnRH-receptor stimulates gonadotrope desensitization, Endocrinol., in press.
25. P.M. Conn, D.C. Rogers, and S.G. Seay, Biphasic regulation of the GnRH receptor by receptor microaggregation and intracellular Ca^{2+} levels, Mol. Pharmacol., in press, (1983).
26. P.M. Conn, and D.C. Rogers, Gonadotropin release from pituitary cultures following activation of endogenous ion channels, Endocrinol. 107:2133, (1980).
27. B.A. White, L.R. Bauerie, and F.C. Bancroft, Calcium specifically stimulates prolactin synthesis and messenger RNA sequences in GH_3 cells. J. Biol. Chem. 256:5942, (1981).
28. L.A. Sternberger, and J.P. Petrali, Quantitative immunocytochemistry of pituitary receptors for luteinizing hormone-releasing hormone. Cell Tiss. Res. 162:141, (1975).
29. M. Zilberstein, H. Zakut, and Z. Naor. Coincidence of down-regulation and desensitization in pituitary gonadotrophs stimulated by gonadotropin releasing hormone. Life Sci. 32:663, (1983).
30. T.M. Nett, M.E. Crowder, G.E. Moss, and T.M. Duello, GnRH-receptor interaction. V. Down-regulation of pituitary receptors for GnRH in ovariectomized ewes by infusion of homologous

hormone. Biol. Reprod. 24:1145, (1981).

31. D. Heber, R. Dodson, C. Stoskopf, M. Peterson, and R.S. Swerdloff, Pituitary desensitization and the regulation of pituitary gonadotropin-releasing hormone (GnRH) receptors following chronic administration of a superactive GnRH analog and testosterone. Life Sci. 30:2301, (1982).
32. G. Keri, K. Nikolics, I. Teplan, and J. Molnar, Desensitization of luteinizing hormone release in cultured pituitary cells by gonadotropin-releasing hormone. Mol. Cell. Endocrinol. 30:109, (1983).
33. M.A. Smith, M.H. Perrin, and W.W. Vale, Desensitization of cultured pituitary cells to gonadotropin-releasing hormone: evidence for a post-receptor mechanism. Mol. Cell. Endocrinol. 30:85, (1983).
34. M.H. Perrin, Y. Haas, J.E. Rivier, and W.W. Vale, Gonadotropin-releasing hormone binding to rat anterior pituitary membrane homogenates. Mol. Pharmacol. 23:44, (1983).
35. A.V. Schally, Current status of antagonistic analogs of LH-RH as a contraceptive method in the female. Res. Frontiers in Fert. Reg. 2:1, (1983).

RECENT PROGRESS IN CELL BIOLOGY OF SECRETORY PROCESS IN ANTERIOR PITUITARY CELLS

Andrée Tixier-Vidal and Claude Tougard

Groupe de Neuroendocrinologie Cellulaire

Collège de France, 75231 Paris Cedex 05

INTRODUCTION

The present concept on the secretory process in anterior pituitary cells is based on a large body of informations among which the contribution of electron microscopy was primordial. This concept follows the model formerly proposed by Palade for the exocrine pancreas and thereafter applied to several endocrine cells which secrete various polypeptides or proteins (see rev. Palade, 1975, Farquhar, 1981, Farquhar and Palade, 1981). There is now a complete agreement that the secretory process is a dynamic phenomenon which involves two main components : 1. the secretory protein itself which undergoes an intracellular transit before to be exported and 2. the intracellular membranes which limit the intracellular compartments where the secretory material is sequestered during its intracellular transit. These two aspects of the secretory process will be briefly reviewed.

Intracellular transit of AP hormones

The morphological basis of the successive steps of the intracellular route of A.P. hormones were first provided for prolactin (PRL) cells by Smith and Farquhar (1966). Their schema has then been extended to other AP cells and has received experimental supports from multidisciplinary approaches. At present, a general schema which integrates the available informations related to AP cells as well as to other protein secreting cells can be proposed (see rev. Tixier-Vidal et al, 1984). The anterior pituitary hormones are synthesized as prehormones on polysomes which attach to the membrane of the rough endoplasmic reticulum (RER) through insertion of an hydrophobic sequence, the "signal sequence", located at the NH2 end of the nascent protein (Lingappa et al, 1977). This is followed by vectorial discharge of the protein into the lumen of the RER and enzymatic cleavage of the signal sequence. This gives rise to the authentic hormones (PRL, growth hormone) or to prohormones (precursor of ACTH and β-endorphin) (Gumbiner and Kelly, 1981) or to the apoproteins of glycoprotein hormone subunits (LH, FSH, TSH)(Counis et al, this book). These proteins then undergo a transit through the Golgi zone where they are concentrated and packaged into membrane bound secretory granules which represent storage organelles. During that intracisternal transit the proteins undergo chemical modifications which occur in a sequential manner during its progression. They consist of glycosylations, enzymatic cleavages, conformational changes, covalent associations, leading to mature hormones. At the same time are added components of secretory granule matrix, such as sulfated macromolecules (Zanini et al, 1980, Moore et al, 1983). The secretory granules are then either released by exocytosis or degraded by crinophagy, which implies their fusion with lysosomes. A pivotal step in this intracisternal transit of AP hormones is located at the Golgi zone. Indeed several other proteins, such as lysosomal hydrolases, are simultaneously synthesized and translocated into the RER. Therefore a mechanism of sorting should exist to direct the proteins towards their final site of insertion, secretory granules or lysosomes (see rev. Farquhar and Palade, 1981, Tartakoff, 1980). Although the mechanism of sorting of AP hormones is still unknown, it obviously occurs in the Golgi zone.

Membrane compartments

The intracellular compartmentalization of the hormone and its transfer from one compartment to another involve a primordial role of the membranes which limit these compartments. Most of the informations available on that question have been obtained on cells other than AP cells. Studies on the composition (lipids, proteins, enzymes) of RER and Golgi membranes indicate that each of these membrane compartments displays a biochemical specificity (see rev. Farquhar and Palade, 1981, Tartakoff, 1980). As concerns the molecular mechanisms by which they interact with secretory proteins, important progress have been recently achieved concerning RER membranes, with the discovery of the docking protein, an integral membrane protein which serves as a receptor for the signal sequence through a cytoplasmic signal recognition particle (Walter and Blobel, 1982, Meyer et al, 1982). In contrast, the mechanisms involved in the function of Golgi membranes are still hypothetical (Farquhar and Palase, 1981, Tartakoff, 1980).

In the case of AP cells most informations on membrane compartments have been obtained by a morphological approach.

Moreover most studies have been concerned with the endocytotic pathway, that is the centripetal route (see rev. Farquhar, 1981, Tixier-Vidal et al, 1984). In contrast, the centrifuge route which is involved in the exportation of AP hormones as well as of plasma membrane proteins has received so far less attention because of the lack of specific probes. Based exclusively on electron microscope observations, it is admitted that the intracellular transit of secretory proteins from the RER to the Golgi zone and from the Golgi zone to the secretory granules is exerted through vesicles which bud from one organelle and fuse with the other as first postulated by Palade for the exocrine pancreas (see rev. 1975). To maintain a biochemical specificity along the successive compartments of the endoplasmic reticulum one have therefore to imagine the existence of mechanisms of regulation which are still hypothetical (see rev. Farquhar and Palade, 1981). Further progress in their analysis first requires a better characterization of membrane components in AP cells.

The present chapter reviews recent studies performed in our laboratory on rat prolactin cells in culture, using new immunological probes and methods, applied to intact cells, with the hope to answer, at least partially, to some critical questions : how is regulated the intracellular transit of PRL ? Are they biochemical or immunological specificity of membrane compartments in PRL cells ? Is there a membrane flow concomitantly to the transit of PRL ?

Two models of PRL cells in culture have been used in these studies : clonal, tumor derived GH3 cells and primary cultures of dispersed normal male rat AP cells prepared as previously described (Tougard et al, 1980). The first model represents an homogenous population of secretory cells which differ from normal cells by the small number and size of secretory granules. The second one retains more or less the in vivo ability to store secretory granules but also the cellular heterogeneity of the AP tissue. In order to modulate the cell secretory activity we used as physiological stimulus the neuropeptide thyroliberin (TRH) or, as inhibitor, monensin, a monovalent carboxylic ionophore which is known to block the intracellular transport of secretory products at the level of the Golgi apparatus (Tartakoff and Vassali, 1978).

INTRACELLULAR TRANSIT OF PROLACTIN

The intracellular transit of PRL could be followed at the electron microscope level thanks to recent improvement of immunoelectron microscope methods which permitted to localize PRL not only in the secretory granules but also along the successive compartments of the endoplasmic reticulum that is the RER cisternae and several subcompartments of the Golgi zone (Tougard et al, 1980, 1982).

PRL immunostaining in cells cultured in basal conditions

In normal PRL cells PRL was visualized in the totality of the RER cisternae, including the perinuclear cisternae. In the Golgi zone the outer saccules were the most strongly stained, whereas the intensity of the staining decreased up to the innermost saccules. Moreover in the core of the Golgi zone some short cisternae as well as several vesicles were also strongly stained. No clear evidence for the existence of immunoreactive transition vesicles between the RER and the cis-face of the Golgi stacks could be found. In all of the positive Golgi cisternae the reaction product was associated to the inner face of the smooth membranes instead of filling the lumen of RER cisternae, which strongly suggests a role of membrane in the concentration procedure and addition of sulfated components before packaging of secretory granules (Zanini et al, 1980).

In GH3 cells which possess very few or even no secretory granules, PRL could be visualized in same compartments as in normal PRL cells, that is RER cisternae, Golgi cisternae, small vesicles and the ground cytoplasm. In the Golgi stacks,the intensity of the staining decreased from the cis-face to the trans-face, as found in normal PRL cells. Similarly to normal PRL cells, the intensity of the immunostaining greatly varied from one compartment to another and from one cell to another, indicating a functional heterogeneity of both the compartments and the cells. Of interest is the fact that in GH3 cells the Golgi cisternae were immunostained, more or less, in all cells, whereas the RER cisternae were unstained in 40% of the cells. This suggests that PRL stays a longer time in the Golgi zone than in the RER cisternae (fig. 1 A).

PRL immunostaining in GH3 cells exposed to thyroliberin (TRH)

It was previously found that TRH exerts a biphasic effect on PRL secretion by GH3 cells : a rapid stimulation of the release of an intracellular PRL store (within the first hour) and a delayed effect on PRL synthesis (starting at 2 hours)(Dannies and Tashjian, 1976, Morin et al, 1975, Morin and Tixier-Vidal, 1983). This could be correlated with a progressive disappearance of PRL reaction product in the RER cisternae and in the Golgi saccules for the first hour. At the same time numerous small vesicles lined with a slight rim of deposit appeared in the Golgi zone and beneath the plasma membrane (fig. 1 B). At 2 hours of exposure onward, a progressive and massive reloading of PRL occurred in both compartments of the endoplasmic reticulum ; this was prevented by simultaneous exposure to cycloheximide. However the cytoplasmic staining persisted in any case in the presence of TRH or cycloheximide or both suggesting that it represents an unmobilizable compartment (Tougard et al, 1982).

PRL immunostaining in GH3 cells exposed to monensin

Monensin (1 µm) was found to decrease strongly the basal release of prolactin in the culture medium, but did not prevent the TRH induced stimulation of PRL release for any preincubation period (Tougard et al, 1983 a). Concomitantly monensin alone induced a rapid dilation of Golgi cisternae into large vacuoles which were lined on their innerface with PRL reaction product (fig. 1 C). Exposure to TRH of monensin pretreated cells induced the formation of small vesicles loaded with PRL, some of them seemed to be derived by budding from the large vacuoles (Tougard et al, 1983 a)(fig. 1 D).

Functional correlates of PRL immunostaining : existence of several intracellular PRL compartments

The subcellular localization of PRL reveals that PRL is distributed into several intracellular compartments which are limited by membranes : the RER cisternae, the Golgi cisternae and the secretory granules (particularly in normal PRL cells). This brings a direct verification of the present concept on the intracellular transit of secretory proteins. In addition, these observations reveal, particularly in GH3 cells, a vesicular compartment which may be the main route for PRL release in those cells. TRH accelerates the transit of PRL along the endoplasmic reticulum and induces the formation of vesicles which serve as carrier for PRL release. Moreover the effects of monensin suggest the existence of two routes for the release of PRL from the Golgi zone, a monensin sensitive one for basal release and a monensin insensitive one for TRH induced release. This implies a functional subcompartmentalization of the Golgi zone. Taken together these findings indicate that the intracellular compartments of PRL are interconnected and that they may be separately regulated in response to modulators of the secretory activity.

These conclusions are consistent with the results of pulse-chase experiments performed on both GH3 cells and normal PRL cells in culture (Morin and Tixier-Vidal, 1983, Morin et al, submitted). Indeed, the decay of the specific activity of PRL released into the medium during the chase period does not follow a first order kinetics indicating that PRL is distributed into several compartments, at least two, which differ by their turnover time. Moreover it was found in both PRL cell types that newly synthesized PRL is preferentially released in basal condition whereas older PRL molecules are preferentially released under exposure to TRH. According to Walker and Farquhar (1980) this is the result of a functional heterogeneity among normal PRL cells. This does not exclude the existence of several intracellular routes as suggested by our immunocytochemical studies in GH3 cells. The possibility of several pathways arising from different levels of the Golgi

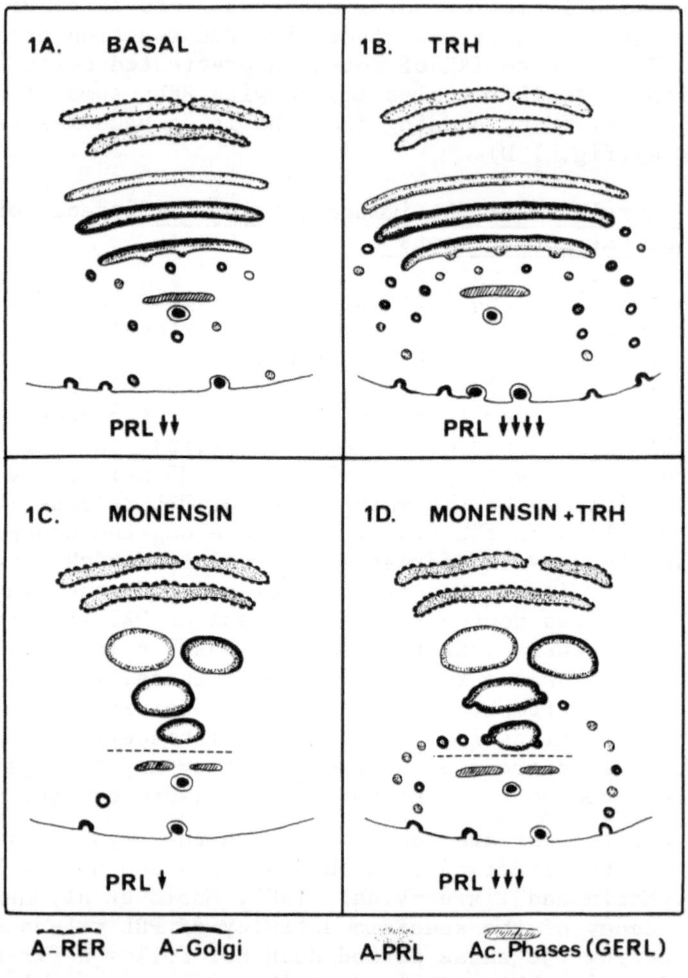

Fig. 1. Schematic representation of the subcellular localizations of the immunostainings with A-RER, A-Golgi and A-PRL, respectively, in GH3 cells, in relation with the secretory activity.

zone has also been proposed from biochemical studies recently performed on the AtT20 pituitary cell line which secretes ACTH and its unprocessed precursor (Gumbiner and Kelly, 1981, 1982, Moore et al, 1983). Such a possibility will be again considered in the light of recent results obtained using membrane immunological probes in same models of PRL cells in culture as above used.

IMMUNOLOGICAL SPECIFICITY OF MEMBRANE COMPARTMENTS

Until recently, data concerning the biochemistry of RER membranes and Golgi membranes were lacking for PRL cells, as well as many other endocrine cells. Decisive progress have been made possible with the availability of specific antibodies directed against several membrane polypeptides of the dog pancreas (29,000, 58,000, 66,000 and 91,000 MW)(A-RER) and against one membrane polypeptide (135,000 MW) of rat liver Golgi light fraction (A-Golgi), recently prepared by Louvard et al (1982). These immunological probes have been applied to intact cells using same procedures as for PRL subcellular localization (Tougard et al, 1983 b).

Subcellular localization of membrane antigens in PRL cells cultured in basal conditions

The A-RER exclusively stained the totality of the membranes of the RER, inclusing those of the perinuclear cisternae, in both normal PRL cells and GH3 cells. Same structures were previously stained with A-PRL, but in contrast to PRL reaction product, the staining with A-RER was exclusively located on membranes. Other cellular structures were totally negative (fig. 1).

The A-Golgi labelled similar structures in both normal PRL cells and GH3 cells. In the Golgi zone it labelled the medial saccules of the stacks with a decreasing intensity up to the inner saccules of the trans-face, as well as some short cisternae in the core of the Golgi zone. In addition, the A-Golgi also labeled small vesicles in the Golgi zone and beneath the plasma membrane, the membranes of lysosome-like structures and in some cells discrete patches of the plasma membrane. In contrast the secretory granule membranes were never stained excepted a very slight staining at the level of a very few segregating granules (Tougard et al, 1983b) (fig. 1 A). It should be mentioned that such subcellular localizations of a Golgi membrane antigen were not restricted to PRL cells. Other glandular cells in the primary culture, particularly gonadotropic cells, displayed same pictures, as illustrated on fig. 2.

As compared to the subcellular localization of PRL, there is only a partial overlapping. Indeed the A-Golgi does not label

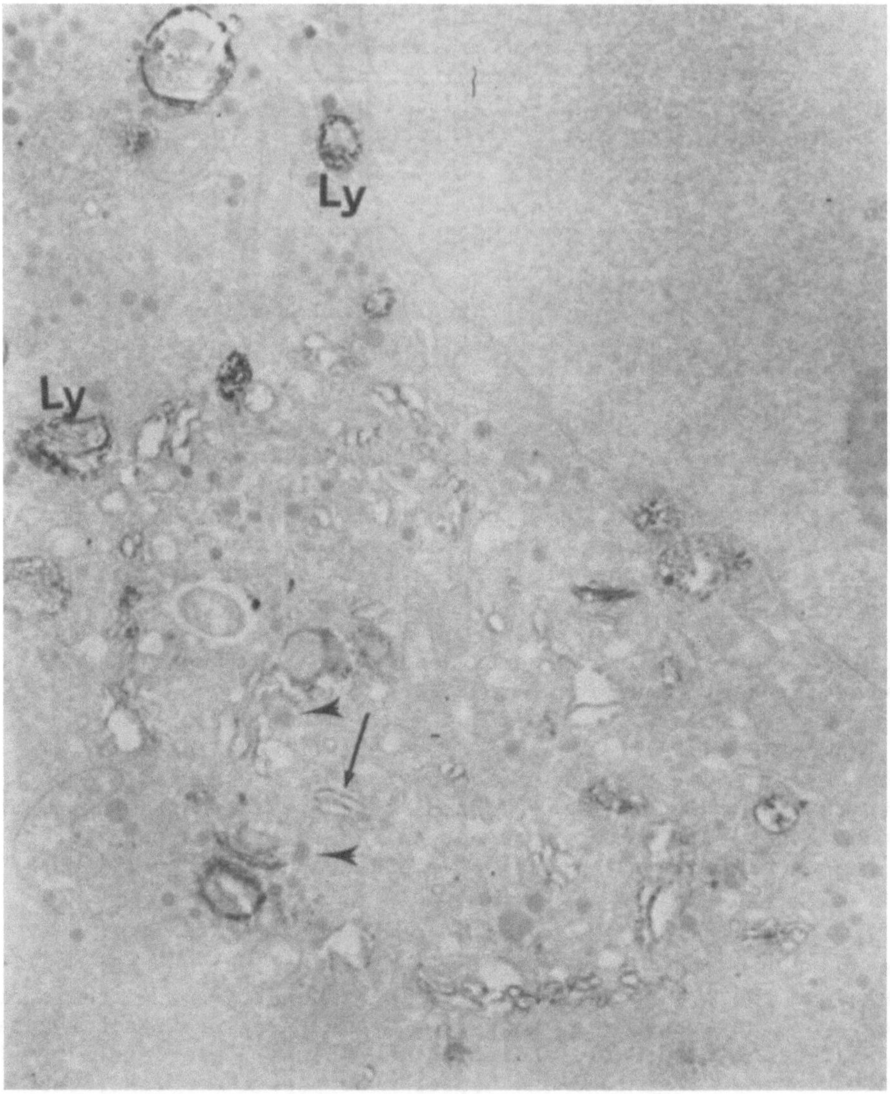

Fig.2. Immunostaining with the A-Golgi of the Golgi zone of a putative gonadotropic cell, identified by its two classes of rounded secretory granules in a primary culture of normal rat anterior pituitary cells. The A-Golgi labels two medial saccules in the peripheral stacks as well as several short cisternae in the center of the Golgi zone (⟶) as well as lysosome-like (Ly) structures which are particularly abundant in cultured gonadotropes (Tougard et al, 1977). The membrane of the secretory granules is unstained, excepted a discrete deposit around two segregating secretory granules (➤). Some vesicles in the core of the Golgi zone are also slightly labeled. The other structures are unstained (x13000).

the membrane of some structures which were filled with PRL : the outer Golgi saccules and the secretory granules. Inversely, it stained the membranes of lysosomes, which are other Golgi derived organelles specialized for the segregation of acid hydrolases, another protein which is known to transit through the Golgi zone. Thus, these observations disclose a biochemical or immunological heterogeneity of Golgi membranes in PRL cells and they demonstrate a relative independance of the traffic of membrane components and of secretory protein respectively.

Subcellular localization of Golgi membrane antigen in relation with the secretory activity

The subcellular distribution of A-RER staining was not affected, neither by TRH nor by monensin, in both normal PRL cells and GH3 cells. In contrast, important modifications of the organization of A-Golgi labeled membranes could be observed (Tougard et al, 1983 b).

TRH treatment for one hour induced in both types of PRL cells an extension of the positive Golgi cisternae and an increase in number of small positive vesicles in the Golgi zone as well as in the cytoplasm beneath the plasma membrane. Some of these vesicles were seen fusing with the plasma membrane which resulted in an increased insertion of Golgi labeled patches in the plasma membrane (Tougard et al, 1983 b)(fig. 1 B). Such modifications of A-Golgi labeled membranes strongly suggest that TRH treatment induced a flow of membrane from the Golgi zone towards the plasma membrane, through the formation of small vesicles. This is consistent with the above described effect of TRH on the formation of PRL loaded vesicles. However it remained to be precised whether same vesicles are labeled with A-Golgi and loaded with PRL.

In monensin treated PRL cells, the A-Golgi labeled most, although not all, of the dilated vacuoles of the Golgi zone. In GH3 cells it also labeled some short elongated cisternae which were previously seen positive for acid phosphatase reaction (Tougard et al, 1983 a). In addition, monensin did not prevent the increase in number of A-Golgi labeled vesicles in response to TRH (Tougard et al, 1983 b)(fig. 1 C, 1 D). These observations provide a direct evidence for a specific site of action of monensin on a large subcompartment of the Golgi zone in PRL cells. They are consistent with the above reviewed effects of monensin alone or in conjonction with TRH on the subcellular distribution of PRL, although it would be of interest to localize simultaneously both antigens, since some monensin induced vacuoles were not labeled with the A-Golgi whereas most of them contained PRL. In any case these observations indicate again an immunological and functional subcompartmentalization of the Golgi zone. They argue in favor of the existence of several routes for membranes arising from the Golgi zone.

CONCLUSION

This chapter has reviewed recent findings obtained using immunological probes specific for a secretory protein (PRL) on the one hand and for membrane antigens (A-RER, A-Golgi), on the other hand, in order to perform a dissection of the secretory process in intact PRL cells in culture (normal PRL cells and GH3 cells).

The visualization of PRL at all steps of its intracellular transit provides a morphological support to the existence of several intracellular compartments of PRL, already put forward by biochemical studies. Moreover it brings new insights into the understanding of the secretory process : 1. the role of small vesicles arising from a subcompartment of the Golgi zone for the stimulated release of PRL has been revealed, 2. the possibility of an independent regulation of PRL compartments has been suggested as well as the existence of several routes arising from Golgi subcompartments for PRL release.

The visualization of membrane antigens specific for RER and Golgi membranes respectively has provided the first evidence for an immunological specificity of membrane domains along the endoplasmic reticulum as well as for an immunological subcompartmentalization of the Golgi zone. These data together with those obtained from PRL localization reveal a partial independence between the traffic of membrane components and the intracellular transit of PRL. Thus they illustrate the role of the Golgi zone in the sorting of secretory products (PRL, acid hydrolases) and of membrane proteins which are directed to their final site of insertion, secretory granules, lysosomes, plasma membrane.

Such an immunological approach still requires further progress, in particular technical progress for the simultaneous localization of several antigens in same sections as well as development of new immunological probes for other membrane compartments (lysosome, secretory granule membrane). This approach is certainly one of the most promizing for the future in the analysis of the secretory process in AP cells.

REFERENCES

Dannies, P.S., and Tashjian, A.H. Jr., 1976, Release and synthesis of prolactin by rat pituitary cell strains are regulated independently by thyrotropin-releasing hormone, Nature, 261: 707-710.

Farquhar, M.G., 1981, Membrane recycling in secretory cells : implications for traffic of products and specialized membranes within the Golgi complex. In : "Basic Mechanisms of Cellular Secretion. Methods in Cell Biology", A. Hand and C. Oliver, eds, Academic Press, N.Y., vol. 23, pp. 339-427.

Farquhar, M.G., and Palade, G., 1981, The Golgi apparatus (complex) - (1954-1981)- from artifact to center stage. J. Cell Biol. , 91: 77s-103s.

Gumbiner, B., and Kelly, R.B., 1981, Secretory granules of an anterior pituitary cell line, AtT-20, contain only mature forms of corticotropin and beta-lipotropin, Proc. Natl. Acad. Sci. USA, 78: 318-322.

Gumbiner, B., and Kelly, R.B., 1982, Two distinct intracellular pathways transport secretory and membrane glycoproteins to the surface of pituitary tumor cells. Cell, 28: 51-59.

Lingappa, V.R., Devillers-Thiery, A., and Blobel, G., 1977, Nascent prehormones are intermediates in the biosynthesis of authentic bovine pituitary growth hormone and prolactin, Proc. Natl. Acad. Sci., USA, 74: 2432-2436.

Louvard, D., Reggio, H., and Warren, G., 1982, Antibodies to the Golgi complex and the rough endoplasmic reticulum, J. Cell Biol. 92: 92-107.

Meyer, D.I., Louvard, D., and Dobberstein, B., 1982, Characterization of molecules involved in protein translocation using a specific antibody, J. Cell Biol., 92: 579-583.

Moore, H.P., Gumbiner, B., and Kelly, R.B., 1983, A subclass of proteins and sulfated macromolecules secreted by AtT-20 (Mouse Pituitary Tumor) cells is sorted with adrenocorticotropin into dense secretory granules. J. Cell Biol., 97: 810-817.

Morin, A., Tixier-Vidal, A., Gourdji, D., Kerdelhué, B., and Grouselle, D., 1975, Effect of thyrotrope releasing hormone (TRH) on prolactin turnover in culture. Mol. Cell. Endocrinol., 3: 351-373.

Morin, A., and Tixier-Vidal, A., 1983, Effect of thyroliberin on prolactin turnover in two systems of rat prolactin cells : clonal GH3B6 cells and normal anterior pituitary cells in primary cultures. In : "Multihormonal Regulations in Neuroendocrine cells", A. Tixier-Vidal, and Ph. Richard, eds, INSERM, p. 593.

Palade, G.E., 1975, Intracellular aspects of the process of protein synthesis, Science, Wash.D.C., 189:347-358.

Smith, R.E., and Farquhar, M.G., 1966, Lysosome function in the regulation of the secretory process in cells of the anterior pituitary gland, J. Cell Biol., 31: 319-349.

Tartakoff, A.M., 1980, The Golgi complex : crossroads for vesicular traffic. Internat. Rev. Exper. Pathol., 22: 227-250.

Tartakoff, A., and Vassali, P., 1978, Comparative studies of intracellular transport of secretory proteins. J. Cell Biol. 79: 694-707.

Tixier-Vidal, A., Tougard, C., and Morin, A., 1984, Cellular events involved in transport, storage and release of pituitary hormones. In : "Pituitary Hyperfunction : Physiopathology and Clinical Aspects", G.M. Molinatti, F. Carmanini, and E.E. Muller, eds, Raven Press, N.Y., pp. 71-83.

Tougard, C., Tixier-Vidal, A., Kerdelhué, B., and Jutisz, M., 1977, Etude immunocytochimique de l'évolution des cellules gonadotropes dans des cultures primaires de cellules antéhypophysaires de rat. Aspects quantitatifs et ultrastructuraux, Biol. Cell., 28: 251-260.

Tougard, C., Picart, R., and Tixier-Vidal, A., 1980, Electron-microscopic cytochemical studies on the secretory process in rat prolactin cells in primary culture, Am. J. Anat., 158: 471-490.

Tougard, C., Picart, R., and Tixier-Vidal, A., 1982, Immunocytochemical localization of prolactin in the endoplasmic reticulum of GH3 cells. Variations in response to thyroliberin. Biol. Cell, 43: 89-102.

Tougard, C., Picart, R., Morin, A., and Tixier-Vidal, A., 1983 a, Effect of monensin on secretory pathway in GH3 prolactin cells. A cytochemical study. J. Histochem. Cytochem., 31: 745-754.

Tougard, C., Louvard, D., Picart, R., and Tixier-Vidal, A., 1983 b, The rough endoplasmic reticulum and the Golgi apparatus visualized using specific antibodies in normal and tumoral prolactin cells in culture. J. Cell Biol., 96: 1197-1207.

Walker, A.M., and Farquhar, M.G., 1980, Preferential release of newly synthesized prolactin granules is the result of functional heterogeneity among mammotrophs, Endocrinology, 107: 1095-1104.

Walter, P., and Blobel, G., 1982, Signal recognition particle contains a 7 S RNA essential for protein translocation across the endoplasmic reticulum, Nature, 299: 691-698.

Zanini, A., Gianattasio, G., Nussdorfer, G., Margolis, R.K., Margolis, R.U., and Meldolesi, J., 1980, Molecular organization of prolactin granules. II. Characterization of glycosaminoglycans and glycoproteins of the bovine prolactin matrix. J. Cell Biol., 86: 260-272.

ACKNOWLEDGEMENTS

We acknowledge the skillful technical assistance of Mrs. Renée Picart , Mr. Pennarun and Miss A. Bayon for their help in the preparation of this manuscript. Works from our laboratory presented in this review have been suppported by grants from CNRS (ER 89).

FLUIDITY OF GONADOTROPIN STORAGE IN CYCLING FEMALE RATS

Gwen V. Childs

Department of Anatomy
The University of Texas Medical Branch
Galveston, Texas

INTRODUCTION

Hormone storage in gonadotropes has been the subject of a debate for over a decade. The cytophysiological evidence for non-parallel secretion of LH and FSH agreed with the early morphological evidence that there were two types of gonadotropes (Farquhar and Rinehart, 1954; Barnes, 1962). Workers postulated that each might be responsible for the secretion of only one gonadotropin (Barnes, 1962; Kurosumi and Oota, 1968). However, in the early 1970's, immunocytochemists showed that both hormones were present in most of the same cells (Nakane, 1970; Phifer, *et al.*, 1972; Tougard, *et al.*, 1971, 1973). Furthermore, the two morphological cell types could not be distinguished on the basis of their gonadotropin content. During the subsequent 10 years a number of studies reported results from serially sectioned pituitaries that included a variety of species. These results showed collectively that most gonadotropes contained both hormones (multihormonal) (Tixier-Vidal *et al.*, 1975; Herbert, 1975; Batten and Hopkins, 1978; Hopkins *et al.*, 1981; Smith and Keefer, 1982). A number of these studies also reported that there were cells that contained only FSH or LH (monohormonal) (Nakane, 1970; Moriarty, 1976a, b; Pelletier, *et al.*, 1976; El Etreby and Fath El Bab, 1977; Purandare, *et al.*, 1978; Bugnon *et al.*, 1977; Dacheux, 1978, 1980; Girod, *et al.*, 1980; Fellmann *et al.*, 1982; Jansen, 1982; Childs, *et al.*, 1980, 1981, 1982a, b, 1983a, b; Dada, *et al.*, 1983).

Most of the above studies were dependent on the use of matched serial fields or cells from serial sections stained for LH or FSH that were either 4-7 μm (paraffin), 1 μm (plastic) or 70-80 nm (ultrathin). The matching process has several potential pitfalls that might affect both the accuracy of the collection process and the interpretation.

These pitfalls are as follows: first, the thicker (4-7 μm) sections may not allow the study of joint storage in cells that are less than 10 μm in diameter. In recent studies of pituitary cell fractions separated by centrifugal elutriation, we showed that a significant number of monohormonal gonadotropes are 7-10 μm in diameter (Childs, *et al.*, 1983b). If this population is eliminated because 7 μm serial sections are used, the data will favor the large multihormonal gonadotropes. Our survey of the literature shows that most studies that use thick paraffin sections report the predominence of multihormonal gonadotropes in the cell population.

Second, the use of 4-7 μm sections prevents the analysis of serial fields through the nucleus which averages 4-5 μm in diameter. Clusters of monohormonal gonadotropes along blood vessels may include adjacent LH and FSH cells. Matching the nuclear region of the LH cell with a process from an FSH cell would cause its misidentification as an LH-FSH cell.

The thinner sections present a sampling problem (Childs, 1983). While they allow multiple sections through the nuclear region of the same cell, their use may prevent the detection of storage of LH and FSH in separate regions especially if they are too widely spaced to allow the serial fields to be matched accurately. For example, if multihormonal gonadotropes dissociate their stores to peripheral processes during a particular physiological state, the cells may be counted erroneously among the monohormonal cell population.

Having recognized this third pitfall in the interpretation of our serial section data, we decided to approach the studies of the female rat gonadotrope differently (Childs, *et al.*, 1983c, d; Childs, 1983). In the immunocytochemical study by Nakane, (1970), the gonadotropes were defined with double peroxidase stains that were applied to the same sections. Each was distinguished with a different colored peroxidase substrate. During the past year, we developed double stains for a biotinylated analog of GnRH and LH or FSH (Childs, *et al.*, 1983d), or LH and FSH (Childs, 1983) and since then have applied them to whole pituitary cells in a 2-3 day monolayer and to 1 μm plastic sections. Not only do they allow the detection of dissociated storage of LH and FSH in the same cell (Childs, 1983), they also allow one to determine the percentages of total gonadotropes in a monolayer, section, or cell fraction. The purpose of this report is to describe the fluidity of the gonadotropin storage pattern in cycling female rats. In the study, data is obtained from serial 1 μm sections from rats in different stages of the estrous cycle, double stains from gonadotrope-enriched elutriation fractions, and double stains applied to GnRH stimulated monolayer cells. There is good correlation between the results from the different preparative techniques. Furthermore, the results show non-parallel changes in the LH and FSH cell populations during the estrous cycle and demonstrate the dynamic nature of the gonadotrope population.

MATERIALS AND METHODS

The methods for these studies are published in our recent papers. Briefly, the ultrathin or 1 μm thick plastic embedded (Araldite 6005 or glycol methacrylate - GMA) sections were stained with the avidin-biotin peroxidase (ABC) complex as described previously (Childs and Unabia, 1982,a, b; Childs, *et al.*,1981, 1982, 1983a, e). The double stains were applied with PAP complexes or ABC complexes as described in our recent papers (Childs, *et al.*, 1983c; Childs, 1983). The first peroxidase substrate in the double stain was nickel intensified diaminobenzidine (black-blue) and the substrate used in the second stain was either diaminobenzidine (DAB-amber) or 3-amino-9-ethyl-carbazole (AEC-red).

The antisera dilutions employed in all post-embedding stains included the following range of working dilutions: 1:10,000-1:50,000 anti bovine LH-beta (from J.G. Pierce) or 1:1000-1:8000 anti human FSH beta (A.F. Parlowe, NIADDK). One-ten μg of rat FSH were added to each ml of diluted anti bLH-beta; similar amounts of LH were added to the diluted anti FSH-beta.

The pre-embedding stains on the monolayer cells were more sensitive because there were more antigens available for the reaction in the whole cells. Therefore, the antisera dilution ranges were 1:40,000-1:60,000 anti LH-beta, or 1:50,000-1:70,000 anti FSH-beta.

The care and handling of the cycling female rats is described elsewhere (Childs, *et al.*, 1983e). In the early studies, the stage of the cycle was determined by vaginal smears and uterine histology; later groups included serum LH and FSH measurements by radioimmunoassay. Different fixatives or embedding media are tested in this study including 1% and 2% glutaraldehyde, 4% p-formaldehyde, or picric acid formaldehyde as fixatives and either Araldite 6005 or GMA as embedding media. The GMA is water soluble and can be polymerized at 4°C under UV light whereas the Araldite is infiltrated with organic solvents after dehydration and is polymerized at 60°C.

The fixatives for the pre-embedding double stains were either 1% or 2.5% glutaraldehyde. One-half of the monolayer was dehydrated after staining and mounted in permount; the other half was mounted in water and glycerol to test the effect of the mounting process on the stains (Childs, *et al.*, 1983c, d; Childs, 1983).

Thus, the above preparative tests were built into this study to determine if any step in the tissue processing affects either the antigens or the stains. Additional controls for the specificity of the methods were run and are described elsewhere (Childs, *et al.*, 1981, 1982, 1983a, b). These include absorption of the diluted antisera with 10-100 ng of homologous antigen prior to staining which resulted in the abolishment of the stain. Controls for the double

Table 1. Percentage of Gonotropes in the cell population (±SEM)

	Diestrus	Proestrus	Estrus
	Female Rats		
LH	9.0 ± 0.4%	7.7 ± 0.4%[a]	9.5 ± 0.3%
FSH	8.5 ± 0.3%[a]	12.7 ± 1.0%	11.0 ± 0.4%
	Male Rats[c]		
	Intact	24 hour post castration	
LH	10.0 ± 0.4%	14 ± 2%[b]	
FSH	8.8 ± 0.4%	15 ± 1%[b]	

[a]Values significantly different from those in the other two stages.
[b]Values significantly different from intact.
[c]Data taken from Childs, *et al.*, 1982b.

Table 2. Hormone Storage in Serially sectioned gonadotropes (±SEM)

	Diestrus	Proestrus	Estrus
	Female Rats		
LH only	46 ± 8%	29 ± 5%[a]	53 ± 8%
FSH only	15 ± 5%[a]	32 ± 10%	31 ± 8%
LH-FSH	37 ± 5%	40 ± 6%	15 ± 4%[a]
	Male Rats[c]		
	Intact	12-24 hour post castration	
LH only	17 ± 3%	4 ± 1% [b]	
FSH only	13 ± 2%	4 ± 1% [b]	
LH-FSH	70 ± 3.6%	92 ± 3% [b]	

Values significantly different from the other two stages.
Values significantly different from intact.
Taken from Childs, *et al.*, 1982b.

Table 3. Volume and area measurements of gonadotropes (±SEM)

Females	Volume (Vv)	Area (μm)
Diestrus		
LH	3.8 ± 0.1%	131 ± 4
FSH	3.8 ± 0.3%	158 ± 10
Proestrus		
LH	3.3 ± 0.1%[b]	134 ± 3
FSH	5.0 ± 0.2%[b]	170 ± 5[b]
Estrus		
LH	4.0 ± 0.1%	142 ± 4[b]
FSH	4.4 ± 0.1%	148 ± 4
Males		
LH	5.0 ± 0.2%	133 ± 12
FSH	5.1 ± 0.1%	179 ± 14

[a]As reported in Childs, *et al.*, 1981, 1983a.
[b]Significantly different from the other two stages.

Figures 1a and b illustrate a field from an estrous rat showing abundant monohormonal FSH cells. The opposite pattern is shown in the field illustrated in Figures 2a and b, from another estrous rat. LH cells are abundant; FSH cells and multihormonal cells are scarce. Finally, the larger size of the monohormonal FSH cell in the proestrous rat is shown in Figure 3a and b which illustrates two large FSH cells near two smaller monohormonal LH cells. Figure 4 shows an electron micrograph illustrating a multihormonal gonadotrope from a proestrous rat.

Application of double stains to elutriation fractions

In a separate series of experiments we applied the double stains to sections of cell fractions and the initial cell suspension (ICS) from the elutriation project (Hyde, *et al.*,1982; Childs, *et al.*, 1983b). These fractions were obtained from six separate experiments each of which included cells from 50 or more female rats in mixed cycles. Table 4 lists the percentage of each gonadotroph cell type in each fraction identified by the average diameter of the cells therein (Childs, *et al.*, 1983b). As was described in the previous studies in which serial fields were examined, the majority of the multihormonal gonadotropes were found in the fractions containing cells 13-14 μm diameter. Large monohormonal FSH cells were found in the wash fraction (16 μm average diameter). Most of the gonadotropes that eluted in fractions with 7-12 μm cells were monohormonal. Note that the use of the double stain shows a greater enrichment of fraction 6A.

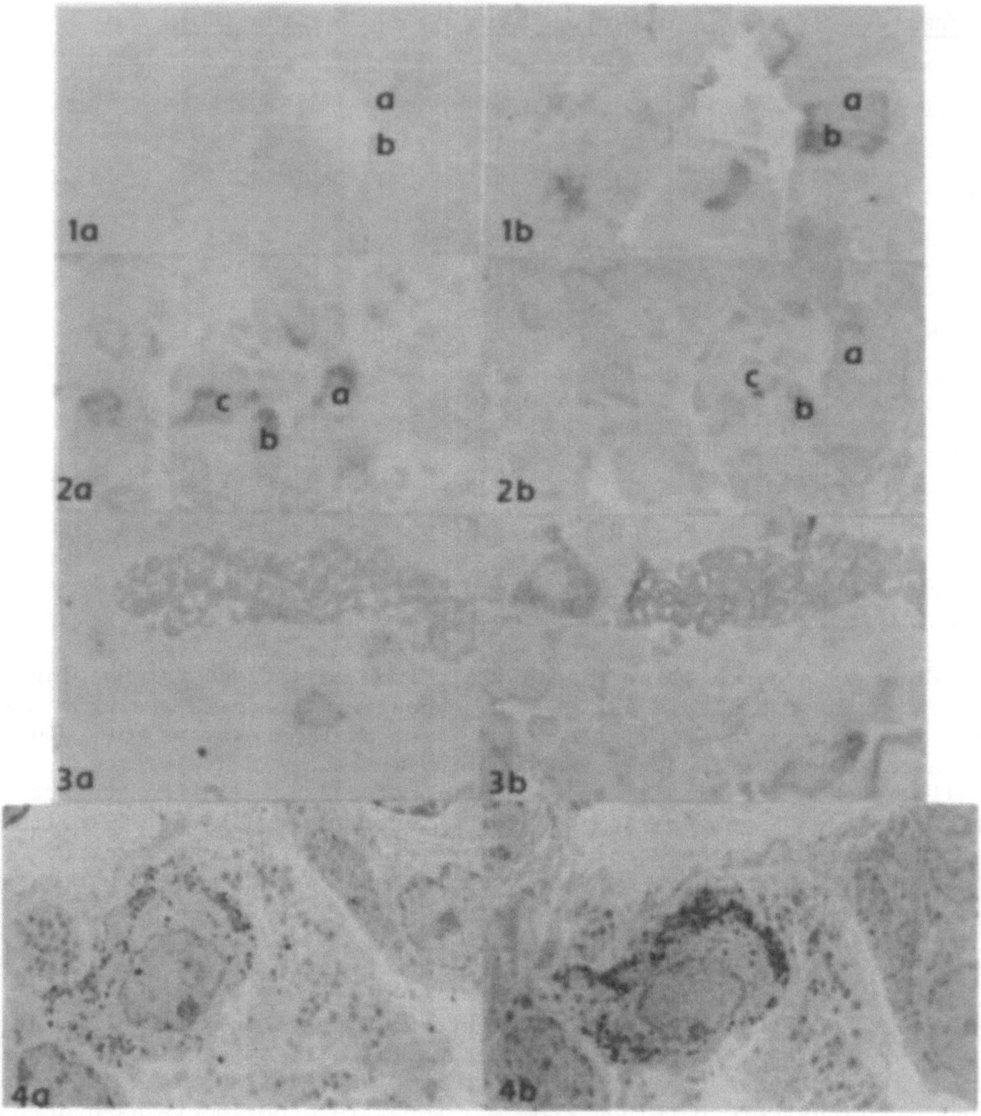

Figures 1-4

Serial fields from cycling female rats; 1-4a stained for LHβ; 1-4b stained for FSHβ. Figs. 1 and 2 show monohormonal cells from estrous rats. Fig. 3 illustrates large monohormonal FSH cells (a,b) from proestrous rat. Fig. 4, serial electron micrographs showing multihormonal cell from proestrous rat. Magnification X 700 Figures 1-3; X 4000 - Fig. 4.

stains included the omission of pituitary antisera in either the first or second sequence proving that both stains were dependent upon two complete staining sequences. All double stains included duplicate or quadruplicate fields for each experimental group in which the sequence of the stains was alternated (Childs, *et al.*, 1983d; Childs, 1983).

As described in our previous studies of the male rat, (Childs, *et al.*, 1980, 1981, 1982a, b, 1983a) the morphometric analysis included a calculation of percentage of LH or FSH cells in the cell population and a calculation of the percent of the volume occupied by LH or FSH gonadotropes. This latter measurement evaluates changes both in cell size and number and is called Vv. Average gonadotrope area was estimated by determining the fraction of the ocular grid area occupied by individual gonadotropes; the ocular grid is calibrated and the area fraction, or $\bar{a}$, is calculated by multiplying the Vv x 10,000 μm^2 (grid area) divided by the number of gonadotropes under the grid.

Individual measurements were averaged for each experimental group and the variance tested by a one way analysis. If the F ratio was significant ($p<.05$), the individual means were compared with the use of Duncan's Multiple Range test at the 1% and 5% levels.

RESULTS

Changes in gonadotropin storage during the estrous cycle.

There were significant differences in percentage, Vv, and area with the stage of the estrous cycle. Table 1 shows that the lowest percentage of LH cells was found in proestrous rats whereas the lowest percentage of FSH cells was found in the diestrous group. These low percentages were significantly different from the higher values found in each population during the other two stages. Table 1 also lists the percentages of gonadotropes in male rats, as reported in previous studies (Childs, *et al.*, 1982b).

Table 2 shows that the drop in percentages of LH cells at proestrus and FSH cells at diestrus correlates with the serial sections. A significant drop in percentage of monohormonal LH cells is seen at proestus and a drop in percentage of monohormonal FSH cells is seen at diestrus. The serial sections also show that the estrus rat has fewer multihormonal gonadotropes and the highest percentage of LH cells.

There were non-parallel changes in Vv and area in the LH and FSH cell population as well (Table 3). The largest LH cells were found in the estrous rat (142 μm) and the largest FSH cells were found in the proestrous rat (170 μm). Both area measurements were significantly different from the areas in the other two groups. The smallest LH cell Vv was found in the proestrous group and the smallest FSH cell Vv was in the diestrous group.

Table 4. Size vs Hormone Storage in Elutriation Fractions Doublestained for LH and FSH

Diameter	7 μm	8 μm	10.5 μm	11.5 μm	12.4 μm	14 μm	16 μm
% LH only	13	8	57	29	43	5.5	0
% FSH only	86	92	32	34	20	5.5	73
% LH-FSH	0	0	10	36	37	89	26
% Total Gon.	4	6	12	22	44	55	25

Fractions collected from 5 experiments including <50 female rats/ experiment; mixed cycles (Hyde, *et al.*,1982).

Initial Cell suspension contained 57% LH-FSH cells; 18% LH cells and 22% FSH cells. Total gonadotropes in ICS-14 ± 1.4%

Average diameter of LH cells = 13.5 μm; of FSH cells = 12.4 μm.

Figures 5 and 6 illustrate a field showing monohormonal and multihormonal gonadotropes from fractions 4 and 6A. Figure 7 shows multihormonal gonadotropes from fraction 7. These do not stain as intensely for either hormone as do those in the lower fractions and they appear dusty brown. In the lower fractions, one can discriminate the black from the amber or red, even in the same cells (Figure 6).

Analysis of Gonadotropin Storage in vitro

Thus far we have illustrated the heterogeneity of the gonadotrope population in the cycling female rat and the non-parallel size, volume and area changes seen during the estrous cycle. The serial sections and double stains suggest that the gonadotrope population includes a number of monohormonal cells.

To examine this population further, we applied the double stains to fixed whole pituitary cells to determine if one could detect monohormonal cells. As reported recently, (Childs, 1983) the double stains demonstrated the presence of 57% LH-FSH cells and 20-22% monohormonal gonadotropes in a 3 day cell monolayer. These values are comparable to the percentages calculated for the initial cell suspension either from serial 1 μm sections (Childs, *et al.*, 1983b), or from double stains.

The next question related to the dynamics of synthesis and storage of the 2 hormones. Will monohormonal cells become multihormonal following GnRH stimulation? We stimulated 3 day monolayers with either biotinylated [D-Lys^6] GnRH or the unlabeled analog and stained for GnRH and LH or FSH; or for LH and FSH. As reported in previous studies, stimulation for up to 4 hours did not alter the percentage of total gonadotropes which was 15.9% (Childs, *et al.*, 1983c, d; Childs, 1983). Furthermore, the percentage of cells labeled with biotinylated GnRH

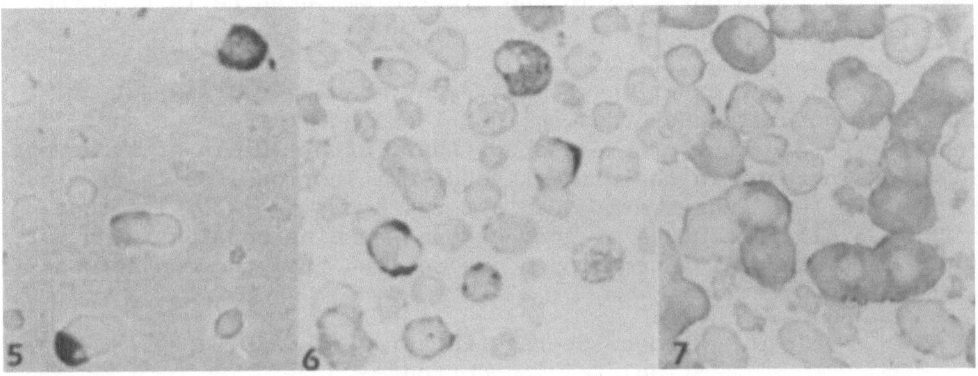

Figures 5-7 show cells from elutriation fractions double stained for LH (black) and FSH (amber). Fig. 5 illustrates monohormonal LH cells (a,b) and an FSH cell (c) from fraction 4 (average diameter 11.5 μm). Fig. 6 illustrates multihormonal cells (a-e); and monohormonal FSH (f) or LH (g) cells from fraction 6A (12.4 m average diameter). Note compartmentalization of gonadotropins in multihormonal cells. Fig. 7 shows multihormonal (dusty brown) gonadotropes from fraction 7 (14 μm diameter) Magnification X 640.

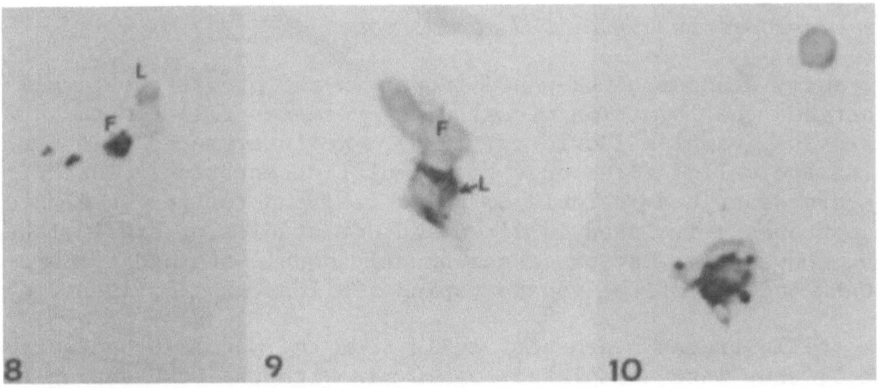

Figures 8-10 illustrate monolayers stimulated with GnRH and double stained for LH and FSH. Figure 8 was stimulated with 0.1 nM [D-Lys^6] GnRH and stained for FSH (black) and LH (orange). Cell has 2 processes, each containing a different gonadotropin. Figures 9 and 10 were stimulated for 4 h with 0.1 nM [D-Lys^6] GnRH and stained for LH (black) and FSH (orange). A multihormonal cell is seen in Fig. 9, next to a monohormonal FSH cell. Fig. 10 shows a stimulated monohormonal LH cell (a) and a round monohormonal FSH cell (b). Magnification X 600.

was 16% after 3-30 minutes of exposure. These percentages are not different from those obtained in the plastic embedded cells from the initial cell suspensions (14 ± 1.2%).

In six separate experiments, the 3 day monolayer cells were treated with unlabeled GnRH analog (0.5-1 nM) and then fixed and stained for LH and FSH. Table 5 shows that, after 30 min of treatment, there is an increase in the percentage of multihormonal cells from 57% to 67%. A further increase is seen after 4 hours to 74%. The fact that the overall percentage of gonadotropes remains constant, suggests that the multihormonal gonadotropes are derived from the monohormonal population.

Table 5. Hormone Storage Patterns in GnRH Stimulated Gonadotropes[a]

Time	0	10 min	30 min	60 min	4 hr
% LH only	21 ± 2%	19 ± 9%	22 ± 1%	17 ± 2%[b]	14 ± 3%[b]
% FSH only	22 ± 3%	19 ± 5%	15 ± 6%	15 ± 3%[b]	12 ± 3%[b]
% LH-FSH	57 ± 2%	62 ± 4%	63 ± 6%	68 ± 2%[b]	74 ± 3%[b]
% Total Gon.	17 ± 1%	22 ± 5%	22 ± 4%	18 ± 2%	18 ± 2%

[a]Three day monolayer cells were stimulated with [D-Lys^6] GnRH--10^{-10}M for 10 min to 4 hr as described in Childs, *et al.*, 1983c, d.
[b]Values significantly different from those at time 0 (± SEM).

Morphological changes in stimulated gonadotropes

In our early studies of LH gonadotropes in the proestrous female rat, we described the formation of cellular processes filled with stained secretion granules (Moriarty, 1976). We interpreted this morphology as the cellular response to stimulated secretion. In the cell monolayers described in Table 5, processes, and ruffles developed in the gonadotropes stimulated in vitro and our studies of biotinylated GnRH binding showed that the processes usually double-stained for biotinylated GnRH and one of the gonadotropins (Childs, *et al.*, 1983c, d).

Figure 8 illustrates a group of cells from the monolayers described in Table 5; they were stimulated for 10 min with the GnRH analog and then fixed and doublestained for FSH and LH. The cells exhibit 2 blebs or processes that are filled with stain. Some of these processes are stained for only one gonadotropin. After 4 hours of stimulation, the multihormonal gonadotropes show a mixed staining pattern (Figure 9). Some areas stain for both hormones while other areas show a clear dissociation of storage sites for LH and FSH. It is evident that a 1 μm (or thinner) serial section through the monohormonal areas might not demonstrate the full storage capacity of the multihormonal cell. The fact that monohormonal cells can be found, even in a stimulated monolayer is illustrated in Figure 10. The LH cell has formed processes as a result of the 4 hour stimulation and is dark blue-black. The FSH cell in this field appears to be unresponsive and remains round. It stains amber-orange.

Figure 11 shows a micrograph of a gonadotrope stimulated for 3 min with biotinylated GnRH, followed by fixation. The GnRH is then localized with avidin-ferritin. Secretion granules fill a process that also contains vesicles that label with the ferritin. This cell illustrates the rapid formation of the process and uptake of the GnRH. It also illustrates that the secretion granules do not contain the GnRH. Our double stains correlate well with these findings and colored photomicrographs can be seen in recent publications (Childs, *et al.*, 1983c, d; Childs, 1983).

The double stains for GnRH and LH or FSH also suggest, that there is a population of monohormonal gonadotropes in the monolayer. In a given double stain, 60-80% of the GnRH labeled cells co-label with one of the gonadotropins. Since the percentage of GnRH labeled cells matches that of the total gonadotrope population, these data suggest that the remaining 20-40% of GnRH labeled cells may contain only the other gonadotropin (Childs, *et al.*, 1983d).

Studies of Different Fixatives and Embedding Media

The population of rat pituitaries that were embedded in water soluble GMA showed identical percentages of LH and FSH cells. The gentler method allowed the use of more dilute antisera. However, the poor preservation of the cells prevented the accurate determination of volume or area. Furthermore, the stain was spread and muddy as if the antigens had diffused outside the cells. Therefore, these data were not included in Tables 1 or 2.

There were no differences in percentage, or size of gonadotropes with the different fixatives. Glutaraldehyde fixation resulted in a weaker stain for FSH,however the cells were as numerous as those fixed in p-formaldehyde. As stated earlier, the pre-embedding stains were 10-20 times more efficient in that they required less concentrated antisera than the post-embedding stains. While these low concentrations were vital to the discrimination of the double stains; our cell counts showed that the LH and FSH cells were as numerous in the monolayers as they are in the intact tissue, or in the initial cell suspensions from 6 elutriation experiments (Tables 1 and 4).

DISCUSSION

These studies were designed to describe the gonadotrope population in the adult female rat with techniques of immunocytochemistry combined with light microscopic morphometry. The counts of stained gonadotropes show that there are 14-16% total gonadotropes in the cell population of normal female rats. These percentages agree with the

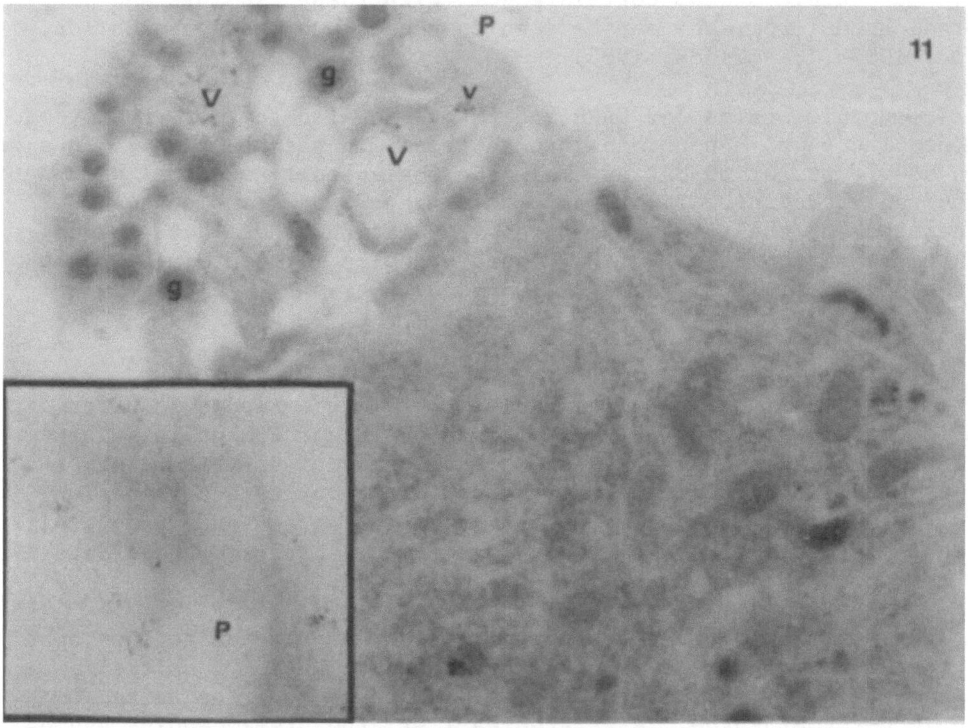

Figure 11 shows a monolayer cell stimulated with 10^{-10}M biotinylated GnRH for 3 min, fixed and then stained with avidin-ferritin. The gonadotrope shows a process (P) that is filled with secretion granules (g) and vacuoles. The ferritin stain shows the biotinylated GnRH in the vacuoles (V), vesicles (v) and not in the secretion granules. Inset shows surface stain on a process 1 min after exposure to the biotinylated GnRH. See Childs *et al.*, 1983 c, d for details of methodology. Magnification X 100,000; inset X 180,000.

values reported by previous workers for the male rat (Fellmann, *et al.*, 1982) and with the percentages of GnRH labeled cells reported by us (Childs, *et al.*, 1983c,d) and others (Naor, *et al.*, 1980). The reliability of these percentages is enhanced by the fact that they were derived from cell populations exposed to different preparative protocols.

Our morphometric studies also show that gonadotropes average 133-170 µm in area. This is also in agreement with measurements of male rat gonadotropes by Fellmann, *et al.*, (1982) who reported a size range of 30-160 µm and Dada, *et al.*, (1983). Our values for the female rat are larger than those reported by Dada, *et al.*, (1983) who show measurements of 100 µm for both LH and FSH cells.

The larger size of the FSH cell population is found in both male and female rats especially the proestrous females. The elutriation data confirm the presence of large monohormonal FSH cells in the wash fraction that average 16 µm in diameter. The data from the cycling female rat suggests that these large FSH cells may be derived from the proestrous rats.

Our area measurements show that LH cells have expanded significantly during estrus. Their failure to show an expansion at proestrus may be due to the rapid loss of stainable LH during the surge and the movement of the LH into small processes that are difficult to detect in the light microscopic fields. The expansion at estrus may correlate with the synthesis of additional LH stores which fill more of the body of the cell.

FSH cells expand most rapidly during proestrus which correlates with the high serum levels that persist until midestrus (Savoy-Moore, *et al.*, 1981; Dada, *et al.*,1983). However, the FSH cells do not degranulate as severely as do the LH cells probably because there is no surge in serum FSH. Therefore, they are easier to identify in the tissue sections. Their reduction in average size during estrus may correlate with the rise in steroids that may reduce secretion and slow further cellular expansion.

The changes in percentages of LH cells during proestrus correlate with their degranulated condition as a result of the LH surge. Electron microscopic studies have demonstrated the presence of poorly granulated LH and FSH cells most of which elute in the fractions with the small cells (Childs, *et al.*, 1983b). These cells are difficult to detect by light microscopy. They may have exhausted their reserves of LH-beta. The return to previous percentages in the estrous rat (9%) suggests that the cells have replenished their stores and can be identified by light microscopy.

The increase in the percentage of FSH cells during proestrus correlates with their stimulated state and probably reflects the fact that the cells are synthesizing sufficient FSH to prevent degranulation. Some degranulated FSH cells are seen in estrous rats.

Our analysis of 1 μm serial sections shows that 37-40% of gonadotropes contain both hormones in the female rat compared with 70% in the male rat. There are changes in the storage pattern with the stage of the estrous cycle. The decrease in percentage of monohormonal LH cells at proestrus suggests that these cells may be primarily responsible for the LH surge. The LH-FSH cells may then respond during estrus. The low percentages of LH-FSH cells at estrus could reflect the secretion of FSH during early estrus; or it could reflect the dissociation of the gonadotropin stores into separate peripheral processes that are impossible to detect accurately in the serial fields. As stated earlier, we are reluctant to match a cellular process with a nucleated area in the serial field recognizing that the two areas could belong to separate, adjacent cells.

A similar drop in percentages of LH-FSH cells was seen in male rat gonadotropes following castration and adrenalectomy or sham adrenalectomy. The latter 2 operations retarded the development of castration cells and decreased the percentage of LH-FSH cells from 92% in the castrate, to 30-40% in the animals exposed to simultaneous, dual operations. This and the estrous cycle data show the fluidity of the gonadotrope cell population. The fact that the percentage of LH-FSH cells increases following castration (70% to 92%) suggests that all gonadotropes are multipotential but that some remain monohormonal until stimulated to synthesize the other gonadotropin. These monohormonal cells may be reserve cells; or, they may have a special set of receptors to facilitate rapid secretion of their gonadotropin, or both.

In order to test the monohormonal cells further, we examined dissociated pituitary cells both after cell fractionation by elutriation, and in a monolayer. The elutriation fractions showed that the monohormonal gonadotropes were most numerous among the cells that were 7-10 μm in diameter. Although these fractions were not enriched with gonadotropes, they contained the highest number of cells. Therefore, the actual numbers of small monohormonal gonadotropes are relatively high. For example, Fraction 4 contained 40-80 million cells/ml and 6% FSH cells or 2.4-5.3 million FSH cells/50 pituitaries or 0.5-1 million small FSH cells/pituitary. In Fraction 6,7 there were 10-18 million cells, and 55% gonadotropes, most of which contained both hormones. This yields 5-10 million multipotential gonadotropes/50 rat pituitaries or 1-2 million/pituitary. Furthermore since there are additional small monohormonal gonadotropes in the lower fractions and Fraction 5, when added together, they may actually outnumber the larger gonadotropes.

Neither Fellmann *et al.*, (1981) nor Dada *et al.*, (1983) report the presence of large monohormonal FSH gonadotropes in their populations. Perhaps this is due to their low numbers. The wash fraction, which is enriched with these cells, contains only 6-13 million cells/ml. Since FSH cells are 20% of this fraction, this yields only 1-2.6 million large FSH cells/50 pituitaries, or 24,000-50,000 per rat. Their presence was detected in the radioimmunoassays of cell fractions by Denef *et al.*, (1978) who reported that the ratio of FSH to LH secretion increased with increasing cell size.

The elutriation data suggests that one might selectively stimulate small and large gonadotropes to learn if there is any difference between populations that are primarily monohormonal and those that are multihormonal. As a prelude to these tests, we developed the preembedding doublestaining methods for use on dissociated cells. We learned that it was possible to detect monohormonal cells in a whole cell preparation. Furthermore, the stains showed that GnRH stimulation affects the pattern of hormone storage in the overall population. There was a significant increase in the percentage of LH-FSH cells after 60 min-4 hr of stimulation with no accompanying changes in the overall percentage of gonadotropes. This suggests that the monohormonal cells are being stimulated to produce the other gonadotropin. The data agree with studies of stimulated 6 day monolayers by Khar *et al.*, (1978) who show significant incorporation of H^3 Proline into cellular and media LH and FSH within 2 hours after stimulation with comparable amounts of GnRH.

The pre-embedding stains also allow the study of fluid changes in hormone storage patterns in gonadotropes stimulated by GnRH. Shortly after stimulation, hormone stores move to the periphery and fill small processes that may develop as a result of the extra membrane added during secretion by exocytosis. There appears to be a regional association between sites of GnRH binding and sites of active secretion of the hormone as if GnRH directed the movement of the gonadotropins. Furthermore, some multihormonal gonadotropes have dissociated the LH and FSH into separate regions and processes of the same cell. This is probably a Golgi complex mediated event and if it occurs *in vivo*, it may add a new mechanism for non-parallel secretion of LH and FSH, and perhaps also serve as a site for separate control of the two hormones.

REFERENCES

Barnes, B.G., 1962, Electron microscopic studies on the secretory cytology of the mouse anterior pituitary. *Endocrinology* , 71:618.

Batten, T.F.C. and Hopkins, C.R., 1978, Discrimination of LH, FSH, TSH and ACTH in dissociated porcine anterior pituitary cells by light and electron microscope immunocytochemistry, *Cell Tiss. Res.*, 192:107.

Bugnon, C., Fellmann, D., Lenys, D., Bloch, B., 1977, Etude cyto-immunologique des cellules gonadotropes et des cellules threotropes de l'adenohypophyse du Rat, *C.R.Soc. Biol.*, 171:907.

Childs, G.V., Ellison, D.G., Garner, L.L., 1980, An immunocytochemist's view of gonadotropin storage in the adult male rat: cytochemical morphological heterogeneity in serially sectioned gonadotropes. *Am. J. Anat.*, 158:397.

Childs, G.V., Ellison, D.G., Foster, L.P., Ramaley, J.A., 1981, Postnatal maturation of gonadotropes in the male rat pituitary, *Endocrinology*, 109:1683.

Childs, G.V., Ellison, D.G., Ramaley, J.A., 1982a, Storage of anterior lobe adrenocorticotropin in corticotropes and a subpopulation of gonadotropes during the stress-nonresponsive period in the neonatal male rat, *Endocrinology*, 110:1676.

Childs, G.V., Ellison, D.G., Lorenzen, J.R., Collins, T.J., and Schwartz, N.B. 1982b, Immunocytochemical studies of gonadotropin storage in developing castration cells, *Endocrinology*, 111:1318.

Childs, G.V., Ellison, D.G., Lorenzen, J.R., Collins, T.J., and Schwartz, N.B., 1983a, Retarded development of castration cells after adrenalectomy or sham-adrenalectomy, *Endocrinology*, 113:166.

Childs, G.V., Hyde, C., Naor, Z., and Catt, K., 1983b, Heterogeneous luteinizing hormone and follicle stimulating hormone storage patterns in subtypes of gonadotropes separated by centrifugal elutriation. *Endocrinology*, 113: in press.

Childs, G.V., Naor, Z., Hazum, E., Tibolt, R., Westlund, K.N. and Hancock, M.B., 1983c, Localization of biotinylated gonadotropin releasing hormone on pituitary monolayer cells with avidin-biotin complexes, *J. Histochem. Cytochem.* 31: in press.

Childs, G.V., Naor, Z., Hazum, E., Tibolt, R. Westlund, K.N. and Hancock, M.B., 1983d, Cytochemical characterization of pituitary target cells for biotinylated gonadotropin releasing hormone. *Peptides*, 4: in press.

Childs, G.V., Hyde, C. and Naor, Z. 1983e, Morphometric analysis of thyrotropes in developing and cycling female rats: studies of intact pituitaries and cell fractions separated by centrifugal elutriation, *Endocrinology*, 113: in press.

Childs, G.V., 1983, Application of dual pre-embedding stains for gonadotropins to pituitary cell monolayers with avidin-biotin (ABC) and peroxidase-antiperoxidase (PAP) complexes: light microscopic studies, *Stain Technology* 58: in press.

Childs, G.V., and Unabia, G., 1982a, The application of the avidin-biotin peroxidase complex (ABC) to the light microscopic localization of pituitary hormones, *J. Histochem. Cytochem.* 30:713.

Childs, G.V., and Unabia, G., 1982b, The application of a rapid avidin peroxidase complex (ABC) technique to the localization of pituitary hormones at the electron microscopic level. *J. Histochem. Cytochem.* 30:1320.

Dacheux, F., 1978, Ultrastructural localization of gonadotropic hormones in the porcine pituitary using the immunoperoxidase technique, *Cell Tiss. Res.*, 191;219.

Dacheux, F., 1980, Ultrastructural localization of LH and FSH in the porcine pituitary. *In, Synthesis and Release of Adenohypophyseal hormones.* M. Jutisz and K.W. McKerns, eds., Plenum Press, p 187.

Dada, M.O., Campbell, G.T., and Blake, C.A., 1983, A quantitative immunocytochemical study of the luteinizing hormone and follicle stimulating hormone cells in the adenohypophysis of adult male rats and adult female rats throughout the estrous cycle. *Endocrinology*, 113:970.

Denef, C., Hautekeete, D., Dewals, R., 1978, Monolayer cultures of gonadotrophs separated by velocity sedimentation: Heterogeneity in response to luteinizing hormone-releasing hormone. *Endocrinology*, 103:736.

El Etreby, M.F., and Fath El Bab, M.R., 1977, Localization of gonadotrophic hormones in the dog pituitary gland. *Cell Tiss. Res.*, 183:167.

Farquhar, M.G., and Rinehart, J.F., 1954, Electron microscope studies of the anterior pituitary of castrated rats, *Endocrinology*, 54:516.

Fellmann, D., Bresson, J.L., Clevequin, M.C., and Bugnon, C., 1982, Quantitative immunocytochemical studies of the gonadotrophs isolated from the pituitary of the male rat. *Cell Tiss. Res.* 224:137.

Girod, C. Dubois, M.P., and Trouillas, J., 1980, Immunohistochemical study of the pars tuberalis of the adenohypophysis in the Monkey, *Macaca irus*, *Cell Tiss. Res.*, 210:191.

Herbert, D.C., 1975, Localization of antisera to LH and FSH in the rat pituitary gland. *Am. J. Anat.* 144:379.

Hyde, C.L., Childs, G., Wahl, L.M., Naor, Z. and Catt, K.J., 1982, Preparation of gonadotropin-enriched cell populations from adult rat pituitary cells by centrifugal elutriation. *Endocrinology*, 111:1421.

Hopkins, C.R., Semoff, S., and Gregory, H., 1981, Regulation of gonadotropin secretion in the anterior pituitary. *Phil. Trans. R. Soc. Lond. B*, 296:73.

Jansen, H.G., 1982, Distribution and Number of gonadotropic cells in the pituitary gland of prepubertal female rats, *J. Endocr.* 94:381.

Khar, A., Debeljuk, L. and Jutisz, M., 1978, Biosynthesis of gonadotropins by rat pituitary cells in culture and in pituitary homogenates: effect of gonadotropin-releasing hormone, *Mol. Cell. Endocrin.* 12:53.

Kurosumi, K. and Oota, Y., 1968, electron microscopy of two types of gonadotrophs in the anterior pituitary of persistent estrous and diestrous rats. *Z. Zellforsch. Mikrosk. Anat.* 85:34.

Moriarty, G.C., 1976a, Immunocytochemistry of the pituitary glycoprotein hormones. *J. Histochem. Cytochem.* 24:846.

Moriarty, G.C., 1976b, Ultrastructural immunocytochemical studies rat pituitary gonadotropes in cycling female rats. *Gunma Symp. Endocrinology*, 13:207.

Nakane, P.K., 1970, Classifications of anterior pituitary cell types with immuno-enzyme histochemistry. *J. Histochem. Cytochem.* 18:9.

Naor, Z., Clayton, R.N., and Catt, K.G., 1980, Characterization of gonadotropin-releasing hormone receptors in cultured rat pituitary cells, *Endocrinology*, 107:1144.

Pelletier, G., Leclerc, R. and Labrie, F., 1976, Identification of gonadotropic cells in the human pituitary by immunoperoxidase techniques, *Mol. Cell. Endocrin.* 6:123.

Phifer, R.F., Midgley, A.R., and Spicer, S.S., 1972, Histology of the human hypophyseal gonadotropin secreting cells. *In: "Gonadotropins"* B.B. Saxena, C.G. Beling, and H.M. Gandy, eds., Wiley-Interscience, New York, p. 9.

Purandare, T. Sar, M. and Stumpf, W.E., 1978, Immunohistochemical localization of FSH and LH in rat pituitary. *Mol. Cell Endocrin.* 10:57.

Savoy-Moore, R.T., Schwartz, N.B., Duncan, J.A., Marshall, J.C., 1981, Pituitary gonadotropin-releasing hormone receptors on proestrus effect of pentobarbitol blockade of ovulation in the rat, *Endocrinology*, 109:1360.

Smith, P.F. and Keefer, D.A., 1982, Immunocytochemical and ultrastructural identification of mitotic cells in the pituitary gland of ovariectomized rats, *J. Reprod. Fert.*, 66:383.

Tixier-Vidal, A., Tougard, C., Kerdelhuè, B., and Jutisz, M., 1975, Light and electron microscopic studies on immunocytochemical localization of gonadotropic hormones in the rat pituitary gland with antisera against ovine FSH, LH, LHα and LHβ, *Ann. N.Y. Acad. Sci.*, 254:433.

Tougard, C., Kerdelhuè, M.B., Tixier-Vidal, A., and Jutisz, M., 1971, Localization par cyto-immunoenzymlolgie de la LH, de ses sous-unites α et β et de la FSH dans l'adenohypophyse de la ratte castree, *C.R. Acad. Sc. Paris*, 273:897.

Tougard, C., Kerdelhue, B., Tixier-Vidal, A., and Jutisz, M., 1973, Light and electron microscope localization of binding sites of antibodies against ovine luteinizing hormone and its two subunits in rat adenohypophysis using peroxidase-labeled antibody technique, *J. Cell Biol.* 58:503.

Tougard, C., 1980, Immunocytochemical identification of LH-β and FSH-β secreting cells at the light and electron microscopic levels. *In: "Synthesis and Release of Adenohypophyseal Hormones"*, M. Jutsiz and K.W. McKerns, Eds., Plenum Press N.Y., p. 15.

Supported by NIH RCDA HD 00395 and NIH RO1 HD-15472.

REGULATION OF PEPTIDE HORMONE RECEPTORS IN THE PITUITARY-GONADAL AXIS: RECEPTORS TO GONADOTROPINS AND GONADOTROPIN RELEASING HORMONE

Abraham Amsterdam

Department of Hormone Research
The Weizmann Institute of Science
Rehovot, 76100, Israel

INTRODUCTION

Most peptide hormones exert their effects on target cells *via* interaction with specific receptors located on the cell membrane (for review see Amsterdam et al., 1981a). This interaction often results in changes in the concentration of the cellular receptors for the homologous hormone. Plasma membrane receptors for hormones and neurotransmitters are usually decreased or "down regulated" by exposure to their respective ligands (Prives et al., 1979; Amsterdam et al., 1979a,b,c, 1980a, 1981a). However, at least three hormones: prolactin (Posner et al., 1975), angiotensin II, (Hauzer et al., 1978), and gonadotropin releasing hormone (GnRH) (Frazer et al., 1981, Amsterdam et al., 1981a), have been found to increase cellular receptors; however, even these ligands can cause receptor loss under appropriate experimental conditions. In gonadal cells, receptor sites to luteinizing hormone (LH)/human chorionic gonadotropin (hCG) were shown to be decreased by exogenous gonadotropins both *in vivo* and *in vitro* (Amsterdam et al., 1979c, 1980a, 1981a; Amsterdam and Lindner, 1983). However, the nature of the ligand (hCG and LH purified from different species) will affect the rate of internalization of the receptor bound hormone (Mock and Niswender, 1983). Interestingly, we also found recently that changes in the amount of sugar on the glycoprotein hormone can affect the rate of internalization (Amsterdam et al., 1983; Zor et al., 1984b). In addition, elevation in the number of LH receptors can be observed under specific experimental conditions prior to their disappearance (Huhtaniemi et al., 1981; Amsterdam et al., 1981a). Recently, receptors to follicular stimulating hormone (FSH) were also shown to be "up-regulated" either by the native or the deglycosylated hormone (Knecht et al., 1983; Zor et al., 1984b).

The major mechanism by which receptor loss occurs is by the internalization of the receptor-ligand complex and its subsequent degradation. However, there is increasing evidence that at least some of the internalized receptors can escape degradation and be recirculated (Steer and Ashwell, 1980; Naor et al., 1983a). Specific internalization may be preceded by lateral migration and aggregation of receptor-hormone complexes on the cell membrane. These clustered receptors are then internalized via endocytosis. Indeed, these phenomena were observed in a variety of membrane antigens including receptors to LH/hCG and GnRH (Amsterdam et al., 1977, 1979c, 1981a; Naor et al., 1980, 1981; Amsterdam and Lindner, 1983; Hazum et al., 1984). Local concentrations of cellular receptors at specific regions of the cell membrane were observed for the low density lypoprotein (LDL) receptors predominantly on coated pits (Goldstein et al., 1979). LH receptors were localized mainly on the microvilli of ovarian granulosa (Amsterdam et al., 1981a; Amsterdam and Lindner, 1983) as well as luteal cells (Anderson et al., 1979), and testicular Leydig cells (Amsterdam et al., 1980b, 1981a). Local concentration of hormone-receptor complexes on the specific area of the cell membrane and their subsequent internalization may be a prerequisite for specific internalization. Interestingly, aggregation of receptors to acetylcholine on the cell surface and their subsequent disappearance can also occur spontaneously without ligand binding (Prives et al., 1976).

Several cell components have been implicated in the internalization of receptor-ligand complex including coated pits, coated vesicles, membrane ruffles, endocytic vesicles, Golgi apparatus and lysosomes. Receptor mediated endocytosis for different ligands may share the same intercellular pathways. However, diversity both in the kinetics of internalization and in some of the intracellular pathways can occur according to the nature of both the ligand and its specific receptors as exemplified by GnRH- and LH-receptor interaction in target cells in the pituitary-gonadal axis.

REGULATION OF OVARIAN FUNCTION BY GONADOTROPIC HORMONE

Gonadotrophic hormones control ovarian function in a sequential manner: FSH is primarily responsible for regulation of follicular development while LH controls the later processes of ovulation and luteinization. Both hormones exert their effects by binding to specific receptors located in the cell membrane, with subsequent stimulation of adenylate cyclase (for review, see Amsterdam, 1980; Amsterdam et al., 1981; Amsterdam and Lindner, 1983). However, the subsequent biochemical and related morphological events are not yet clear.

An important step in understanding the gonadotropin receptor function is to study receptor hormonal complex localization and possible redistribution and correlate these events with the cellular response to the hormone. The site of LH binding to its receptor can be visualized by autoradiography in the preovulatory follicles using ^{125}I-human chorionic gonadotropin (hCG), which binds specifically to LH receptors (Amsterdam et al., 1975; Lindner et al., 1977; Rajaniemi et al., 1977). Subsequent to *in vivo* administration of the hormone to pro-estrous rats, labeled molecules could be demonstrated only in the periphery of the follicle, in the theca and mural granulosa cells (Amsterdam et al., 1975). No significant labeling was found over the oocyte and the granulosa cells bordering the ovum (corona radiata). Following *in vitro* incubation of isolated compartments of the follicles with the labeled hormone, we observed (Amsterdam and Tsafriri, 1979; Amsterdam, 1982; Amsterdam and Lindner, 1983) that the number of LH receptor sites in the outer granulosa cell layers (membrana granulosa) was 7 to 10 times greater than in the inner layers (cumulus oophorus); the oocyte and zona pellucida showed no specific labeling. It is, therefore, conceivable that only those cells that bind LH or hCG respond to the hormone, and that the signal generated by the primary cell-hormone interaction might be translated into a chemical message or electric impulse which is propagated toward the interior of the follicle and oocyte.

Gap junctions have been characterized between follicular cells (Amsterdam et al., 1974, 1976; Albertini and Anderson, 1974; Amsterdam and Lindner, 1978) and we have identified similar junctions also between follicular cells and the oocyte (Amsterdam et al., 1976). Such junctional elements may permit intercellular transfer of ions and small molecules such as cyclic AMP (Sheridan 1971). Therefore, the network of follicular gap junctions may provide a structural basis for a flow of electrical or chemical information from follicular cells to the oocyte. This transfer of information may be modified by LH, permitting the hormone to control ovum maturation, in spite of the lack of LH receptors on the oocyte. We recently found that in cultured granulosa cells obtained from hypophysectomized immature rats, formation of LH receptors coincides with the appearance of junctional elements between the cultured cells following FSH stimulation (Amsterdam et al., 1981b). A causal relationship between these two developmental events has not been established, but both appear to depend on the action of FSH, as does the formation of a follicular antrum (Goldenberg et al., 1980; Richards, 1980). *In vivo*, follicular gap junctions are largely confined to the more mature follicles, viz. the antral follicles (Amsterdam et al., 1974, 1976; Albertini and Anderson, 1974).

THE MECHANISM OF GRANULOSA CELLS DIFFERENTIATION: EFFECTS OF FSH, ESTRADIOL AND GnRH

The regulation of ovarian follicular cell maturation *in vivo* is believed to be controlled by the dual action of estrogens and FSH

(Richards, 1980). The differentiation process which is a prerequisite for the responsiveness of the matured follicle to the preovulatory LH surge is characterized by the appearance of various structural and biochemical markers. The differentiation process *in vivo*, involves production of progesterone as well as development of receptors to LH and prolactin (Channing and Kammerman, 1973; Zeleznik et al., 1974; Goldenberg, 1980; Hillier, 1980; Richards, 1980). We and others have shown that initiation of differentiation by FSH can also be achieved *in vitro* in cultured granulosa cells (Erickson et al., 1979, Nimrod and Lindner, 1980; Amsterdam et al., 1981a) and that the biochemical aspects of differentiation are apparent *in vitro* in the absence of serum from the culture medium. Moreover, we have shown that the morphological transformation that occurred in the cultured cells during differentiation resembles those observed *in vivo* (Amsterdam et al., 1981b). We found that most of the FSH-treated cells in culture became highly aggregated and grew in multilayered clusters. Numerous gap junctions were seen between cells, indicating the formation of significant intercellular communication. Microvilli densely covered the surface of the hormone-stimulated cells, which contained enlarged mitochondria with convoluted cristae, characteristic of steroidogenic cells. LH-receptors, identified by autoradiography with ^{125}I-labeled hCG, were mainly associated with aggregated cells, whereas single cells were usually free of the labeled hormone (Amsterdam et al., 1981b).

In the last few years it was shown that ovarian tissue contains receptors to GnRH (Clayton et al., 1979) and that GnRH agonists block gonadotropin-induced formation of LH receptors and progesterone production in both granulosa cells (Hsueh and Erickson 1979; Hsueh et al., 1980) and luteal cells (Clayton et al., 1979; Harwood et al., 1980a,b). These findings indicate that the hypothalamic peptide hormone can exert a direct effect on ovarian function. However the exact mechanism of LH receptor induction and differentiation of granulosa cells by FSH and its inhibition by GnRH remain to be defined. Addition of a GnRH agonist to cultures of dissociated granulosa cells prevented the appearance of LH receptors and markedly impaired cyclic AMP and progesterone production, as well as the morphological changes induced by FSH (Amsterdam et al., 1981b; Knecht et al., 1982). The majority of the granulosa cells assumed a flattened, smooth shape and grew primarily in monolayers. The maintenance of cellular aggregation and intercellular communication by FSH, and its inhibition by GnRH or an ovarian peptide with similar properties (Ying et al., 1981), may play an important role in the cytodifferentiation of ovarian granulosa cells. However, GnRH has not yet been identified in significant concentrations in the ovary. It is of interest that epidermal growth factor too has been shown to inhibit the formation of LH receptors in granulosa cells (Mondschein and Schomberg, 1981).

In searching for the mechanism of induction by FSH of granulosa cell differentiation, we found that both 8-Bromo cyclic AMP and cholera toxin are potent stimulants for differentiation in culture and that the accompanying biochemical and morphological events are essentially similar to those obtained with FSH (Amsterdam et al., 1981b; Knecht et al., 1981a). This would suggest that the acute cellular response to FSH as well as the differentiative effect of the hormone is mediated by cAMP. The accumulation of cAMP during the entire course of differentiation would further support this hypothesis (Knecht et al., 1981b).

SPATIAL DISTRIBUTION OF LH RECEPTORS AND CELLULAR RESPONSE TO THE HORMONE

Prolonged exposure of ovarian tissue to LH or hCG, both of which bind to the same receptor, causes prompt stimulation of adenylate cyclase followed by desensitization of the enzyme to renewed hormonal challenge in vitro (for review see Lindner et al., 1977; Zor, 1983). A similar phenomenon is also observed in other systems in which hormones exert their effects via adenylate cyclase. The mechanisms responsible for this refractoriness are not as yet clear, but several alternative explanations have been suggested. These include the process of agonist-induced depletion of receptor sites, referred to as 'down-regulation', decreased activity of the catalytic enzyme unit (Catt et al., 1979) and impaired receptor-cyclase coupling (Amsterdam et al., 1979a,b,c; 1980a, 1981a).

We have studied the temporal relationship between redistribution of receptors to LH/hCG in cultured granulosa cells and the cellular response to hormonal challenge (Amsterdam et al., 1979a,b,c; 1980a; Amsterdam and Lindner, 1983). Visualization of receptor-bound hCG by indirect immunofluorescence, utilizing hormone-specific antibodies after fixation with 2% formaldehyde, revealed the existence of small clusters around the entire cell circumference 5-20 min after exposure to the hormone at 37°C. Larger clusters were evident following prolonged (2-4 h) incubation at 37°C. The latter change coincided with diminished cAMP accumulation in response to challenge with fresh hormone (Amsterdam et al., 1980a). When the fixation step was omitted and antibodies to hCG were applied following hormonal binding, acceleration of both receptor clustering and the desensitization process was observed. This manoeuvre also induced capping of the hormone receptors. In contrast, monovalent Fab' fragments of the specific antibodies were without effect (Amsterdam et al., 1980a). These observations suggest that clustering of the luteinizing hormone receptors may play a role in cellular responsiveness to the hormone. Massive aggregation of the receptors may desensitize the cell by interfering with coupling to adenylate cyclase (Fig. 1). However, it now appears that a number of disparate mechanisms may underlie the phenomena which have been observed under different experimental conditions and which are subsumed under the term desensitization. Biochemical uncoupling of the receptor-cyclase system, possibly by autophosphorylation, may be important in certain of these circumstances (Amir-Zaltzman et al., 1980).

Radiolabeled hormone-receptor complexes were shown by high resolution autoradiography to be internalized, accounting for the loss of surface receptors or 'down-regulation' observed after prolonged hormonal stimulation. However, desensitization of the adenylate cyclase system preceded extensive receptor internalization (Amsterdam et al., 1979c). This uncoupling of receptor and cyclase may be due to immobilization of receptor molecules by aggregation (Schlessinger et al., 1978). Internalization of these clusters seemed to be initiated by cytoskeletal elements, since microfilaments were found to be associated with invaginations of the plasma membrane at clustered regions of the receptor molecules (Amsterdam et al., 1979c). Pharmacological manipulation of cytoskeletal function has recently been shown to modify the desensitization process in granulosa cells with respect to prostaglandins and the primary response of these cells to gonadotropins (Zor et al., 1978, 1979; Zor, 1983).

We recently observed that the LH receptors newly synthesized after FSH stimulation are mainly localized to microvillous processes, which are loaded with microfilaments (Amsterdam et al., 1981a; Amsterdam and Lindner, 1983; Fig. 1). Perhaps microfilaments participate in the control of vertical receptor movement (insertion into membrane and internalization) as well as lateral movement (within the plane of the membrane). Much of the internalized hormone-receptor complex was incorporated into lysosomes (Fig. 1), and evidence of hormone degradation was obtained (Amsterdam et al., 1979c). Limited labeling over the Golgi area suggests the possibility of receptor recycling. Significant labeling was also found over the nuclei 8 h after introduction of the labeled hormone (Amsterdam et al., 1979c) but it is not clear whether this represented intact hormone, a peptide fragment, or recycled radio-tyrosine. The penetration of protein hormones into the interior of the cell opens the possibility that these hormones, believed to interact exclusively with cell surface receptors, may have additional sites of action unrelated to adenylate cyclase. Rao and Mitra (1979) found significant binding of hCG in nuclear fractions obtained from homogenates of bovine corpora lutea. Specific binding sites in nuclei and Golgi cisternae were also demonstrated recently in bovine corpora lutea slices (Cheqini et al., 1984a, b).

Internalization of receptor-bound hCG was described in the luteinized sheep and rat ovary *in vivo* (Chen et al., 1977; Conn et al., 1978). However, the rate of internalization *in vivo* is significantly lower than that observed in cultured cells. Significant loss of receptors after *in vivo* administration of hCG was found

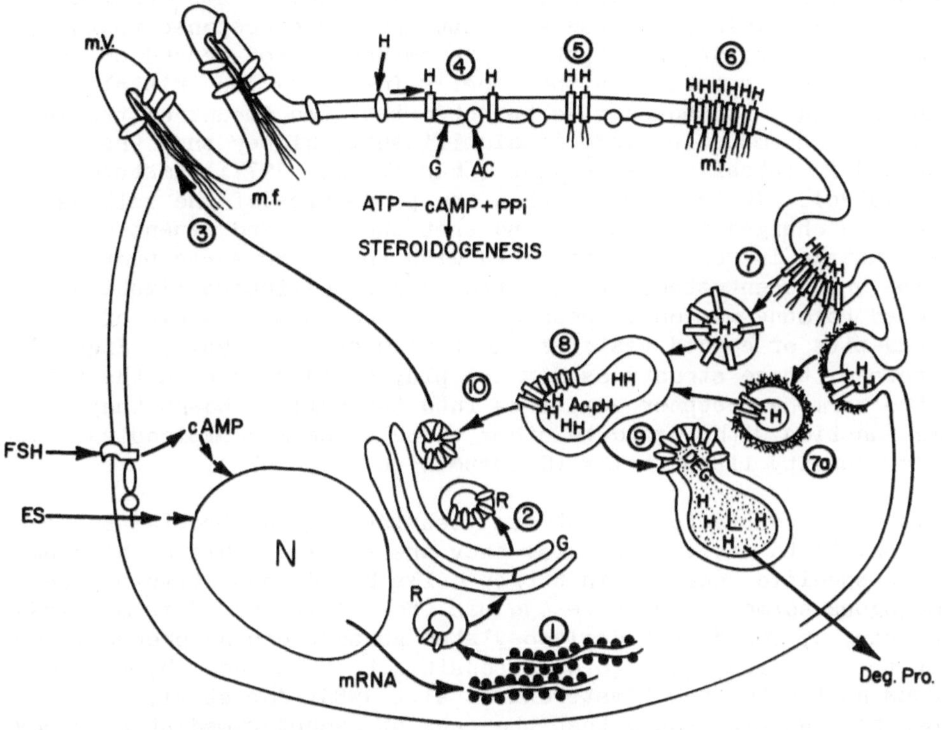

Fig. 1. Proposed model of LH receptor biosynthesis function and turnover in the granulosa cell. 1. Synthesis of receptor molecule (R) or its precurser, stimulated by FSH (via cyclic AMP production) and by estrogen. 2. Post-translational processing (e.g. glycosylation) and emergence of receptor containing vesicles from Golgi complex. 3. Fusion with the cell membrane predominantly in microvilli loaded with thin filaments. 4. LH binding (H) and induction of receptor conformational changes leading to coupling of adenylate cyclase (AC) via the regulatory complex (G). 5. Microclustering of receptors, anchorage to the cytoskeleton (microfilaments and microtubules). 6. Macroclustering coincides with desensitization to hormone response. 7. Receptor induced endocytosis via non coated areas of the plasmalemma (major route) and via coated pits (7a) (minor route). 8. Fusion with receptosomes and possible dissociation of the hormone receptor complex in acidic (Ac) pH. 9. Degradation of the hormone or hormone receptor complexes in lysosomes. DP = degradation products. 10. Alternatively, receptor recycling.

only after 24 h of administration of the hormone, i.e. long after the onset of desensitization (Conti et al., 1977; Amsterdam et al., 1981a). This would suggest that the acute response to the hormone, and the desensitization phenomenon do not depend on internalization of receptors in these cells following the initial hormone binding. It should also be noted that the amount of the internalized hormone in vitro is significantly higher than that detected in luteal cells in vivo (Chen et al., 1977; Amsterdam et al., 1979c). It is possible that the properties of the cell membrane are changed in culture, and that the rate and extent of membrane uptake in regions associated with the hormone-receptor complexes are accentuated. During the process of internalization, labeled hormone was only occasionally found to be associated with coated pits or coated vesicles (Amsterdam et al., 1981a; Fig. 1). Therefore, these structures may not play a major role in the uptake of the hormone-receptor complexes into the cells, though they have this function with regard to other circulating macromolecules, such as low density lipoproteins (Goldstein et al., 1979).

It was recently found that deglycosylated gonadotropins serve as antagonists to native hormones; they are still capable of binding to the specific receptor in target cells but do not stimulate the homologous hormone sensitive cyclase (for review see Sairam, 1983). Moreover, we found that deglycosylated gonadotrophins probably protect the cell from undergoing desensitization induced by the homologous native hormone (Amsterdam et al., 1983; Zor et al., 1984a,b). We also found that the rate of receptor-mediated endocytosis and degradation of the deglycosylated hCG is significantly lower compared to the native hormone (Amsterdam et al., 1983; Zor et al., 1984b). We are currently investigating whether the deglycosylated hormone is able to induce receptor aggregation which may be an important step in regulating the cellular response to the hormone. It is hoped that these experiments will shed light on the role of the sugar moiety in the gonadotropin molecules in transduction of the hormonal signal in target cells.

LH RECEPTORS IN LEYDIG CELLS

Testicular binding sites for LH (and hCG) are localized in the Leydig cells. Both LH and hCG bind to specific cell membrane receptors of the Leydig cell, acutely stimulating cyclic AMP formation and testosterone production (for review see Amsterdam et al., 1981a; Amsterdam and Lindner, 1983).

High resolution techniques have revealed that most of the receptors occupied by the hormone are located over the microvillous area at the circumference of these cells. Moreover, application of antibodies to hCG with the immunoferritin technique results in massive aggregation of the receptor bound hormone with accumulation of microfilaments and microtubules beneath such aggregates (Amsterdam et al., 1980b, 1981a; Amsterdam and Lindner, 1983). This would suggest (as for the ovarian LH receptor) an association of cytoskeletal elements with the receptor molecule. Indeed, several studies have implicated cytoplasmic contractile elements in receptor mobility (Silverstein et al., 1977). It was found that LH can acutely increase its own receptors in the Leydig cells and that up-regulation observed 1 h after LH administration is blocked by cytochalasin B (Huhtaniemi et al., 1981; Amsterdam et al., 1981a). This finding suggests that the mechanism of receptor insertion or exposure on the cell surface may require the involvement of microfilaments.

Internalization of the LH receptors after saturation with the hormone is a relatively slow process. A significant loss of total binding sites can be observed only after 18 h of hormonal administration, while after the first hour there is a significant rise in the number of Leydig cell receptors (for review see Amsterdam et al., 1981a). It is, therefore, apparent that the reduction in the rate of cAMP accumulation observed after 6 h of incubation with the hormone is not due to loss of binding sites to the hormone. When Leydig cells were incubated for 6 h with saturating doses of ^{125}I-hCG *in vitro* and examined by high resolution radioautography, most of the labeled protein was localized on the cell surface, while only a small fraction of the tracer hormone was found within the cells. The labeled hormone internalized by the cells was mainly associated with intracellular vesicles, some of them still bearing the microvillous processes. On occasion, radioactive material was found to be associated with coated pits or coated vesicles (Amsterdam et al., 1980b, 1981a; Amsterdam and Lindner, 1983). This would suggest that the major pathway of internalization of the receptor-hormone complex is not via the coated area, but that other parts of the membrane (e.g. microvilli and membrane ruffles) where the receptor molecules are predominantly concentrated, may be involved in the internalization process.

The preceding observations indicate that ovarian and testicular LH receptors share several common features at the molecular and cellular levels:

1. The rate of dissociation of the receptor-hormone complex is very slow.

2. Structural and pharmacological evidence suggests that the receptor may be associated with cytoskeletal elements (microfilaments) in the intact cells.

3. Uptake of the receptor-hormone complexes after hormonal binding is not essential for the acute cellular response to the hormone, but may serve as a mechanism for metabolizing the bound hormone and recycling the receptor molecules.

4. Coated pits and vesicles are probably not the major cellular components responsible for receptor aggregation and internalization.

RECEPTORS TO GnRH IN PITUITARY GONADOTROPHS

Gonadotropin releasing hormone (GnRH) stimulates pituitary gonadotropin release. The first step in GnRH action is believed to depend on specific binding to plasma membrane receptors located exclusively on pituitary gonadotrophs (for review see Amsterdam et al., 1981a; Naor et al., 1982; Catt et al., 1983).

The mechanism by which GnRH exerts its effect on the release of LH and FSH located within the secretory granules in pituitary gonadotrophs is not completely clear. A model of our current thinking regarding the mechanism of action of GnRH in the pituitary was recently suggested (Naor et al., 1983a), and is summarized in Fig. 2. Following the binding, GnRH activates conversion of phosphatidyl inositol (PI) to phosphatidic acid (PA) and calcium channels are activated. Among the several enzymes that might be activated by a calcium-calmodulin complex is phospholipase A_2. Activation of this enzyme leads to the accumulation of free arachidonic acid (AA) in the cell. Activation of the Ca^{++} channels and the PI response may lead to the appropriate change in the plasma membrane inducing fusion of the granule membrane with the cell membrane leading to prompt release of the granule content from the cell by exocytosis. There is suggestive evidence that AA and/or one of its metabolized products in the lipoxygenase route may have an important role in GnRH action on pituitary gonadotropin release (Naor et al., 1983a,b). Clustering of the receptor molecules induced by the hormone may also play a part in the transduction of the hormonal signal (Conn, 1982; Fig. 2).

MODULATION OF GnRH RECEPTOR NUMBERS

The phenomenon of homologous regulation of cellular receptors by the ligand is well-known (Catt et al., 1979). This process is apparently responsible for target cell sensitivity in the face of variations in hormone concentration. Pituitary responsiveness to pulsatile secretion of hypothalamic GnRH is influenced by the number of GnRH binding sites and the hormonal mileau in a given physiological condition. Fluctuation in GnRH receptors and cell responsiveness was observed in the rat estrous cycle, pregnancy and lactation (Savoy-Moore et al., 1980; Clayton and Catt, 1981a,b). Non-physiological modifications, such as castration, hypothalamic lesions or administration of GnRH antagonists or antibodies, resulted in changes in GnRH binding sites in accordance with the postulate that endogenous GnRH exerts a regulatory action on the maintenance of its own receptors (Clayton and Catt, 1981a, b; Clayton et al., 1982a, b; Frazer et al., 1981; Marian et al., 1981; Piper et al., 1982; Fig. 2). Further support for this above proposal was derived from in vitro studies in which the direct effect of GnRH on its own receptors was investigated (Loumaye and Catt, 1981; Zilberstein et al., 1983). As demonstrated, exposure of cultured rat pituitary cells to low concentrations of GnRH, or one of its potent agonists, caused a dose-related increase in GnRH binding sites (up-regulation) that was followed by a decline at higher concentrations of the peptides (Loumaye and Catt, 1981). Changes in the binding capacity resulted from alterations in the number of the binding sites rather than changes in affinity. The sequence of events of receptor regulation by GnRH seems to be initiated by a rapid loss in GnRH binding sites which is not dependent on protein synthesis (Loumaye and Catt, 1981; Catt et al., 1983). Following the decline in binding sites, GnRH (at near physiological concentrations) increases the number of its own receptors probably via protein synthesis (Catt et al., 1983). The increase in the number of binding sites is linked to post-receptor activation processes since the effect can be mimicked by 50 mM KCl but not by a potent GnRH antagonist (Loumaye and Catt, 1981; Catt et al., 1983). On the other hand, high concentrations of GnRH ($> 10^{-7}$ M) caused down-regulation of GnRH receptors, probably due to massive internalization and processing of the hormone-receptor complex (Zilberstein et al., 1983 and Fig. 2).

LOCALIZATION OF PITUITARY GnRH RECEPTORS WITH HIGH RESOLUTION TECHNIQUES

We have demonstrated, by light microscopic autoradiography and fluorescent microscopy that following the binding to specific receptors, analogs of GnRH are rapidly internalized into pituitary gonadotrophs in vivo and in cultured cells (Amsterdam et al., 1981a; Naor et al., 1981; 1983; Catt et al., 1983; Hazum et al., 1982; 1984). To further characterize the intracellular distribution of the internalized hormone we have used the technique of high-resolution autoradiography.

To determine the fate of the internalized GnRH in pituitary gonadotrophs, we injected [^{125}I]iodo-(D-Ala^{6})des-Gly^{10}-GnRH N ethylamide (2 mM, intracardial) into mature female rats and followed the uptake of the agonist by high resolution autoradiography (Naor et al., 1983a). Maximal specific uptake in the pituitary was reached between 15 and 30 min; thereafter the amount of bound hormone declined by 50% within 30 min. Following the agonist injection (30 min) the labeled hormone was found almost exclusively over the gonadotrophs. Analysis of electron microscope autoradiograms revealed about 24% of the grains associated with the cell membrane, while the rest of the labeling was mainly distributed over intracellular smooth-membrane vesicles (29%) over secretory granules (23%) and over lysosome-like structures (12%). Some of the labeled secretory granules were found in proximity to the cell membrane.

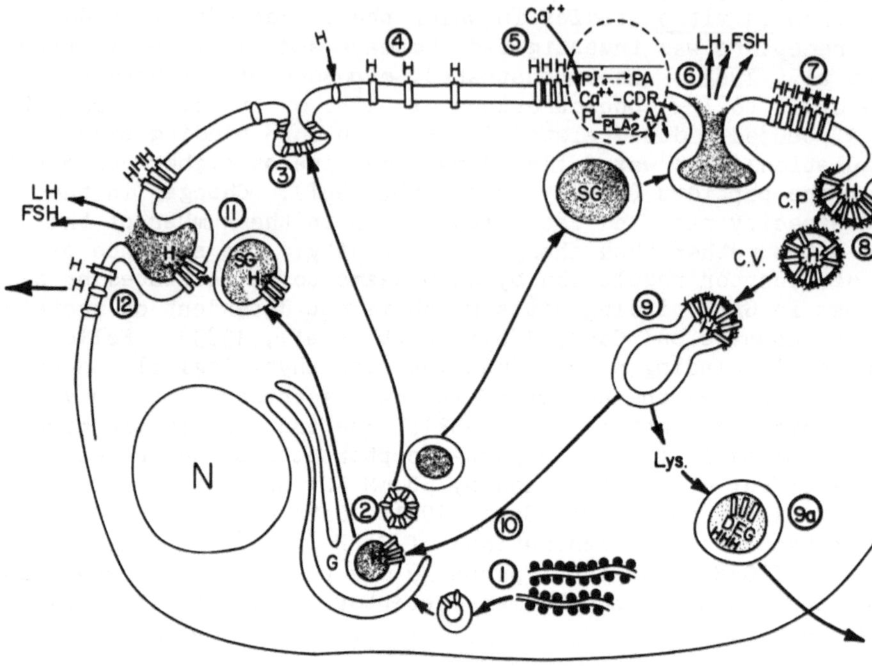

Fig. 2. Proposed model for GnRH receptor biosynthesis, function and turnover in pituitary gonadotrophs. 1. Synthesis of GnRH receptor (R) on the rough endoplasmic reticulum. 2. Post-translational processing and emergence of receptor containing vesicles from Golgi complex (G). 3. Insertion of R to the cell membrane. 4. GnRH (H) binding and induction of conformational changes in the receptor molecule. 5. Microclustering of receptor hormone complexes, conversion of phosphatidyl inositol (PI) to phosphatidic acid (PA), opening of Ca^{++} channels, interaction of Ca++ with calmodulin (CDR), activation of phospholipase A_2 (PLA_2) which catalysed conversion of phospholipids (PL) to arachidonic acid (AA). 6. AA and/or one of its metabolites induce fusion of gonadotropin containing secretory vesicles with the cell membrane and release of the hormone to the extracellular space (exocytosis). 7. Macroclustering. 8. Concentration of hormone receptor complex in coated area of the cell membranes, internalization via coated pits. 9. Fusion of coated vesicle with receptosomes. 10. Receptor recycling through insertion to secretory granule membrane. 11. Fusion of secretory granules containing LH and FSH and exposing of recycled receptor molecule on the cell membrane. 12. Dissociation of hormone from previously occupied receptor.

The results demonstrate the intracellular localization of the internalized GnRH-analog and indicate that aside from the lysosomal degradative pathway, GnRH can be rapidly taken up by the secretory granules containing LH and FSH (Fig. 2).

We found that, although DAla^6 analog was a suitable marker for localization of GnRH in vivo, binding of this labeled analog in cell suspension or in monolayers of pituitary gonadotrophs, was followed by dissociation of labeled hormone from the cells. Therefore, in order to follow the distribution of GnRH receptors after their binding to target cells in vitro (Naor et al., 1982) it was most desirable to use hormone analogs which can be covalently bound to the receptor and thus minimize possible dissociation of the hormone-receptor complexes (for review see Hazum, 1983). Two ^{125}I-labeled analogs of GnRH, (azidobenzoyl-D-Lys^6)GnRH (I) and (D-Lys^6)GnRH (II), were used for the localization of GnRH receptors in pituitary gonadotropes (Hazum et al., 1982; 1984). The analogs retained high binding affinity to a single class of receptors and, after photoactivation (analog I) or crosslinking with glutaraldehyde (analog II), are bound covalently to pituitary cells. The distribution of the labeled hormones by electron microscopic autoradiography indicated that after exposure of pituitary cells to the ^{125}I -labeled hormones at 4°C (90 min), most of the labeled hormones were associated with the cell surface membrane, while at 37°C (15 min) about 25% of the cell-bound labeled hormones were internalized. After 45 min of incubation at 37°C, only half of the label was associated with the plasma membrane, while the rest was found in lysosome-like structures (21%), in secretory granules (20%) and in the Golgi complex (3%). The incidence of clustered grains over the cell membrane was high after 15 min and 45 min of incubation, and a significant fraction of the grains was associated with coated pits of the cell membrane. It is suggested that the mechanism of internalization of the hormone-receptor complexes involves aggregation of the receptor molecules and removal from the cell surface by coated pits. The association of the hormone receptor complexes with the secretory granules may be part of a recycling mechanism of the receptor molecules for GnRH (Fig. 2).

SUMMARY

Membrane receptors for LH can be visualized on target cells in the ovary and testis by immunofluorescence, immunoferritin and High Resolution autoradiography. After the initial binding step, redistribution of the receptor bound hormone is followed by internalization to lysosomes and degradation. Evidence is presented to suggest that the internalization process does not play a part in the acute response to the hormone. Instead this process may be involved in the long-term regulation of the number of receptors on target cells, and possibly in some of the trophic effects of the hormone. Early desensitization of the cells to the hormone may be associated with rearrangement of the receptor molecule in clusters on the cell membrane rather than with internalization. The glycosidic part of the gonadotropin molecule may play an important part in the induction of the biological response to the hormone and in the initiation of receptor internalization in target cells.

FSH was shown to induce both biochemical and morphological differentiation in cultured granulosa cells. Our data suggest that cellular contact and intercellular communication may play a role in the differentiation process. cAMP mediates both the acute and the differentiation response to FSH, and GnRH inhibits the stimulatory effects of FSH on granulosa cell differentiation, probably by preventing cyclic AMP accumulation.

Receptors to GnRH were visualized on target cells in the pituitary by fluoroscinated analogs of the hormone and by high resolution autoradiography. In order to avoid dissociation of the ligand receptor complex after aldehyde fixation, a photoffinity derivative was used. GnRH analogs exclusively bind to gonadotrophs both *in vivo* and in cultured cells. At $4^{\circ}C$ the radioligand bound exclusively to the cell membrane. Clustering of the receptor molecules and rapid internalization was shown to occur mainly *via* coated pits. Radiolabeled internalized ligand could be found within lysosomes and also within LH and FSH containing secretory granules. It is suggested that some of the internalized receptor molecules can escape degradation and be recirculated to the cell membranes via the secretory granules. Thus, GnRH and gonadotropins play an important role in the regulation of pituitary-gonadal function, and exert their effects after binding to specific receptors located on the cell membrane of the respective target cells. Internalization of the receptor hormone complexes following hormone binding occurs at different rates in different cell types, and the extent of internalization may also vary. The internalized hormone receptor complexes may serve as part of the mechanism by which these hormones exert their long-term biological effects including regulation of the receptor number on target cells.

ACKNOWLEDGEMENTS

I thank Dr. A. Dunn for helpful discussions and Mrs. M. Kopelowitz for excellent secretarial assistance.

REFERENCES

Albertini, D.F. and Anderson, A., 1974, The appearance and structure of intercellular connections during the ontogeny of the rabbit ovarian follicle with particular reference to gap junctions, *J. Cell. Biol.*, 63:234.

Amir-Zaltsman, Y., Ezra, E., Walker, N., Lindner, H.R. and Salomon, Y., 1980, Labeling of specific proteins in rat ovarian plasma membranes with [^{32}P] GTP, FEBS Lett., 122:166.

Amsterdam, A., 1980, Regulation of follicular gonadotropin receptors in the mammalian ovary, Proc. Australian Acad. Sci. (VI International Congress Endocrinology, Melbourne) pp. 587-590.

Amsterdam, A., 1982, Function, turnover and distribution analyses of plasma membrane-associated receptors, Fresenius Z. Anal. Chem., 311:338.

Amsterdam, A. and Lindner, H.R., 1978, Incidence of gap junctions in the Graafian follicle, in: "Ovarian Follicular Development and Function", A.R. Midgley, Jr. and W.A. Sadler, eds., Raven Press, New York. pp. 137-138.

Amsterdam, A. and Tsafriri, S., 1979, In vitro binding of ^{125}I-human chorionic gonadotrophin (hCG) in the preovulatory follicle: Absence of receptor sites on oocyte, J. Cell Biol., 83:255a.

Amsterdam, A. and Lindner, H.R., 1983, Localization of gonadotropin receptors in the gonads, in: "Electron Microscopy in Biology and Medicine: Current Topics in Ultrastructural Research", P.M. Motta, ed., The Hague, The Netherlands, Martinus Nijhoff Publ., pp. 253-262.

Amsterdam, A., Josephs, R., Lieberman, M.E. and Lindner, H.R., 1974, Organization of intramembrane particles of granulosa cell gap junctions in rat ovarian follicle, J. Cell Biol. 63:8a.

Amsterdam, A., Koch Y., Lieberman, M.E. and Lindner, H.R., 1975, Distribution of binding sites for human chorionic gonadotropin in the preovulatory follicle of the rat, J. Cell Biol., 67:894.

Amsterdam, A., Josephs, R., Lieberman, M.E. and Lindner, H.R., 1976, Organization of intramembrane particles in freeze-cleaved gap junctions of rat Graafian follicles: optical diffraction analysis, J. Cell Sci., 21:93.

Amsterdam, A., Hollander, Z., Nimrod, A., Riesel, R. and Kohen, F., 1977, Lateral mobility and internalization and luteinizing hormone (LH) receptors in granulosa cells shown by immunofluorescence, J. Cell Biol., 75:222a.

Amsterdam, A., Kohen, F., Nimrod, A. and Lindner, H.R., 1979a, Lateral mobility and internalization of hormone receptors to human chorionic gonadotropin in cultured rat granulosa cells, Adv. Exp. Med. Biol., 112:69.

Amsterdam, A., Nimrod, A., Kohen, F. and Lindner, H.R., 1979b, Redistribution of receptor for human chorionic gonadotropin in cultured rat granulosa cells in relation to the cellular response to the hormone, in: "Molecular Mechanisms of Biological Recognition", M. Balaban, ed., Elsevier/North-Holland Biomedical Press, pp. 419-428.

Amsterdam, A., Nimrod, A., Lamprecht, S.A., Burstein, Y. and Lindner, H.R., 1979c, Internalization and degradation of receptor-bound human chorionic gonadotrophin in granulosa cell cultures, Am. J. Physiol., 5:E129.

Amsterdam, A., Berkowitz, A., Nimrod, A. and Kohen, F., 1980a, Aggregation of luteinizing hormone receptors in granulosa cells: A possible mechanism of desensitization to the hormone. Proc. Natl. Acad. Sci. (U.S.A.), 77:3440.

Amsterdam, A., Dufau, M.L. and Catt, K.J., 1980b, Regional distribution of receptors to luteinizing hormone in dispersed testicular Leydig cells. J. Cell Biol., 87:160a.

Amsterdam, A., Naor, Z., Knecht, M., Dufau, M. and Catt, K.J., 1981a, Hormone action and receptor redistribution in endocrine target cells: gonadotropins and gonadotropin-releasing hormone, in: "Receptor-mediated Binding in Internalization of Toxins and Hormones", J.L. Middlebrook and L.D. Kohn, eds., Academic Press, pp. 283-310.

Amsterdam, A., Knecht, M. and Catt, K.J., 1981b, Hormonal regulation of cytodifferentiation and intercellular communication in cultured granulosa cells, Proc. Natl. Acad. Sci. (U.S.A.), 78:3000.

Amsterdam, A., Sairam, M.R. and Zor, U., 1983, Deglycosylated human chorionic gonadotropin retards the down-regulation of luteinizing hormone receptors in granulosa cells, J. Cell Biol. 97:407a.

Anderson, W., Kaney, H., Perroti, M.E., Bramley, T.A. and Ryan, R.J., 1979, Interactions of gonadotropins with corpus luteum membranes. III. Electron microscopic localization of [^{125}I]-hCG binding to sensitive and desensitized ovaries seven days after PMSG-hCG, Biol. Reprod. 20:362.

Catt, K.J., Harwood, J.P., Aguilera, G. and Dufau, M.L., 1979, Hormonal regulation of peptide receptors and target cell responses, Nature, 280:109.

Catt, K.J., Loumaye, E., Katikineni, M., Hyde, C.L., Childs, G., Amsterdam, A. and Naor, N., 1983, Receptors and actions of gonadotropin releasing hormone (GnRH) on pituitary gonadotrophs. in: "Role of Peptides and Proteins in Control of Reproduction", (McCann and Dhindsa, eds.) The Netherlands, Elsevier. pp. 33-61.

Channing, C.P. and Kammerman, S., 1973, Characteristics of gonadotropin receptors of porcine granulosa cells during follicle maturation, Endocrinology, 92:531.

Chegini, N., Rao, Ch.V. and Carman, Jr., F.R., 1984a, Internalization of ^{125}I-human choriogonadotropin in bovine luteal slices. A biochemical study. Exp. Cell Res., in press.

Chegini, N., Rao, Ch.V. and Cobbs, G., 1984b, A quantitative electron microscope autoradiographic study on ^{125}I-human choriogonadotropin internalization in bovine luteal slices. Exp. Cell Res., in press.

Chen, T.T., Abel, Jr., J.A., McCellan, M.I., Sawyer, H.R., Diekman, M.A. and Niswender, G.D., 1977, Localization of gonadotropic hormones in lysosomes of ovine luteal cells, Cytobiologie, 14:412.

Clayton, R.N. and Catt, K.J., 1981a, Gonadotropin releasing hormone receptors: characterization, physiological regulation and relationship to reproductive function, Endocr. Rev., 2:186.

Clayton, R.N. and Catt, K.J., 1981b, Regulation of pituitary gonadotropin releasing hormone receptors by gonadal hormones, Endocrinology, 108:887.

Clayton, R.N., Harwood, J.P. and Catt, K.J., 1979, Gonadotropin-releasing hormone analogue binds to luteal cells and inhibits progesterone production, Nature, 282:90.

Clayton, R.N., Channabasavaiah, K., Stewart, J.M. and Catt, K.J., 1982a, Hypothalamic regulation of pituitary GnRH receptors: Effects of hypothalamic lesions and a GnRH antagonist, Endocrinology, 110:1108.

Clayton, R.N., Popkin, R.M. and Fraser, H.M., 1982b, Hypothalamic regulation of pituitary GnRH receptors: effects of GnRH immunoneutralization, Endocrinology, 110:1116.

Conn, P.M., Conti, M., Harwood, J.P., Dufau, M.L. and Catt, K.J., 1978, Internalization of gonadtrophin-receptor complex in ovarian luteal cells, Nature, 274:598.

Conn, P.M., Rogers, D.C., Stewart, J.M., Niedel, J., and Sheffield, T., 1982, Conversion of a gonadotropin releasing hormone antagonist to an agonist, Nature, 296:653.

Conti, M., Harwood, J.P., Dufau, M.L. and Catt, K.J., 1977, Regulation of luteinizing hormone receptors and adenylate cyclase activity by gonadotropin in the rat ovary, Mol. Pharmacol., 13:1024.

Erickson, G.F., Wang, C. and Hsueh, A.J.W., 1979, FSH induction of functional LH receptors in granulosa cells cultured in a chemically defined medium, Nature, 279:336.

Frazer, M.S., Pieper, D.R., Tonetta, S.A., Duncan, J.A. and Marshall, J.C., 1981, Pituitary GnRH receptors: effects of castration, steroid replacement and the role of GnRH in modulating receptors in the rat. J. Clin. Invest. 67:615.

Goldenberg, R.L., Vaitukaitis, J.L. and Ross, G.T., 1980, Estrogen and follicle stimulating hormone interactions on follicle growth in rats, Endocrinology, 90:1492.

Goldstein, J.L., Anderson,R.G.W. and Brown, M.S., 1979, Coated pits, coated vesicles and receptor-mediated endocytosis, Nature, 279:679.

Harwood, J.P., Clayton, R.N., and Catt, K.J., 1980a, Ovarian gonadotropin-releasing hormone receptors. I. Properties and inhibition of luteal cell function, Endocrinology, 107:407.

Harwood, J.P., Clayton, R.N., Chen, T.T., Knox, G., and Catt, K.J., 1980b, Ovarian gonadotropin-releasing hormone receptors. II. Regulation and effects on ovarian development, Endocrinology, 107:414.

Hauzer, R.L., Aguilera, G. and Catt, K.J., 1978, Angiotensin II regulates its receptor sites in the adrenal glomerulosa zone. Nature (London), 271:176.

Hazum, E., 1983, Photoaffinity labeling of peptide hormone receptors. Endocr. Rev., 4:352.

Hazum, E., Meidan, R., Keinan, D., Okon, E., Koch, Y., Lindner, H.R. and Amsterdam, A., 1982, A novel method for localization of gonadotropin releasing hormone receptors, Endocrinology, 111:2135.

Hazum, E., Koch, Y., Liscovitch, M. and Amsterdam, A., 1984, Intracellular pathway of receptor-bound GnRH agonist in pituitary gonadotropes, Submitted.

Hillier, S.G., Zeleznik, A.J., Knazak, R.A. and Ross, G.T., 1980, Hormonal regulation of preovulatory follicle maturation in the rat, J. Rep. Fert., 60:219.

Hsueh, A.J.W. and Erickson, G.F., 1979, Extrapituitary action of gonadotropin-releasing hormone: direct inhibition of ovarian steroidogenesis, Science, 204:854.

Hsueh, A.J.W., Wang, C. and Erickson, G.F., 1980, Direct inhibitory effect of gonadotropin-releasing hormone upon follicle-stimulating hormone induction of luteinizing hormone receptor and aromatase activity in rat granulosa cells, Endocrinology, 106:1697.

Huhtaniemi, I., Katikineni, M., Chan, V. and Catt, K.J., 1981, Gonadotropin-induced positive regulation of testicular luteinizing hormone receptors. Endocrinology, 108:58.

Knecht, M., Amsterdam, A. and Catt, K.J., 1981a, The regulatory role of cyclic AMP in hormone induced granulosa cell differentiation, J. Biol. Chem. 256:10628.

Knecht, M., Katz, M.S. and Catt, K.J., 1981b, Gonadotropin-releasing hormone inhibits cyclic nucleotide accumulation in cultured rat granulosa cells, J. Biol. Chem., 256:34.

Knecht, M., Amsterdam, A. and Catt, K.J., 1982, Inhibition of granulosa cell differentiation by gonadotropin-releasing hormone, Endocrinology, 110:865.

Knecht, M.,Ranta, T. and Catt, K.J., 1983, Granulosa cell differentiation in vitro: Induction and maintenance of follicle-stimulating hormone receptors by adenosine 3',5'-monophosphate. Endocrinology, 113:949.

Lindner, H.R., Amsterdam, A., Salomon, Y., Tsafriri, A., Nimrod, A., Lamprecht, S.A., Zor, U. and Koch, Y., 1977, Intraovarian factors in ovulation: determinants of follicular response to gonadotropins, J. Reprod. Fert., 51:215.

Loumaye, E. and Catt, K.J., 1981, Homologous regulation of gonadotropin releasing hormone receptors in cultured pituitary cells. Science, 215:983.

Marian, J., Cooper, R.L. and Conn, P.M., 1981, Regulation of the rat pituitary GnRH receptor, Mol. Pharmacol., 19:319.

Mock, E.J., and Niswender, G.D., 1983, Differences in the rates of internalization of ^{125}I-labeled human chorionic gonadotropin, luteinizing hormone, and epidermal growth factor by ovine luteal cells, Endocrinology, 113:259.

Mondschein, J.S., and Schomberg, D.W., 1981, Growth factors modulate gonadotropin receptor induction in granulosa cell cultures, Science, 211:1179.

Naor, Z., Atlas, D., Clayton, R.N., Forman, D.S., Amsterdam, A., and Catt, K.J., 1980, Fluorescent derivative of gonadotropin releasing hormone: visualization of hormone-receptor interaction in cultured pituitary cells, J. Cell Biol., 87:159a.

Naor, Z., Atlas, D., Clayton, R.N., Forman, D.S., Amsterdam, A. and Catt, R.J., 1981, Interaction of fluorescent gonadotropin-releasing hormone with receptors in cultured pituitary cells, J. Biol. Chem., 256:3049.

Naor, Z., Childs, G.V., Leifer, A.M., Clayton, R.N., Amsterdam, A. and Catt, K.J., 1982, Gonadotropin-releasing hormone binding and activation of enriched population of pituitary gonadotrophs, Mol. Cell. Endocrinol., 25:85.

Naor, Z., Amsterdam, A. and Catt, K.J., 1983a, Binding and activation of gonadotropin-releasing hormone receptors in pituitary gonadotrophs, in: "Hormone Receptors in Growth and Reproduction", B.B. Saxen, K.J. Catt, L. Birnbaumer and L. Martini, eds., New York, Raven Press, vol. 9, pp. 1-19.

Naor, Z., Vanderhoek, J.Y., Lindner, H.R. and Catt, K.J., 1983b, Arachidonic acid products as possible mediators of the action of gonadotropin-releasing hormone, Advances in Prostaglandin, Thromboxane and Leukotriene Research, 12:259.

Nimrod, A. and Lindner, H.R., 1980, Heparin facilitates the induction of LH receptors by FSH in granulosa cells cultured in serum-enriched medium, FEBS Lett., 119:155.

Pastan, I.H. and Willingham, M.C., 1981, Receptor-mediated endocytosis of hormones in cultured cells, Ann. Rev. Physiol, 43:239.

Pieper, D.R., Gala, R.R., Regiani, R. and Marshall, J.C., 1982, Dependence of pituitary gonadotropin-releasing hormone (GnRH) receptors on GnRH secretion from the hypothalamus, Endocrinology, 110:749.

Posner, B.I., Kelly, P.A. and Friesen, H.G., 1975, Prolactin receptors in rat liver: Possible induction by prolactin, Science, 188:57.

Prives, J., Silman, I., and Amsterdam, A., 1976, Appearance and disappearance of acetylcholine receptor during differentiation of chick skeletal muscle in vitro. Cell, 7:543.

Prives, J., Hoffman, L., Tarrab-Hazdai, R., Fuchs, S. and Amsterdam, A., 1979, Ligand induced changes in stability and distribution of acetylcholine receptors on surface membranes of muscle cells, Life Sci., 24:1713.

Rajaniemi, H.J., Midgley, Jr., A., Duncan, J.A. and Reichert, Jr., L.E., 1977, Gonadotrophin receptors in rat ovarian tissue; III. Binding sites for luteinizing hormone and differentiation of granulosa cells to luteal cells, Endocrinology, 101:898.

Rao, Ch.V. and Mitra, S., 1979, Gonadotropin and prostaglandins binding sites in nuclei of bovine corpora lutea, Biochim. Biophys. Acta, 584:454.

Richards, J-A.S., 1980, Maturation of ovarian follicles: Actions and interactions of pituitary and ovarian hormones on follicular cell differentiation, Physiol. Revs. 60:51.

Savoy-Moore, R.T., Schwartz, N.B., Duncan, J. and Marshall, J.C., 1980, Pituitary gonadotropin releasing hormone receptors during the rat estrous cycle, Science, 209:942.

Schlessinger, Y., Shechter, Y., Cuatrecasas, P., Willingham, M.C. and Pastan, I., 1978, Quantitative determination of the lateral diffusion coefficients of the hormone-receptor complexes of insulin and epidermal growth factor on the plasma membrane of cultured fibroblasts. Proc. Natl. Acad. Sci. U.S.A., 75:5353.

Sheridan, J.D., 1971, Dye movement and low resistance junctions between reaggregated embryonic cells, Devl. Biol.., 26:627.

Silverstein, S.C., Steinman, R.M. and Conn, Z.A., 1977, Endocytosis, Ann. Rev. Biochem. 46:699.

Steer, C., and Ashwell, G., 1980, Studies on a hepatic binding protein specific for asialoglycoproteins. Evidence for receptor recycling in isolated rat hepatocytes, J. Biol. Chem., 225:3008.

Ying, S-Y., Ling, N., Bohlen, P. and Guillemin, R., 1981, Gonadocrinins: Peptides in ovarian follicular fluid stimulating the secretion of pituitary gonadotropins, Endocrinology, 108:1206.

Zeleznik, A.J., Midgley, Jr. A.R. and Reichert, Jr., L.E., 1974, Granulosa cell maturation in the rat: Increased binding of human chorionic gonadotropin following treatment with follicle-stimulating hormone in vivo, Endocrinology, 95:818.

Zilberstein, M., Zakut, H., and Naor, Z., 1983, Coincidence of down regulation and desensitization in pituitary gonadotrophs stimulated by GnRH, Life Sci., 32:663.

Zor, U., 1983, Role of cytoskeleton organization in the regulation of adenylate cyclase-cyclic adenosine monophosphate by hormones, Endocr. Rev., 4:1.

Zor, U., Strulovici, B. and Lindner, H.R., 1978, Implication of microtubules and microfilaments in the response to the ovarian adenylate cyclase-cyclic AMP system to gonadotropins and postaglandin E_2, Biochem. Biophys. Res. Commun., 80:983.

Zor, U., Strulovici, B., Lamprecht, S.A., Oplatka, A., Amsterdam, A. and Lindner, H.R., 1979, Effect of modulators of cytoskeletal function on prostaglandin E_2-induced desensitization of ovarian adenylate cyclase, Prostaglandins, 18:869.

Zor, U., Shentzer, P., Azrad, A., Sairam, M.R. and Amsterdam, A., 1983a, Deglycosylated lutropin prevents desensitization of cyclic AMP response by lutropin: Dissociation between receptor uncoupling and down regulation, Endocrinology, in press.

Zor, U., Sairam, M.R., Shentzer, P., Azrad, A., and Amsterdam, A., 1983b, The role of carbohydrate moiety in the gonadotropin molecule in evoking cellular response to the hormone, Submitted.

STRATEGIES FOR THE INHIBITION OF GONADOTROPIN ACTION

M.R. Sairam

Reproduction Research Laboratory
Clinical Research Institute Laboratory
110 Pine Avenue West
Montreal, Quebec H2W 1R7 Canada

INTRODUCTION

The growth and maintenance of gonadal functions are directly under the control of pituitary gonadotropins. In special events such as pregnancy the placenta also provides important gonadotropic support by secreting highly active choriogonadotropins. In view of this various approaches for curtailing their action have been constantly sought as suitable points of attack to control reproduction. The isolation, characterization and structure of the gonadotropic hormones and the hypothalamic releasing factor LH-RH and the synthesis of numerous analogs of the latter with differing and well defined biological activity have intensified research in this direction.

For the purposes of discussion of the theme of this article, the present knowledge of the hypothalamo-pituitary-gonadal axis can be depicted as shown in figure 1. Based on this scheme four principal strategies that have the net effect of preventing the action of gonadotropins can be considered. These are 1) inhibition of the secretion of pituitary gonadotropins by compounds such as LH-RH analogs, gonadal steroids and non-steroidal substances (inhibin). Except for inhibin(s) which is still in its developmental stages there are extensive and decisive data describing the development of potent and long acting compounds related to LH-RH (1) and steroids (2). 2) Neutralization of the circulating gonadotropins by passive or active immunization using highly purified gonadotropins, subunits or their synthetic fragments coupled to suitable carriers (3). In this regard we can expect interesting developments by the application of hybridoma technology. 3) The selective inhibition of binding of gonadotropins to their cellular

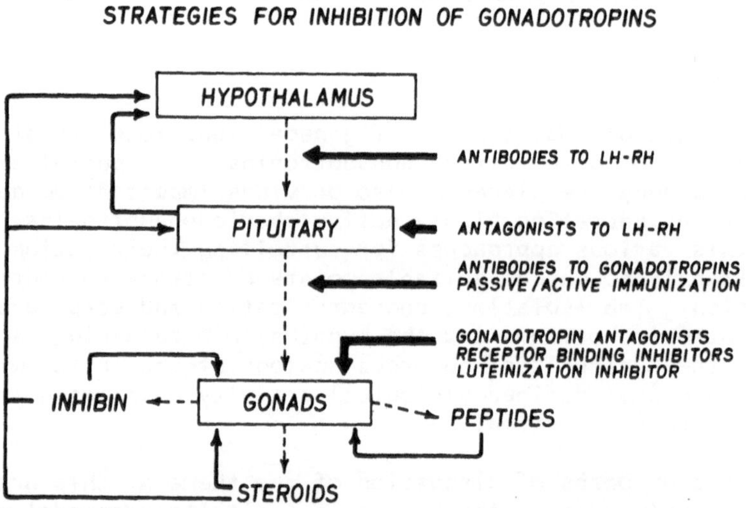

Fig. 1. Strategies for inhibition of gonadotropins.

receptors and 4) by other substances such as steroids, prostaglandins, LH-RH like factors or other pharmacological drugs which exert an intracellular action in the ovary and testis.

The third approach has been of considerable interest to us in recent years and I wish to focus attention on these aspects. The localization of gonadotropin receptors principally in the gonads and the highly specific nature of the hormone-receptor interaction suggests that an inhibitor of hormone binding may have the potential of preventing gonadotropin action at the target level. The development of rapid radioreceptor assays and analysis of hormone effects in dispersed or cultured gonadal cells have stimulated interest in the pursuit of these inhibitors. This article evaluates the presently available data on gonadotropin receptor binding inhibitors and shows that the chemically deglycosylated gonadotropin antagonists are the most well characterized among this group of compounds.

<u>Gonadotropin receptor binding inhibitors (RBI)</u>.

A substance binding to the receptor may either be an agonist or antagonist capable of stimulating or inhibiting the cells response. Since our interest is in the latter further discussion on the receptor binding inhibitors will be considered with this in view. Gonadotropin receptor binding inhibitors have been reported to be present in serum, ovarian follicular fluid, extracts of the corpus luteum, testis, semen and urine. They have also been prepared recently by specific chemical modification of highly purified pituitary and placental gonadotropin preparations.

The compounds which are reported to act as blocking agents at the gonadotropin receptor can be calssified into 3 categories as shown in fig. 2. Their discussion leads to a number of questions such as the following:

1. Problem of isolation.

2. What is their chemical nature and structure?

3. Any relation to gonadotropin?

4. Are there any sex differences in nature and action?

5. What is their efficacy and specificity-tissue and hormone?

6. Do they have any intrinsic agonistic activity. If so, how much compared to the hormone?

7. Do they inhibit hormone action? Specificity?

8. Immunological problems. Is antibody formation induced?

9. Are they active *in vivo?*

At present none of the gonadotropin RBI substances in biological fluids or extracts have been isolated in a highly purified state sufficient for detailed chemical characterization and hence most data are based on the use of raw or partially purified fractions. Such data are to be viewed with some caution as receptor assays can be influenced by many non specific factors.

Follitropin binding inhibitors (FSHRBI) found in serum appear to be of different types. FSHRBI activity is associated with a small molecular weight compound of less than 1000 daltons (6) and a large molecule behaving like an IgG (7). The latter present in sera of patients are thought to be antibodies directed at or near the FSH receptor and could be responsible for their clinical FSH resistance. Small molecular weight compounds with FSHRBI have also been detected in testis extracts (8) and follicular fluid (9). Data from our own studies suggest large molecular weight fractions similar to pituitary FSH (perhaps not identical) may be present in bovine and porcine follicular fluid (M.R. Sairam & Ranganathan, M.R., unpublished results) and bull seminal plasma (10). They effectively

BLOCKING AGENTS ACTING AT THE RECEPTOR

Receptor Binding Inhibitors	Modified Gonadotropins	Other
A. Lutropin binding Inhibitor LH-RBI-rat, bovine, ovine, porcine, human ovary, rat & calf testis.	A. Deglycosylated hormones DG-LH, DG-FSH, DG-hCG	LH & hCGβ subunits DAPA
	B. Nitroguanidyl oLH	
B. Follitropin binding Inhibitor FSH-RBI, rat, calf, sheep and primate testis, bovine and porcine ovary. Serum, seminal plasma.	C. Urinary Gonadotropin inhibiting materials (LH-GIM, FSH-GIM?)	

Fig. 2. Classification of gonadotropin receptor blocking agents. Small molecules such as steroids and prostaglandins are not included in this category. Reference for β subunit see (4) and DAPA-dansyl-arginyl-(4'-ethyl) piperidine amide see (5).

compete for binding to FSH receptor sites in the testis but their biological properties viz. ability to induce FSH type of response have not been studied in detail to warrant tests for antagonistic behavior.

Reports on the presence of Lutropin binding inhibitor in the ovary are more numerous. These have been found in extracts of corpora lutea of rats (11), pig (12), sheep (13) and human (14). The precise molecular size of these factor(s) is not known but appear to greatly vary ranging from 3800 to greater than 30,000. The rat luteal LHRBI is apparently sex specific because it does not affect the binding of LH to testicular receptors (11). Consequently, the rat luteal inhibitor inhibits LH stimulated progesterone synthesis in the ovarian slices of pseudopregnant rats but no such effects are seen in testicular cells *in vitro* (15). Similar data on LHRBI of other species are not available to conclude if this is a typical characteristic of the molecule(s).

It is difficult to predict the physiological significance of these receptor binding inhibitors of gonadal or other origin because the most important and crucial step of isolating the active substance(s) has not been successfully completed. Whether some of them represent fragments of the membrane (receptor) or the hormone is unknown. We need more conclusive data to evaluate their potential role in normal physiology or pathology and contraception. Their isolation is complicated by the accompanying presence of the so called receptor binding stimulators in the crude extracts (16). With the application of the more highly resolving purification methods of recent years we may expect significant advances in their isolation and characterization.

Modified gonadotropins as receptor binding inhibitors

Available data show that at present the modified gonadotropin preparations represent the best form of gonadotropin receptor binding inhibitors. These preparations arose from the systematic investigations on the structure-function relationships of the gonadotropic hormones (17). Treatment of highly purified gonadotropins which contain 15-40% carbohydrate with reagents such as anhydrous hydrogen fluoride (16,18) results in the specific and quick removal of up to 80% of the sugar residues within 60 mins. The resulting product, called deglycosylated hormone in the following discussion has properties that interest both biochemists as well as physiologists and prompt their use as antagonists.

We have now successfully applied the technique of chemical deglycosylation in four instances (Fig. 3) to obtain the four DG-hormones. Their preparation and properties have been described in detail and complete references may be found in the recent review (17) on this subject. The specific removal of carbohydrate has no

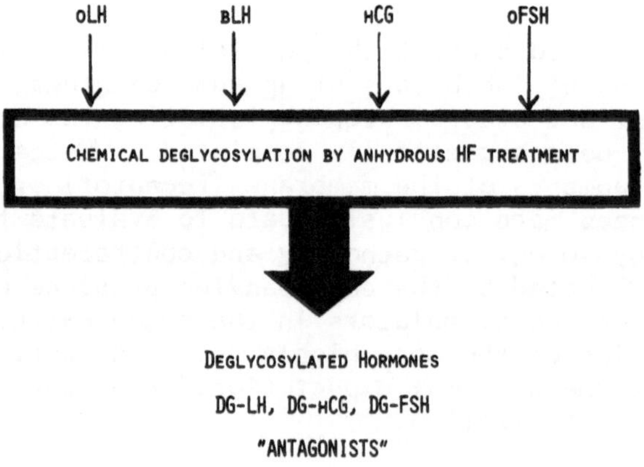

Fig. 3. Preparation of deglycosylated (DG) gonadotropins as receptor binding inhibitors.

effect on the integrity of the polypeptide backbone of the hormones including the maintenance of the quaternary structure. Their physico-chemical characteristics are known (17) and adequate quantities can be easily produced in any biochemical laboratory (19).

Specific removal of nearly 3/4ths of the carbohydrate moiety does not reduce receptor binding activity. On the other hand as illustrated for DG-hCG in table 1 below, this activity is increased with all the four receptor systems investigated thus far. This is clearly due to the increased affinity of the DG-hCG to the membrane receptors. Hormone binding specificity is not also altered by deglycosylation because DG-hCG like hCG itself remains very weakly active in its ability to bind to FSH receptors either in the ovary or testis.

Table 1. Receptor binding activity of deglycosylated hCG (DG-hCG).

Receptor preparation	% Binding Activity*
Rat testis	186 ± 10
Rat ovary	179 ± 18
Porcine ovary	200 ± 6
Human testis	300-500

* Binding activity in each instance is compared with hCG as 100%. The ability of DG-hCG to compete with ^{125}I-hCG was assessed in the respective membrane receptor assays with an incubation period of 2-6 hrs at 37°C.

Similar data are available with DG-FSH which shows an increased affinity to all the membrane receptors of the ovary and testis but with DG-oLH and DG-bLH (Fig. 3) their affinities are about the same as that of the native hormone. The kinetics of hormone binding to the receptor are similar for both hCG and DG-hCG. When this is examined with receptor preparations from the pig ovary maximal binding is attained in about 4 hrs. There is virtually no difference between hCG and DG-hCG in their ability to effectively prevent further binding of ^{125}I-labeled hCG after the initiation of the reaction (Fig. 4). Both preparations inhibit binding provided the additions of the unlabeled samples are made before the receptor-

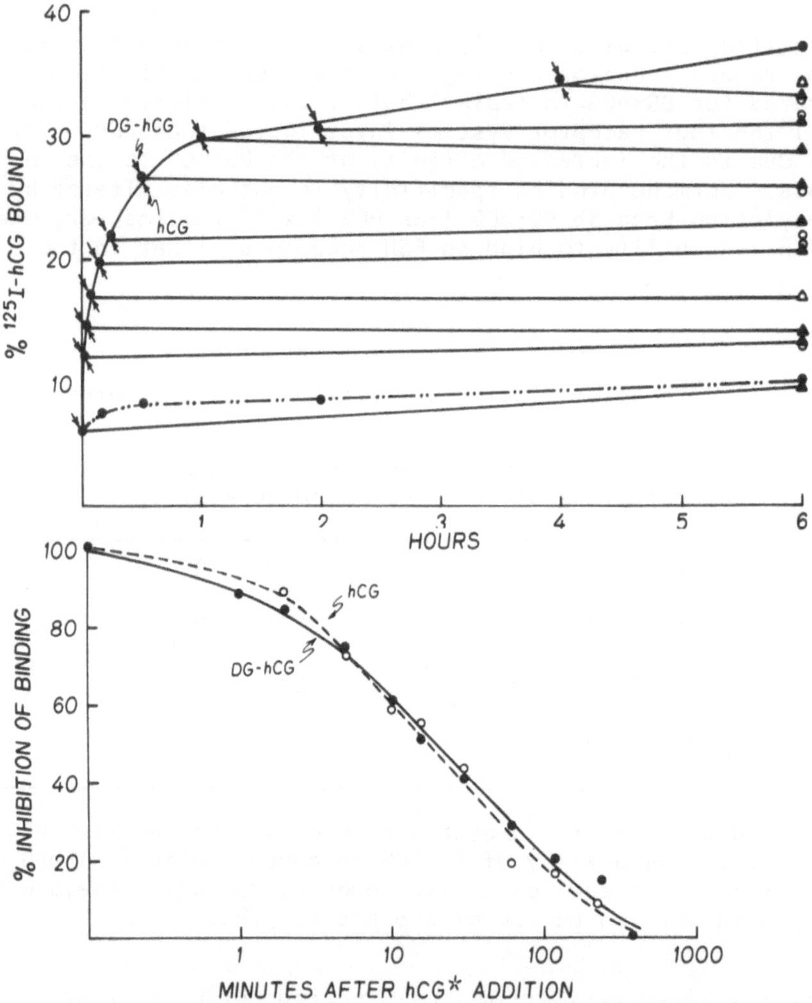

Fig. 4. Competition by hCG and DG-hCG for binding to the porcine ovarian receptor. In the top panel unlabeled DG-hCG & hCG were added at different times (shown by arrows) after the initiation of binding with ^{125}I-hCG at zero hr. The reaction was terminated at 6 hr and % bound ^{125}I-hCG was determined. In the bottom panel the data are shown depicting inhibition vs time-50% inhibition can still be seen after a delay of 20 mins.

hormone complex(es) attains a state of irreversibility. This illustrates that hormone binding *in vitro* seems to be one of a very tight nature in the isolated membranes.

Tissue specificity of binding of the hormone is not altered by deglycosylation because both labeled preparations bind only to the testicular and ovarian membranes from where they are effectively displaced by respective unlabeled preparations. However, their binding to non-target tissues such as liver and kidney under identical conditions remains low and non specific.

An important characteristic of the subunit nature of the gonadotropins is that their appropriate union is required for effective hormone binding to the receptor and biological activity. Removal of 3/4ths of carbohydrate from either the α and β subunits or both has no effect on the formation of a recombinant which effectively inhibits binding of labeled gonadotropin to the receptor. This has been demonstrated using subunits of oLH, oFSH and hCG (17). As discussed elsewhere (17), the biological profile of the recombinant depends on the crucial and complete integrity of the α-subunit.

Immunological properties

In specific radioimmunoassays using antiserum prepared against the native hormone the respective DG-gonadotropins are fully reactive indicating that the carbohydrate units are not too important for immunological activity. Similar data are available with individual deglycosylated subunits (eg. of oLH ref. 20).

Cellular actions of modified gonadotropins

Gonadotropins act on their target organs producing acute as well as long term effects. The acute responses such as cyclic AMP accumulation and stimulation of steroidogenesis can be easily measured in dispersed gonadal cells incubated *in vitro*. The long term effects which include growth, development of receptors and differentiation can also be studied by maintaining cells in tissue culture.

We have now accumulated considerable amount of data on the acute effects of deglycosylated gonadotropins *in vitro*. Unlike the native hormones, the DG preparations are in general very poor stimulators of intracellular responses such as cyclic AMP accumulation and steroidogenesis. Such contrasting profiles in activity is illustrated in fig. 5 for hCG and DG-hCG. The phenomenon is similar with other DG-hormones in ovarian and/or testicular cells incubated *in vitro*. These activity data considered together with the results on receptor binding shown in table 1 clearly suggest a dissociation of events in the biological action of DG-hCG. Thus, the modified hormone once bound to the external membrane receptor becomes incapable of catalyzing intracellular metabolic events that lead to a

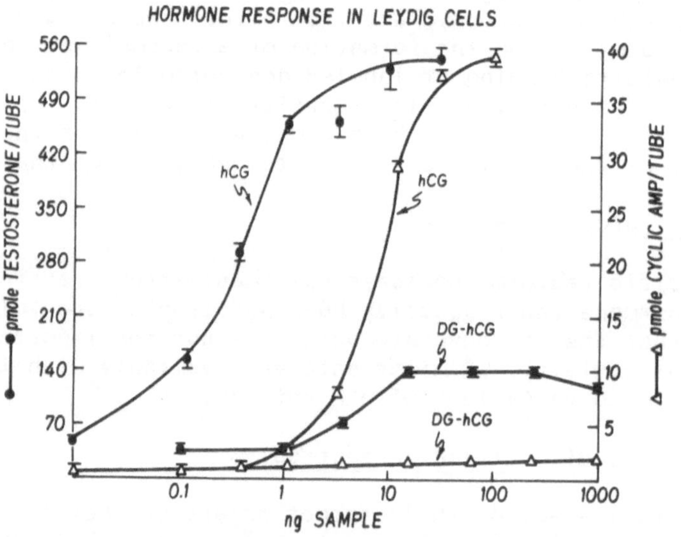

Fig. 5. Response of rat interstitial cells to the action of hCG and DG-hCG. Taken from ref. 21.

full complement of hormone response(s). This would imply that adenylate cyclase activity in the cell is not activated in the presence of DG-hCG or the modified gonadotropin induces an uncoupling of the receptor-adenylate cyclase system.

Hormonal antagonistic activity *in vitro*

It is logical for molecules such as DG-gonadotropins which bind with high affinity to the receptor without evoking full hormonal response to display considerable degree of hormonal antagonistic activity. This expectation if fulfilled by all the DG-gonadotropic preparations examined thus far (17). The inhibition of hormone action is both dose dependent and virtually complete. For example DG-hCG has no effect on FSH action on its own target cells in the ovary or testis. Similarly, it does not inhibit the action of TSH on thyroid cells. These results are fully consistent with the receptor binding specificity of DG-hCG. DG-hCG has no inhibitory action on non-hormonal or non-gonadotropin stimuli that can act on gonadal cells eg: choleragen, inducing cyclic AMP accumulation (21). Thus, in the presence of DG-gonadotropins, the coupling between hormone-receptor complex on the exterior and the adenylate cyclase in the interior of the cell membrane appears to be disrupted. The exact manner in which this effect is brought about has not yet been understood and is the subject of further studies.

Competition for receptor binding *in vivo*

The assessment of the ability of an unlabeled antagonist to compete with ^{125}I-labeled gonadotropin for binding sites in the target tissue is useful in evaluating its potential efficacy *in vivo*. In pseudopregnant rats which have a high number of LH receptors in the ovary, injection of ^{125}I-labeled hCG leads to maximal accumulation of radioactivity in about 120 mins. In such instances simultaneous administration of unlabeled DG-hCG (Table 2) can effectively block the uptake of radioactivity (hCG). In marked contrast to this, up to 25 µg of asialo hCG, a form of the hormone which can also bind effectively to the receptor *in vitro* but has no *in vivo* biological activity because it is cleared rapidly cannot compete with ^{125}I-hCG. These comparative data reveal that adequate quantities of DG-hCG can reach the target tissue to compete with ^{125}I-hCG for the binding sites.

It appears that the antagonist reaching the ovary remains bound to the receptor for a much longer time (Table 3). We have speculated that this could be due to the differential metabolism of DG-hCG as compared to hCG once it is bound to the ovarian receptor sites. Indeed, more recent data have revealed that DG-hCG is internalized and metabolized at a rate much slower than hCG (A. Amsterdam, personal communication).

Table 2. Inhibition of uptake of ^{125}I-hCG in the pseudopregnant rat ovary.

Group	Treatment ^{125}I-hCG plus	Ratio of radioactivity in 100 mg ovary/ 100 μl blood Mean ± SEM	
1	vehicle	120.0 ± 6.0	
2	hCG 5 μg	23.0 ± 0.6	$P < 0.05$
3	DG-hCG 5.7 μg	111.0 ± 2.3	NS
4	DG-hCG 11.4 μg	19.0 ± 3.6	$P < 0.05$
5	DG-hCG 45.6 μg	18.1 ± 0.7	$P < 0.05$
6	Asialo hCG 25 μg	101.6 ± 9.8	NS

Approximately 3 ng equivalent of ^{125}I-hCG (specific activity 60-90 μCi/μg) was injected into pseudopregnant rats (n = 5 per group). ^{125}I-hCG and other unlabeled hormone solutions were injected intracardiac in 0.2 ml vehicle which consisted of 1% bovine serum albumin in 0.9% saline. Rats were sacrificed 2 hrs after injection, a time at which uptake of ^{125}I-hCG was maximum. A decrease in the ratio of radioactivity in the ovary: Blood denotes effective competition. Statistical significance is compared with group 1. NS = Not significant.

Antagonistic activity of receptor binding inhibitors *in vivo*

There are virtually no reports of the *in vivo* antagonistic properties (if any) of substances identified as gonadotropin receptor binding inhibitors, although some (22) have been attributed to their presence. Since the data were derived from the use of very crude extracts the conclusions must be regarded as tentative. In contrast to this there have been numerous reports over the last 20 years of the so called urinary gonadotropin inhibiting substances exhibiting *in vivo* antagonistic effects against circulating LH in rats and mice (see 17 for review). The identification of the active ingredients in these partially purified extracts awaits further studies.

Table 3. Fate of bound ^{125}I-hCG and ^{125}I-hCG in the ovary.

Time	hCG* % Maximum	DG-hCG* % Maximum
15 mins	23	96
30 mins	53	85
60 mins	87	100
120 mins	100	83
240 mins	59	59
360 mins	23	54

* Experimental protocol similar to Table 2. Data at each time are expressed as % of radioactivity remaining bound to the ovary as compared to the maximum uptake attained for ^{125}I-hCG (2 hrs) and ^{125}I-DG-hCG (1 hr).

Table 4. Termination of pregnancy by hCG antagonist.

Treatment	Implantation sites	% fetal mortality	Serum progesterone ng/ml Mean ± SEM
Vehicle control	13.4	7.5	120.1 ± 13.6
DG-hCG, 10 μg (5)	11.4	22.9	96.8 ± 12.8
DG-hCG, 30 μg (5)	12.0	96.7	56.5 ± 16.7[a]
DG-hCG, 50 μg (7)[b]	11.0	100.0	15.5 ± 4.0[a]

Animals were laparotomized on day 8. After noting the number of sites, treatment was initiated once daily until day 11. The animals were autopsied on day 16. The number of animals per group is shown in parentheses.

[a] $P < 0.05$ as compared to control.

[b] The animals in this group had resorbing fetuses on day 16.

Table 5. Properties of gonadotropin antagonists and GIM.

Property	DG-gonadotropins	GIM
Characteristics	Well defined	Incomplete, to be isolated & identified
Carbohydrate content	Residual	Perhaps residual
Specificity		
binding	Yes	Yes
sex	No	No
species	No	No
Inhibitory activity *in vitro* & *in vivo*	Yes	Yes
Immuno reactivity v/s gonadotropic antisera	Yes	Unknown
Stability	Highly stable including heat treatment	Highly stable including heat treatment

Besides such reports, the use of deglycosylated hormones as antagonists provides the first successful demonstration of blockade of gonadotropin action at the receptor level by well defined chemical entities. Encouraged by the antagonistic activity of DG-hCG *in vitro* and uptake studies *in vivo*, we have used the rat as a model to test the *in vivo* efficacy of DG-hCG as an inhibitor of circulating LH. It is well established that hypophysectomy or neutralization of circulating LH in the rat before midpregnancy results in the inhibition of implantation as well termination of an established pregnancy. The ability of appropriately administered DG-hCG in inhibiting implantation and pregnancy (Table 4) is in complete agreement with these conclusions. The drastic fall in serum progesterone in the treated animals as compared to control pregnant rats (Table 4) must be responsible for the termination of gestation. Interestingly, if the antagonist DG-hCG is administered during the second half of pregnancy i.e. beyond day 13, there is no detrimental effect on pregnancy or parturition as all animals deliver at the expected time (23). These are again in complete accord with the well known fact that LH is not required in the rat after day 12 for the maintenance of pregnancy.

In other studies (24) DG-hCG has been shown to inhibit ovulation in immature and cycling rats. Such evidence have led us to conclude that DG-hCG is an inhibitor of gonadotropin action *in vivo* by virtue of its exerting a blockade at the receptor level.

Parallels in the nature and action of human urinary GIM and deglycosylated gonadotropins

Although they were not classified as such then, the gonadotropin inhibiting materials(s) (GIM) reported in human urine since 1960's (see 17) were the first receptor binding inhibitors to be described. As gonadotropin receptor binding assays were not available then, such activity had not been recognized. With the development of deglycosylated gonadotropins as antagonists, one can recognize many similarities in their nature and mechanism of action and those of GIM (see table 5). As discussed elsewhere, this has given rise to the speculation that GIM(s) may indeed be some form of a modified gonadotropin produced *in vivo* during metabolism and excreted in the urine (17). Renewed studies are required to substantiate and clarify these possibilities.

Concluding Comments

The idea of interfering with the action of gonadotropins at the local level by means of receptor binding inhibitors specific for lutropin and follitropin is interesting and gaining ground. Among the host of substances described in the recent literature the modified gonadotropins generated by specific alteration of highly purified hormone preparations are the most well defined and potent. They have been shown to be active *in vitro* and *in vivo* by exerting a specific blockade at the receptor level by an uncoupling of the receptor-adenylate cyclase complex. Our data on deglycosylated gonadotropins first reported in 1979 has been confirmed in many laboratories. In view of the evidence that specific removal of a substantial part of the carbohydrate which is presumed to be on the periphery, induces profound changes in the biological profile of the molecule, we pose the question whether such a mechanism(s) operates *in vivo*, if so at what level and their potential physiological significance for the regulation of hormone action (17). Such metabolic alterations have been identified in examples such as adrenocorticotropin and parathyroid hormone. A vigorous pursuit of the many gonadotropin receptor binding inhibitors in variety of fluids or extracts, would provide us a new class of regulators. Identification and synthesis of small molecular weight compounds and/or methods to deliver the antagonists to the site of action will have important practical implications. Undoubtedly these specific gonadotropin antagonists will serve as excellent tools in exploring the mechanism of action of LH, hCG and FSH. Some of these aspects are discussed in the accompanying chapter by Zor *et al.* (25).

ACKNOLEDGEMENTS

This investigation was supported in part by MRC of Canada, WHO special program and Ford Foundation. I appreciate the collaboration of Drs. K. Kato and P. Manjunath in certain phases of this work and N. Valiquette for typing the manuscript.

REFERENCES

1. A.V. Schally, D.H. Coy and A. Arimura, Int. J. Gynaecol. Obstet. 18:318 (1980).
2. E. Diczfalusy, J. Steroid. Biochem. 11:443 (1979).
3. C. Sheela Rani, N.R. Moudgal, in: "Hormonal proteins and peptides. Gonadotropins", vol. 11, ed., C.H. Li, Acad. Press, pp. 135-184 (1983).
4. N.R. Moudgal and C.H. Li, Proc. Natl. Acad. Sci. (USA) 79:2500 (1982).
5. P. McIlroy, E.R. Bergert and R.J. Ryan, Endocrinol. 113:222, (1983).
6. L.E. Reichert, M.A. Sanzo and N.S. Darga, J. Clin. Endo. Metab. 49:866 (1979).
7. V. Chiauzzi, S. Cigorraga, M.E. Escobar, M.A. Rivarola and E.H. Charreau, J. Clin. Endo. Metab. 54:1221 (1982).
8. L.E. Reichert and H. Abbou-Issa, Biol. Reprod. 17:614 (1977).
9. P.W. Fletcher, J.A. Dias, M.E. Sanzo and L.E. Reichert, Mol. Cell. Endo. 25:303 (1982).
10. M.R. Sairam, M.R. Ranganathan and P. Lamothe, J. Endo. 84:17 (1980).
11. K.P. Yang, N.A. Samaan and D.N. Ward, Endocrinol. 98:233 (1976).
12. C.N. Sakai, B. Engel and C.P. Channing, Proc. Soc. Exptl. Biol. Med. 155:373 (1977).
13. G.L. Kumari, Ind. J. Exptl. Biol. 19:16 (1981).
14. G.L. Kumari, S. Vohra, L. Joshi and S. Roy, Hormone Res. 13:57 (1980).
15. K.P. Yang, N.A. Samaan and D.N. Ward, Endocrinol. 104:552 (1979).
16. D.N. Ward, W.K. Liu and S.D. Glenn, Adv. Exptl. Biol. Med. 147:263 (1982).
17. M.R. Sairam, in: "Hormonal proteins and peptides. Gonadotropins", vol. 11, ed., C.H. Li, Acad. Press, pp. 1-79 (1983).
18. M.R. Sairam and P.W. Schiller, Arch. Biochem. Biophys. 197:294 (1979).
19. P. Manjunath and M.R. Sairam, in: "Methods in Enzymology. Hormone Action", eds., L. Birnbaumer and B. O'Malley, Acad. Press, (In Press).
20. M.R. Sairam, Arch. Biochem. Biophys. 204:199 (1980).
21. M.R. Sairam and P. Manjunath, J. Biol. Chem. 258:445 (1983).
22. C.P. Channing, S.K. Batta and I.H. Bae, Proc. Soc. Exptl. Biol. Med. 166:479 (1981).
23. K. Kato, M.R. Sairam and P. Manjunath, Endocrinol. 113:195 (1983).
24. K. Kato and M.R. Sairam, Contraception 27:515 (1983).
25. U. Zor, M.R. Sairam and A. Amsterdam, see this volume.

THE ROLE OF CARBOHYDRATE MOIETY OF GONADOTROPIN MOLECULE IN TRANSDUCTION OF BIOLOGICAL SIGNAL

Uriel Zor, *M.R. Sairam, Pnina Shentzer, Anat Azrad and Abraham Amsterdam

Department of Hormone Research, The Weizmann Institute of Science, Rehovot, 76100, Israel, and
*Reproduction Research Laboratory, Clinical Research Institute of Montreal, Montreal, Quebec, Canada

INTRODUCTION

Antagonists to small peptide hormones such as vasopressin, oxytocin, gonadotropin-releasing hormone (GnRH) and even to protein hormones such as adrenocorticotropin-hormone (ACTH) or glucagon have been known for many years. These antagonists were useful to establish the mode of action of these hormones. However, until recently, no clearly identified antagonists to glycoprotein hormones such as luteinizing hormone (LH), human chorionic gonadotropin (hCG), follicle stimulating hormone (FSH) and pregnant mare serum gonadotropin (PMSG) were available (for review see Sairam, 1983).

Several investigators, using chemical and enzymatic techniques, have succeeded in removing most (80%) of the various sugar moieties from different gonadotropins (Moyle et al., 1975; Channing et al., 1978; Chen et al., 1982; Goverman et al., 1982; Manjunath and Sairam, 1982; Sairam, 1983; Rebois and Fishman, 1983; Sairam and Munjunath, 1983). The protein core of these derivatives is not modified during these procedures (Sairam, 1983). All these deglycosylated (DG) hormone derivatives (DGLH, DGhCG, DGFSH) bind specifically to the receptor of the homologous native hormone and have in general higher affinity (Chen et al., 1982; Sairam, 1983; Zor et al., 1984). However, all the DG hormones have very weak (if any) agonist activity with regard to stimulation of cyclic AMP formation by the gonads (Moyle et al., 1975; Channing et al., 1978; Chen et al., 1982; Goverman et al., 1982; Manjunath and Sairam, 1982; Rebois and Fishman, 1983; Sairam, 1983; Sairam and Manjunath, 1983;

Zor et al., 1984). DGLH, DGhCG and DGFSH do however behave as selective and strong antagonists, preventing the stimulatory effects of the homologous intact agonist on cyclic AMP and steroid hormone production (Moyle et al., 1975; Channing et al., 1978; Chen et al., 1982; Goverman et al., 1982; Manjunath and Sairam, 1982; Rebois and Fishman, 1983; Sairam, 1983; Sairam and Manjunath, 1983; Zor et al., 1984). Furthermore, in vivo administration of DGhCG to pregnant rats antagonized the action of pituitary LH and induced fetal mortality (Kato et al., 1983).

A decade ago, we first demonstrated that prolonged culture of ovarian follicles with LH reduced cyclic AMP formation in response to the hormonal challenge (Zor et al., 1972; Lamprecht et al., 1973; see also Fig. 1). This phenomenon was later shown to be hormone-specific (homologous desensitization), developing with relatively high concentrations of the agonist (Zor et al., 1976). An early hypothesis proposed by various groups suggested that massive loss of receptors from plasma membrane (receptor "down regulation") which sometimes occurred following chronic administration of hormones, may lead to desensitization of cyclic AMP response (Mukherjee et al., 1976). However, the discrepancy between the kinetics of development of desensitization and the reduction in binding sites by administration of various hormones, suggests that these events are separate and may be unrelated phenomena. In fact, desensitization occurs even though most (if not all) of the receptors can still be detected on the cell surface (Lamprecht et al., 1977; Amsterdam et al., 1979; 1980; 1981; Su et al., 1979; Zor, 1983; Zor et al., 1984). Therefore, the mechanism suggested for hormone induced-desensitization is based on macroaggregation of hormone-receptor complexes on the cell surface, followed by uncoupling of the occupied receptor from the adenylate cyclase moiety (Lamprecht et al., 1977; Amsterdam et al., 1979; 1980; 1981; Su et al., 1979; Zor, 1983; Zor et al., 1984).

In this article we discuss the role of the carbohydrate moiety in the gonadotropin molecule in transduction of the hormonal signal in the gonads. The DG gonadotropins are useful to differentiate between receptor occupancy and subsequent biological responses such as stimulation of cyclic AMP formation, and to investigate the phenomenon of desensitization (Zor et al., 1984).

RESULTS

The relationship between receptor loss and desensitization of cyclic AMP response induced by LH and DGLH were examined. Granulosa cells (GC) cultured for 20 h with LH retained only 10% of their maximal response to fresh LH (Fig. 1 and Table 1). Pretreatment with DGLH alone resulted in 55% retention of sensitivity to LH challenge (Fig. 1). Receptor binding capacity in GC was examined

Culture (20 h)	Washing	Challenge
DGLH or LH	pH 3.0	^{125}I-hCG or LH

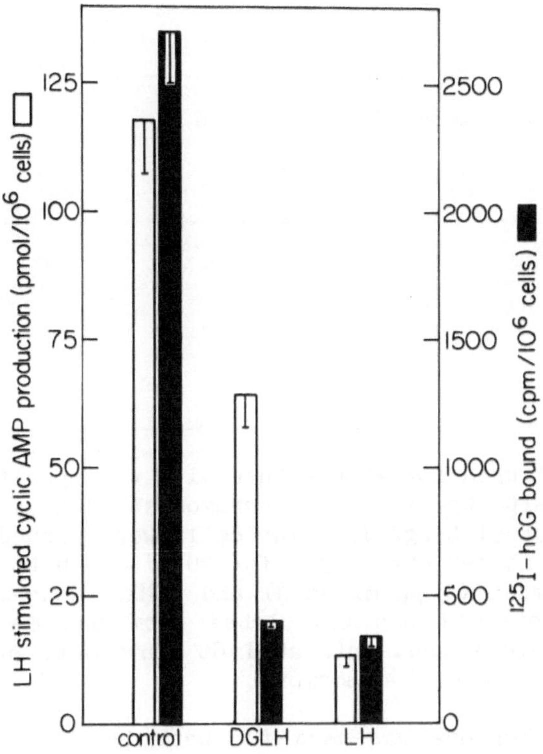

Fig. 1. Induction of receptor loss and desensitization of cyclic AMP response by DGLH and LH. Rat granulosa cells (GC) were prepared from PMSG-treated animals as described previously (Zor et al., 1984). GC were cultured for 20 h with DGLH (1.0 µg/ml), LH (1.0 µg/ml) or in a plain medium (control). The cells were washed for 3 min at 4°C with acidic medium (pH 3.0), in order to remove the bound hormones (Zor et al., 1984). GC then challenged either with ^{125}I-hCG for binding studies ▬ (for more experimental conditions see Amsterdam et al., 1979; 1980; 1983) or with unlabelled LH (1.0 µg/ml) + IBMX (0.45 mM) for examination of cyclic AMP formation ▭ during 30 min of incubation (for more experimental details see Lamprecht et al., 1977; Zor et al., 1984). Bars represent S.E.M.

by using labelled ^{125}I-hCG. During 20 h of culture with LH or DGLH, 85% of the receptors disappeared from the cell surface

Table 1: Prevention by DG hormones of gonadotropin-induced desensitization of cyclic AMP response.

	Retention of cyclic AMP response (%)			
Culture \ Challenge	LH	hCG	FSH	PMSG
Hormone[1]	10	10	10	5
DG hormone + hormone[2]	55	55	60	57

GC were cultured for 20 h either with the specified hormone (1.0 µg/ml) or with the specified antagonist (1.0 µg/ml) + the specified agonist (1.0 µg/ml). The cells were washed in acidic medium and thereafter challenged for 30 min with the specified homologous hormone (1 µg/ml each) and IBMX. Percent of cyclic AMP response retained was calculated from the maximal (100%) response obtained when untreated GC were only challenged for 30 min with the specified hormone.

1 Homologous hormone was used for both induction of desensitization during culture and for challenge.

2 DG homologous hormone was used together with the same homologous hormone. Only in the case of PMSG, DGhCG was added during culture together with PMSG.

(Fig. 1). Concomitant addition of DGLH with LH to cultured GC, prevented them by 55% from desensitization induced by LH (Table 1).

GC cultured for 20 h with hCG retained only 10% of their maximal response to challenge with hCG (Fig. 2). However, 50% of the receptors still remained on the plasma membrane. Pretreatment with DGhCG alone resulted in 55% retention of sensitivity to hCG challenge and a 15% reduction in number of surface receptors (Fig. 2). Concomitant addition of DGhCG with hCG to cultured GC, prevented them by 55% from desensitization induced by hCG (Table 1).

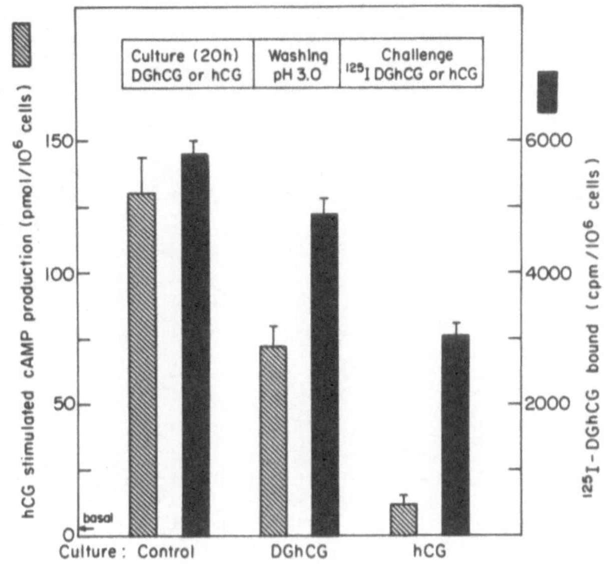

Fig. 2. Induction of receptor loss and desensitization of cyclic AMP response by DGhCG and hCG. GC were cultured for 20 h with DGhCG (1.0 µg/ml) or hCG (1.0 µg/ml) or in a plain medium (control). The cells were washed in acidic medium and thereafter challenged either with ^{125}I-DGhCG ▬ or with unlabelled hCG ▨ (1.0 µg/ml) + IBMX. (From Zor et al., in preparation.)

Hormone internalization and degradation was analyzed and compared using DGhCG and the native hormone. The intracellular fate of ^{125}I-labeled ligands was detected by high resolution autoradiography. The degraded product of the internalized hormones was assayed after precipitation of cells and media proteins by 10% trichloroacetic acid (TCA) (Amsterdam et al., 1979).

Eight hours after pulse with ^{125}I-DGhCG (60 min, at 37°C), 61% of the total specific binding of the ligand was retained on the cell membrane. In contrast, only 28% of the labelled hormone was retained when the cells were pulsed with ^{125}I-hCG. The reverse picture was obtained when the intracellular distribution of the labeled ligands was examined. Only 5% of ^{125}I-DGhCG, but about 25% of ^{125}I-hCG had accumulated in the lysosomes. The rate of degradation of ^{125}I-DGhCG was 40-50% to that of ^{125}I-hCG during 8 hr of incubation (Fig. 3).

Since the differentiated GC responded equally well to LH and FSH, we compared the ability of DGFSH to induce FSH receptor internalization and desensitization.

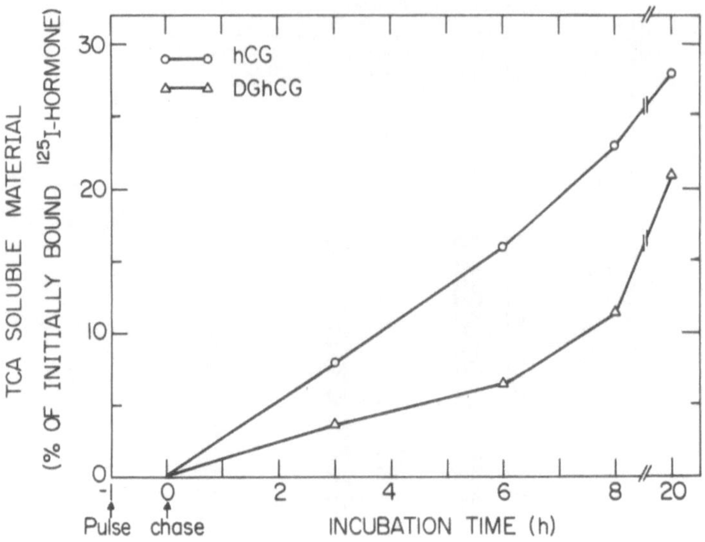

Fig. 3. Time course of degradation of receptor bound ^{125}I-hCG or ^{125}I-DGhCG by granulosa cell cultures. Granulosa cell cultures were pulse labeled with the radioactive ligands (4.10^6 cpm/ml) for 1 h and then chased in a hormone-free medium. Media were collected at different intervals, and precipitated in 10% TCA. The radioactivity in TCA soluble material which represents the degraded hormone was counted. The data are expressed as % of radioactivity bound to the cells at the end of the pulse (from Amsterdam et al., in preparation).

GC cultured for 20 h with FSH retained only 10% of the maximal response to challenge with the hormone (Fig. 4), while most (65%) of the receptors still remained on the cell surface. Pretreatment with DGFSH alone resulted in 60% retention of sensitivity to FSH challenge (Fig. 4). Not only was there no receptor loss but DGFSH actually induced a 25% increase in density of surface receptors above control level. Concomitant addition of DGFSH with FSH to cultured GC, prevented them by 60% from desensitization induced by FSH (Table 1).

Purified PMSG has the intrinsic activity of both FSH and LH. We used DGFSH and DGhCG in order to evaluate the relative activity of each gonadotropin in the PMSG molecule on stimulation of cyclic AMP formation (Fig. 5). Incubation of DGFSH with GC reduced by 20% the response to PMSG. However, this effect was reduced to a much greater extent (70%) by DGhCG. Concomitant addition of both DGFSH and DGhCG reduced by 95% the stimulatory effect of PMSG (Fig. 5).

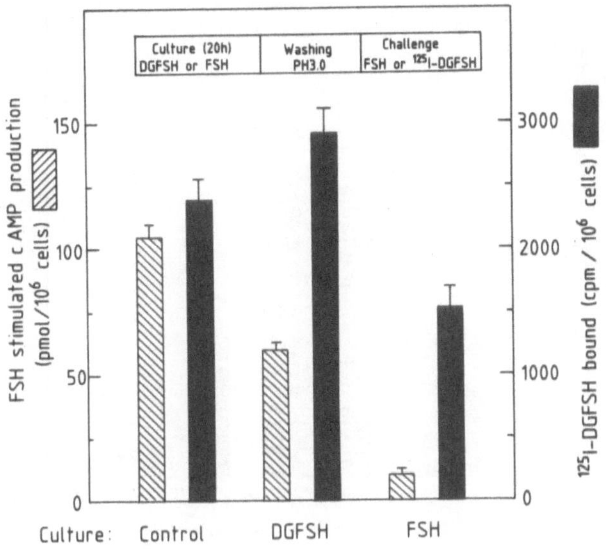

Fig. 4. Induction of receptor gain by DGFSH and receptor loss by FSH as well as desensitization of cyclic AMP response by both agonist and antagonist. GC were cultured for 20 h with DGFSH (1.0 µg/ml) or FSH (1.0 µg/ml) or in a plain medium (control). The cells were washed in acidic medium and thereafter challenged either with ^{125}I-DGFSH ▬ or with unlabelled FSH (1.0 µg/ml) + IBMX ▨ (Zor et al., in preparation).

GC culture for 20 h with PMSG retained only 5% of their maximal response to challenge with fresh PMSG (Table 1). When DGhCG was added with PMSG for 20 h they retained 57% of the sensitivity to PMSG (Table 1). With DGFSH, GC retained 23% of the sensitivity to PMSG. With concomitant addition of DGhCG + DGFSH + PMSG 75% of the sensitivity to PMSG challenge was retained.

DISCUSSION

The present study demonstrates that deglycosylated gonadotropins specifically prevent desensitization induced by the homologous native hormones, LH, hCG and FSH (Table 1). It should be noted that even after 20 h culture with the antagonists, a moderate reduction (about 40%) is observed in the maximal cyclic AMP response to challenge by the appropriate hormone agonist (Figs. 1, 2 and 4). Nev-

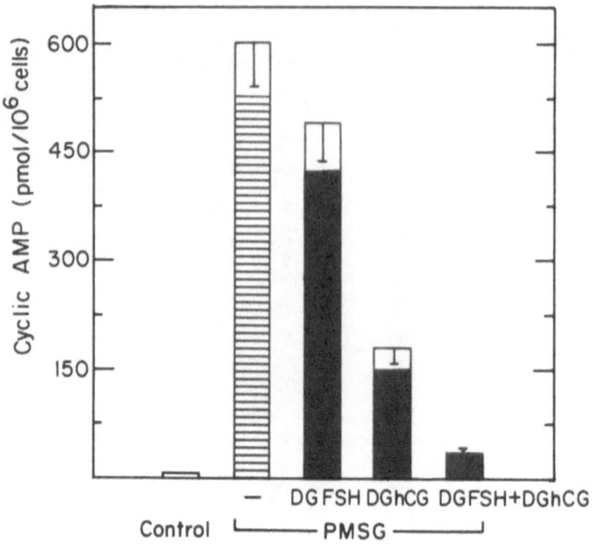

Fig. 5. Effect of DGFSH and/or DGhCG on the stimulatory effect of purified PMSG on cyclic AMP formation by GC. DGFSH (1.0 µg/ml) and/or DGhCG (1.0 µg/ml) added 30 min before PMSG. PMSG (1.0 ug/ml) + IBMX were added for another 30 min (Zor et al., in preparation).

ertheless, the desensitization induced by the native gonadotropins is far greater (about 90%) than that observed with the antagonists (Table 1 and Figs. 1, 2 and 4). It is possible that DG hormones induce sustained conformational changes in the receptor molecule. These interfere with the agonist-induced coupling mechanism between receptor and adenylate cyclase moiety, even after complete removal of the antagonists from the receptors. With regard to receptor disappearance, it was found that DGLH induces substantial (90%) reduction in receptor number, similar to that observed with LH. DGhCG, however, has no such effect (15% reduction only) and DGFSH even induces a significant increase in receptor density on the cell surface.

In a general comparison of binding of agonist or antagonist to receptor and induction of biological responses, several features may be noted. First, both agonist and antagonist bind to the same receptors, although generally there is higher affinity for antagonists (Moyle et al., 1975; Chen et al., 1982; Munjunath and Sairam, 1982; Sairam, 1983). Second, the rate of association and dissociation of agonists and antagonists is not influenced to the same extent under different experimental conditions (Hazum, 1981).

Third, agonists can induce fast coupling between receptor and effector. Antagonists in general do not induce coupling and so are devoid of biological activity. Moreover, prolonged administration of agonist may induce uncoupling, while antagonist cannot modulate the coupling/uncoupling mechanism (Mukherjee et al., 1976; Smith and Vale, 1981). Fourth, agonists induce lateral mobility and aggregation of receptors, while antagonists may be inactive in this respect (Conn et al., 1982). However, under certain conditions, antagonists could be transformed to agonists by attaching antagonist antibodies to the receptor-bound antagonist (Shechter et al., 1979; Conn et al., 1982). Fifth, receptor-bound antagonist was internalized and degraded, in vivo and in vitro at a slower rate than the agonist (Amsterdam et al., 1983; Kato et al., 1983, and Fig. 3).

DGhCG was retained on surface receptors of the cultured granulosa cell to a greater extent than that of hCG. These results are in accordance with those obtained in rat ovary in vivo (Kato et al., 1983). This may suggest that the rate of disappearance of the bound ligand and consequently degradation by the lysozomes, is somehow related to the carbohydrate moiety of the ligand. However, it was recently found that ovine LH internalized about 40 times faster than human LH (Mock and Niswender, 1983; Mock et al., 1983), although the contents of carbohydrate moiety are about the same in both. While Mock and Niswender (1983) compared glycoprotein hormone from two different species, our study deals with the same hormone molecule but with an altered sugar content. It should be noted that the decreased receptor loss from the cell surface induced by DGhCG as compared to the native hormone, coincides with the low rate of degradation of the bound ligand.

Two main mechanisms for hormone-induced desensitization are suggested. 1) Upon prolonged incubation of a hormone with cells, the hormone-receptor complex gradually becomes uncoupled from the GTP-regulatory unit and/or from the catalytic unit of adenylate cyclase (Lamprecht et al., 1977; Amsterdam et al., 1979; Su et al., 1979; Zor, 1983). The hormone is bound by the receptors and induces massive aggregation of hormone-receptor complexes at the cell surface. This can lead to uncoupling and consequently to desensitization (Amsterdam et al., 1980; 1981). We suggest therefore, that the inability of the DG gonadotropins to induce complete desensitization is related to their failure to induce massive receptor aggregation. 2) The hormone induces translocation of receptors from the cell surface, or sequestration of receptors in such a way as to render them inaccessible to free hormones. This phenomenon is termed receptor "down regulation" (Mukherjee et al., 1976; Krupp and Lane, 1981). Different cell types may exhibit the two different mechanisms of desensitization with regard to the same hormone: thus, catecholamines induce receptor uncoupling in turkey erythrocytes (Stadel et al., 1982) but receptor "down regulation" in frog erythrocytes (Mukherjee et al., 1976).

By using ovine DGLH, DGhCG and ovine DGFSH we have been able to differentiate between induction of desensitization and receptor loss. Culture of GC with DGLH for 20 h causes a loss of 85% of receptors from the cell surface, while the response to LH challenge is not severely affected. These results are in accordance with recent observations that the β-adrenergic antagonists markedly reduce the number of β adrenergic binding sites, but adenylate cyclase activity remains fully responsive to the adrenergic agonist (Giudicelli et al., 1979). In contrast to DGLH, DGhCG had only a marginal effect on receptor disappearance. This difference between DGLH and DGhCG is not yet understood. It may be significant, however, that native ovine LH is internalized at a rate about 60 times faster than that of native hCG (Mock and Niswender, 1983; Mock et al., 1983). The present study also suggests, at least in the case of DGLH, that loss of binding sites is probably not a rate limiting step in hormonal responsiveness, and that transduction of hormonal signal, is not a prerequisite for receptor internalization.

It is interesting to note that the antagonist of gonadotropin releasing hormone (GnRH), unlike the agonist, is not able to induce desensitization as assessed by stimulation of LH release (Smith and Vale, 1981). The ability of DGLH, DGhCG and DGFSH to induce partial desensitization, in contrast to the ineffectiveness of β adrenergic antagonists (Mukherjee et al., 1976; Giudicelli et al., 1979) or GnRH antagonists (Smith and Vale, 1981), may be related to the fact that the protein core of the DG gonadotropins are unimpaired, while the other antagonists are significantly altered both in chemical structure and conformation compared to native agonist.

It is not yet clear what role the carbohydrate moiety on the two subunits of the gonadotropin molecules play in the biological activity of the hormone. It seems however, that the carbohydrate moiety is important mainly for the α subunit of LH, since the recombinant native α + DGβ keeps full biological agonistic activity, while DGα + native β in contrast, has substantial antagonistic activity (Sairam, 1983).

Recent studies suggest that cytoskeletal elements are involved in activation of adenylate cyclase by hormones (for review see Zor, 1983). In addition, it was found that the LH receptor is initially associated with microvilli which are loaded with microfilaments (Amsterdam et al., 1981; Amsterdam and Lindner, 1983). Hormone antagonists may not be able to release the receptor which is constrained by the cytoskeleton, and so, it is possible in the case of LH, hCG and FSH, that the sugar moiety on the protein hormone essential for lateral mobility of the hormone-receptor complex (Amsterdam et al., 1980). Another possibility is that the receptor-GTP regulatory protein complex is formed only with the agonist and not when the receptor is unoccupied or occupied by antagonist (Limbird et al., 1980). LH can increase the binding of guanyl nucleotides to the plasma membrane (Dufau et al., 1980). It would be most interesting to examine whether DG gonadotropins are also active in this respect. The ability of the intact hormone to activate adenylate cyclase, in contrast to the inability of DG gonadotropins to do so, may suggest that the sugar part on a subunit of the hormone molecule is involved in coupling.

PMSG is used successfully for the induction of follicular development and maturation. It was believed that PMSG mainly resembled FSH-like activity. Our study, however, using either the antagonists of LH or FSH, clearly shows that the intrinsic biological activity in the PMSG molecule is mainly LH-like activity. The ratio between LH:FSH activity seems to be 3:1. This ratio is in agreement with the study of Combarnous et al. (1978). We therefore suggest that the high potency of PMSG in inducing follicular development may be related to its unique molecule that contains LH and FSH activity together, and with a very long half life in vivo.

It is obvious that gonadotropin antagonists such as deglycosylated hCG, FSH and possibly PMSG (when this will become available), serve as important tools in basic research for evaluation of the mechanism of gonadotropin action. Not less important, is the potential use of these antagonists in the interruption of human pregnancy, and also in the clinical treatment of increased production and release of gonadotropins during postnatal development. It will be highly interesting to examine whether DGhCG can prevent precocious puberty in children and interrupt pregnancy in adult humans.

SUMMARY AND CONCLUDING REMARKS

We have examined whether various deglycosylated gonadotropins (DGLH, DGhCG and DGFSH), which are hormone antagonists, could affect desensitization of cyclic AMP response induced by continuous exposure to homologous agonists (LH, hCG, FSH), and whether they induce receptor internalization.

We found that a) receptor occupancy alone without activation, for a long period, is essential, but not sufficient to induce complete hormone desensitization. b) The gonadotropin antagonists (DGLH, DGhCG, DGFSH) largely protect the bound receptors from being uncoupled by the homologous gonadotropin agonists, and thus prevent desensitization of the cyclic AMP response. c) Receptor-bound DGhCG internalized and degraded at a much slower rate than hCG. d) DGLH and DGhCG compete for the same receptors, but vary tremendously in their ability to induce receptor loss from the cell surface. e) No correlation exists between the ability of agonists or even antagonists to induce receptor loss and to induce desensitization of the response to agonist. f) Desensitization to gonadotropins results mainly from uncoupling of the hormone-receptor complex from the GTP regulatory protein and/or adenylate cyclase moiety.

ACKNOWLEDGMENT

This study was supported by grants from the Ford Foundation and the Rockefeller Foundation (to the late Prof. H.R. Lindner). We are grateful to Mrs. M. Kopelowitz and R. Levin for typing the manuscript. We thank Dr. S. Shoham-Moshonov for reading and editing the manuscript. U. Zor holds the W.B. Graham Professorial Chair in Pharmacology. This investigation was partially supported by the MRC of Canada (to M.R.S.).

REFERENCES

Amsterdam, A., and Lindner, H.R., 1983, Localization of gonadotropin receptors in the gonads, in: "Electron Microscopy in Biology and Medicine: Current Topics in Ultrastructural Research", P.M. Motta, ed., The Hague, The Netherlands, Martinus Nijhoff Publ., pp. 253-262.

Amsterdam, A., Berkowitz, A., Nimrod, A. and Kohen, F., 1980, Aggregation of luteinizing hormone receptors in granulosa cells: A possible mechanism of desensitization to the hormone, Proc. Natl. Acad. Sci. U.S.A. 77:3440.

Amsterdam, A., Naor, Z., Knecht, M., Dufau, M.L. and Catt, K.J., 1981, Hormone action and receptor redistribution in endocrine target cells: Gonadotropins and gonadotropin-releasing hormone, In: "Receptor-mediated Binding and Internalization of Toxins and Hormones", J.L. Middlebrook and L.D. Kohn, eds., Academic Press, Inc., p. 283.

Amsterdam, A., Nimrod, A., Lamprecht, S.A., Burstein, Y. and Lindner, H.R., 1979, Internalization and degradation of receptor-bound hCG in granulosa cell cultures, Am. J. Physiol. 236(2):E129.

Amsterdam, A., Sairam, M.R., and Zor, U., 1983, Deglycosylated human chorionic gonadotropin retards the down-regulation of luteinizing hormone receptors in granulosa cells, J. Cell Biol., 97:407a.

Channing, C.P., Sakai, C.N. and Bahl, O.P., 1978, Role of the carbohydrate residues of human chorionic gonadotropin in binding and stimulation of adenosine 3',8'-monophosphate accumulation by porcine granulosa cells, Endocrinology, 103:341.

Chen, H-C., Shimohigashi, Y., Dufau, M.L., and Catt, K.J., 1982, Characterization and biological properties of chemically deglycosylated human chorionic gonadotropin. Role of carbohydrate moieties in adenylate cyclase activation, J. Biol. Chem. 257:14446.

Combarnous, Y., Hennen, G., and Ketelslegers, J.M., 1978, Pregnant mare serum gonadotropin exhibits higher affinity for lutropin than for follitropin receptors of porcine testis, FEBS Lett. 90:65.

Conn, P.M., Rogers, D.C., Stewart, J.M., Niedel, J. and Sheffield, T., 1982, Conversion of a gonadotropin-releasing hormone antagonist to an agonist, Nature, 296:653.

Dufau, M.L., Baukal, A.J. and Catt, K.J., 1980, Hormone-induced guanyl nucleotide binding and activation of adenylate cyclase in the Leydig cell, Proc. Natl. Acad. Sci. U.S.A. 77:5837.

Giudicelli, Y., Lacasa, D. and Agli, B., 1979, Evidence for a second desensitized state of β-adrenergic receptor with low affinity for β-antagonists and normal reactivity towards β-agonists in adipocyte membranes previously exposed to β-antagonists, Eur. J. Biochem. 99:457.

Goverman, J.M., Parsons, T.F. and Pierce, J.G., 1982, Enzymatic deglycosylation of the subunits of chorionic gonadotropin. Effects on formation of tertiary structure and biological activity, J. Biol. Chem. 257:15059.

Hazum, E., 1981, Some characteristics of GnRH receptors in rat pituitary membranes: differences between an agonist and an antagonist, Mol. Cell. Endocr. 23:275.

Kato, K., Sairam, M.R. and Manjunath, P., 1983, Inhibition of implantation and termination of pregnancy in the rat by a human chorionic gonadotropin antagonist, Endocrinology, 113:195.

Krupp, M. and Lane, M.D., 1981, On the mechanism of ligand-induced down-regulation of insulin receptor level in the liver cell, J. Biol. Chem. 256:1689.

Lamprecht, S.A., Zor, U., Tsafriri, A. and Lindner, H.R., 1973, Action of prostaglandin E_2 and of luteinizing hormone on ovarian adenylate cyclase, protein kinase and ornithine decarboxylase activity during postnatal development and maturity in the rat, J. Endocr. 57:217.

Lamprecht, S.A., Zor, U., Salomon, Y., Koch, Y., Ahrén, K. and Lindner, H.R., 1977, Mechanism of hormonally induced refractoriness of ovarian adenylate cyclase to luteinizing hormone and prostaglandin E, J. Cyclic Nucl. Res. 3:69.

Limbird, L.E., Gill, D.M. and Lefkowitz, R.J., 1980, Agonist-promoted coupling of the β-adrenergic receptor with the guanine nucleotide regulatory protein of the adenylate cyclase system, Proc. Natl. Acad. Sci. U.S.A. 77:775.

Manjunath, P. and Sairam, M.R., 1982, Biochemical, biological, and immunological properties of chemically deglycosylated human choriogonadotropin, J. Biol. Chem. 257:7109.

Mock, E.J. and Niswender, G.D., 1983, Differences in the rates of internalization of ^{125}I-labeled human chorionic gonadotropin, luteinizing hormone, and epidermal growth factor by ovine luteal cells, Endocrinology, 113:259.

Mock, E.J., Papkoff, H. and Niswender, G.D., 1983, Internalization of ovine luteinizing hormone/human chorionic gonadotropin recombinants: Differential effects of the α- and β-subunits, Endocrinology, 113:265.

Moyle, W.R., Bahl, O.P. and März, L., 1975, Role of the carbohydrate of human chorionic gonadotropin in the mechanism of hormone action, J. Biol. Chem. 250:9163.

Mukherjee, C., Caron, M.G. and Lefkowitz, R.J., 1976, Regulation of adenylate cyclase coupled β-adrenergic receptors by β-adrenergic catecholamines, Endocrinology, 99:347.

Rebois, V.R., and Fishman, P.H., 1983, Deglycosylated human chorionic gonadotropin. An antagonist to desensitization and down-regulation of the gonadotropin receptor-adenylate cyclase system, J. Biol. Chem. 258:12775.

Sairam, M.R., 1983, Gonadotropic hormones: Relationship between structure and function with emphasis on antagonists, Hormonal Proteins and Peptides, XI:1.

Sairam, M.R. and Manjunath, P., 1983, Hormonal antagonistic properties of chemically deglycosylated human choriogonadotropin, J. Biol. Chem. 258:445.

Shechter, Y., Hernaez, L., Schlessinger, J. and Cuatrecasas. P. 1979, Local aggregation of hormone-receptor complexes is required for activation by epidermal growth factor, Nature, 278:835.

Smith, M.A. and Vale, W.W., 1981, Desensitization to gonadotropin-releasing hormone observed in superfused pituitary cells on cytodex beads, Endocrinology, 108:752.

Stadel, J.M., Nambi, P., Lavin, T.N., Heald, S.L., Caron, G. and Lefkowitz, R.J., 1982, Catecholamine-induced desensitization of turkey erythrocyte adenylate cyclase. Structural alterations in the β-adrenergic receptor revealed by photoaffinity labeling, J. Biol. Chem. 257:9242.

Su, Y-F., Harden, K.T. and Perkins, J.P., 1979, Isoproterenol-induced desensitization of adenylate cyclase in human astrocytoma cells. Relation of loss of hormonal responsiveness and decrement in β-adrenergic receptors, J. Biol. Chem. 254:38.

Zor, U., Lamprecht, S.A., Kaneko, T., Schneider, H.P.G., McCann, S.M., Field, J.B., Tsafriri, A. and Lindner, H.R., 1972, Functional relations between cyclic AMP, prostaglandins and luteinizing hormone in rat pituitary and ovary, Adv. Cyclic. Nucl. Res. 1:503.

Zor, U., Lamprecht, S.A., Misulovin, Z., Koch, Y. and Lindner, H.R., 1976, Refractoriness of ovarian adenylate cyclase to continued hormonal stimulation, Biochim. Biophys. Acta, 428:761.

Zor, U., Shentzer, P., Azrad, A., Sairam, M.R. and Amsterdam, A., 1984, Deglycosylated lutropin prevents desensitization of cyclic AMP response by lutropin: Dissociation between receptor uncoupling and down regulation, Endocrinology (in press).

Zor, U., 1983, Role of cytoskeletal organization in the regulation of adenylate cyclase-cyclic adenosine monophosphate by hormones, Endocrine Rev. 4:1.

INTRAOVARIAN REGULATION OF FOLLICULAR GRANULOSA CELL DIFFERENTIATION

Joseph Orly, Patricia Weinberger-Ohana and Ronit Shoshani

Department of Biological Chemistry, Institute of Life Sciences, The Hebrew University of Jerusalem
91904 Jerusalem, Israel

INTRODUCTION

The cytodifferentiation process of follicular granulosa cells from immature rat ovaries is mainly regulated by FSH. Previous studies have shown that in response to *in vivo* or *in vitro* treatment with FSH, the granulosa cells produce progestins[1,2], develop new receptors for LH[3] and acquire aromatase enzyme complex which converts androgen substrate to estrogen[4,5]. Since FSH binding to the cell receptors results in stimulation of adenylate cyclase and accumulation of cAMP[6,7], recent studies have tried to demonstrate that all the FSH induced effects mentioned above are cAMP mediated phenomena[8-11].

The intensive biochemical examination carried out during the past few years on the cytodifferentiation process of ovarian granulosa cells was made possible due to culture techniques which allowed the maintenance of functional cells in the absence of serum[12-16]. For that purpose we used a defined medium to maintain the rat granulosa cells in long-term cultures. This medium (4F medium) consisted of a 1:1, vol/vol, mixture of DME and Ham's F-12 media, supplemented with insulin, transferrin, hydrocortisone and fibronectin[12,17]. The various supplements were essential for the maintenance of the cells in culture for periods of three weeks or more. Using 4F medium we started to search for possible intraovarian substances that might regulate the response of the follicular granulosa cells to FSH. We have thus recently found an apparently low molecular weight substance which exists in the rat ovary and can mimic the stimulatory action of FSH on progestin production in cultured granulosa cells[18]. The present study further characterizes the various effects of the ovarian substance (OS) on the granulosa cytodifferentiation.

MATERIALS AND METHODS

Culture media

Serum-free medium (4F medium) consisted of a DME:F-12 mixture, supplemented by 2 μg/ml insulin, 5 μg/ml transferrin, 0.2 μM hydrocortisone and 1.5 μg/cm^2 fibronectin, as previously described[12].

Animals

Immature female rats (Wistar-derived strain, 22-25 days old) were neither hypophysectomized nor treated with diethylstilbestrol.

Granulosa cell culture

Granulosa cells were collected by needle puncturing, as previously described[12]. About 5 x 10^4 viable cells were plated into each well (2 cm^2) of a 24 multiwell plate (Nunc, Denmark), containing 0.5 ml of 4F medium.

OS preparation

The ovarian substance was released into the culture medium (conditioned medium) while puncturing the ovaries to express the granulosa cells, as described above. A standard preparation of OS contained activity produced by puncturing 12 ovaries in 8 ml of 4F medium. OS conditioned medium was ultrafiltered through PM-10 Diaflo membranes (Amicon stirring cell) and filter sterilized before storage at 4°C.

Steroid measurements

The 20α-hydroxypregn-4-ene-3-one (20α-OH-P) content in the culture medium was measured by radioimmunoassay (RIA) as previously described[12,18]. The data present the mean steroid content in duplicate or triplicate wells for each treatment. Each RIA sample was assayed in duplicate determinations. Anti-20α-OH-P was a generous gift from Dr. F. Kohen of The Weizmann Institute of Science, Rehovot.

Aromatase assay

Aromatase activity was determined by measuring the stereospecific release of tritium to produce ^3H_2O when [1β,2β-^{3}H]testosterone is aromatized to 17β-estradiol[19-21]. Briefly, the cells were primed for two days with OS and/or 100 ng/ml FSH. After thorough washing with warm medium, the cells were further incubated in 0.2 ml of 4F medium containing 150,000 dpm [1β,2β-^{3}H]testosterone (0.25 μM). At the indicated times, the culture medium was transfered into plastic RIA tube, treated with charcoal, and the content of ^3H_2O in the charcoal supernatant was measured after centrifugation[21].

Cyclic AMP determinations

Accumulation of cAMP in intact cells was measured as previously described[18]. Prior to addition of agonists, the cell monolayers were incubated in 0.2 ml of 4F medium containing 2 μCi of [^{3}H]adenine (2 μM). After 2 hours of incubation at 37°C, the monolayers were washed twice with warm 4F medium, and agonists were added at zero time. After 50 minutes with agonist, the cells were lysed by addition of 0.3 ml ethanol solution (70%) and 0.2 ml "stop solution." The content of the stop solution and the procedure for determination of [^{3}H]cAMP, using sequential chromatography on Dowex (BioRad Laboratories, Richmond, CA) AG 50W-X4 and aluminum oxide columns, were as described in a previous report[28]. The counts corresponding to purified [^{3}H]cAMP were normalized when expressed as percentage of conversion of tritium cpm to [^{3}H]cAMP (% of conversion).

RESULTS

Morphological response to OS

We first observed that OS is released into the culture medium from cultured ovaries which had been freed from their granulosa cell content[18]. This report, however, characterizes the biological activity of OS which is released from the rat ovaries during the processing procedure to express the content of the follicular granulosa cells into culture. The two preparations of OS were indistinguishable by all criteria.

OS conditioned medium caused dramatic morphological changes when added to long-term culture of granulosa cells. The well-spread cells (Fig. 1A) rounded-up, and many acquired a spherical shape (Fig. 1B). This temporal shape change reversed after 2-3 hours of incubation. Similar morphological responses have been described before also for FSH action[22]. In addition, prolonged incubation with OS for a few days resulted in morphological luteinization of the cells, as shown in Fig. 1C.

OS induced progestin production

The effects of OS on progestin production meet all the criteria to be considered for a putative hormone action. OS induction of 20α-OH-P synthesis was time dependent (Fig. 2), concentration dependent (Fig. 7C), reversible[23], and sensitive to inhibitors of mRNA and protein synthesis[23]. Moreover, Fig. 3 shows that OS did not alter the metabolic pathway of progesterone reductions known to occur in cultures of FSH induced granulosa cells[24]. Therefore, it is highly unlikely that OS might be an intermediary substrate for progestin synthesis.

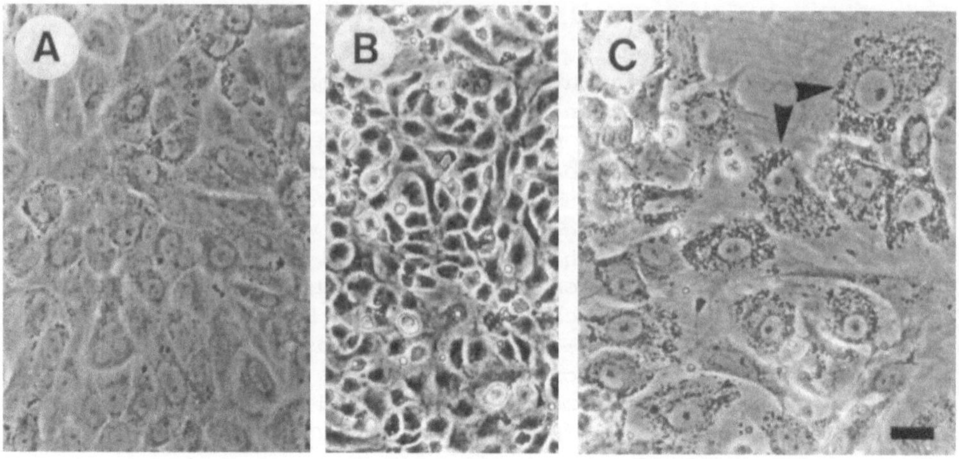

Fig. 1. Morphological luteinization and short-term morphological changes induced by OS. Phase contrast micrographs were taken 8 days after inoculation. A. control without OS. Note the confluent monolayer of the cells. B. Cells exposed to OS for 45 minutes at 37°C. Note the dramatic cell rounding. C. Cells incubated for 8 days in the presence of OS. Note the round nuclei with prominent nucleoli and the lipid droplets scattered in the cytoplasm. Bar = 40 μm.

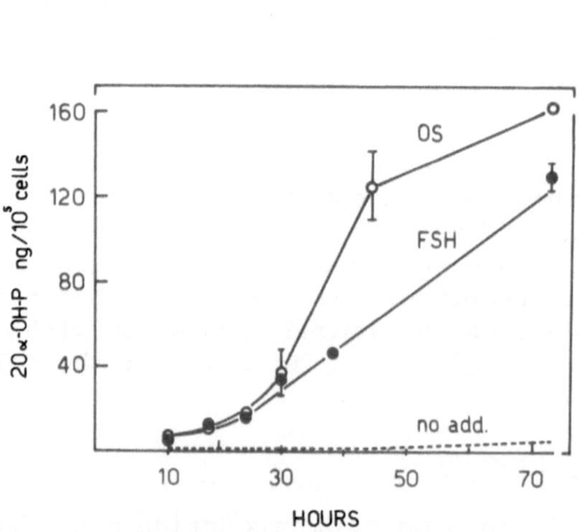

Fig. 2. Time dependent accumulation of 20α-OH-P in response to OS or FSH. After 11 days in culture, cells (1.64 x 10^5/well) were incubated with 0.5 ml 4F medium containing OS (o-o) or 100 ng/ml FSH (●-●). At each time point, 50 μl aliquots were removed from 4 wells of each treatment and stored until 20α-OH-P content was determined by RIA. Dashed line (---) represents control wells without added agonist.

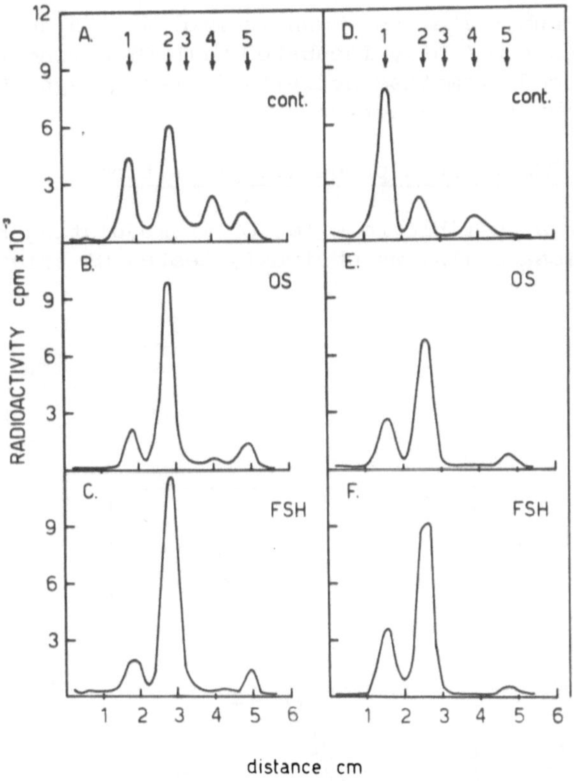

Fig. 3. Pregnenolone metabolism in stimulated cells. After 10 days in culture, cells were incubated with OS (B, e) or 100 ng/ml FSH (C, F) for 48 hours. The monolayers were then thoroughly washed and further incubated with [^{3}H]pregnenolone (19 Ci/m-mole, 50 nM). Control cells (cont.) were not treated with agonist (A, D). After 3 hours (A-C) and 8 hours (D-F), the culture media were extracted with ether[24] for analysis by thin layer chromatography. Steroid markers were: (1) 5α-pregnane-3α-20α-diol; (2) 20α-OH-P; (3) pregnenolone; (4) 20α-hydroxy-5α-pregnan-3-one; (5) progesterone. Note that (a) in all treatments no [^{3}H]pregnenolone was left unmodified in the culture medium, and (b) progesterone reduction occurred with time in all treatments. 20α-OH-P is clearly the major reduced metabolite under FSH and OS stimuli.

OS induced aromatase activity

Induction of androgen aromatizing enzyme is an additional quality shared by OS and FSH. After a 2-day priming period with either OS or FSH, granulosa cells from both treatments produced estrogen from testosterone substrate, as shown in Fig. 4. In addition, when the androgen was concomitantly incubated with OS during the priming period[23], the induced aromatase activity increased synergistically, as reported to occur for FSH action[25].

OS enhancement of FSH-induced progestin production

Searching for a possible role for OS in modulating FSH action on cultured granulosa cells, we obviously tested OS effects on FSH

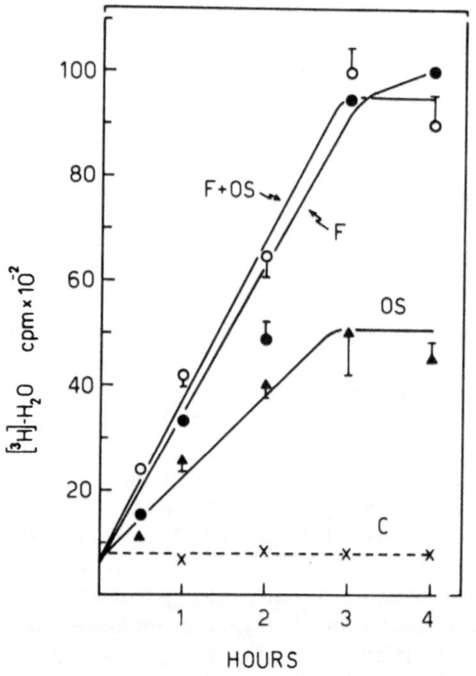

Fig. 4. Induction of aromatase enzyme by OS. After 11 days in culture, cells (1.15 x 10^5/well) were primed with either 100 ng/ml FSH (●), OS preparation (▲) or the two agonists added together (o). Control cells (x---x) were not primed with either agonist. After priming for 48 hours, the cells were thoroughly washed and further incubated in 4F medium containing 60,000 cpm of [1β,2β-^{3}H]testosterone (0.25 μM). At the indicated times, the culture medium was removed and the content of ^3H_2O, generated as a result of aromatase action, was determined as described in Materials and Methods.

induced progestin secretion. Fig. 5 demonstrates that graded doses of OS markedly augmented the FSH-induced 20α-OH-P production. It should be noted that this experiment was conducted using freshly inoculated cells instead of long-term cultured monolayers. Such cells responded poorly to OS when plated at high densities (> 10^5 cells/well, data not shown). Nevertheless, OS synergistically increased up to 4-fold the FSH induced responsiveness over their additive responses when tested separately.

<u>OS induction of LH receptors</u>

The third biochemical marker which we chose to compare OS and FSH action on granulosa cells involves the induction of LH receptors. Fig. 6 shows that, unlike FSH, OS-primed cells failed to express new functional LH receptors since no LH steroidogenic responsiveness could be detected following OS treatment.

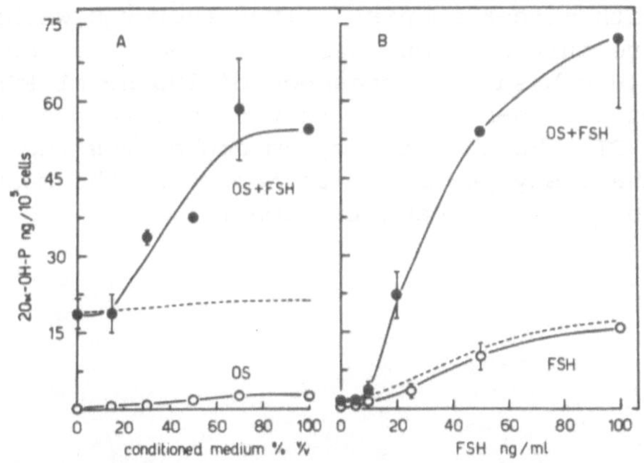

Fig. 5. OS augments FSH action in freshly inoculated cells. After 24 hours in culture, two sets of cells (1.35 x 10^5/well) were challenged with OS and FSH respectively. A. Cells in duplicate wells were incubated with the indicated dilutions of OS conditioned medium in the absence (o) or presence of 100 ng/ml FSH (•). After 48 hours of incubation, 20α-OH-P content in the culture medium was determined by RIA. B. Alternatively, cells were similarly incubated to determine 20α-OH-P production in response to graded doses of FSH, in the absence (o) or presence of maximal concentrations of OS (•). Dahsed line (---) indicates the calculated sum of individual effects of FSH and OS.

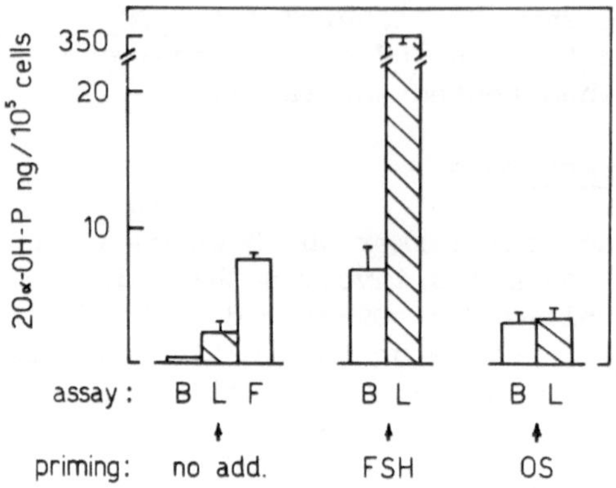

Fig. 6. Effect of OS on induction of LH responsiveness in freshly inoculated cells. Following 24 hours in culture, cells (7 x 10^4/well) were primed for 48 hours with either OS preparation or 100 ng/ml FSH. Control (no add.) cultures were not primed with either agonist. After thorough washing, the cells were further incubated for 48 hours (assay) in the absence (B = basal) or presence of 100 ng/ml FSH (F) or LH (L). The 20α-OH-P content in the culture medium was determined by RIA. Hatched histogram emphasizes the LH treatments during the assay period. Data represent the mean ± S.E. of duplicate wells for each treatment

Apparent lack of cAMP involvement in the OS mechanism of action

It is now accepted that hormonally induced steroid formation is mediated by cAMP as the intracellular messenger[6,7]. Therefore, we have first ruled out the possibility that OS is nothing but cAMP itself[18]. Moreover, when dose-dependent responsiveness of granulosa cells was compared in both progestin production and cAMP accumulation, OS clearly failed to elicit cAMP formation above basal levels (Fig. 7). Two preparations of OS (OS_1 and OS_2) which, at maximal concentrations stimulated 2-3 times more progestin production than FSH, did not cause a significant increase in the intracellular cyclic nucleotide content.

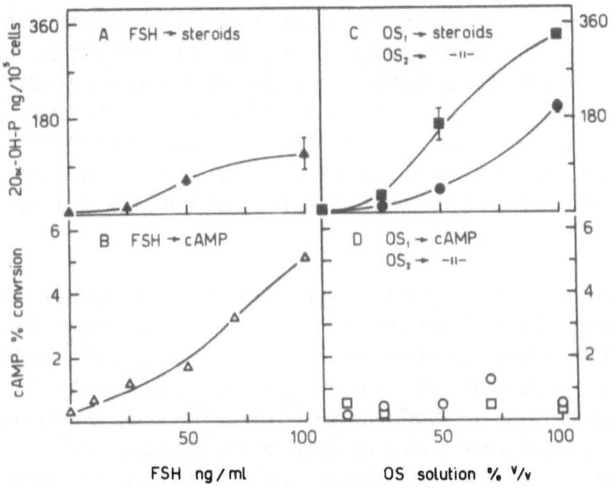

Fig. 7. Accumulation of cAMP and 20α-OH-P in response to graded doses of OS or FSH. Following 11 days in culture, cells (1.2×10^5/well) were exposed to graded doses of either FSH (Panels A, B) or OS (panels C, D). In one set of wells, cells were treated to determine cAMP accumulation (panels B, D) as described in Materials and Methods, while in the second group of wells the cells were incubated for 48 hours to produce 20α-OH-P (panels A, D). 3-Isobutyl-1-methylxanthine was not included in the culture medium in either assay. OS_1 (●,o) and OS_2(■,□) were prepared by puncturing 24 and 48 ovaries in 8 ml of 4F medium respectively (see Materials and Methods). OS solution was diluted with 4F medium to achieve the indicated concentrations (%, vol/vol).

DISCUSSION

As large quantities of purified OS are not yet available, we have characterized its biological activity using crude conditioned medium which had been freed from large proteins by ultracentrifugation. OS activity could not be detected in the conditioned medium of the cultured cells themselves, not even after 48 hours of exposure to FSH. We may thus conclude that probably ovarian cells, other than granulosa, produce the OS activity.

Although OS may be considered as a putative hormone, it apparently does not stimulate progestin production via a cAMP-mediated mechanism. Numerous studies have recently accumulated using 8-Br-cAMP and $(Bu)_2$-cAMP to support a unifying concept concerning the obligatory role of cAMP in FSH induction of progestins[6-8] and LH receptors[9-11]. Our data are consistent with this view, since the ED_{50} values for FSH induced steroidogenesis and the gonadotropin-dependent cAMP formation are almost identical. In contrast, OS seems to activate the granulosa cells in a fashion more like ACTH acts in the adrenal where physiological concentrations of ACTH, which stimulated maximal steroidogenesis, elicited only marginal increases in cAMP levels[26]. Similar disparities between the hormone induced physiological responses and cAMP formation were also reported for LH action on luteal[27] and testicular cells[8].

Since a marked steroidogenic response can be achieved with OS concentrations which do not evoke cAMP formation above basal levels, we also examined the possibility that OS affects Ca^{2+} mobilization or alters the turnover rate of phosphatidyl-inositides in the cultured granulosa cell membranes. Studies using Ca^{2+}-free medium, Ca^{2+} ionophore or $CoCl_2$, did not reveal any alterations of OS-induced effects (not shown). Hence, calcium mobilization did not seem to correlate with OS action. We also verified that OS did not act via induction of prostaglandin synthesis because indomethacine was unable to block OS activity (not shown). Consequently, we are currently seeking for mechanisms that may provide an explanation for OS action independently of cAMP formation. Activation of a protein kinase resulting from the interaction of cells with OS is one such possibility.

When OS responsiveness was studied using freshly inoculated cells, a marked difference was revealed between OS and FSH induction of progestin synthesis. As the inoculum size decreased, the cell responsiveness to OS surprisingly increased (not shown). The fact that FSH responsiveness contrastingly increased with higher cell densities, may provide a clue concerning the physiological target cell of OS action in the ovary. If an analogy can be made between an *in vitro* monolayer of sparsely populated granulosa cells and a single layer of granulosa cells comprising the primordial follicle *in vivo*, it may be hypothesized that OS is meant to act on such primitive follicular cells which might not yet have responsiveness to FSH. Furthermore, although OS seems poorly active in high density inoculi (Fig. 5), it still synergistically augments FSH induced steroidogenesis. If the high density cells in culture presumably represent a stratified granulosa epithelium in growing primary follicles, OS is therefore suggested to substitute or increase FSH action as a trophic hormone during early stages of the follicular development, when the hypophysal trophic hormone levels in the circulation are very low and ineffective.

ACKNOWLEDGEMENTS

We wish to thank Dr. F. Kohen from the Department of Hormone Research, The Weizmann Institute of Science, Rehovot, Israel, for providing us with the anti-20α-OH-P serum. We are also grateful to Mrs. E. Dicker for her excellent editorial and secretarial assistance.

J.O. is an incumbent for the Charles H. Revson Career Development Chair.

This work was supported by the United States - Israel Binational Science Foundation, Grant #2656/81, and by the Bat-Sheva de Rothschild Fund for the Encouragement of Science and Technology.

REFERENCES

1. C.P. Channing, Influence of the *in vivo* and *in vitro* hormonal environment upon luteinization of granulosa cells in tissue culture, Rec. Prog. Horm. Res. 26:589 (1970).
2. J.H. Dorrington and D.T. Armstrong, Effects of FSH on gonadal functions, Rec. Prog. Horm. Res. 35:301 (1979).
3. A.J. Zeleznik, A.R. Midgley, Jr. and L.E. Reichert, Granulosa cell maturation in the rat: Increased binding of human chorionic gonadotropin following treatment with follicle stimulating hormone *in vivo*, Endocrinology 95:818 (1974).
4. J.H. Dorrington, D.T. Armstrong and Y.S. Moon, Estradiol-17β Biosynthesis in cultured granulosa cells from hypophysectomized rats: Stimulation by follicle stimulating hormone, Endocrinology 97:1328 (1975).
5. D.T. Armstrong and H. Papkoff, Stimulation of aromatization of exogenous androgen in ovaries of hypophysectomized rats *in vivo* by follicule stimulating hormone, Endocrinology 99:1144 (1976).
6. J. Kolena and C.P. Channing, Stimulatory effect of LH, FSH and prostaglandin upon 3',5'-cyclic AMP levels in porcine granulosa cells, Endocrinology 90:1543 (1972).
7. A.K. Goff and D.T. Armstrong, Stimulatory action of gonadotropins and prostaglandins on adenosine-3',5'-monophosphate production by isolated rat granulosa cells, Endocrinology 101:1461 (1977).
8. G.B. Sala, M.L. Dufau and K.J. Catt, Gonadotropin action on isolated ovarian luteal cells: The intermediate role of adenosine 3',5'-monophosphate in hormonal stimulation of progesterone synthesis, J. Biol. Chem. 254:2077 (1977).
9. A. Nimrod, The induction of ovarian LH-receptors by FSH is mediated by cyclic AMP, FEBS Lett. 131:31 (1981).
10. M. Knecht, A. Amsterdam and K.J. Catt, The regulatory role of cyclic AMP in hormone induced granulosa cell differentiation, J. Biol. Chem. 256:10628 (1981).
11. M.M. Sanders and A.R. Midgley, Jr., Cyclic nucleotides can induce luteinizing hormone receptors in cultured granulosa cells, Endocrinology 112:1382 (1983).

12. J. Orly, G.H. Sato and G.F. Erickson, Serum suppresses the expression of hormonally induced functions in cultured granulosa cells, Cell 20:817 (1980).
13. G.F. Erickson, Primary cultures of ovarian cells in serum-free medium as models of hormone dependent differentiation, Mol. Cell Endocrinol. 29:21 (1983).
14. R.E. Gore-Langton, M. Lacroix and J.H. Dorrington, Differential effects of luteinizing hormone releasing hormone on follicle stimulating hormone dependent responses in rat granulosa and Sertoli cells *in vitro*, Endocrinology 108:812 (1981).
15. A. Amsterdam, M. Knecht and K.J. Catt, Hormonal regulation of cytodifferentiation and intercellular communication in cultured granulosa cells, Proc. Natl. Acad. Sci. USA 78:3000 (1981).
16. M.M. Sanders and A.R. Midgley, Jr., Rat granulosa cell differentiation: An *in vitro* model, Endocrinology 111:614 (1982).
17. J. Orly, Methods for growth of functional primary and established rat ovary cultures in serum-free medium, in: "Cell Culture Methods," D. Barnes, D. Sirbasku and G. Sato, eds., Vol. 2, Alan R. Liss, New York (1984), in press.
18. J. Orly, Y. Farkash, N. Hershkovits, L. Mizrahi and P. Weinberger, Ovarian substance induces steroid production in cultured granulosa cells, In Vitro 18:980 (1982).
19. E.A. Thompson, Jr. and P.K. Siiteri, Utilization of oxygen and reduced nicotinamide adenine dinucleotide phosphate by human placental microsomes during aromatization of androstenedione, J. Biol. Chem. 249:5364 (1974).
20. K.C. Reed and S. Ohno, Kinetic properties of human placental aromatase, J. Biol. Chem.251:1625 (1976).
21. R. Gore-Langton, H. McKeracher and J.H. Dorrington, An alternative method for the study of follicle-stimulating hormone effect on aromatase activity in Sertoli cell cultures, Endocrinology 107:464 (1980).
22. T.S. Lawrence, R.D. Ginzberg, N.B. Gilula and W.H. Beers, Hormonally induced cell shape changes in cultured rat ovarian granulosa cells, J. Cell Biol. 80:21 (1979)
23. P. Weinberger-Ohana, R. Shoshani, Y. Farkash, N. Hershkovits, N.B. Goldring, R. Epstein-Almog and J. Orly, Low molecular weight substance from rat ovary induces steroidogenesis in cultured granulosa cells (1983), submitted for publication.
24. A. Nimrod, Studies on the synergistic effect of androgen on the stimulation of progestin secretion by FSH in cultured rat granulosa cells: Progesterone metabolism and the effect of androgens, Mol. Cell. Endocrinol. 8:189 (1977).
25. S.A.J. Daniel and D.T. Armstrong, Enhancement of follicle-stimulating hormone-induced aromatase activity by androgen in cultured rat granulosa cells, Endocrinology 197:1027 (1980).
26. D.I. Buckley and J. Ramachandran, Characterization of corticotropin receptors on adrenocrotical cells, Proc. Natl. Acad. Sci. USA 78:7431 (1981).

27. M.R. Clark and K.M.J. Menon, Regulation of ovarian steroidogenesis: The disparity between ^{125}I-labeled choriogonadotropin binding, cyclic adenosine 3',5'-monophosphate formation and progesterone synthesis in the rat ovary, Biochim. Biophys. Acta 444:23 (1976).

28. D. Schulster, J. Orly, G. Seidel and M. Schramm, Intracellular cyclic AMP production enhanced by a hormone-receptor transferred from a different cell, J. Biol. Chem. 253:1201 (1978).

CALCIUM: A CELLULAR MEDIATOR OF LUTEOLYSIS

Harold R. Behrman, Peter J. Albert, Steven D. Gore and Laneta J. Dorflinger

Reproductive Biology Section, Departments of Obstetrics/ Gynecology and Pharmacology, Yale University School of Medicine, New Haven, CT 06510

INTRODUCTION

Regression of the corpus luteum with the consequent loss of ovarian progesterone secretion appears to be an induced response which is necessary for the re-occurrence of ovulation. Conversely, prevention of corpus luteum regression is essential for the continuation of pregnancy. The pivotal role of the corpus luteum in the reproductive cycle with its poorly understood functional regulation and control has generated interest in this organ for many years. Although progress has been made, the nature, origin and mechanism of action of agents which prolong corpus luteum function during early pregnancy have not been resolved. Moreover, the nature, origin and mechanism of action of luteolytic hormones are poorly understood in lower animals, and are completely unknown in the human. It is to these areas that we have directed our attention.

In this paper we will present a general overview of recent results obtained in our laboratory on the cellular mechanisms of luteolysis in the rat. For these studies we utilized prostaglandin (PGF2a), gonadotropin releasing hormone (GnRH), and ion-active drugs - agents which induce functional luteolysis in isolated cells and/or luteal regression in vivo. In brief, our results implicate calcium (Ca2+) as an intracellular mediator of these luteolytic agents. The site of action of Ca2+ appears to be within the plasma membrane on, or near, the adenylate cyclase-LH receptor complex. The response in either intact cells or isolated membranes to an increase in Ca2+ is a functional uncoupling of the receptor complex, an effect which occurs independently of hormone binding.

OVERVIEW OF FUNCTIONAL REGULATION OF THE CORPUS LUTEUM

The corpus luteum is an endocrine controlled, end-differentiated gland composed of cells derived from the follicle. Differentiation of the luteal cell from the follicular granulosa cell is characterized by a marked increase in cytoplasmic elements necessary for cholesterol-dependent progesterone synthesis and a shift of endocrine control from FSH to LH. Since the corpus luteum is dependent on gonadotropin for its function, we suggested some time ago that luteolysis may be linked to an interruption of gonadotropin support (1). One possibility is that luteolysis may be caused by reduced gonadotropin secretion because it has long been known that hypophysectomy results in a prompt loss of corpus luteum function. However, direct measurement of circulating levels of gonadotropin, although low in the luteal phase, show that no decrease preceeds luteal regression. The first evidence that interruption of gonadotropin support may be involved in the initiation of luteolysis was obtained from studies with the rat in which we showed that PGF2a inhibited the steroidogenic response of an acute injection of LH (1). Since this early report, we have shown that the action of PGF2a is directly on the ovary (1,2), that it does not compromize blood flow (i.e. gonadotropin delivery) to the ovary (1,3), and that it directly antagonizes the action of LH in intact hamster corpora lutea (4) and isolated luteal cells (5). Evidence that PGF2a may be the physiological luteolysin has been previously reviewed (6,7).

Some progress has been made on the cellular mechanisms involved in luteal regression. It was shown several years ago that a decrease in the number of LH receptors (i.e. receptor downregulation) in luteal tissue is associated with luteolysis (8,9). We showed that LH receptor downregulation occurred several hours after treatment of the rat with a luteolytic dose of PGF2a (10). Others have since shown that a similar effect occurs in the monkey (11) and the ewe (12). However, we found that the loss of LH receptors followed, rather than preceeded the decrease in function of the corpus luteum (10). Consequently, we presently view downregulation as a mechanism to insure that regression is irreversible, but conclude that it is not a cause of luteolysis. To more closely examine early events in functional luteolysis, we used two approaches: studies in the intact animal and studies with isolated luteal cells. In the animal studies, it was found that PGF2a caused a prompt and marked decrease in the specific uptake of radiolabelled hCG, a ligand for the LH receptor, in parallel with a decrease in progesterone secretion (13). However, PGF2a did not inhibit hCG-uptake in isolated luteal cells (14), which led us to suggest that the response in vivo was due either to a PGF2a-induced impairment of ovarian capillary transfer of hCG (since no effect on blood flow was seen), or that PGF2a produced secondary effects in vivo which reduces LH receptor binding activity. With in vitro studies we showed that PGF2a directly inhibits the acute steroidogenic response of luteal cells to LH (4, 14,15). This effect occurs within minutes at physiological levels of PGF2a, it is unrelated to an action on LH receptor binding activity, and it is specific for the luteal cell since no effect occurs in Leydig cells.

Progress has also been made on the intracellular events associated with functional luteolysis. In minces of rat luteal tissue, it was shown that PGF2a inhibited stimulation of cyclic AMP accumulation by LH (16). We confirmed these results in isolated luteal cells and showed that this effect was linked to a simultaneous inhibition of progesterone biosynthesis (4,14,15). In addition, we showed that PGF2a did not stimulate cyclic AMP degradation in luteal cells or interfere with binding of LH by the cells. From these studies we concluded that PGF2a inhibits activation of adenylate cyclase by LH (14,15). However, PGF2a did not inhibit adenylate cyclase activity in isolated luteal membranes, which indicates that an intracellular agent probably mediates the action of PGF2a (14,15). This conclusion is also supported by evidence which describes specific membrane receptors for PGF2a in rat luteal cells (17,18). Luteal PGF2a receptors had previously been described in human and ruminant luteal tissue (19-21).

We recently found that adenine-derived purines have a pro-gonadotropic action in luteal cells from the rat and the human (22). These purines rapidly amplify the response to LH by an ATP-linked mechanism (23,24), and they competitively inhibit the action of PGF2a in the luteal cell (25). The role of purines appears to be intimately involved in acute regulation of ovarian cells; these studies have recently been reviewed (26).

EFFECT OF ION-ACTIVE DRUGS ON THE LUTEAL CELL

Our interest in the effect of ion active drugs on the luteal cell arose from studies in which it was shown that GnRH produced effects similar to, but independent of, PGF2a (27). Since both GnRH and PGF2a appear to interact with the rat luteal cell via specific membrane receptors, the similar action of these luteolysins implies that they probably share a common intracellular mediator. To assess if ionic shifts may be involved in initiation of functional regression, several ion-active drugs were used. These were ouabain - an inhibitor of Na+-K+-ATPase, monesin - a monovalent cation ionophore with high selectivity for Na+,

A-23187 - a Ca2+ ionophore, verapamil - a Ca2+ channel blocker, and tetrodotoxin - a Na+ channel blocker. The results of these studies have been described in detail (28,29) and the major findings will be summarized herein.

Both ouabain and monensin would be expected to increase intracellular levels of Na+ by inhibition of Na+ extrusion and by a direct ionophore effect, respectively. Both of these drugs produce a marked and dose-related inhibition of LH-stimulated cyclic AMP accumulation and progesterone secretion very similar to that described earlier for GnRH and PGF2a. The IC-50 for both responses by these drugs was 50 and 0.1 uM, respectively. Both drugs elicited effects only in the intact cell; they showed no nonspecific effects, no effect on LH receptor binding activity, and inhibition was not affected by isobutyl methyl xanthine (MIX, a cyclic AMP phoshodiesterase inhibitor). Removal of Na+ from the extracellular medium completely prevented inhibition by both ouabain and monensin. However, reducing extracellular Na+ to 32 Meq/L, increasing extacellular K+ to 66 Meq/L, or treatment of the cells with a wide range of concentrations of tetrodotoxin had no effect on the stimulation of cyclic AMP accumulation by LH. On the other hand, removal of extracellular Ca2+ completely blocked the inhibition of cyclic AMP accumulation produced by ouabain and monensin. From these studies, we concluded that the inhibitory effect of ouabain and monensin was due to an influx of Na+ into the luteal cell. The increase of Na+ in the cell did not directly inhibit LH-sensitive adenylate cyclase activity but it induced a secondary influx of extracellular Ca2+ (Na+-Ca2+ antiport system) which secondarily inhibited activation of adenylate cyclase at a site involved in coupling of the occupied receptor to the enzyme. It is interesting that a decrease in Na+-K+ ATPase activity is associated with luteal regression in the rat (30), and PGF2a has also been shown to produce a similar effect in this species (31).

Since these studies strongly implicated Ca2+ as the inhibitory ion which mediated the action of ouabain, monensin, and possibly GnRH and PGF2a, we examined the effects of Ca2+ on the luteal cell (29). It was found that treatment of luteal cells with a Ca2+ ionophore (A-23187) caused a marked and dose-related decrease in LH-stimulated cyclic AMP accumulation and progesterone synthesis. This effect of A-23187 was completely dependent on the presence of extracellular Ca2+, which is consistent with the action of this drug as a Ca2+ ionophore. No direct effect of A-23187 was seen on LH receptor binding activity, LH-sensitive adenylate cyclase activity or cyclic AMP degradation. From these studies we concluded that A-23187 caused an increase in intracellular Ca2+ and it was this response which interruupted the luteal cell function.

and it was this response which interrupted the luteal cell function.

To evaluate if extracellular Ca2+ is necessary for the action of natural luteolysins, several approaches were used which included the removal of extracellular Ca2+ and the use of a Ca2+-channel blocker (verapamil). It was found that removal of extracellular Ca2+ had no effect on the action of PGF2a and only a slight attenuation of the action of GnRH was seen. In addition, verapamil had no effect over a wide range of concentrations on the action of PGF2a or GnRH. Therefore, it was concluded that extracellular Ca2+ was probably not involved in the acute antigonadotropic response of the luteal cell to PGF2a, and to only a minor extent to GnRH. However, the results with ouabain, monensin, and A-23187 all indicated that an increase of intracellular Ca2+ inhibits the response to LH in a manner very similar to that produced by the natural luteolysins.

EFFECT OF CALCIUM ON LH-SENSITIVE ADENYLATE CYCLASE

To directly evaluate the effect of Ca2+ on intracellular events essential for the expression of LH, studies in isolated luteal membranes were conducted (29). In this manner, physiological concentrations of Ca2+ could be examined. It was found that Ca2+ dramatically inhibited activation of adenylate cyclase by LH in a dose-dependent manner. Inhibition of this response showed an IC-50 of free Ca2+ in the low micromolar range and inhibition was evident with concentrations of Ca2+ less than 1 uM, a level which is well within the physiological range. This action of Ca2+ was shown to be independent of an effect of Ca2+ on LH receptor binding activity or on cyclic AMP degradation. These results led us to conclude that Ca2+ prevents interaction of the occupied receptor with adenylate cyclase in a manner identical to that produced by PGF2a and GnRH. The major difference between the action of Ca2+ and the natural luteolysins is that Ca2+ produces this effect directly in isolated membranes whereas PGF2a and GnRH require an intact cell. Therefore, it appears reasonable to propose that if Ca2+ is the mediator, changes in activity or concentration of this ion inside the cell occur independently of the extracellular pool, at least under acute conditions.

Although the antigonadotropic site of action of Ca2+ is in the plasma membrane of the luteal cell, the mechanism of action of Ca2+ in abrogation of adenylate cyclase activity is not known. We have recently found, however, that Ca2+ may interact with the GTP-binding protein which is involved in activation of adenylate cyclase by hormones (32). This evidence is based on the observation that fluoride, a GTP analog (GppNHp), and GTP at nanomolar concentrations all block the direct inhibition of adenylate cyclase by Ca2+. The nature of the interaction of Ca2+ with the GTP-binding protein is not resolved.

SUMMARY AND CONCLUSIONS

Based on investigations over the past few years, we suggest that regression of the corpus luteum is an active process induced by natural agents which serve a killer role. PGF2a and possibly GnRH, or some peptide whose action is mimicked by GnRH, serve this role in the rat and probably in other species. With the use of the rat luteal model, we have shown that the initial events involved in functional regression of the corpus luteum (that occur within minutes) are intimately linked to inhibition of the cellular response to LH. The action of this gonadotropic hormone, in concert with other progonadotropic agents (possibly adenine-derived purines), appears to be essential for the continued function of the corpus luteum.

The site of the initial action of natural luteolytic agents appears to be directly in the plasma membrane of the luteal cell in which specific receptors for these agents have been identified. We suggest that interaction of the luteolytic agents with their respective receptors produces secondary, but as yet unidentified, actions inside the cell which lead to an increase in intracellular levels of free Ca2+ in the immediate environment surrounding the LH receptor-adenylate cyclase complex. This increase in Ca2+ does not appear to be due to an influx of extracellular Ca2+; however, an induced influx of Ca2+ produced by inhibition of the membrane Na+-K+ pump, increasing intracellular levels of Na+ or treatment with a Ca2+ ionophore, will completely mimic the action of the luteolytic hormones. Ca2+ directly blocks activation of adenylate cyclase at a site in the plasma membrane by a mechanism which appears to involve GTP because the inhibitory action of Ca2+ is reversed ty GTP, analogs of GTP, or fluoride, all which interact with the GTP-binding protein of adenylate cyclase in the plasma membrane.

Although the present evidence is consistent with the above scenario, several questions remain. First, no direct evidence that PGF2a or GnRH increase intracellular Ca2+ has been shown. The link between these luteolytic agents and Ca2+ is based on the use of pharmacologic agents whose actions were shown to be Ca2+-dependent, and results which showed that Ca2+ mimics the action of the natural luteolysins in isolated membranes. Direct studies which show that an increase in intracellular Ca2+ occurs with exposure of intact cells to luteolytic hormones, are necessary in order to conclude that Ca2+ is the mediator of these agents.

Second, the mechanism involved in elevation of intracellular Ca2+ in the luteal cell is not known. However, we have obtained preliminary evidence that luteolytic hormones may block Ca2+ extrusion from the cytoplasm by inhibition of a high affinity Ca2+-ATPase (33) - a putative Ca2+-extrusion pump previously described by others in the rat corpus luteum (34). Third, the mechanism of the inhibitory action of Ca2+ on adenylate cyclase in the luteal cell plasma membrane has not been resolved. Results from these and other areas of investigation with the corpus luteum will possibly yield a greater understanding of the cellular events of luteal regression and perhaps lead to important insights into the processes of cell and tissue death in general, for which the luteal cell appears to be an interesting model.

ACKNOWLEDGEMENTS

[Supported by grants from the NIH; HD-10718 and HD-15403.]

REFERENCES

1. H.R. Behrman, K. Yoshinaga and R.O. Greep, Extraluteal effects of prostaglandins, Ann. N.Y. Acad. Sci. 180:426 (1972).
2. H.R. Behrman, G.J. Macdonald and R.O. Greep, Regulation of ovarian cholesterol esters: evidence fof the enzymatic sites of prostaglandin-induced loss of corpus luteum function, Lipids 6:791 (1971).
3. C.Y. Pang and H.R. Behrman, Acute effects of PGF2a on ovarian and luteal blood flow, luteal gonadotropin uptake *in vivo* and gonadotropin binding *in vitro*, Endocrinology 108:2239 (1981).
4. H.R. Behrman, T.S. Ng and G.P. Orczyk, Interactions between prostaglandins and gonadotropins on corpus luteum function, *in*: "Gonadotropins and Gonadal Function", N.R. Moudgal, ed., Academic Press, N.Y. (1974).
5. C.Y. Pang and H.R. Behrman, Acute effects of PGF2a on ovarian and luteal blood flow, luteal gonadotropin uptake *in vivo* and gonadotropin binding *in vitro*, Endocrinogy 108:2239 (1981).
6. E.W. Horton and N.L. Poyser, Uterine luteolytic hormone: a physiological role for PGF2a , Physiol. Rev. 56:595 (1976).
7. H.R. Behrman, Prostaglandins in hypothalamo-pituitary and ovarian function, Ann. Rev. Physiol. 41:685 (1979).
8. C.Y. Lee, K. Tateishi, R.J. Ryan and N.S. Jiang, Binding of human chorionic gonadotropin by rat ovarian slices: dependence on the functional state of the ovary, Proc. Soc. Exp. Biol. Med. 148:505 (1975).

9. M. Hichens, D.L. Grinwich and H.R. Behrman, PGF2a-induced loss of corpus luteum gonadotropin receptors, Prostaglandins 7:449 (1974).

10. D.L. Grinwich, M. Hichens and H.R. Behrman, Control of the LH receptor by prolactin and prostaglandin F2a in rat corpora lutea, Biol. Reprod. 14:1212 (1974).

11. J.L. Cameron and R.L. Stouffer, Gonadotroopin receptors of the primate corpus luteum. II. Changes in available luteinizing hormone- and chorionic gonadotropin-binding sites in macaque luteal membranes during the nonfertile menstrual cycle, Endocrinology 110:228 (1982).

12. M.A. Dickman, P.O'Callaghan, T.M. Nett and G.D. Niswender, Effect of prostaglandin F2 on the number of LH receptors in ovine corpora lutea. Biol Reprod. 19:1010 (1978).

13. H.R. Behrman and M. Hichens, Rapid block of gonadotropin uptake by corpora lutea *in vivo* induced by prostaglandin F2a, Prostaglandins 12:83 (1976).

14. J.P. Thomas, L.J. Dorflinger and H.R. Behrman, Mechanism of the rapid antigonadotropic action of prostaglandins in cultured luteal cells, Proc. Nat. Acad. Sci. (USA) 75:1344 (1978).

15. L.J. Dorflinger, J.L. Luborsky, S.D. Gore and H.R. Behrman, Inhibitory characteristics of prostaglandin F2a in the rat luteal cell, Mol. Cell. Endocrinology 33:225 (1983).

16. M. Lahav, A. Freud, and H. Lindner, Abrogation by prostaglandin F2a of LH stimulated cyclic AMP accumulation in isolated rat corpora lutea of pregnancy, Biochem. Biophys. Res. Commun. 68:1294 (19976).

17. K. Wright, C.Y. Pang and H.R. Behrman, Luteal membrane binding of prostaglandin F2a and sensitivity of corpora lutea to prostaglandin F2a-induced luteolysis in pseudopregnant rats, Endocrinology 106:1333 (1980).

18. K. Wright, J.L. Luborsky and H.R. Behrman, Specific binding of prostaglandin F2a to membranes of rat corpora lutea, Mol. Cell. Endocrinology 13:25 (1979).

19. W.S. Powell, S. Hammarstrom, V. Kylden, B. Samuelsson and B. Sjoberg, Prostaglandin F2a receptor in human corpora lutea, Lancet 1:120 (1974).

20. W.S. Powell, S. Hammarstrom and B. Samuelsson, Prostaglandin F2a receptor in ovine corpora lutea, Eur. J. Biochem. 41:103 (1974).

21. W.S. Powell, S. Hammarstrom and B. Samuelsson, Occurrence and properties of prostaglandin F2a receptor in bovine corpora lutea, Eur. J. Biochem 56:73 (1975).

22. A.K. Hall, S.L. Preston and H.R. Behrman, Purine amplification of luteinizing hormone actions in ovarian luteal cells, J. Biol. Chem. 256:10390 (1981).

23. H.R. Behrman, R. Ohkawa and S.L. Preston, Transport and selective utilization of adenosine as a prosubstrte for LH-sensitive adenylate cyclase in the luteal cell, Endocrinology 113:1132 (1983).

24. T. Brennan, R. Ohkawa, S.D. Gore and H.R. Behrman, Adenine-derived purines increase ATP levels in the luteal cell: Evidence that cell levels of ATP may limit the stimulation of cyclic AMP accumulation by LH, Endocrinology 112:4999 (1983).

25. H.R. Behrman, A.K. Hall, S.L. Preston and S.D. Gore, Antagonistic interactions of adenosine and prostaglandin F2a modulate acute responses of luteal cells to luteinizing hormone, Endocrinology 110:38 (1982).

26. H.R. Behrman, M.L. Polan, R. Ohkawa, N. Laufer, J.L. Luborsky, A.T. Williams and S.D. Gore, Purine modulation of LH action in gonadal cells, J. Steroid. Biochem. 19:789 (1983).

27. H.R. Behrman, S.L. Preston and A.K. Hall, Cellular mechanism of the antigonadotropic action of LHRH in the corpus luteum, Endocrinology 107:6546 (1980).

28. S.D. Gore and H.R. Behrman, Alteration of transmembrane sodium and potassium gradients inhibits the action of LH in the luteal cell, Endocrinology (In Press 1984).

29. L.J. Dorflinger, P.J. Albert, A.T. Williams and H.R. Behrman, Calcium is an inhibitor of LH-sensitive adenylate cyclase in the luteal cell, Endocrinology (In Press 1984).

30. T.A. Bramley and R.J. Ryan, Interactions of gonadotropins with corpus luteum membranes. IX Changes in the specific activities of some plasma-membrane marker enzymes in rat ovarian homogenates and purified membrane fractions at various times of the priming with PMSG and hCG, Mol. Cell. Endocrinology 19:33 (1980).

31. I. Kim and D.S. Yeoun, Effect of prostaglandin F2a on Na+-K+-ATPase activity in luteal membranes, Biol. Reprod. 29:48 (1983).

32. H.R. Behrman, Unpublished observations.

33. P.J. Albert, S.L. Preston and H.R. Behrman, Prostaglandin-induced luteolysis linked to inhibition of calcium pump activity, 7th Int. Cong. Endocrinology (1984).

34. A.K. Verma and J.T. Penniston, A high affinity Ca2+-stimulated and Mg2+-dependent ATPase in rat corpus luteum plasma membrane fractions, J. Biol. Chem. 256:1269 (1981).

29. L.J. Dorflinger, P.J. Albert, A.T. Williams and H.R. Behrman, Calcium is an inhibitor of LH-sensitive adenylate cyclase in the luteal cell, Endocrinology (In Press 1984).

30. T.A. Bramley and R.J. Ryan, Interactions of gonadotropins with corpus luteum membranes. IX Changes in the specific activities of some plasma-membrane marker enzymes in rat ovarian homogenates and purified membrane fractions at various

times of the priming with PMSG and hCG, Mol. Cell. Endocrinology 19:33 (1980).
31. I. Kim and D.S. Yeoun, Effect of prostaglandin F2a on Na+-K+-ATPase activity in luteal membranes, Biol. Reprod. 29:48 (1983).
32. H.R. Behrman, Unpublished observations.
33. P.J. Albert, S.L. Preston and H.R. Behrman, Prostaglandin-induced luteolysis linked to inhibition of calcium pump activity, 7th Int. Cong. Endocrinology (1984).
34. A.K. Verma and J.T. Penniston, A high affinity Ca2+-stimulated and Mg2+-dependent ATPase in rat corpus luteum plasma membrane fractions, J. Biol. Chem. 256:1269 (1981).

NEW PERSPECTIVES ON THE ENDOCRINE REGULATION OF THE RABBIT CORPUS LUTEUM

P. Landis Keyes,[1] Khe-Ching M. Yuh, Charles H. Bill II, and John E. Gadsby

Department of Physiology and Reproductive Endocrinology Program
The University of Michigan
Ann Arbor, Michigan 48109

Department of Physiology and Biophysics
Colorado State University
Fort Collins, Colorado 80523

INTRODUCTION

In many species a luteotrophic hormone has been identified which maintains the morphological and functional integrity of the corpus luteum. For example, in large domestic animals and in primates LH is thought to have the preeminent role as the luteotrophic hormone (Hansel et al., 1973; Niswender et al., 1980; Knobil, 1973), and prolactin is recognized as the major luteotrophic hormone in the rat (Rothchild, 1981). However, it has become evident that other hormones can act upon the corpus luteum, and thus potentially have a significant influence upon steroidogenic activity as well as lifespan of the gland. To illustrate this feature, progesterone synthesis can be stimulated in cow and sheep corpora lutea by catecholamines *in vitro*, and this action, at least in sheep, is directly upon steroidogenic luteal cells (Jordan et al., 1978; Condon and Black, 1976). The ultimate control of steroidogenesis in sheep luteal cells is unclear in view of the recent observation that the large luteal cells, which

---

[1]Visiting Scientist, Department of Physiology and Biophysics, Colorado State University, 1983-84.

comprise the major progesterone secretory component of the ovine corpus luteum *in vivo*, exhibit no steroidogenic response either to LH or to elevated cyclic AMP (Fitz et al., 1982; Hoyer et al., 1983). The rat corpus luteum passes through an LH-sensitive period which is thought to be mediated by estrogen produced within the corpus luteum (Gibori et al., 1977; 1978). In the rabbit, 17β-estradiol of follicular origin is considered the essential luteotrophic hormone (Keyes et al., 1983), although the luteal tissue is clearly responsive to LH (Dorrington and Kilpatrick, 1969; Hunzicker-Dunn and Birnbaumer, 1976) and also possesses a catecholamine sensitive adenylyl cyclase (Hunzicker-Dunn, 1982).

In the experiments to follow, we have sought to determine if 17β-estradiol can serve as a complete luteotrophic hormone in the absence of LH. A forthright approach is to determine if the action of estradiol is sufficient to promote a normal luteal phase, i.e. a normal profile of progesterone in blood, after hypophysectomy. The luteotrophic activity of estrogen in hypophysectomized rabbits is well established (Robson, 1937), and Spies and colleagues (1968a) found that estradiol benzoate would maintain normal concentrations of progesterone in ovarian vein plasma when measured 7 to 8 days after hypophysectomy. The question addressed here is whether estradiol is assisted by LH or other pituitary hormones at any stage throughout the normal life span of the corpus luteum of pseudopregnancy, a period of about 17 days (see Fig. 1). Also, the requirement for extrinsic hormonal support has been investigated by placing the corpus luteum in organ culture.

METHODS AND PROCEDURES

Dutch-belted rabbits were mated to sterile males to induce ovulation and initiate pseudopregnancy. On the day after sterile mating, hypophysectomy was performed by the parapharyngeal approach (Bill and Keyes, 1983). At the time of hypophysectomy or sham hypophysectomy, a silastic capsule containing 17β-estradiol was placed subcutaneously. This implant maintained mean concentrations of estradiol in peripheral serum at 6 to 9 pg/ml; these concentrations are at the upper end of the physiological range in normal pseudopregnant rabbits (Holt et al., 1975; Browning et al., 1980). Blood samples were taken from the marginal ear vein. Completeness of hypophysectomy was determined by inspection of the sella turcica with a dissecting microscope for pituitary fragments, and/or by injection of GnRH and measurement of serum LH (Bill and Keyes, 1983). Incompletely hypophysectomized animals were excluded from the studies. Progesterone and 17β-estradiol were measured in serum extracts and in unextracted culture medium and incubation medium by radioimmunoassays (Holt et al., 1975; Yuh and Keyes, 1981); 20α-dihydroprogesterone was measured in unextracted culture medium and incubation medium by radioimmunoassay (Bender et al., 1978).

Corpora lutea to be incubated were removed on day 10 of pseudopregnancy from hypophysectomized, estradiol-treated and sham-hypophysectomized, estradiol-treated rabbits. The rabbits were anesthetized with xylazine (12 mg/kg, i.m.) and ketamine hydrochloride (60 mg/kg, i.m.), and the corpora lutea, from which interstitial tissue had been removed, were sliced using a razor blade. For each animal, incubations of luteal tissue (approximately 10 mg/flask) were performed in triplicate, and for each animal a mean of steroid produced in the 3 flasks was determined; this value was then considered a single (N=1) observation. The corpora lutea were incubated for 12 hours and the medium changed completely every 3 hours under conditions described previously (Bill and Keyes, 1983).

Corpora lutea to be cultured were removed the day after ovulation induced by mating to a sterile male. With the aid of a microscope, and using fine forceps the fresh corpora lutea were isolated and the adhering interstitial tissue removed. A single corpus luteum was placed on a stainless steel grid in a plastic culture dish containing 2 ml of Dulbecco's Modified Eagle Medium: Ham's F-12 nutrient mixture (1:1), 10 mM HEPES, 100 IU/ml penicillin and 100 μg/ml streptomycin. In some dishes testosterone (10 ng/ml) was added. The corpora lutea were cultured in 95% air and 5% CO_2 with high humidity at 37°C; the medium was changed completely every 24 hours. Protein content of the corpora lutea on the day of isolation (day 0) and at the end of culture (day 10) was determined by the method of Lowry et al. (1951).

RESULTS

Effect of Hypophysectomy on Serum Progesterone in Estradiol-treated Rabbits

Figure 1 shows the profiles of serum progesterone in rabbits either hypophysectomized or sham hypophysectomized and treated continuously with 17β-estradiol from day 1 through day 20. The serum concentrations of progesterone were essentially the same in both groups throughout pseudopregnancy, and in both groups of animals progesterone had returned to estrous values by days 17 to 18. The mean number (±SEM) of corpora lutea in hypophysectomized rabbits was 8.2 ± 0.6, and in sham-hypophysectomized animals 7.6 ± 0.3.

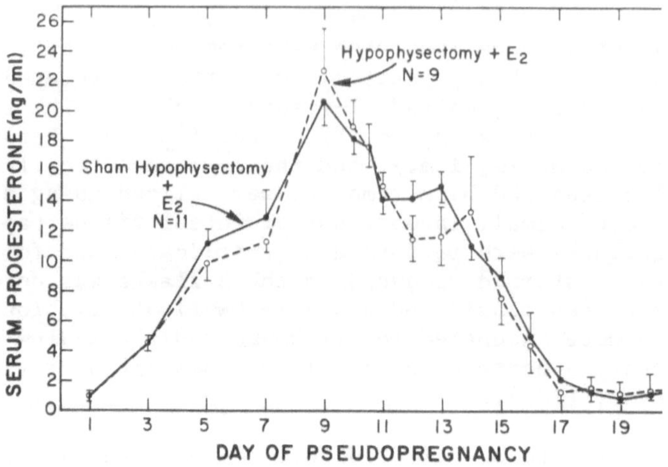

Fig. 1. Progesterone concentration in serum throughout pseudopregnancy in rabbits either sham-hypophysectomized (solid line) or hypophysectomized (broken line) and treated with 17β-estradiol (E_2) via a silastic capsule placed s.c. on day 1. Sham hypophysectomy or hypophysectomy was performed on day 1, the day after sterile mating. Data expressed as mean ± SEM; N=number of animals (From Keyes et al., 1983 with permission).

Effect of Removal and Replacement of Estradiol on Serum Progesterone in Hypophysectomized Rabbits

To determine the dependence of the corpus luteum upon estradiol, the estradiol implant was either sham-removed (removal followed by immediate replacement) or removed and replaced 18 hours later using a local anesthetic on day 10 in hypophysectomized rabbits. Figure 2 shows the changes in serum progesterone in these animals. Removal of the implant caused a precipitous decline in progesterone, from 14 ng/ml to 2 ng/ml within 18 hours. A temporary decline in progesterone was also seen in controls (sham removal); the act of removing and immediately replacing the implant may have reduced transiently serum estradiol concentrations. When the implant was replaced, serum progesterone increased and

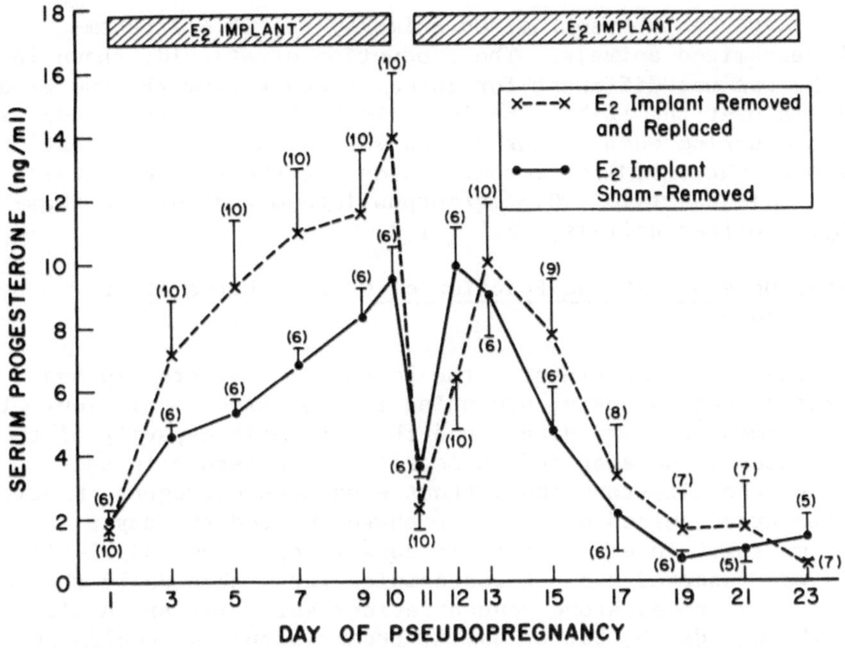

Fig. 2. Serum progesterone concentration after removal and replacement of an estradiol implant (silastic capsule containing 17β-estradiol) in rabbits hypophysectomized on day 1. The estradiol implant was removed on day 10 and replaced s.c. 18 hours later; sham removal consisted of removing the implant followed by immediate replacement. Data expressed as mean ± SEM; ()number of animals.

returned toward normal values. In both groups, the gradual decline in progesterone that heralds the natural course of regression was observed beginning around day 15.

In Vitro Production of Progesterone and 20α-Dihydroprogesterone by Corpora Lutea of Hypophysectomized and Sham hypophysectomized Rabbits

To assess the capacity of luteal tissue to produce progesterone and the metabolite 20α-dihydroprogesterone, corpora lutea were removed from hypophysectomized and sham-hypophysectomized rabbits that had been treated continuously with estradiol as described above. The conditions for the incubation are described in Methods. The initial tissue content of progesterone measured by radioimmunoassay, after petroleum ether extraction and sephadex LH-20 chromatography of extract, was 10 ± 2 ng/mg wet luteal tissue (hypophysectomized animals) and 15 ± 2 (sham-hypophysectomized animals. The production of steroid, shown in Figure 3, was not different for luteal tissues from the two groups of animals over the 12-hour period. In both groups the production of steroid during each 3-hour period was essentially constant. The mean weight (±SEM) of corpora lutea for the hypophysectomized animals was 13.0 + 0.9 mg/corpus luteum and for the sham-hypophysectomized animals, 12.5 ± 1.2.

Transient Development and Function of Corpora Lutea After Hypophysectomy

In the above experiments, the corpora lutea were exposed to estradiol continuously, beginning the day after ovulation. In this experiment we have determined the intrinsic capacity of the corpora lutea to develop and to secrete progesterone in the absence of the pituitary and without exogenous estrogen. Rabbits were hypophysectomized or sham-hypophysectomized the day after sterile mating. An empty silastic capsule or an estradiol-filled capsule was inserted s.c. Blood samples were taken daily through day 6. Serum progesterone concentrations were similar in all groups through day 3, but by day 4, progesterone was declining in the hypophysectomized animals without estradiol treatment (Fig. 4). On days 5 and 6, serum progesterone in this group was less than 0.5 ng/ml. With estradiol treatment, the corpora lutea of hypophysectomized rabbits appeared normal as reflected by the normal values for serum progesterone through day 6. The normal, though brief, development of corpora lutea in the hypophysectomized animals without estradiol treatment is attested by the similarity in wet weights (mean ± SEM) of corpora lutea on day 4: hypophysectomy - 4.0 ± 0.4 mg/corpus luteum; sham-hypophysectomy - 5.3 ± 0.2; hypophysectomy plus estradiol - 6.0 ± 0.5; sham-hypophysectomy plus estradiol - 5.8 ± 0.4. By day 6, the corpora lutea of the hypophysectomized animals without estradiol treatment had regressed.

Function of Corpora Lutea in Organ Culture

In the preceding section, evidence was presented that newly formed corpora lutea persist for 3 to 4 days after hypophysectomy, produce progesterone during this period, then regress prematurely if estrogen is not administered. Our objective in the following experiments was to develop an *in vitro* approach that might allow us to investigate the differentiation and premature demise of the corpus luteum under defined conditions. The conditions for the culture of corpora lutea removed the day after ovulation are described in the Methods section. Figure 5 shows the profile of progesterone and 20α-dihydroprogesterone produced daily by cultured corpora lutea from 7 rabbits. The production of both

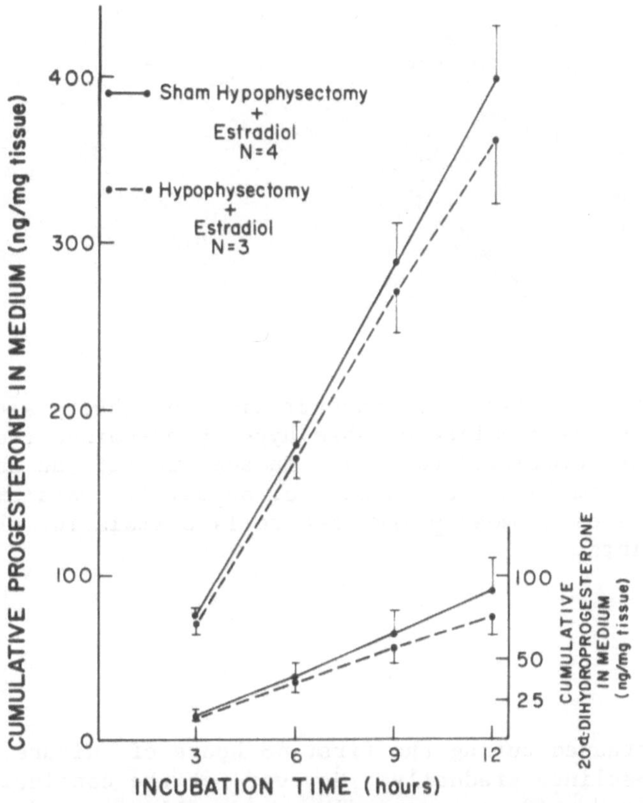

Fig. 3. *In vitro* production of progesterone and 20α-dihydroprogesterone by sliced corpora lutea removed from sham-hypophysectomized, estradiol-treated and hypophysectomized, estradiol-treated rabbits on day 10 of pseudopregnancy. The medium was changed completely every 3 hours. The data are plotted as cumulative values, mean ± SEM; N=number of animals. (From Bill and Keyes, 1983 with permission).

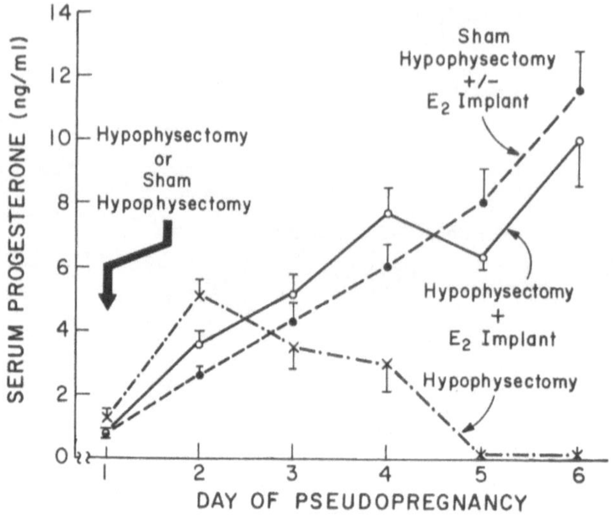

Fig. 4. Serum progesterone concentration in rabbits either hypophysectomized or sham hypophysectomized the day after ovulation (day 1). In some rabbits an estradiol (E_2) implant was placed s.c. on day 1. Data expressed as mean $\pm$ SEM; N=4 to 14 animals for all points.

steroids increased during the first 48 hours of culture, then plateaued and declined gradually. However, at the conclusion of the experiment on day 10 (corresponding to day 11 of pseudopregnancy) the production of both steroids was still elevated. The presence of testosterone in the medium had no effect on the production of progesterone and 20α-dihydroprogesterone (data not shown). The mean ($\pm$SEM) initial content of progesterone in corpora lutea removed the day after ovulation was 10 $\pm$ 1 ng/corpus luteum (n=4). Figure 6 shows the production of 17β-estradiol by corpora lutea from 6 of these rabbits. In the absence of added testosterone, the corpora lutea produced estradiol for 4 days in declining quantities. This represents synthesis, since the mean ($\pm$SEM) initial content of estradiol in corpora lutea removed the day after ovulation was 9 $\pm$ 4 pg/corpus luteum (n=5). In the presence of testosterone added to the medium, the corpora lutea produced substantially more estradiol on each day, but by day 7 and on subsequent days (not shown) of culture, no estradiol formation was detected. The content of protein in corpora lutea removed the day

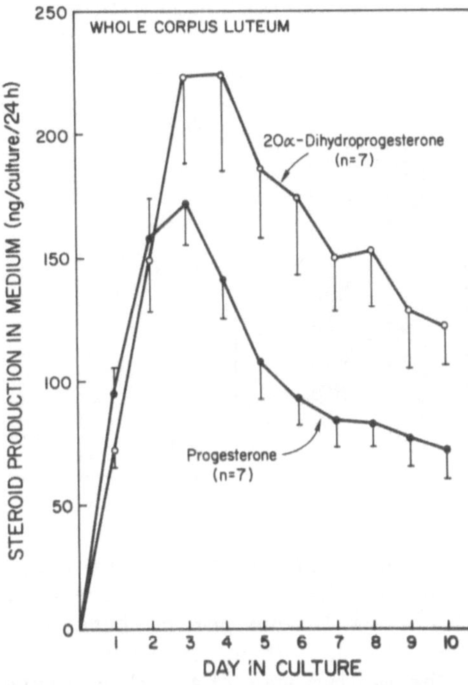

Fig. 5. Daily production of progesterone and 20α-dihydroprogesterone by corpora lutea in culture (1 corpus luteum per culture dish; corpora lutea removed the day after ovulation, i.e. day 0 of culture). The medium was changed completely every 24 hours. Data expressed as mean ± SEM; N=number of animals.

after ovulation (before culture) was 125 μg/corpus luteum; the protein content after 10 days of culture was 65 μg/corpus luteum. Figure 7 shows the histological appearance of a corpus luteum after 13 days of culture. The cells are enlarged relative to cells of corpora lutea removed the day after ovulation, and they are similar in appearance to luteal cells of normal corpora lutea. In the photomicrograph shown here, the thecal or capsular cells appear to be interior. This may be due to gradual eversion of the structure during culture; each corpus luteum was "opened" with fine forceps before it was placed in culture.

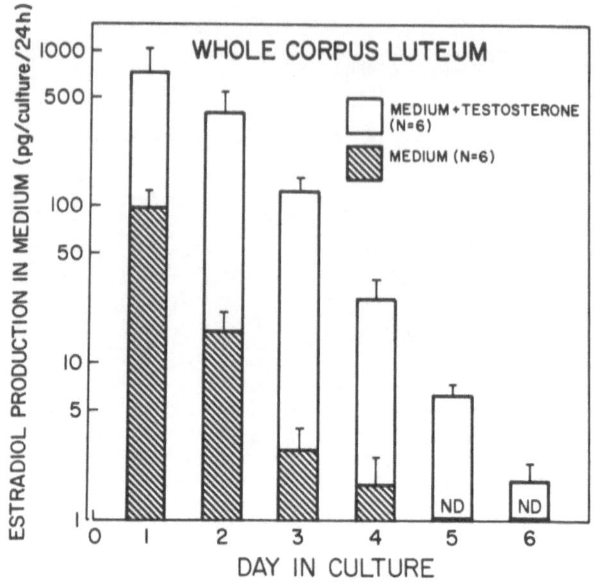

Fig. 6. Daily production of 17β-estradiol by corpora lutea in culture in the absence or presence of testosterone, 10 ng/ml (1 corpus luteum per culture dish; corpora lutea removed the day after ovulation, i.e. day 0 of culture). The medium was changed completely every 24 hours. Data expressed as mean ± SEM; N=number of animals; ND=not detectable.

DISCUSSION

The hypothesis was tested that 17β-estradiol is a sufficient luteotrophic hormone for a normal luteal phase in the absence of the pituitary. The results disclose that the formation, maintenance and regression of the corpora lutea are normal by the major criterion of progesterone concentration in blood. The validity of a comparison of serum progesterone values in hypophysectomized and sham hypophysectomized animals is strengthened by the observations that numbers of corpora lutea and wet weight of individual corpora lutea were not different for the two groups. Further indication of normal steroidogenesis after hypophysectomy is seen in the rates of production of progesterone and 20α-dihydroprogesterone by the luteal tissues in vitro. The results of removal and replacement of estradiol reveal the acute dependence of steroidogenesis upon estradiol and reveal the capacity for

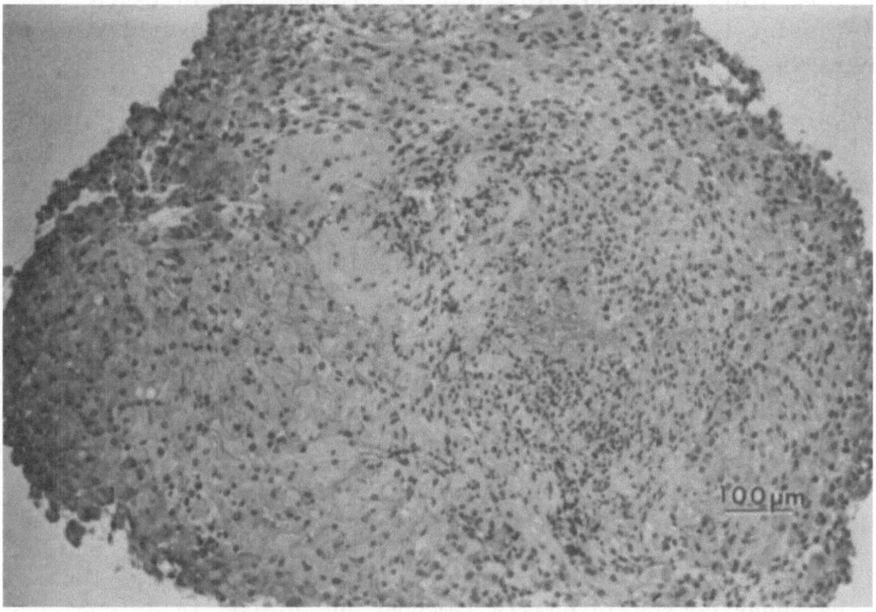

Fig. 7. Histological appearance of corpus luteum after 13 days in culture (stained with hematoxylin and eosin).

renewed response after temporary withdrawal of estradiol as reported previously in intact rabbits (Bender et al., 1978). If estradiol is removed and not replaced, serum progesterone declines to values typical of estrous rabbits, and the corpora lutea regress prematurely (Holt et al., 1975; Bill and Keyes, 1983).

From the above observations and interpretations, we are led to the conclusion that beyond the day after ovulation, the corpora lutea do not require direct stimulation by LH or other pituitary hormones. Indirectly, LH has an essential role, which is the stimulation of estradiol secretion by ovarian follicles that develop to maturity within 4 to 6 days after ovulation (Hilliard and Eaton, 1971). As shown in the present study, estradiol must be in the circulation by day 4, otherwise the corpora lutea collapse and die by day 6. A similar fate was observed for ectopic corpora lutea developing from preovulatory follicles autotransplanted beneath the kidney capsule in ovariectomized rabbits (Miller and Keyes, 1975). The nature of the regulation of the initial post-ovulatory growth and differentiation of the corpus luteum remains obscure. A limited period (approximately 4 days) of development and function of the corpus luteum in the absence of the pituitary has been reported in women after ovulation induced by LH (Vande Wiele et al., 1970). In rabbits, LH released during the preovulatory gonadotropin surge is presumed to initiate luteinization (Keyes, 1969) which can proceed for several days in the absence of the pituitary gland (Deanesly et al., 1930; Smith and White, 1931), and without any requirement for exogenous estrogen to promote steroidogenesis (Fig. 4). The corpus luteum itself may produce estradiol for a brief period after ovulation, as indicated by the waning capacity of the corpus luteum in culture to produce estradiol. However, in a preliminary experiment, we did not detect aromatase activity in corpora lutea removed from rabbits 4 days after ovulation.

Unexpectedly, the corpus luteum in culture exhibited prolonged survival in striking contrast to the premature death of corpora lutea deprived of estrogen in vivo. How are we to interpret these observations? One explanation is that prolonged estradiol production in vitro has prolonged the secretion of progesterone. But, to counter this argument, progesterone synthesis continued well beyond day 4, the last day of detection of estradiol in the medium in the absence of testosterone. Another possibility to consider is that estrogen is essential for the maintenance of the vascular system in the corpus luteum. Thus, when the young corpus luteum is removed and placed in an enriched medium, the luteal cells can survive and produce progesterone for extended periods. In the hypophysectomized animal, deprived of estrogen, the collapse of the vascular system of the young corpora lutea might be the immediate cause of premature luteal regression.

Whether the corpus luteum in culture ultimately undergoes a process resembling "physiological" regression remains an intriguing question. In the animal, it is clear that regression of the corpora lutea is normal and predictable after hypophysectomy and with estradiol present, ruling out any direct role of pituitary hormones (Bill and Keyes, 1983; also see Fig. 1). It has been known for some time that regression of corpora lutea in this species does not require withdrawal of estradiol (Spies et al., 1968b; Miller and Keyes, 1976); in fact, estradiol secretion appears to rise as the corpus luteum regresses (Browning et al., 1980). A concept that emerges, is that the corpus luteum gradually loses its response to estrogen, although it is not known if access of estradiol to the luteal cell and subsequent uptake is progressively diminished.

Whatever the mechanism of regression, it is forestalled by the conceptus. In this species, the placenta does not produce progesterone (Thau and Lanman, 1974); therefore, the corpora lutea must remain active throughout gestation aided by a putative factor of placental origin (Holt and Ewing, 1974). Although the biological activity is unknown, the placental factor is not luteotrophic alone; if follicular estrogen synthesis is eliminated and fetal viability is maintained by exogenous progestin, the corpora lutea regress (Gadsby et al., in press). On the other hand, the effectiveness of estradiol as a luteotrophic hormone is rapidly lost after hysterectomy in the second half of pregnancy (Gadsby and Keyes, unpublished). These observations are interpreted to mean that the corpora lutea continue to function during the second half of pregnancy through the combined actions of estradiol produced by ovarian follicles and a placental factor that maintains luteal responsiveness to estrogen or access of estrogen to luteal tissue.

CONCLUSION

From these experiments we have gleaned new evidence for the central role of 17β-estradiol as the luteotrophic hormone in the rabbit. Through the action of this hormone, the corpus luteum reaches its zenith of activity and then regresses in orderly fashion. The remarkable feature is that LH has no obvious direct luteotrophic action throughout pseudopregnancy, other than to initiate luteinization of the Graafian follicle. The longevity of corpora lutea in tissue culture raises questions as to the site of action of estrogen in vivo. A tempting hypothesis is that estrogen acts primarily to maintain the vascular system in the corpus luteum. However, enthusiasm for this hypothesis is tempered by the knowledge that the estrogen receptor, which appears to mediate the steroidogenic response to estradiol (Yuh and Keyes, 1981, 1982; Holt et al., 1981), is located in the luteal cells proper, not in adjacent stromal or endothelial cells (Holt et al., 1982).

ACKNOWLEDGMENTS

This research and preparation of manuscript were supported by NIH grants HD-07127, HD-13645, and HD-11311, by National Research Service Awards F33-HD06493 (P.L.K.), F32-HD06001 (C.H.B.), and by a grant from the Mellon Foundation (J.E.G.). We thank R. M. Possley for technical assistance and J. Sterkel for typing the manuscript.

REFERENCES

Bender, E. M., Miller, J. B., Possley, R. M. and Keyes, P. L., 1978, Steroidogenic effect of 17β-estradiol in the rabbit: stimulation of progesterone synthesis in prematurely regressing corpora lutea, Endocrinology, 103:1937.

Bill, C. H., II and Keyes, P. L., 1983, 17β-estradiol maintains normal function of corpora lutea throughout pseudopregnancy in hypophysectomized rabbits, Biol. Reprod., 28:608.

Browning, J. Y., Keyes, P. L. and Wolf, R. C., 1980, Comparison of serum progesterone, 20α-dihydroprogesterone, and estradiol-17β in pregnant and pseudopregnant rabbits: evidence for postimplantation recognition of pregnancy, Biol. Reprod., 23:1014.

Condon, W. A. and Black, D. L., 1976, Catecholamine-induced stimulation of progesterone by the bovine corpus luteum in vitro, Biol. Reprod., 15:573.

Deanesly, R., Fee, A. R., and Parkes, A. S., 1930, Studies on ovulation. II. The effect of hypophysectomy on the formation of the corpus luteum, J. Physiol (Lond.), 70:38.

Dorrington, J. H. and Kilpatrick, R., 1969, The synthesis of progestational steroids by the rabbit ovary, in: "The Gonads", K. W. McKerns, ed., Appleton-Century-Crofts, N.Y.

Fitz, T. A., Mayan, M. H., Sawyer, H. R., and Niswender, G. D., 1982, Characterization of two steroidogenic cell types in the ovine corpus luteum, Biol. Reprod., 27:703.

Gadsby, J. E., Keyes, P. L., and Bill, C. H., II, Control of corpus luteum function in the pregnant rabbit: role of estrogen and lack of a direct luteotrophic role of the placenta, Endocrinology (in press).

Gibori, G., Keyes, P. L., and Richards, J. S., 1978, A role for intraluteal estrogen in the mediation of luteinizing hormone action on the rat corpus luteum during pregnancy, Endocrinology, 103:162.

Gibori, G., Rodway, R., and Rothchild, I., 1977, The luteotrophic effect of estrogen in the rat: prevention by estradiol of the luteolytic effect of an antiserum to luteinizing hormone in the pregnant rat, Endocrinology, 101:1683.

Hansel, W., Concannon, P. W., and Lukaszewska, J. H., 1973, Corpora lutea of the large domestic animals, Biol. Reprod., 8:222.

Hilliard, J., and Eaton, L. W., Jr., 1971, Estradiol-17 , progesterone and 20α-hydroxypregn-4-en-3-one in rabbit ovarian venous plasma, Endocrinology, 89:522.

Holt, J. A., Dinerstein, R. J. and Lorincz, M. A., 1982, Site of estrogen action in rabbit ovarian tissue, Am. J. Physiol., 243:E188.

Holt, J. A. and Ewing, L. L., 1974, Acute dependence of ovarian progesterone output on the presence of placentas in 21-day pregnant rabbits, Endocrinology, 94:1438.

Holt, J. A., Keyes, P. L., Brown, J. M., and Miller, J. B., 1975, Premature regression of corpora lutea in pseudopregnant rabbits following the removal of polydimethylsiloxane capsules containing 17β-estradiol, Endocrinology, 97:76.

Holt, J. A., Lorincz, M. A., and Lyttle, C. R., 1981, Estrogen receptor in rabbit ovaries and effects of antiestrogen on progesterone production, Endocrinology, 108:2308.

Hoyer, P. B., Fitz, T. A., and Niswender, G. D., 1983, Progesterone secretion by large ovine luteal cells is not regulated by 3'5'-cyclic adenosine monophosphate (cAMP), Biol. Reprod., 28:34 (Abstract).

Hunzicker-Dunn, M., 1982, Epinephrine-sensitive adenylyl cyclase activity in rabbit ovarian tissues, Endocrinology, 110:233.

Hunzicker-Dunn, M., and Birnbaumer, L., 1976, Adenylyl cyclase activities in ovarian tissues. IV. Gonadotrophin-induced desensitization of the luteal adenylyl cyclase throughout pregnancy and pseudopregnancy in the rabbit and rat, Endocrinology, 99:211.

Jordan, A. W., III, Caffrey, J. L. and Niswender, G. D., 1978, Catecholamine-induced stimulation of progesterone and adenosine 3'5'-monophosphate production by dispersed ovine luteal cells, Endocrinology, 103:385.

Keyes, P. L., 1969, Luteinizing hormone: Action on the Graafian follicle in vitro, Science, 164:846.

Keyes, P. L., Gadsby, J. E., Yuh, K-C. M., and Bill, C. H., 1983, The corpus luteum, in: "Reproductive Physiology, IV, International Review of Physiology", Vol. 27, R. O. Greep, ed., University Park Press, Baltimore.

Knobil, E., 1973, On the regulation of the primate corpus luteum, Biol. Reprod., 8:246.

Lowry, O. H., Rosebrough, N. J., Farr, A. L., and Randall, R. J., 1951, Protein measurement with the Folin phenol reagent, J. Biol. Chem., 193:265.

Miller, J. B., and Keyes, P. L., 1975, Progesterone synthesis in developing rabbit corpora lutea in the absence of follicular estrogens, Endocrinology, 97:83.

Miller, J. B., and Keyes, P. L., 1976, A mechanism for regression of the rabbit corpus luteum: uterine-induced loss of luteal responsiveness to 17β-estradiol, Biol. Reprod., 15:511.

Niswender, G. D., Sawyer, H. R., Chen, T. T., and Endres, D. B., 1980, Action of luteinizing hormone at the luteal cell level, Adv. Sex Horm. Res., 4:153.

Robson, J. M., 1937, Maintenance by oestrin of the luteal function in hypophysectomized rabbits, J. Physiol. (Lond.), 90:435.

Rothchild, I., 1981, The regulation of the mammalian corpus luteum, Rec. Prog. Horm. Res., 37:183.

Smith, P. E. and White, W. E., 1931, The effect of hypophysectomy on ovulation and corpus luteum formation in the rabbit, J. Am. Med. Assoc., 97:1861.

Spies, H. G., Hilliard, J., and Sawyer, C. H., 1968a, Maintenance of corpora lutea and pregnancy in hypophysectomized rabbits, Endocrinology, 83:354.

Spies, H. G., Hilliard, J., and Sawyer, C. H., 1968b, Pituitary and uterine factors controlling regression of corpora lutea in intact and hypophysectomized rabbits, Endocrinology, 83:291.

Thau, R., and Lanman, J. T., 1974, Evaluation of progesterone synthesis in rabbit placentas, Endocrinology, 94:925.

Vande Wiele, R. L., Boqumil, J., Dyrenfurth, I., Ferin, M., Jewelewicz, R., Warren, M., Rizkallah, T., and Mikhail, G., 1970, Mechanisms regulating the menstrual cycle in women, Rec. Prog. Horm. Res., 26:63.

Yuh, K-C. M., and Keyes, P. L., 1981, Effects of human chorionic gonadotropin in the rabbit corpus luteum: loss of estrogen receptor and decreased steroidogenic response to estradiol, Endocrinology, 108:1321.

Yuh, K-C. M. and Keyes, P. L., 1982, Relationships between estrogen receptor and estradiol-stimulated progesterone synthesis in the rabbit corpus luteum, Biol. Reprod., 27:1049.

SECRETION AND ACTION OF STEROIDS IN THE LUTEAL CELL

Geula Gibori[1], M. Iqbal Khan[1], Rajagopala Sridaran[1], Y-D. Ida Chen[2], Salman Azhar,[2] Mrinalini C. Rao[1], Pondicherry Jayatilak[1] and J. Randy Gruber[1]

[1]Department of Physiology and Biophysics, College of Medicine, University of Illinois, Chicago, IL 60612, and [2]Department of Medicine, Stanford University School of Medicine, Palo Alto, CA 94304.

INTRODUCTION

The corpus luteum (CL) is a transient endocrine gland that synthesizes the steroid(s) necessary for ovum implantation and development of both placenta and fetus. In some species, such as primate and rat, the CL secretes both progesterone (P) and estradiol (E). However, luteal production of steroids is required for fetal survival throughout pregnancy in rats, while the CL is necessary only during early pregnancy in primates.

One of the most exciting aspects of luteal regulation and P secretion concerns the necessity of more than one luteotropic hormone. Why are different hormones necessary to produce only one effect and what is the specific role of each luteotropic hormone? In the pregnant rat, activation and maintenance of CL function involves the interplay of PRL, LH (or their counterparts from the placenta) and E. A major aim of the research in this laboratory has been to try to elucidate the respective roles of each luteotropin and to understand how the multitude of hormones involved in steroidogenesis interact. Our studies have assigned increasing importance to luteal E and have strongly indicated that LH and PRL act indirectly through this mechanism. That is, PRL, from either the pituitary or placenta maintains both LH and E receptors (Gibori and Richards, 1978; Gibori et al., 1979; Basuray et al., 1983) and LH stimulates ovarian production of androgen substrate for luteal cell production of E (Sridaran et al., 1981; Kalison and Gibori, 1983). There is no question that LH acutely enhances P synthesis by rat luteal cells and the mechanism of action of this process is presently under intense investigation. However, results of our investigations strongly suggest that the sustained effect of LH on P synthesis in the pregnant rat is mediated by luteal E (Gibori et al., 1978). When CL are deprived of LH by administration of LH-antiserum or hypophysectomy on either day 10 or 11 of pregnancy and intraluteal concentrations of E are maintained at physiological levels by the administration of low amounts of testosterone (T), P synthesis is maintained at normal levels (Gibori et al., 1979). Furthermore, CL with desensitized adenylate cyclase are capable of secreting P if provided with aromatizable androgen (Sridaran et al., 1983). Therefore, the sustained role of LH on luteal cell production of P appears to be indirect: LH stimulates the ovarian production of androgen (Sridaran and Gibori, 1982) which is converted locally to E by the active aromatase system (Elbaum and Keyes, 1976; Gibori et al., (1982). E then acts to stimulate P synthesis and luteal growth (Takayama and Greenwald, 1973; Gibori et al., 1977; Gibori and Richards, 1978; Gibori and Keyes, 1978; Ochiai and Rotchild, 1981; Rodway and Garris, 1982; Goldsmith et al., 1982).

Neutralization of LH with LH-antiserum before day 8 of pregnancy is not followed by abortion (Morishige and Rothchild, 1974) and results in only a partial decline in P production (Gibori and Keyes, 1980). However, the same treatment between days 8-11 causes an immediate cessation of luteal cell function (Madhwa Raj and Mougdal, 1970; Morishige and Rothchild, 1974). These results have been interpreted to mean that LH, and thus E, are not necessary for luteal cell function in the first week of pregnancy. Similar observations have been reported in the rabbit, a species in which P secretion is also controlled by E (Bender et al., 1978). Rabbit CL remain capable of secreting P for several days after ovulation even after E has been experimentally reduced or eliminated (Miller and Keyes, 1978). This indicates a degree of autonomy from estrogen before day seven. However, recent investigations by P.L. Keyes and collaborators (personal communication) have revealed that this "estradiol independency" may be more apparent than real. CL of rabbits obtained on day 1 of pregnancy and maintained in organ culture produce E for several days in the absence of any stimuli.

The ability of the CL to make androgen and estrogen is probably directly related to the extent to which theca cells take part in the composition of the CL. In the rat, LH induces and activates the 17α-hydroxylase and 17,20 lyase enzymes in theca cells of preovulatory follicles (Bogovich and Richards, 1982). After ovulation and luteinization, the theca cells of the CL may produce enough androgenic precursor for E biosynthesis and the E formed *in situ* may sustain luteal function in conjuction with PRL. With time, theca cells may degenerate and the limited number of cells remaining may be unable to produce enough androgen for E biosynthesis unless stimulated by sustained levels of LH. Alternatively, the theca cell number may remain constant but the enzyme responsible for the conversion of P to T may decay after day 7. The sustained presence of LH may then become necessary for the induction/activation of these enzymes.

From mid-pregnancy, CL secrete P independently. The loss of a specific dependence on LH, however, is not equivalent to a loss of dependence on estrogen. The marked increase in P secretion and luteal weight after day 12 of pregnancy is almost certainly a response to estrogen (Gibori et al., 1977; Nakamura and Ichikawa, 1978; Rodway and Garris, 1982). A LH-like hormone, rat chorionic gonadotropin (rCG), has been found in the peripheral circulation (Blank et al., 1979). RCG may bind to the LH receptor in the luteal cell and stimulate T production. However, desensitization of luteal adenylate cyclase after day 12 of pregnancy does not diminish P production (Sridaran, et al; 1983). The findings that the placentas secrete significant amounts of T throughout the second half of pregnancy (Gibori and Sridaran, 1981; Sridaran et al., 1981) and that T sustains P synthesis by luteal cells with low LH receptor content and desensitized adenylate cyclase (Sridaran et al., 1983), strongly suggest that the absence of a requirement for LH after day 12 may be due to the availability of sufficient androgen in the circulation derived from the placentas.

The effect of either LH or E on luteal function requires previous prolonged exposure to PRL or PRL-like hormones of placental origin. In the absence of PRl both LH receptor and E receptor content in luteal cells drop dramatically (Gibori and Richards, 1978; Gibori et al., 1979). The source of PRL varies throughout pregnancy. Until day 8, the continual presence of pituitary PRL is crucial for luteal cell function (Morishige and Rothchild, 1974). From day 8, the decidual tissue secretes a PRL-like material, decidual luteotropin (Gibori et al., 1974; Basuray and Gibori, 1980; Gibori et al., 1981; Basuray et al., 1983), which can maintain luteal cell production of P if PRL secretion is impaired. Between days 11-14, the trophoblast secretes yet another PRL-like material, rat placental luteotropin (rPL) (Kelly et al., 1975), a highly potent hormone with a longer half-life than PRL (Glaser et al., in preparation). RPL sustains luteal cell responsiveness to both LH and E for at least 4 days after its disappearance from the circulation (Gibori and Richards, 1978; Khan et al., 1983). The placenta also produces a lactogen late in pregnancy which binds to luteal PRL receptors but has no luteotropic activity (Kelly et al., 1975; Glaser et al., in preparation).

It has been previously suggested that the luteotropic requirements of the CL in the rat change during gestation (Morishige and Rothchild, 1974; Smith et al., 1976; Behrman et al., 1979) and that CL function is controlled by PRL until day 8, by LH and placental lactogen between days 8-11 and by placental lactogen from day 12. However, recent observations strongly suggest that the regulatory signals involved in CL growth and function do not vary throughout pregnancy but rather that the <u>source</u> of PRL and androgenic precursors for E biosynthesis changes, and that throughout pregnancy both luteal E and PRL activate the machinery necessary for steroid production and growth.

It is well established that luteal cells of pregnant rats possess an active aromatase (Alloiteau and Mayer, 1967; Gibori and Kraicer, 1973; Elbaum and Keyes, 1976; Gibori et al., 1982). A tremendous increase in E occurs when CL are provided with T (Elbaum and Keyes, 1976; Gibori et al., 1983). However, because luteal cells secrete only small amounts of T (Taya and Greenwald, 1981) and E (Elbaum and Keyes, 1976) when incubated in vitro and convert negligible amounts of [^{3}H]-P to [^{3}H]-E (Zmigrod and Lindner, 1972), luteal cells of rats were considered to possess a weak 17α-hydroxylase and 17,20 lyase system. Utilizing uterine weight changes and vaginal cornification as indicators of estrogen secretion, earlier reports (MacDonald et al., 1966) have shown that ovaries of hypophysectomized rats containing CL secrete estrogen in response to injections of LH, while ovaries devoid of CL do not. However, it was not possible to determine from these investigations whether LH stimulates T production by the non-luteal tissue which is then converted to E by the luteal cells or whether the effect of LH is directly on the CL. Because luteal cells of pregnant rats possess LH receptors coupled to adenylate cyclase (Gibori and Richards, 1978; Hunzicker-Dunn and Birnbaumer, 1976; Sridaran et al., 1983) and because LH stimulates T production by Leydig cells and follicular theca cells, we first sought to determine what effect LH might have on luteal production of T. Specifically, we attempted to determine whether LH might play a direct role in the induction and/or activation of the enzymes responsible for the conversion of P to E.

Although the necessity of E in the maintenance of luteal steroidogenesis has been well documented in both rats and rabbits, very little is currently known about on the biochemical mechanisms that subserve estrogen action. Cholesterol is the obligatory precursor of P and changes in either its cellular concentration or metabolism might be expected to play a central role in regulating P biosynthesis. Several recent studies (Schuler et al., 1981; McNamara et al., 1981; Azhar and Menon, 1981; Bruot et al., 1982) have suggested that high density lipoprotein (HDL) serves as the major source of cholesterol for rat steroidogenic tissues. E has been reported to either increase (Fillios et al., 1958; Kelner et al., 1977) or decrease (Kovanen et al., 1979) plasma cholesterol levels and to increase both lipoprotein receptors and lipoprotein uptake in the liver (Kovanen et al., 1979; Chao et al., 1979; Windler et al., 1980). Estrogen may stimulate steroidogenesis by modulating cellular uptake of lipoprotein substrate, regulating intracellular cholesterol utilization and/or altering steroidogenic enzyme activity. Thus, the second objective of this investigation was aimed at defining the mechanisms by which E is able to affect luteal steroidogenesis and growth.

EFFECT OF LH ON LUTEAL CELL PRODUCTION OF TESTOSTERONE AND ESTRADIOL

To determine whether LH/hCG stimulates luteal cell synthesis of T and E, pregnant rats were injected with different doses of hCG twice daily from day 12 until day 14. Rats were bled from the ovarian vein and CL were isolated and incubated in Medium 199 for 4 h. As shown in Tables I and II, hCG increased the ovarian secretion of both T and E tremendously and greatly enhanced the capacity of luteal cells to produce T and E *in vitro*. The greatest increase in basal T and E production was observed following treatment with the smallest dose of hCG. An inverse dose-response relationship was observed with higher doses of hCG. Since all doses of hCG caused a dramatic decrease in luteal hCG binding and LH-stimulated adenylate cyclase (Table II), it appears that the decreased ability of high doses of hCG to stimulate T and E synthesis is not due solely to a desensitizing effect.

Table I. Effect of various doses of hCG on ovarian secretion of T and E. Rats were injected sc twice daily with hCG on days 12 and 13. On day 14, rats were treated with a single injection and were bled 2 h later from the ovarian vein. Steroids were measured by RIA.

TREATMENT	OVARIAN SECRETION	
HCG (IU)	Testosterone PG/ML	Estradiol PG/ML
0	645 ± 0	591 ± 34
3	12526 ± 3535	4897 ± 1324
6	13864 ± 6322	6733 ± 1709
18	11689 ± 2179	2771 ± 502
60	7416 ± 1355	3513 ± 691

To determine whether hCG rapidly stimulates ovarian production of T and E, both *in vivo* and *in vitro* approaches were used. 3 IU of hCG were administered at 24 h intervals to rats on day 14 of pregnancy. Levels of T and E in the ovarian vein and the capacity of luteal cells to secrete both steroids were determined at different times following hCG administration (Table III). No increase in either ovarian secretion or luteal cell production of T and E was observed until 4 h after hCG administration. A dramatic increase in the formation of both steroids occurred thereafter.

HCG selectively increased luteal cell synthesis of T and E without enhancing P production (Fig. 1). This selective effect of hCG indicates that P substrate is certainly not the rate-limiting step for T synthesis and that the locus of hCG action is on the 17α-hydroxylase and/or 17,20 lyase enyzme. To examine this possibility 1.5 IU of hCG were administered to rats twice daily between days 12-14 of pregnancy and both enzyme activities were determined. hCG increased 17α-hydroxylase activity 2.5 fold. The effect of hCG on 17,20 lyase activity was even more dramatic. Lyase activity was barely detectable in CL of normal pregnant rats yet was enhanced 40 fold by hCG (Gibori and Johnson, in preparation). LH/hCG appears to stimulate the synthesis of enzymes involved in the conversion of P to androgen in the luteal cell rather than stimulate the activation of existing enzymes. A delay of at least 4 h was observed between hCG administration and the first observable

Table II. Effect of various doses of hCG on luteal cell production of T and E and on luteal content of LH receptors and LH-stimulated adenylate cyclase. Rats were treated as described in Fig. legend 1. CL were incubated for 4 h at 37°C in Medium 199. E and T accumulation in the media were measured by RIA. (Data on LH receptor's and adenylate cyclase from Sridaran et al., 1983).

TREATMENT	LUTEAL PRODUCTION OF STEROIDS	
HCG (IU)	Testosterone (PG/CL/4H)	Estradiol (PG/CL/4H)
0	24 ± 5	45 ± 6
3	356 ± 110	4718 ± 627
6	212 ± 55	984 ± 31
18	118 ± 33	573 ± 239
60	74 ± 19	466 ± 50

TREATMENT	LUTEAL LH RECEPTORS AND ADENYLATE CYCLASE		
HCG (IU)	^{125}I-HCG Bound (CPM/CL)	Adenylate Cyclase Activity (Pmol cAMP min.$^{-1}$ Prot.$^{-1}$)	
		-LH	+LH
0	27995 ± 8938	17 ± 1	106 ± 11
3	9870 ± 1394	14 ± 5	19 ± 7
6	1939 ± 316	19 ± 3	20 ± 2
18	1218 ± 408	14 ± 2	15 ± 4
60	1716 ± 188	22 ± 3	28 ± 6

increase in T and E production. This finding may explain why LH does not acutely stimulate androgen and estrogen production by luteal cells *in vitro* (Gibori and Kalison, unpublished).

It remains to be determined whether all luteal cells secrete T when stimulated by LH or whether only luteal cells of thecal origin retain this capacity. CL of rats are formed by two cell types (Wilkinson et al., 1976; Khan and Gibori, in progress) which may originate from the granulosa and theca cells. In the follicle of the rat, only the theca secrete androgen when stimulated by LH, whereas granulosa cells aromatize androgen to E (Fortune and Armstrong, 1978). Therefore, it is possible that luteinized theca cells retain the 17α-hydroxylase and the 17,20 lyase responsible for the conversion of P to androgen whereas the enzyme(s) involved in aromatization could be limited to the granulosa-luteinized cells.

Table III. Time dependent effect of hCG administration on production of T and E. 3 IU of hCG were administered on day 14 and 15 of pregnancy and ovarian blood and CL were obtained at different times thereafter. T and E were measured in the ovarian vein plasma (*in vivo*) and in the incubates (*in vitro*).

HOURS AFTER HCG	STEROIDS PRODUCTION			
	IN VITRO (PG/CL/4H)		IN VIVO (NG/ML)	
	Testosterone	Estradiol	Testosterone	Estradiol
0	43 ± 11	45 ± 6	0.78 ± 0.8	0.23 ± 0.2
0.5	67 ± 7	58 ± 10	0.72 ± 0.8	0.23 ± 0.2
2.0	82 ± 12	72 ± 21	0.72 ± 0.1	0.28 ± 0.7
4.0	90 ± 20	120 ± 64	1.19 ± 0.3	0.33 ± 0.1
12.0	261 ± 9	3010 ± 111	6.10 ± 0.3	2.70 ± 0.2
24.0	311 ± 11	3820 ± 119	8.21 ± 1.0	3.40 ± 0.2
48.0	342 ± 49	4803 ± 389	10.0 ± 1.0	4.78 ± 1.0

It is not clear whether hCG also enhances aromatase activity in luteal cells. CL of pregnant rats are able to convert T to E in the absence of any luteotropin. In fact, CL which have ceased to secrete P retain their aromatase system and continue to produce P when provided with T (Alloiteau and Mayer, 1967; Gibori et al.,

1982). Consequently, it appears that the capacity and ability of the luteal cell to produce E are independent of the functional state of the cell.

In summary, from mid-pregnancy, CL appear to secrete P at full capacity and no further increase can be obtained with an increase in LH/hCG activity. However, secretion of T and E by luteal cells of pregnant rats is submaximal and can be vastly increased by hCG stimulation. Thus, in the final analysis, luteal production of E is tightly controlled by LH.

ESTRADIOL ACTION ON LUTEAL CELL STEROIDOGENESIS

To determine whether E stimulates P synthesis in the pregnant rat by affecting plasma levels of cholesterol and/or by modulating the cellular uptake of lipoprotein and cholesterol metabolism, rats that were hypophysectomized and hysterectomized on day 12 of pregnancy were used. In this experimental model, luteal cells contain low levels of estrogen but remain responsive to E (Gibori et al., 1977; Gibori and Keyes, 1978; Rodway and Garris, 1982).

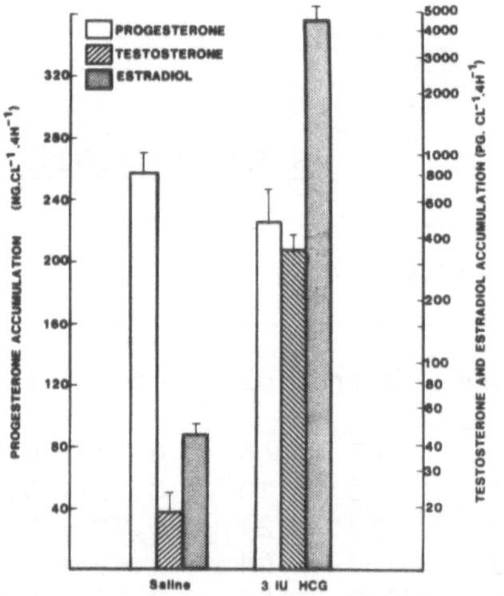

Fig. 1. Luteal cell production of P, T and E after hCG stimulation. Rats were treated with 1.5 IU hCG twice daily on day 12 and 13. On day 14 rats were treated with a single injection. CL were incubated for 4 h in Medium 199. Steroid accumulation in the media was measured by RIA.

They are also rich in aromatase (Gibori et al., 1982) and several lines of evidence (Gibori and Keyes, 1978; Gibori, 1979) suggest that T can be effective in enhancing P synthesis and luteal weight after it is converted to E. Thus, luteal concentrations of E are maintained at physiological levels with the exogenous administration of either E or aromatizable androgen.

To investigate the effect of luteal E on the binding activity of ^{125}[I]-HDL we first had to determine whether luteal cells of pregnant rats possess receptors for HDL. Therefore, ^{125}[I]-HDL binding activity was measured in luteal membranes. The data in Fig. 2 show the characterization of HDL receptors in luteal cells of pregnant rats. ^{125}[I]-HDL binding reached equilibrium as early as 45 min and approached saturation as the HDL substrate concentration increased. Analysis of the specific binding by Scatchard plots demonstrated an apparent single class of binding sites. The specific binding capacity in this experiment was 8.15 pg/cell with an apparent Kd of 29.4 μg HDL-protein/ml.

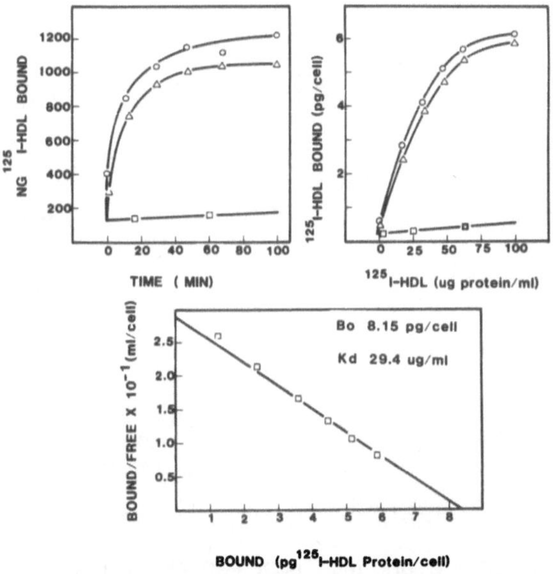

Fig. 2. Characterization of HDL receptors in luteal cells of pregnant rats. Luteal membranes (35 μg protein) prepared from CL of day 15 pregnant rats were incubated with different amounts of [^{125}I]-rat HDL for various periods of time in the absence or presence of a 100 fold excess of unlabelled human lipoprotein. 0-----0: total binding; Δ---Δ : specific binding; ⊟-----⊟: non specific binding.

The administration of either E or T to day 12 hypophysectomized and hysterectomized pregnant rats markedly increased the HDL binding activity in luteal cell membranes (Fig. 3). Since there was no change in binding affinity, the increase in binding activities was a result of increased binding sites. The same binding experiment and Scatchard analysis was carried out for 8 to 11 animals per group and the mean binding and statistical data are shown in Fig. 4 together with LH receptor levels. The results clearly show that E and T treatment elicited a dramatic increase in the luteal cell content of lipoprotein receptor and was not accompanied by any changes in hCG binding capacity.

The mechanism by which E increases lipoprotein receptors in luteal membranes remains unknown. Lipoprotein receptors in

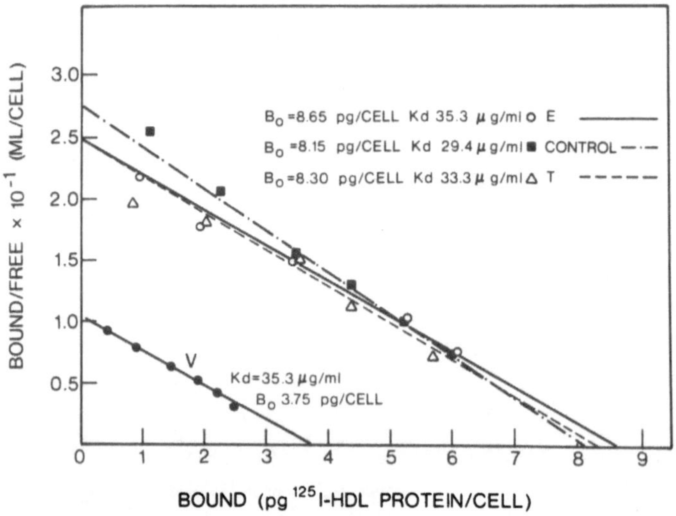

Fig. 3. Scatchard analysis of [^{125}I]-HDL binding to luteal membranes obtained from day 12 hypophysectomized and hysterectomized rats treated with T, E, or vehicle (V) between days 12-15 of pregnancy. C represents control pregnant rats. Bound/free represents the amount of specifically bound lipoprotein (µg protein /ml) divided by the concentration of unbound lipoprotein in the reaction mixture.

fibroblasts can be increased by hormones that stimulate cell growth, including insulin, thyroxine and platelet-derived growth factors (Chait et al., 1978, 1979; 1980 Witte and Cormicelli, 1980). In addition, ACTH increases the lipoprotein binding capacity of adrenal cells. In human skin fibroblasts, low intracellular concentrations of cholesterol lead to an increase in the number of binding sites on the cell surface. Therefore, it is possible that luteal E, which stimulates both luteal growth and luteal steroidogenesis, increases the number of receptors by decreasing intracellular levels of cholesterol. Indeed, treatment with E and with aromatizable androgen depleted the luteal cell content of cholesterol ester (Fig. 5). LH, which stimulates steroidogenesis and depletes cholesterol ester in luteal cells (Behrman amd Armstrong, 1969) has also been shown to enhance lipoprotein receptors in CL of both humans (Ohashi et al., 1982) and immature pseudopregnant rats (Azhar et al., 1983). It also remains possible that the effect of E on lipoprotein receptors is not directly related to changes in intracellular cholesterol. In nonsteroidogenic tissues, such as the liver, E elicits an increase in the number of high affinity lipoprotein receptors without mediating a decrease in intracellular cholesterol (Kovanen et al., 1979; Windler et al., 1980). E may act directly on both liver and luteal cell genes to stimulate the production of such receptors. Recently, Carr and Simpson, 1981, have also suggested that the action of ACTH to increase the number of LDL receptors in human fetal adrenal gland may be mediated, in part, by mechanisms that do not involve changes in intracellular cholesterol levels.

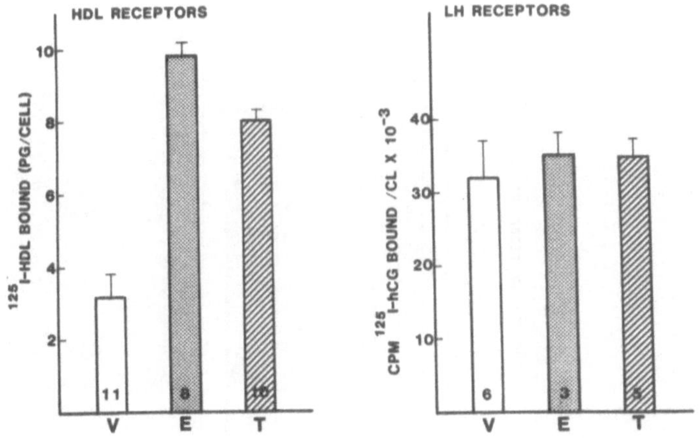

Fig. 4. Effect of T and E on [^{125}I]-HDL and [^{125}I]-hCG binding to luteal cells. Rats were treated as described in Fig. legend 3.

To ascertain whether E stimulates luteal cell steroidogenesis by increasing the delivery of cholesterol substrate through a receptor mediated process, CL obtained from day 12 hypophysectomized and hysterectomized pregnant rats treated with either E, T or vehicle were incubated for 3 h in Medium 199 in the presence of 500 μg of HDL. Addition of HDL to the medium had little effect on P production by CL of rats treated with vehicle (Fig. 6). In contrast, HDL dramatically increased P production by CL of steroid-treated animals. Therefore, it appears that E stimulates P production by affecting the incorporation and utilization of cholesterol from HDL into the cells and thus allowing increased substrate delivery for steroidogenesis.

Luteal E not only affected lipoprotein substrate incorporation into the cells but also enhanced de novo synthesis of cholesterol. We evaluated de novo cholesterol synthesis by determining the specific activity of 3-hydroxy-3-methyl-glutaryl coenzyme A (HMGCoA) reductase, the rate limiting enzyme in cholesterol biosynthesis and by measuring the incorporation of ^{14}[C] acetate into cholesterol. We found that E treatment caused a marked stimulation of de novo synthesis of cholesterol, as measured by both of these techniques (Table IV). Since HMGCoA reductase activity has been shown to exist in both phosphorylated (inactive) and dephosphorylated (active) forms (Brown et al., 1979; Ingebritsen et al., 1979; Beg and Brewer, 1981), we attempted to see if the E-induced stimulation in enzyme activity was due to a change in the total amount of enzyme or in the phosphorylated state of the enzyme.

In order to examine this question, we isolated luteal microsomes in the presence of sodium fluoride. This treatment blocks the conversion of the inactive to active form of HMGCoA. The results in Table IV indicate that HMGCoA reductase activity was

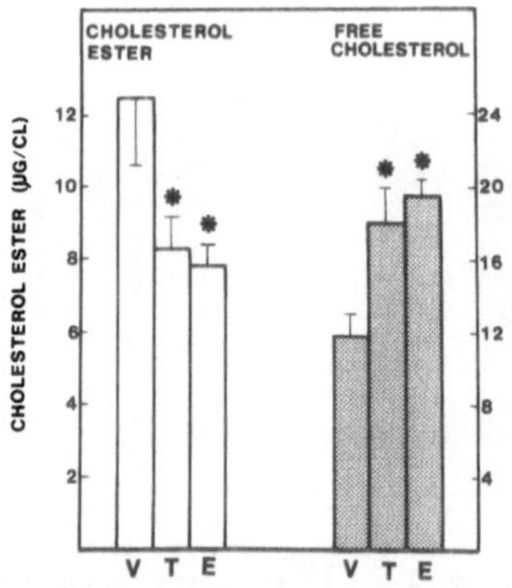

Fig. 5 Effect of T and E on luteal content of choslesteryl ester and free cholesterol. Rats were treated as described in Fig. legend 3.

markedly reduced when microsomes were isolated in the presence of NaF, suggesting that much of the HMGCoA reductase in the luteal cell of the pregnant rat is present in an inactive, i.e. phosphorylated form in vivo. However, the relative ability of luteal E to elevate HMGCoA reductase activity was not reduced when microsomes were isolated in the presence of NaF. The E-induced rise in HMGCoA reductase activity appears, therefore, to be due to a net increase in total amount of enzyme protein.

In recent experiments we have begun to explore the molecular mechanisms by which E might increase P synthesis. The action of E appears to be independent of exogenous gonadotropins and increased intracellular concentration of cAMP. One plausible candidate is calcium since Ca^{2+} ions are known to be involved in steroidogenesis (Veldhuis and Klase, 1982). Ca^{2+}-specific protein kinases and phophoproteins have been identified in a number of tissues, and one possible route for E action is by the alteration of the Ca^{2+}-specific phosphorylation systems: the kinase and/or substrates (some of which may be enzymes necessary for P biosynthesis).

In preliminary studies we examined whether E pretreatment causes any changes in Ca^{2+}-dependent protein phosphorylation in vitro. CL were obtained from day 12 hypophysectomized-hysterectomized pregnant rats treated for 3 days with vehicle or E.

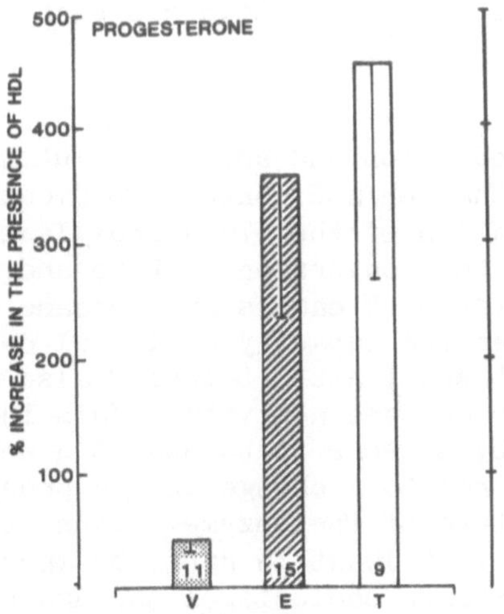

Fig. 6. Effect of HDL on P production by CL of rats treated with steroids. Rats were treated as described in Fig. legend 3. CL were incubated for 3 h in Medium 199 in the presence or absence of 500 μg HDL.

Table IV. Effect of Estradiol and Testosterone on HMGCoA Reductase Activity and Rate of Incorporation of ^{14}[C] Acetate into Cholesterol

TREATMENT	HMGCoA REDUCTASE ACTIVITY (pmol.min^{-1}.mg protein^{-1})		^{14}[C]-ACETATE CHOLESTEROL (DPM/CL)
	NaF (50 mM)	NaCl (50 mM)	
Testosterone	110 ± 19	351 + 57	1780 ± 406
Estradiol	61 ± 7	183 ± 21	1600 ± 276
Vehicle	16 ± 3	62 ± 9	920 ± 108

Controls were intact pregnant rats. Homogenates of isolated CL were incubated with ^{32}[P]-ATP (25 mM) for 1 min at 30°C in the presence or absence of 1.25 mM Ca^{2+}. Proteins were separated by SDS-polyacrylamide gel electrophoresis and phosphoproteins were visualized by autoradiography. A major Ca^{2+}-dependent phosphoprotein in luteal cells of pregnant rats was a cytosolic protein with an approximate Mr of 100,000. This phosphoprotein was poorly visible in luteal cells of vehicle treated animals. E treatment markedly restored the appearance of this phosphoprotein. Ca^{2+}-dependent substrates of similar molecular weight have been reported in CL by Maizels and Jungmann (1982) and in other mammalian tissues (Palfrey, 1983). However, this is the first time that hormonal-dependent regulation of this protein has been reported.

SUMMARY

Studies on E production and action in luteal cells of pregnant rats have revealed that LH/hCG controls E production by inducing the synthesis/activation of the 17α-hydroxylase and 17,20 lyase enzymes involved in the conversion of P to androgen in the luteal cell. The locally formed E causes an increase in HDL receptors and markedly enhances the capacity of luteal cells to produce P from cholesterol-HDL substrate. Luteal E also stimulates the activity of HMGCoA reductase activity. This increase in HMGCoA reductase activity by E seems to be due to a net increase in enzyme activity and not to a change in the phosphorylation/dephosphorylation state of the enzyme. Thus, E regulates luteal cell steroidogenesis, at least in part, by increasing the availability of substrate cholesterol through both a receptor mediated process and _de novo_ synthesis. It is tempting, albeit premature, to speculate that the molecular mechanism by which E increases steroidogenesis may involve Ca^{2+}-dependent phosphorylation of specific proteins.

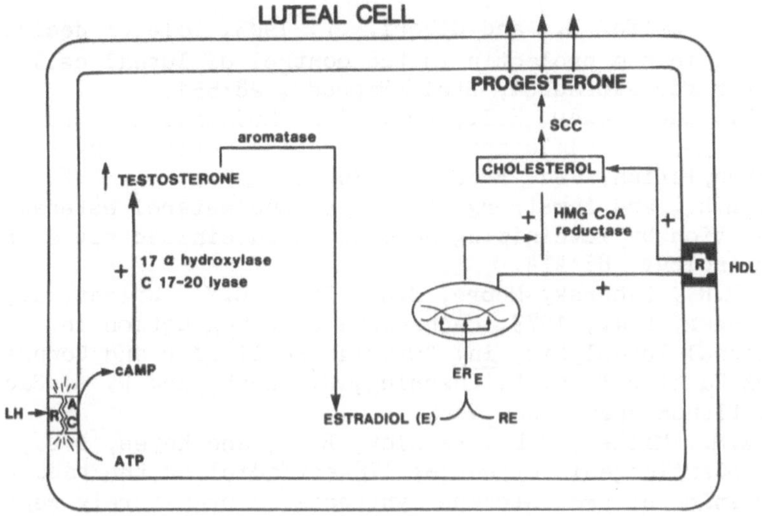

Fig. 7. Schematic drawing of possible sites of action of LH and estradiol on steroidegenesis within the luteal cell of pregnant rat.

ACKNOWLEDGEMENTS

Supported by NIH grants HD-11119 and HD-12356 and NSF grant PCM-811225. The expert editorial assistance of Linda Glaser is gratefully appreciated.

REFERENCES

Alloiteau, J.J., and Mayer, G., 1967, Problems concernant la formation, le maintien et la regression des corps jaunes chez le rat, Arch. Anat. Microsc. Morphol. Exp., 56:189.

Azhar, S., Chen, Y-D. I., and Reaven, G. M., 1983, Stimulation of lipoprotein receptors and role of lipoprotein and cellular cholesterol during gonadotropin induced desensitization of steroidogenic response in luteinized rat ovary, J. Biol. Chem., 258:3735.

Azhar, S., and Menon, K.M.J., 1981, Receptor-mediated gonadotropin action in the ovary. Rat luteal cells preferentially utilize and are acutely dependent upon the plasma lipoprotein-supplied sterols in gonadotropins-stimulated steroid production, J. Biol. Chem., 256:6548.

Basuray, R., and Gibori, G., 1980, Luteotropic action of the decidual tissue in the pregnant rat, Biol. Reprod., 23:507.

Basuray, R., Jaffe, R., and Gibori, G., 1983, Role of decidual-luteotropin and prolactin in the control of luteal cell receptor for estradiol, Biol. Reprod., 28:551.

Beg, Z. H., and Brewer, H.B., Jr., 1982, Modulation of rat liver 3-hydroxy-3-methylglutaryl-CoA reductase activity by reversible phosphorylation, Fed. Proc., 41:2634.

Behrman, H.R., and Armstrong, D., 1969, Cholesterol esterase stimulation by luteinizing hormone in luteinized rat ovaries, Endocrinology, 85:474.

Behrman, H.R., Luborsky-Moore, J.L., Pang, C.Y., Wright, K., and Dorflinger, L.J., 1979, Mechanisms of $PGF_{2\alpha}$ action in functional luteolysis, in: "Ovarian Follicular and Corpus Luteum Function", C. P. Channing, J. Marsh, and W. A. Sadler, eds., Plenum Press, New York.

Bender, E.M., Miller, J.B., Possley, R.M., and Keyes, P.L., 1978, Steroidogenic effect of 17β-estradiol in the rabbit: Stimulation of progesterone synthesis in prematurely regressing corpora lutea, Endocrinology, 103:1937.

Blank, M.S., Dufau, M.L., and Friesen, H.G., 1979, Demonstration of potent gonadotropin-like biological activity in the serum of rats during mid-pregnancy, Life Sci., 92:1527.

Bogovich, K., and Richards, J.S., 1982, Androgen biosynthesis in developing ovarian follicles: Evidence that luteinizing hormone regulates thecal 17α-hydroxylase and C 17,20-lyase activities, Endocrinology, 111:120.

Brown, M.S., Goldstein, J.L., and Dietschy, J.F.M, 1979, Active and inactive forms of 3-hydroxy-3 methylglutaryl coenzyme a reductase in the liver of the rat, J. Biol. Chem., 254:5144.

Bruot, B.C., Wiest, W.G., and Collins, D.C., 1982, Effect of low density and high density lipoproteins on progesterone secretion by dispersed corpora luteal cells from rats treated with aminopyrazolo-(3,4-d) pyrimidine, Endocrinology, 110:1572.

Carr, B.R., and Simpson, E.R., 1981, Lipoprotein utilization and cholesterol synthesis by the human fetal adrenal gland, Endocrine Reviews, 2:306.

Chait, A., Bierman, E.L., and Albers, J. J., 1978, Regulatory role of insulin in the degradation of low density lipoprotein by cultured human skin fibroblasts, Biochim. Biophys. Acta., 529:292.

Chait, A., Bierman, E.L., and Albers, J. J., 1979, Regulatory role of triiodothyronine in the degradation of low density lipoprotein by cultured human skin fibroblasts, J. Clin Endocrinol. Metab. 48:887.

Chao, Y.S., Windler, E.E., Chen, G.C., and Havel, R.J., 1979, Hepatic catabolism of rat and human lipoprotein in rats treated with 17α-ethinyl estradiol, J. Biol. Chem., 254:11360.

Elbaum, D.J., and Keyes, P.L., 1976, Synthesis of 17β-estradiol by isolated ovarian tissues of the pregnant rat: Aromatization in the corpus luteum, Endocrinology, 99:573.

Fillios, L.C., Kaplan, R., Marlin, R.S., and Stare, F.J., 1958, Some aspects of the gonadal regulation of cholesterol metabolism, Am. J. Physiol., 193:47.

Fortune, J.E., and Armstrong, D.T., 1978, Hormonal control of 17β-estradiol biosynthesis in proestrous rat follicles: Estradiol production by isolated theca verus granulosa, Endocrinology, 102:227.

Gibori, G., 1979, Steroidal regulation of luteal tissue function in pregnant rat, Endocrinology, 104:A585.

Gibori, G., Antczak, E., and Rothchild, I., 1977, The role of estrogen in the regulation of luteal progesterone secretion in the rat after day 12 of pregnancy, Endocrinology, 100:1483.

Gibori, G., Basuray, R., and McReynolds, B., 1981, Luteotropic role of the decidual tissue in the rat: Dependency on intraluteal estradiol, Endocrinology, 108:2060.

Gibori, G., and Keyes, P.L., 1978, Role of intraluteal estrogen in the regulation of the rat corpus luteum during pregnancy, Endocrinology, 102:1176.

Gibori, G., and Keyes, P.L., 1980, Luteotropic role of estrogen in early pregnancy in the rat, Endocrinology, 106:1584.

Gibori, G., Keyes, P.L., and Richards, J.S., 1978, A role for intraluteal estrogen in the mediation of LH action on the rat corpus luteum during pregnancy, Endocrinology, 103:162.

Gibori, G., and Kraicer, P.F., 1973, Conversion of testosterone to estrogen by isolated corpora lutea of pregnancy in the rat, Biol. Reprod, 9:309.

Gibori, G., and Richards, J.S., 1978, Dissociation of two distinct luteotropic effects of prolactin: Regulation of luteinizing hormone-receptor content and progesterone secretion during pregnancy, Endocrinology, 102:767.

Gibori, G., Richards, J.S., and Keyes, P.L., 1979, Synergistic effect of prolactin and estradiol in the luteotropic process in the pregnant rat: Regulation of estradiol receptor by prolactin, Biol. Reprod., 21:419.

Gibori, G., Rothchild, I., Pepe, G.J., Morishige, W.K., and Lam, P., 1974, Luteotrophic action of decidual tissue in the rat, Endocrinology, 95:1113.

Gibori, G., and Sridaran, R., 1981, Sites of androgen and estradiol production in the second half of pregnancy in the rat, Biol. Reprod., 24:249.

Gibori, G., Sridaran, R., and Basuray, R., 1982, Control of aromatase activity in luteal and non luteal cells of pregnant rats, Endocrinology, 111:781.

Goldsmith, L.T., De La Cruz, J.L., Weiss, G., and Castracane, V. D., 1982, Steroid effects on relaxin secretion in the rat, Biol. Reprod., 27:886.

Hunzicker-Dunn, M., and Birnbaumer, L., 1976, Adenyl cyclase activities in ovarian tissues. IV. Gonadotropin-induced desensitization of the luteal adenyl cyclase throughout pregnancy and pseudopregnancy in the rabbit and rat, Endocrinology, 99:211.

Ingebritsen, T.S., Geelen, M.S.H., Parker, R.A., Evenson, K. J., and Gibson, D. M., 1979, Modulation of hydroxymethyl-CoA reductase activity, reductase kinase activity, and cholesterol synthesis in rat hepatocytes in response to insulin and glucagon, J. Biol. Chem., 254:9986.

Kalison, B., and Gibori, G., 1983, Role of prolactin in hCG stimulation of luteal cell production of testosterone and estradiol in the rat. in: "Factors Regulating Ovarian Function" G.S. Greenwald, and P.F. Terranova, eds., Raven Press, New York.

Kelly, P.A., Shiu, R.P.C., Robertson, M.C., and Friesen, H.G., 1975, Characterization of rat chorionic mammotropin, Endocrinology, 96:1187.

Kelner, K., Malinow, R., and Anderson, W., 1977, Effect of estradiol-17β on cholesterol metabolism in the rat: A study using a deuterium label and mass spectrometry, Steroids, 29:1.

Khan, M.I., Glaser, L., and Gibori, G., 1983, Reactivation of regressing corpora lutea by estradiol: Dependence on rat placental lactogen, Fed. Proc., 42:A143.

Kovanen, P.T., Brown, M.S., and Goldstein, J.L., 1979, Increased binding of low density lipoprotein to liver membranes from rats treated with 17α-ethinyl estradiol, J. Biol. Chem., 245:11367.

MacDonald, G.J., Armstrong, D.T., and Greep, R.O., 1966, Stimulation of estrogen secretion from normal rat corpora lutea by luteinizing hormone, Endocrinology, 79:289.

Madhwa Raj, H.G., and Moudgal, N.R., 1970, Hormonal control of gestation in the intact rat, Endocrinology, 84:874.

Maizels, E.T., and Jungmann, R.A., 1982, Ca^{2+}-dependent phosphorylation of rat ovary proteins, Biochem. Biophys. Res. Comm., 107:32.

McNamara, B.C., Booth, R., and Stansfield, D.A., 1981, Evidence for an essential role for high density lipoprotein in progesterone synthesis by rat corpus luteum, FEBS Lett., 134:79.

Morishige, W.K., and Rothchild, I., 1974, Temporal aspects of the regulation of corpus luteum function by luteinizing hormone, prolactin and placental luteotrophin during the first half of pregnancy in the rat, Endocrinology, 95:260.

Nakamura, Y., and Ichikawa, S., 1978, Effect of the placental luteotropin and estrogen on the growth of artificially formed secondary corpora lutea of pregnancy in rats, Biol. Reprod., 19:1014.

Ochiai, A., and Rothchild, I., 1981, The relation between conceptus number and the luteotropic effect of estrogen in rats after hypophysectomy and hysterectomy on day 12 of pregnancy, Endocrinology, 109:1111.

Ohashi, M., Carr, B.R., and Simpson, E.R., 1982, Lipoprotein-binding sites in human corpus luteum membrane fractions, Endocrinology, 110:1477.

Palfrey, H.C., 1983, Presence in many mammalian tissues of an identical major cytosolic substrate (Mr 100,000) for calmodulin-dependent protein kinase, FEBS Lett., 157:183.

Rodway, R.G., and Garris, D.R., 1982, Potentiation by prolactin of the luteotrophic effect of estradiol in the pregnant rat, Acta. Endocrinol., 101:287.

Schuler, L.A., Scavo, L., Kirsch, T.M., Flickinger, G. L., and Strauss, J. F., III, 1979, Regulation of de novo biosynthesis of cholesterol and progestogens and formation of cholesteryl ester in rat corpus luteum by exogenous sterol, J. Biol. Chem., 245:8662.

Smith, M.S., McLean, B.K., and Neill, J.D., 1976, Prolactin the initial luteotropic stimulus of pseudopregnancy in the rat, Endocrinology, 98:1370.

Sridaran, R., Basuray, R., and Gibori, G., 1981, Source and regulation of testosterone secretion in pregnant and pseudopregnant rats, Endocrinology, 108:855.

Sridaran, R., Hunzicker-Dunn, M., and Gibori, G., 1983, Testosterone stimulation of progesterone synthesis by gonadotropin desensitized corpora lutea, Endocrinology, 112:610.

Takayama, M., and Greenwald, G.S., 1973, Direct luteotropic action of estrogen in the hypophysectomized hysterectomized rat, Endocrinology, 92:1405.

Taya, K., and Greenwald, G.S., 1981, In vivo and in vitro ovarian steroidogenesis in the pregnant rat, Biol. Reprod., 25:683.

Wilkinson, R. F., Anderson, E., and Aalberg, J., 1976, Cytological observations of dissociated rat corpus luteum, J. Ultrastruct., 57:168.

Windler, T., Kovanen, P.T., Chao, Y.S., Brown, M.S., Havel, R.J., and Goldstein, J.L., 1980, The estradiol-stimulated lipoprotein receptor of rat liver, J. Biol. Chem., 255:10464.

Witte, L. D., and Cormicelli, J. A., 1980, Platelet derived growth factor stimulates low density lipoprotein receptor activity in cultured human fibroblasts, Proc. Natl. Acad. Sci. USA, 77:5962.

Veldhuis, J.D., and Klase, P.A., 1982, Role of calcium ions in the stimulatory actions of luteinizing hormone in isolated ovarian cells: Studies with divalent cation ionophores, Biochem. Biophys. Res. Commun., 104:603.

Zmigrod, A., and Lindner, H. R., 1972, Oestrogen biosynthesis by the rat ovary in early pregnancy, Acta. Endocrinol. (Copenh), 69:127.

HORMONES IN ANTRAL FLUID AND THE REGULATION OF OVARIAN FUNCTION

Griff T. Ross

Professor of Medicine
Sections of Endocrinology and General Internal Medicine
Director, Division of Reproductive Sciences
Dept. of Obstetrics, Gynecology, and Reproductive Sciences
University of Texas Medical School at Houston
Houston, Texas 77030

INTRODUCTION

At a symposium on ovulation held under the auspices of the Society for the Study of Fertility in July 1976, Hans Lindner presented a paper entitled, "Intraovarian Factors in Ovulation: Determinants of Follicular Response to Gonadotropins." In addition to a critical scholarly review, the paper contained a summary of contributions made by his associates in the Department of Hormone Research at the Weizmann Institute of Science. The paper reflected not only the breadth of Hans' scholarship but the diversity of skills of the group of younger scientists whom he had attracted and motivated to work so productively on various aspects of hormonal regulation of ovulation and atresia in mammalian ovarian follicles.

In concluding his remarks, he said, "Ultimately, one would like to understand in molecular terms what distinguishes the follicle that has joined the limited set of growing follicles from the multitude of resting follicles, and what makes this 'cohort' enter a final spurt of accelerated growth that will end for most of its members in atresia but culminates for the lucky, or selected, few in ovulation. We are far from such understanding." I shall review the largely phenomenological data which have accrued to studies of selection of the ovulatory follicles in the human ovary.

HORMONES IN THE MICROENVIRONMENT OF THE FOLLICLE

During each spontaneous menstrual cycle in women and higher primates only one follicle ovulates while the remaining ones of its developmental vintage in both ipsilateral and contralateral ovaries degenerate. Since both ovulation and degeneration (atresia) are catalyzed by gonadotropins, it is difficult to explain these discrepancies without postulating differences in either the quality or the quantity of hormones to which cells in the follicle complexes are exposed. However, concentrations of gonadotropins are uniform in arterial blood perfusing the two ovaries, so that maintaining differences in exposure to these hormones requires some mechanism for regulating the process in the microenvironment of individual follicles. Moreover, if the source of trophic substances be extrinsic to the follicle, the process must depend in part upon diffusion since the interior of the follicle remains avascular until either ovulation or atresia destroys the lamina basalis.

How can the hypothesis, that hormonal concentrations in its microenvironment are determinants of the fate of a developing follicle, be tested? Antral fluid is the only practical site for sampling the microenvironment of an individual follicle. However, in women and higher primates aspirating antral fluid requires anesthesia. Prior to the introduction of in vitro fertilization and embryo transfer into clinical practice, the risks of the procedure were unacceptable in women with normal ovarian function and access to follicle fluid was limited to samples recovered during surgery for diseases not affecting ovarian function (McNatty et al., 1975, 1978) (Bomsel-Helmreich, 1979). Among these latter were women undergoing unilateral oophorectomy as a part of tuboplasties performed in treating infertility due to mechanical obstruction of the Fallopian tubes (Van Hall and Trimbos-Kemper, 1980). In such instances of elective surgery, operation could be scheduled in relation to onset of menses and hormonal markers of time in cycle relative to the preovulatory LH surge in women ovulating spontaneously. Since examination required disruption of its growth, each preovulatory follicle could be examined only once. How then could one be certain as to whether it would ovulate or degenerate? Making this distinction required some criteria for stratifying results of examination in relation to the destiny of the follicle.

Criteria for Differentiating Healthy and Atretic Follicles

The first criterion, useful in the second half of the follicular phase, is follicle size. Serial sonographic studies during spontaneous and induced ovulatory cycles have resulted in definition of rates of growth and sizes achieved by dominant follicles prior to spontaneous and induced ovulation (Fleming & Coutts, 1981; Jones et al., 1982; Quigley et al., 1983). Moreover, comparisons of estrogen levels in the venous effluent of ovaries of women (Baird and Fraser,

1975) and monkeys (di Zerega and Hodgen, 1981) cycling spontaneously showed higher concentrations in blood from the ovary containing the largest follicle in mid-follicular phase. These observations, coupled with the observation of precipitous reductions in peripheral blood estradiol levels and failure of ovulation to occur at the expected time following mid-follicular phase ablation of the largest follicle in women (Aedo et al., 1980; Nilsson et al., 1982) and monkeys (Goodman et al., 1977) validated size as a criterion for identifying the preovulatory follicle destined to ovulate.

A second set of criteria is based upon comparative properties of granulosa cells and oocytes in ovulating and degenerating follicles. These were derived from studies of follicular components during ovulation and atresia in other mammalian ovaries: rodents (Byskov, 1978), sheep (Moor et al., 1978) and rhesus monkeys (Koering, 1969) and adapted for human ovarian follicles (Peters & McNatty, 1980). The incidence of pycnosis in nuclei of granulosa cells, is higher in degenerating than in ovulating follicles. The incidence of mitoses among granulosa cells of degenerating follicles is reduced when compared to that in ovulating follicles. This latter property would predict that numbers of granulosa cells would be greater in ovulating than degenerating follicles. This phenomenon is particularly significant in the light of the fact that, along with increases in antral fluid volume and thecal hypertrophy, granulosa cell proliferation contributes to the rapid growth of the preovulatory follicle late in the follicular phase in mice (Byskov, 1978), rats (Hirshfield and Midgley, 1978), sheep (Moor et al., 1978), and in women (McNatty et al., 1979).

In view of the fact that the oocyte undergoes necrosis in degenerating follicles, it might be expected that some properties of this component would differ depending upon the status of the follicle when the oocyte is removed. In addition to immediate direct examination of the nuclei under phase microscopy, changes following incubation _in vitro_ have been used to compare oocytes from ovulating and degenerating follicles. These changes include germinal vesicle breakdown and extrusion of the first polar body during incubation (McNatty et al., 1979).

The criteria of follicle size, numbers of granulosa cells, the incidence of pycnosis and mitosis among them, and morphology and maturational potential of the oocyte have been coupled with determinations of antral fluid hormone concentrations to describe properties of ovulating, healthy non-ovulating, and degenerating follicles. As one might expect, a combination of these criteria provides more discrimination than any of them taken singly.

An examination of results obtained from these studies will provide evidence of correlations of hormone concentrations with these morphologic markers of ovulation and degeneration at least and possibly suggest studies to determine whether these intrafollicular hormonal properties may be etiologically important in producing differences in the course of follicular maturation.

Morphologic Correlates of Hormones in Antral Fluid

The careful and well-documented study of follicles recovered late in the follicular phase reported by Bomsel-Helmreich et al. (1979) and Brailly et al. (1981) will be paraphrased in some detail. These studies included morphologic and hormonal characterization of follicles recovered at surgery done in the interval between day 8 of the last menses and spontaneous or hCG induced ovulations. Peripheral blood concentrations of FSH, LH, estradiol and progesterone were determined in specimens collected 1 and 2 days before, on the day of, and the day following surgery. At operation antral contents of the one or two largest follicles were aspirated, these follicles excised partially or totally and prepared for examination. Oocytes and granulosa cells were removed from the antral fluid which was then weighed and frozen. Thicknesses of the granulosa layers were measured, an estimate made of the number of granulosa cells, and determinations made of mitotic and pycnotic indices among these cells.

On the basis of measurements of sex steroid and gonadotropic hormone concentrations in peripheral blood, the late follicular phase was sub-divided into 3 parts: phase I: from the beginning of the estrogen surge to its peak; phase II: from estrogen peak to LH peak; phase III: from LH peak to ovulation. For comparisons, results were stratified according to these times. Healthy preovulatory follicles were larger than their nonovulatory counterparts, healthy or atretic, during each of these three preovulatory phases based on temporal relation to hormonal events. The granulosa was thicker in healthy than in atretic follicles, and the pycnotic index remained constant but on the average, an order of magnitude lower in healthy than in atretic follicles. The mitotic index, long known to decline just prior to ovulation, was higher in healthy than in atretic follicles which had a thinner granulosa.

Antral fluid hormone concentrations varied widely among follicles classified morphologically as either healthy or atretic. Levels of estradiol-17β, Δ_4-androstenedione (Δ_4), testosterone and dihydrotestosterone, high in ovulatory follicles during phases I to II, declined as ovulation approached in phase III, whereas progesterone levels rose and ratios of Δ_4/17-OH progesterone declined. These observations were tentatively interpreted to be consistent with a reduction in 17-20 lyase activity (Brailly et al., 1982).

In contrast, in follicles showing more advanced stages of atresia, estradiol and progesterone levels were remarkably reduced when compared with healthy follicles, destined to ovulate or not. Furthermore, levels of Δ_4, testosterone and dihydrotestosterone were higher both absolutely and relative to levels of estrogens and progestogens in atretic follicles. Thus, in follicles examined late in the follicular phase, higher levels of estradiol and progesterone were found in antral fluid from healthy than from atretic preovulatory follicles.

The comprehensive studies on antral fluid hormone composition done by McNatty and his colleagues since 1975 have been summarized recently (McNatty, 1982). These workers began with studies in which sex steroid and gonadotropic hormone levels were measured in antral fluid from ovarian follicles in surgical specimens removed during operations for diseases unrelated to the ovary. Time in cycle on the day of surgery was not controlled as critically as in the studies of Bomsel-Helmreich et al. (1979) and Brailly et al. (1981), and results were stratified on the basis of early, middle and late follicular and luteal phases. Antral follicles were removed, their diameters measured, antral fluid and oocytes removed by pipetting and granulosa cells recovered by scraping the interiors of incised follicles with a platinum loop. Initial oocyte morphology was examined using phase optics and apparently normal oocytes with intact germinal vesicles incubated for 48 hours and examined again. Antral fluid concentrations of estrogens, androgens and progestogens and of FSH, LH and prolactin (PRL) were determined. Granulosa cells were enumerated and in some instances their ability to synthesize estrogens and progestogens with and without additions of gonadotropins monitored for periods of up to 10 days in tissue culture. Results were analyzed initially on the basis of time in cycle when the tissue was removed, size of follicles and antral fluid hormone composition (McNatty et al., 1975). Subsequently correlations were made with numbers of granulosa cells and oocyte morphology as markers of healthy and atretic follicles (McNatty et al., 1979). To facilitate comparing effects of other variables on numbers of granulosa cells per antral follicle over the range of sizes from 2 mm to maturity, numbers were normalized in relation to the maximal numbers of granulosa cells recovered from a follicle of a given diameter. The values for individual follicles could be expressed as a percentage of this maximal number and follicles of the same diameter classified on this basis.

Results can be summarized as follows:

1. As follicular diameter increased from 1 mm to 25 mm, maximal numbers of granulosa cells increased from approximately 5×10^5 (500,000) to 5×10^7 (50,000,000). (Fig. 1)

2. Total antral fluid sex steroid hormone concentrations did not vary significantly with numbers of granulosa cells. However, follicles in each size class with the highest numbers of granulosa cells tended to have higher antral fluid levels of estradiol and progesterone. Since antral fluid androgen concentrations (Δ_4-androstenedione, testosterone and dihydrotestosterone) remained relatively constant, the ratio of androgens to estrogens increased as numbers of

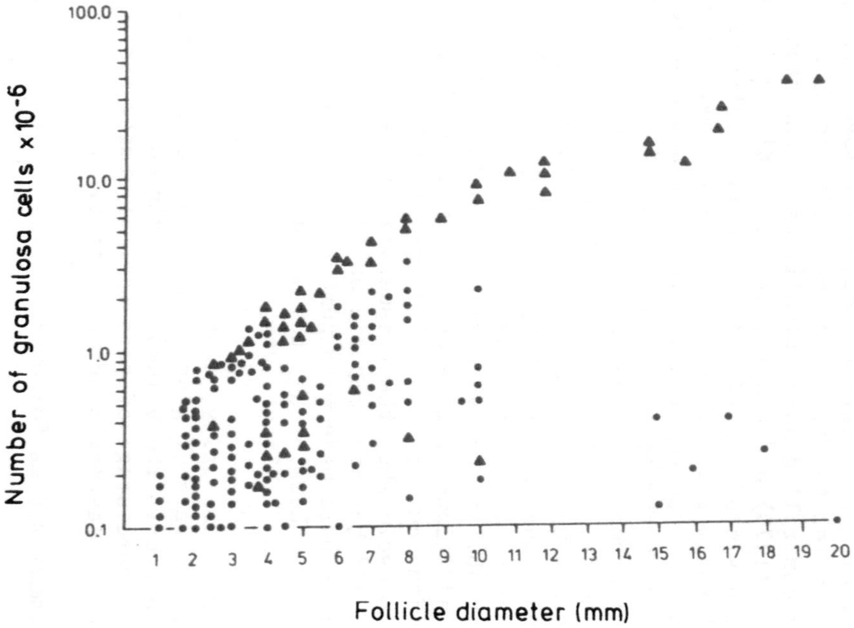

Fig. 1. Numbers of granulosa cells (ordinate) in follicles ranging from 1 to 20 mm in diameter (abscissa) in relation to antral fluid estradiol 17 beta concentrations shown by filled circles: less than 200 ng/ml, and by filled triangles: more than 200 ng/ml. Note that antral fluid from all follicles equal to or less than 2 mm in diameter contained less than 200 ng/ml. (Reproduced with kind permission of authors and publishers of "Follicular Maturation and Ovulation.")

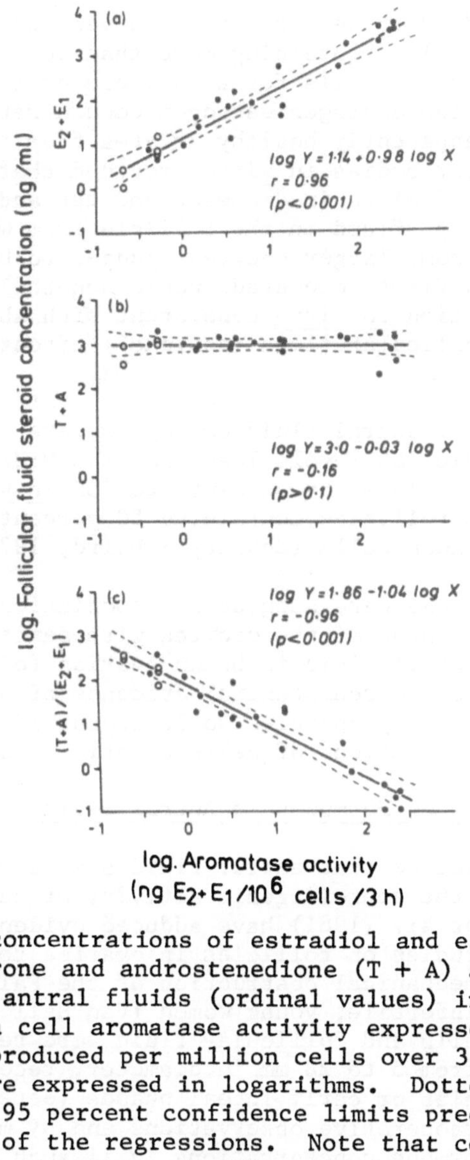

Fig. 2. Sums of concentrations of estradiol and estrone ($E_2 + E_1$), testosterone and androstenedione (T + A) and ratios of these in antral fluids (ordinal values) in relation to granulosa cell aromatase activity expressed as N6 of $E_2 + E_1$ produced per million cells over 3 hours. All values are expressed in logarithms. Dotted lines represent the 95 percent confidence limits predicted by analysis of the regressions. Note that concentrations T + A do not change significantly in relation to aromatase activities. (Reproduced with kind permission of the authors and publishers of the paper by Hillier et al., 1981.)

granulosa cells decreased (McNatty et al., 1979b). Moreover, granulosa cells from follicles judged to be healthy produced more estradiol *in vitro* than cells from follicles judged to be atretic.

3. Oocytes judged to be healthy at harvest were recovered more frequently from follicles containing more than 50 percent of the maximal numbers of granulosa cells for a follicle of its size, and thus from follicles with low androgen:estrogen concentration ratios. It is noteworthy that apparently healthy oocytes from follicles of all sizes would form polar bodies *in vitro* provided that the oocyte ranged from 109 to 127 micra in diameter and the androgen:estrogen ratio was low in antral fluid in the follicle from which these were removed. Moreover, some larger oocytes, judged to be showing signs of degeneration when first recovered, would nonetheless extrude polar bodies during incubation *in vitro* consistent with ability to recover when removed from follicular fluid (noxious?) effects (McNatty et al., 1979b).

4. Low levels of antral fluid estrogens were generally associated with antral fluid FSH levels less than 1.3 MIU/ml but aromatase activity could be stimulated by exposure to FSH *in vitro* in granulosa cells recovered from follicles containing 50 percent or more of the maximal numbers of these cells (McNatty & Baird, 1978).

Collectively, these data suggest an association of numbers of granulosa cells and status of the oocytes with sex steroid hormone composition of the antral fluid in human ovarian follicles. While not constituting proof, circumstantial evidence of a cause-effect relationship among these properties would accrue if it could be shown that these reflected functions of cells comprising a given follicle.

Functional Correlates of Hormones in Antral Fluid

What is the evidence that antral fluid sex steroid hormone concentrations reflect the steroidogenic activity of cells in that follicle? Hillier et al. (1981) have adduced evidence bearing on this problem from studies on follicles in ovaries removed during surgery to correct mechanical obstruction of the Fallopian tubes in otherwise healthy, infertile, young women (Van Hall and Trimbos, 1980). Granulosa cells and follicular fluid were removed from 39 follicles, ranging from 5 to 28 mm in diameter, recovered at surgery done in late follicular or early luteal phases (determined by menstrual history, intraoperative observations and by measurements of blood sex steroid hormone concentrations in 11 such women. Results of granulosa cell aromatase activity determinations were correlated with antral fluid levels of estradiol-17β (E_2) and of testosterone and androstenedione (the aromatase substrates). (Fig. 2). Levels of E_2 correlated positively and levels of aromatizable androgens negatively with granulosa cell aromatase activity. It is noteworthy that androgen levels remained relatively constant in all follicles so that substrate concentration does not appear to be rate-limiting in estrogen synthesis in preovulatory follicles. Hillier's observation that antral fluid androgen levels are similar irrespective of whether a follicle is judged to be preovulatory or degenerating has been confirmed often (Bomsel-Helmreich et al., 1979; Brailly et al., 1981; McNatty et al., 1983; Lobo et al., 1983). This is not surprising since McNatty et al. (1979) observed that thecal androgen synthesis *in vitro* was similar irrespective of the status of the follicle from which the tissue had been recovered. While basal activity was low, exposure to FSH *in vitro* enhanced aromatase activity in granulosa cells recovered from 6-8 mm follicles removed during the luteal phase.

These observations were interpreted to be consistent with the hypothesis that granulosa cell aromatase activity, "controlled by FSH, is a critical determinant of intrafollicular sex steroid content of developing preovulatory follicles and that the granulosa may be the main biosynthetic source of estrogen in the dominant follicle."

McNatty et al. (1983) have extended the studies of Hillier et al. (1981) on 215 follicles recovered from 16 ovaries, 4 removed in the late follicular phase and 12 removed in the luteal phase during surgical correction of Fallopian tube obstruction. Time in cycle was estimated from menstrual history, daily measurements of basal body temperatures and measurements of plasma estradiol and progesterone concentrations on 1-2 days before, on the day of and the day following surgery. Granulosa cells were enumerated and their ability to synthesize estradiol over a 3-hour period determined in the presence and absence of added testosterone. In addition, these cells were maintained in monolayer cultures for 48 hours and the medium assayed for estradiol and progesterone. Oocyte morphology was assessed before and after incubation for 48 hours. Granulosa cell numbers and oocyte viability were used to classify follicles as healthy or atretic. On the basis of these criteria, luteal phase ovaries contained from 0-4 healthy antral follicles and the largest of these was less than 5 mm in diameter.

No significant differences in the sum of androstenedione and testosterone concentrations were observed with respect to status of follicle (healthy or atretic) or time in the luteal phase (early, middle or late). Furthermore, there were no significant differences in antral fluid estradiol concentrations related to status of follicles in luteal phase ovaries. However, basal aromatase activity correlated with follicular diameter for granulosa cells from healthy but not from atretic follicles irrespective of time in cycle. As a measure of granulosa cell aromatase response to FSH, the amounts of estradiol produced when both FSH and testosterone were added to the incubation medium were compared to those produced when only testosterone was added. Responses in granulosa cells removed during middle and late luteal phases were greater than those of granulosa cells removed during late follicular and early luteal phases.

In summary then, antral fluid steroid hormone concentrations did not distinguish luteal phase follicles less than 5 mm in diameter judged to be healthy from similar follicles judged to be atretic on the basis of numbers of granulosa cells or the morphology and maturational potential of the oocyte in vitro. Antral fluid from all these small luteal phase follicles contained low levels of estradiol and high levels of aromatizable androgens, suggesting that the low basal granulosa cell aromatase activity was the limiting factor in the production of estradiol. The observation that exposure to FSH induced aromatase activity in these cells in vitro suggests that a relative deficiency of FSH, consistent with low luteal phase blood levels of the hormone, could account for the low antral fluid estradiol levels in vivo. These data are consistent with Hillier's conclusions quoted above and moreover, it is tempting to speculate that all follicles pass through a stage early in development during which androgen concentrations are high relative to estradiol concentrations in antral fluid so that access to FSH becomes an important determinant of the course of subsequent development.

Although no correlations were made with the status of the follicle, McNatty (1978) measured FSH, LH and prolactin in antral fluid specimens in which steroid hormone levels were also determined. Data were analyzed in relation to size of follicle (<8 mm or ≥ 8 mm) and to time in cycle (early, middle and late follicular and luteal phases). Results demonstrated higher levels of FSH in antral fluid from larger follicles sampled late in the follicular phase. Fluid from these same follicles contained more estrogen and progesterone than did smaller follicles containing less FSH. (Figs. 3 & 4)

These data provide evidence consistent with the concept that the peptide hormones are not uniformly distributed among all follicles sampled at either the same or at different times in the cycle. This is a condition which one would require to be fulfilled in validating the hypothesis that local (follicle by follicle) regulation of exposure to gonadotropins is a determinant of the course of follicular maturation. Moreover, these data are consistent with the concept that access to FSH is a major determinant of the fate of a developing follicle. The time over which a follicle can remain deficient in FSH and still produce a healthy oocyte and an adequate corpus luteum remains to be determined. Reference to Fig. 1 suggests that, judged on the basis of numbers of granulosa cells and antral fluid E_2 levels, this usually occurs when the follicle is less than 4 mm in diameter.

The demonstration that in vitro fertilization and embryo transfer could be used in treating infertility in women with incorrectable mechanical obstruction of the Fallopian tubes (Steptoe et al., 1980) provided an ethically acceptable basis for studying preovulatory follicles in women with normal ovarian function. Moreover, after it became apparent that transferring more than one embryo increased the likelihood of achieving pregnancies following in vitro fertilization

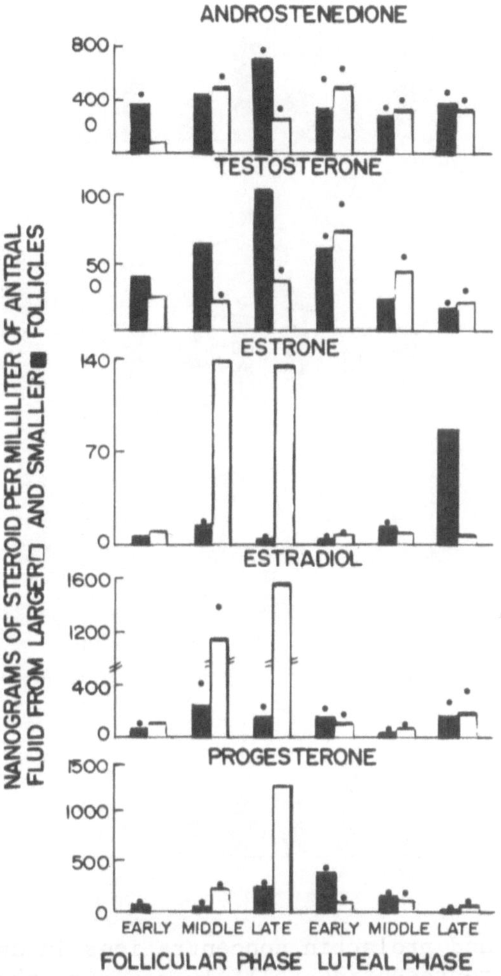

Fig. 3. Steroid hormone concentrations in antral fluid from follicles greater than (clear bars) or smaller than (solid bars) 8 mm in diameter sampled at time in cycle indicated on the abscissa. Note that estrogen and progestogen concentrations were elevated in larger follicles sampled during mid- and late follicular phase. (Reproduced with kind permission of W. B. Saunders Co. from Williams Textbook of Endocrinology.)

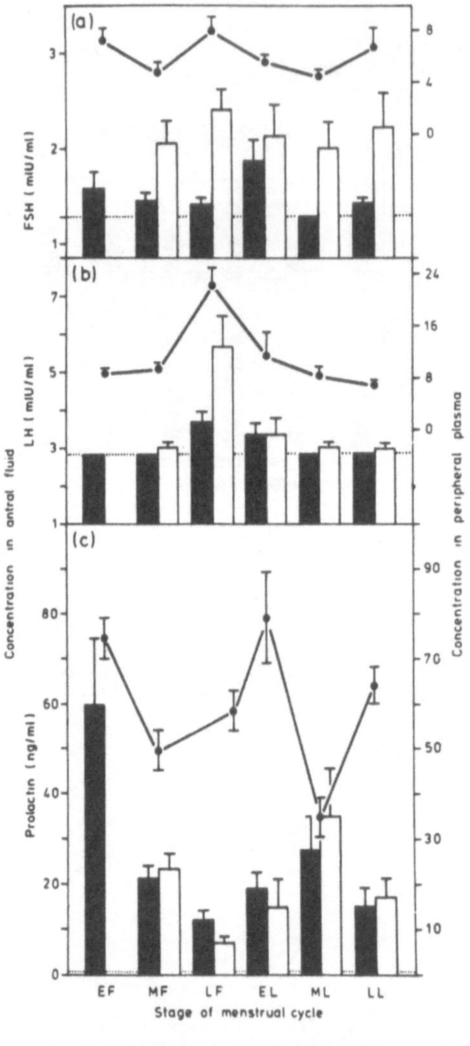

Fig. 4. FSH, LH and prolactin concentrations in antral fluid. Symbols representing follicle size are the same as those shown in Fig. 3. Note that FSH levels were higher in larger preovulatory follicles containing higher concentrations of estrogens and progestogens. (Reproduced from Williams Textbook of Endocrinology with kind permission of W. B. Saunders Co.)

(Spiers et al., 1983) (Lopata, 1983) aspiration of multiple follicles during the late follicular phase became common practice. These practices provided opportunities to add the ability to be fertilized and to undergo cleavage in vitro and in some instances the ability to implant and produce a normal infant at term to the criteria for determining the status of oocytes removed from preovulatory follicles. Furthermore, it provided access to some granulosa cells from the same follicle and opportunities, largely unexploited to date, to characterize these cells in relation to hormonal composition of antral fluid and status of the oocyte.

There are now at least two published accounts of attempts to make correlations of antral fluid steroid concentrations with these properties of the oocyte (Carson et al., 1982; Lobo et al., 1983). In the experience of Carson et al. (1982), oocytes which were fertilized and cleaved in vitro and implanted following transfer were removed from follicles with highest antral fluid E_2 concentrations in 10/156 instances. Lobo et al. (1983) correlated oocyte maturity and fertilizability in vitro with antral fluid levels of androgens, estradiol and progesterone in single follicular aspirates from 7 women ovulating spontaneously, in 23 follicles from 8 ovulatory women hyperstimulated with clomiphene, menopausal gonadotropins or both, and from 11 anovulatory women given the same ovulatory stimulants. Only follicular fluid progesterone and progesterone/estradiol ratios distinguished follicles producing mature from follicles producing immature or "atretic" oocytes. Moreover, the progesterone/estradiol ratio was significantly higher in follicles from ovulatory patients receiving stimulants and achieving pregnancies. Based upon follicular fluid androgen levels, no differences could be discerned, an observation consistent with many observations that antral fluid androgen levels are the same in healthy and atretic follicles. The timing of changes in antral fluid steroid hormone concentrations relative to the LH peak in the studies of Bomsel-Helmreich et al. (1979) and Brailly et al. (1981, 1982) suggests that rising progesterone and declining estradiol concentrations would be satisfactory markers of oocyte maturity. The observations of Lobo et al. (1983) are consistent with this view.

Caution must be exercised in interpreting results of such studies. While failures cannot be attributed to the quality of the oocyte in all cases, it seems probable that not every oocyte produced during spontaneous ovulatory cycles becomes fertilized, not all of those fertilized implant and not all of those implanting produce normal infants. Indeed, failure to establish pregnancies after embryo transfers has not been shown to be related to the quality of the oocyte in experience to date.

CONCLUSION

The data reviewed here are consistent with the hypothesis that acquiring the capacity to aromatize which depends in turn upon exposure to FSH is a determinant of concentrations and indirectly of the proportions of estrogens, androgens and progestogens (?) in antral fluid of individual human ovarian follicles. These, in turn, may be determinants of whether the follicle ovulates or degenerates (becomes atretic), by acting directly or indirectly on cells in the follicle complex. It remains to be determined how gonadotropins and sex steroid hormones modulate the production of other substances which act locally to coordinate cell-cell interactions required for producing a mature oocyte and optimizing for its fertilization, implantation, and gestation. The mystery persists and its denouement "in molecular terms" awaits the efforts of persons with Lindner's ability to phrase the questions and support the necessary experiments.

REFERENCES

Aedo, A. R., Pedersen, P. H., Pedersen, S. C. and Diczfalusy, E., 1980, Ovarian steroid secretion in normally menstruating women, I. Contribution of the developing follicle, Acta Endocrinol. (KBH), 95:212.

Baird, D. T. and Fraser, I. S., 1975, Concentrations of estrone and estradiol in follicular fluid and ovarian venous blood in women, Clin. Endocrinol., 4:259.

Bomsel-Helmreich, O., Gougeon, A., Thebault, A., Saltarelli, D., Milgrom, E., Frydman, R., and Papiernik, E., 1979, Healthy and atretic human follicles in the preovulatory phase: Differences in evolution of follicular morphology and steroid content of follicular fluid, J. Clin. Endocrinol. Metab., 48:686.

Brailly, S., Gougeon, A., Milgrom, E., Bomsel-Helmreich, O., and Papiernik, E., 1981, Androgens and progestins in the human ovarian follicle: Differences in evolution of preovulatory, healthy nonovulatory and atretic follicles, J. Clin. Endocrinol. Metab., 53:128.

Brailly, S., Gougeon, A., Milgrom, E., Bomsel-Helmreich, O., and Papiernik, E., Importance of changes in the transformation of progestin into androgen during preovulatory development and atresia of human follicles, in: "Follicular Maturation and Ovulation," R. Rolland, E. V. Van Hall, S. G. Hillier, K. P. McNatty and J. Schoemaker, eds., Excerpta Medica, Amsterdam, Oxford-Princeton (1982).

Byskov, A. G., Follicular atresia, in: "The Vertebrate Ovary," R. E. Jones, ed., Plenum Press, New York and London (1978).

Carson, R. S., Trounson, A. O., and Findlay, J. K., 1982, Successful fertilization of human oocytes in vitro: Concentration of estradiol-17 beta, progesterone and androstenedione in the antral fluid of donor follicles, J. Clin. Endocrinol. Metab., 55:798.

di Zerega, G. S. and Hodgen, G. D., 1981, Folliculogenesis in the primate ovarian cycle, Endo. Rev., 2:26.

Fleming, R. and Coutts, J. R. T., Oestrogen levels during follicular maturation in women, in: "Functional Morphology of the Human Ovary," J. R. T. Coutts, ed., University Park Press, Baltimore (1981).

Goodman, A. L., Nixon, W. E., Johnson, D. K., and Hodgen, G. D., 1977, Regulation of folliculogenesis in the cycling rhesus monkey: Selection of the dominant follicle, Endocrinology, 100:155.

Hillier, S. G., Van den Boogaard, A. M. J., Reichers, L. E., Jr., Van Hall, G. V., 1981, Control of preovulatory follicular estrogen biosynthesis in the human ovary, J. Clin. Endocrinol. Metab., 52:847.

Hirshfield, A. N., Midgley, A. R., Jr., 1978, Morphometric analysis of follicular development in the rat, Biol. Reprod., 19:597.

Jones, H. W., Seegar-Jones, G., Andrews, M. C., Acosta, A., Bundren, C., Garcia, J., Sandow, B., Veeck, L., Wilkes, C., Witmyer, J., Wortham, J. E., Wright, G., 1982, The program for in vitro fertilization at Norfolk, Fertil. Steril., 38:14.

Koering, M. J., 1969, Cyclic changes in ovarian morphology during the menstrual cycle in Macaca mulatta, Am. J. Anat., 126:73.

Lindner, H. R., Amsterdam, A., Salomon, Y., Tsafriri, A., Nimrod, A., Lamprecht, S. A., Zor, U., and Koch, Y., 1977, Intraovarian factors in ovulation: Determinants of follicular response to gonadotropins, J. Reprod. Fertil., 51:215.

Lopata, A., 1983, Concepts in human in vitro fertilization and embryo transfer, Fertil. Steril., 40:289.

McNatty, K. P., Ovarian follicular development from the onset of luteal regression in humans and sheep, in: "Follicular Maturation and Ovulation," R. Rolland, E. V. Van Hall, S. G. Hillier, K. P. McNatty, and J. Schoemaker, eds., Excerpta Medica, Amsterdam, Oxford-Princeton (1982).

McNatty, K. P. and Baird, D. T., 1978, Relationship between follicle-stimulating hormone, androstenedione and estradiol in human follicular fluid, J. Endocrinol., 76:527.

McNatty, K. P., Hillier, S. G., Van den Boogaard, A. M. J., Trimbos-Kemper, T. C. M., Reichert, L. E., Jr., and Van Hall, E. V., 1983, Follicular development during the luteal phase of the human menstrual cycle, J. Clin. Endocrinol. Metab., 52:1022.

McNatty, K. P., Hunter, W. M., McNeilly, A. S., and Sawers, R. S., 1975, Changes in the concentration of pituitary and steroid hormones in the follicular fluid of human Graafian follicles throughout the menstrual cycle, J. Endocrinol., 64:555.

McNatty, K. P., Makris, A., De Grazia, C., Osathanondh, R., and Ryan, K. J., 1979a, The production of progesterone, androgens, and estrogens by granulosa cells, thecal tissue, and stromal tissue from human ovaries in vitro. J. Clin. Endocrinol. Metab., 49:687.

McNatty, K. P., Smith, D. M., Makris, A., Osathanondh, R. and Ryan, K. J., 1979b, The microenvironment of the human antral follicle: Interrelationships among the steroid levels in antral fluid, the population of granulosa cells and the status of the oocyte in vivo and in vitro, J. Clin. Endocrinol. Metab., 49:851.

Moor, R. M., Hay, M. F., Dott, H. M. and Cran, D. G., 1978, Macroscopic identification and steroidogenic function of atretic follicles in sheep, J. Endocrinol., 77:309.

Nilsson, L., Wikland, M., and Hamberger, L., 1982, Recruitment of an ovulatory follicle in the human following follicle-ectomy and luteectomy, Fertil. Steril., 37:30.

Peters, H. and McNatty, K. P., "The Ovary," University of California Press, Berkeley and Los Angeles (1980).

Quigley, M. M., Maklad, N. F., and Wolf, D. P., 1983, Comparison of two clomiphene citrate dosage regimens for follicular recruitment in an in vitro fertilization program, Fertil. Steril., 40:178.

Spiers, A. L., Lopata, A., Gronow, M. J., Kellow, G. N., Johnston, W. I. H., 1983, Analysis of the benefits and risks of multiple embryo transfer, Fertil. Steril., 39:468.

Steptoe, P. C., Edwards, R. G., and Purdy, J. M., 1980, Clinical aspects of pregnancies established with cleaving embryos grown in vitro, Br. J. Obstet. Gynecol. 87:757.

Van Hall, E. V., Trimbos-Kemper, T. P. M., The surgical management of tubal infertility, in: "Gynecology and Obstetrics, Proceedings of the IXth World Congress of Obstetrics and Gynecology," S. Sakamoto, S. Tojo, T. Nakayama, eds., Excerpta Medica, Amsterdam (1980).

Webb, R. and England, B. G., 1982, Identification of the ovulatory follicle in the ewe: Associated changes in follicular size, thecal and granulosa cell luteinizing hormone receptors, antral fluid steroids, and circulating hormones during the preovulatory period, Endocrinol., 110:873.

REGULATION OF OOCYTE MATURATION

Nava Dekel

The Weizmann Institute of Science
Department of Hormone Research
Rehovot 76100, Israel

Meiotic maturation in the mammalian oocyte is initiated during fetal life. It proceeds through the prophase of the first meiotic division and is arrested at the diplotene stage. The arrest of meiosis is maintained until shortly before ovulation. By this time meiosis is reinitiated and oocyte maturation is resumed. Reinitiation of meiosis in the oocyte is morphologically indicated by the disappearance of the nuclear structure known as the germinal vesicle (germinal vesicle breakdown - GVB).

When meiotically arrested oocytes are removed from the antral follicles they resume maturation spontaneously (Pincus and Enzmann, 1935; Edwards, 1965). However, either in vivo or in vitro, in explanted intact follicles, maturation of the oocytes will not take place unless exposure to gonadotropins had occurred (Ayalon et al., 1972; Tsafriri, 1978; Dekel et al., 1979). These observations led to the generally held conclusion that the antral follicle inhibits oocyte maturation and that this inhibition is reversed as a result of gonadotropins action. This idea gained support later when inhibition of maturation by follicular components cocultured with the isolated oocyte has been demonstrated (Foote and Thibault, 1969; Tsafriri et al., 1975).

Although it is clearly evident that resumption of meiosis in the follicular oocyte is under the control of gonadotropins, the mechanism responsible for regulation of oocyte maturation is one of the major puzzles of reproductive physiology. In the present review, the studies conducted in an attempt to resolve this puzzle, in ours and other laboratories, will be presented. Combining the available information a possible mechanistic model for the hormonal regulation of oocyte maturation will be presented.

The overall mechanism of regulation of oocyte maturation can be divided into two phases. Maintenance of meiotic arrest should be the result of the processes included under the first phase of this regulatory mechanism. Secondly, the whole cascade of events generated following the LH surge should lead to induction of meiosis resumption. The present review will dissociate between these two phases and each one of them will be separately discussed.

Maintenance of meiotic arrest

As stated in the introduction, meiosis is resumed spontaneously in oocytes removed from their follicles and placed in culture. It was shortly after Cho et al. (1974) had demonstrated that the spontaneous maturation *in vitro* of the mouse oocyte is blocked by dibutyryl cAMP that the idea that this cyclic nucleotide could serve as the intrafollicular inhibitor of oocyte maturation has initially been raised (Lindner et al., 1974; Anderson and Albertini, 1976; Dekel and Beers, 1978). These findings in the mouse were later extended to the rat and the complete dose and time dependency of the inhibitory effect of either dibutyryl cAMP or the cyclic nucleotide phosphodiesterase inhibitor, methylisobutylxanthine (MIX), has been established (Magnusson and Hillensjo, 1977; Dekel and Beers, 1978). The fact that not only the spontaneous maturation but also LH-induced meiosis resumption in follicle-enclosed oocytes was found to be inhibited by both dibutyryl cAMP and MIX (Hillensjo et al., 1978; Dekel et al., 1981) provided support to the idea that cAMP could be physiologically involved in the maintenance of meiotic arrest.

The effect on oocyte maturation obtained by administration of either dibutyryl cAMP or MIX could be considered pharmacological until very recently when two reports, both showing a clear correlation between cAMP levels within the oocyte and its stage of development have been published. Schultz et al. (1983) showed that the levels of cAMP in mouse oocytes significantly decrease shortly before meiosis resumption both *in vivo* and *in vitro*, and that this decrease is not observed in oocytes inhibited from resuming meiosis by MIX. Similarly, Vivarelli et al. (1983) have also demonstrated that spontaneous oocyte maturation is associated with a drop in cAMP content within the oocyte, while either maintenance or elevation of cAMP levels results in substantial delay in meiosis resumption.

It should be mentioned, in this respect, that regulation of oocyte maturation by modulation of cAMP levels within the oocyte is not unique to mammals. In the amphibia, it has been well established that prophase arrest of the oocyte is maintained by cAMP and that meiosis resumption is correlated with a decrease in cAMP levels (Maller and Krebs, 1980).

If cAMP is involved in meiotic arrest in vivo, incubation of the oocyte under conditions which stimulate adenylate cyclase should result in inhibition of the spontaneous maturation. Indeed, a dose-dependent inhibition of the spontaneous maturation is obtained when isolated rat cumulus-oocyte complexes are incubated in the presence of choleratoxin (CT; Dekel and Beers, 1980). However, the inhibitory effect of CT on oocyte maturation can only be demonstrated in the presence of the cumulus cells while maturation of cumulus-free oocytes is not affected by this agent. This CT experiment not only provided supportive evidence for the role of cAMP in the maintenance of meiotic arrest, but also raised some ideas concerning the origin of the inhibitory signal. The fact that CT could affect the oocyte only in the presence of the cumulus cells clearly suggests that the source of the inhibitory cAMP is not the oocyte but rather the cells of the cumulus oophorus.

As the oocyte seems to respond to cAMP generated by the cumulus cells, a mechanism responsible for transmission of the nucleotide should be involved in the regulation of oocyte maturation. The possibility that the oocyte is affected by cAMP secreted into the follicular fluid must be eliminated since, as apposed to cAMP derivatives, non-derivitized cAMP cannot penetrate cell membranes failing therefore to elicit an inhibitory action on maturation of isolated oocytes (Magnusson and Hillensjo, 1977; Dekel and Beers, 1978). Alternatively, cAMP can be transmitted from the cumulus cells to the oocyte via intercellular communication.

Communication between the oocyte and the cumulus cells has been suggested since 1890 (Paladino) when the projections of the cumulus cells, which traverse the zona pellucida and contact the oocyte surface, were initially observed. The provision of tropic, metabolic or regulatory factors by the cumulus cells to the developing oocyte was demonstrated later (Biggers, 1972; Donahue, 1972; Eppig, 1977). Moreover, the presence of gap junctions on the regions of contact between the cumulus cells and the oocyte was observed (Amsterdam et al., 1976; Anderson and Albertini, 1976; Gilula et al., 1978), and transfer of ions and small molecules has been demonstrated (Gilula et al., 1978; Moor et al., 1980; Eppig, 1982).

Transmission of cAMP between communicating cells has already been suggested by Lawrence et al. (1978). These investigators demonstrated that exposure of coupled cocultures to a hormone specific for one cell type causes the heterologous cells to respond. They suggested that this cross stimulation results from intercellular communication of a common mediator for both cell types, which is probably cAMP.

In a series of experiments recently performed in our laboratory, we have demonstrated again that an inhibitory signal, apparently cAMP, generated by the cumulus cells, is transmitted to the oocyte to inhibit meiosis resumption. For these experiments the diterpene forskolin, which has recently been shown to act as a potent activator of adenylate cyclase (Seaman and Daly, 1981) has been used. Forskolin not only differs from CT by being a more potent activator of the cyclase system. As apposed to CT stimulation, which is characterized by a lag period of at least 60 min, accumulation of cAMP in response to forskolin is immediate. The rapid action of forskolin is of great importance when inhibition of the spontaneous maturation is studied, since it has been demonstrated that at 45 min after isolation into inhibitor-free medium, the oocytes are irreversibly committed to undergo maturation (Dekel and Beers, 1980). Thus, the failure of CT to maintain meiotic arrest in cumulus-free oocytes could possibly be due to its inability to cause generation of sufficient cAMP to inhibit maturation during the first hour after isolation from the follicle. In fact, even in cumulus-enclosed oocytes the inclusion of MIX (in low concentrations) was necessary to observe the CT-dependent arrest.

Using forskolin we could confirm that in the absence of the cumulus cells rat oocytes fail to respond to activation of the cyclase system by maintaining meiosis arrest while cumulus-enclosed oocytes are fully responsive (Fig. 1). The inhibitory action of forskolin on cumulus-enclosed oocytes is dose-dependent (Dekel et al., 1983) and can be potentiated by inhibition of cAMP degradation (Fig. 2).

Even though indirect, our and other studies mentioned seem to provide strong indications that cAMP could be communicated in the cumulus-oocyte complex. However, very recently Schultz et al. (1983) reported that they failed to demonstrate transfer of cAMP from the cumulus cells to the oocyte. These investigators did get cumulus cell-dependent inhibition of oocyte maturation by cAMP modulators. They also demonstrated that the inhibitory effect correlates with increase in cAMP levels in the cumulus-oocyte complex. However, no difference in cAMP levels was found in oocytes derived from either stimulated or unstimulated complexes. These investigators suggest therefore that the inhibitory effect is directly mediated by an agent other than cAMP, although cAMP generation is required for its action.

The presence of a cAMP-dependent inhibitory mediator which is not cAMP itself can not be excluded by our results obtained with either CT or forskolin. However, before the possibility that cAMP is the inhibitory signal is ruled out, it should be mentioned that in the amphibia it is no more than 10% difference in the content of cAMP within the oocyte which is responsible for alternation between arrest and resumption of meiosis (Schorderet-Slatkine and Baulieu, 1982). As it is possible that the major fraction of cAMP produced by the cumulus cells is protein bound, only a small number of free molecules of the nucleotide can freely pass the gap junctions.

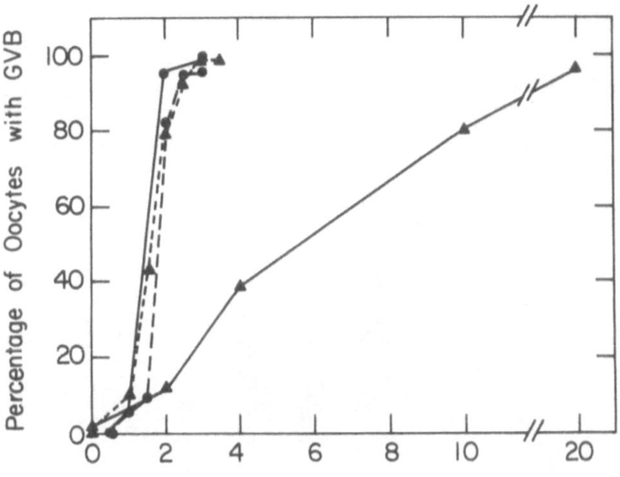

Fig. 1: Effect of forskolin on the spontaneous maturation of isolated oocytes in vitro. Either cumulus-enclosed (full lines) or cumulus-free (broken lines) oocytes were isolated and incubated in the presence (▲) or absence (●) of 100 μM of forskolin. The presence of GV in the oocytes was analyzed at the indicated time-points by Nomarski Interference Contrast microscopy.

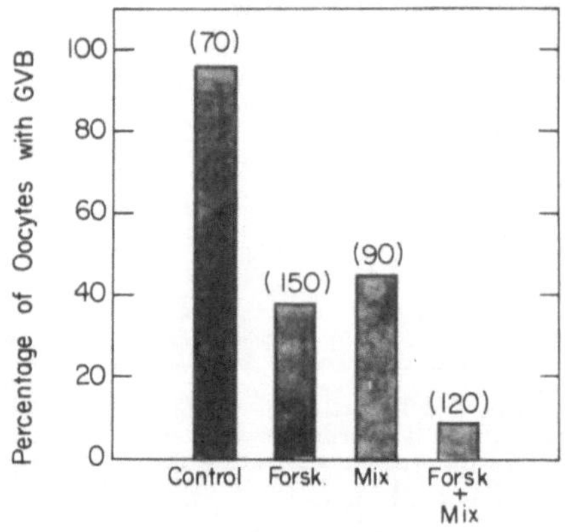

Fig. 2: Potentiation of forskolin-induced inhibition of the spontaneous maturation of cumulus-enclosed oocytes by MIX. Isolated cumulus-enclosed oocytes were incubated in the absence or presence of either forskolin (100 μM), MIX (10 μM) or a combination of these agents. After 2 h of incubation oocytes were examined for the presence of GV by Nomarski Interference Contrast microscopy.

Like in the amphibian oocyte, these low amounts of cAMP available for transfer can maintain meiotic arrest being undetectable by the available techniques for cAMP determination.

As administration of high cAMP levels to the oocyte has been shown to inhibit maturation (Cho et al., 1974), the inability of both cyclase activators to affect the naked oocyte may indicate that the rat oolemma lacks the adenylate cyclase system. The definitive answer to this intriguing possibility can be provided only by direct biochemical analyses. Our studies, however, indicate that in response to both CT and forskolin rat oocytes cannot generate sufficient levels of cAMP required for maintenance of meiotic arrest.

Induction of oocyte maturation

As mentioned in the introduction meiosis resumption in the mammalian oocyte is triggered by LH. The mechanism by which LH induces oocyte maturation is not yet elucidated. As a predominant effect of LH is to elevate cAMP levels in the ovary the first question to be addressed is whether LH-induced oocyte maturation is a cAMP-mediated response. Follicle-enclosed oocytes were used to study the mechanism of maturation induction since isolated oocytes resume meiosis spontaneously. Forskolin, which triggers the cAMP generating system thus mimics hormone action, was considered the most suitable agent for this investigation. We found that forskolin can mimic the effect of LH on the ovarian follicle stimulating both cAMP accumulation and oocyte maturation (Dekel and Sherizly, 1983). Elevation of cAMP levels which could be detected as soon as 5 min after exposure to forskolin was the earliest event demonstrated. A minimal exposure of 30 min was sufficient to induce meiosis resumption in 50% of the oocytes while the actual response as indicated by GVB in the oocytes was obtained at 90 min of culture (Fig. 3). This sequence of events suggests that the induction of oocyte maturation is probably coupled to the elevation of follicular cAMP levels. The significant potentiation of the effect of forskolin on the oocytes, obtained by exposure of the follicles to the cyclic nucleotide phosphodiesterase inhibitor MIX, strongly supports this conclusion.

Taken together these last findings with the studies described earlier, an apparent paradox seems to be present - i.e. if LH-induced oocyte maturation is a cAMP-mediated response, since cAMP inhibits oocyte maturation, what mechanism allows the oocyte to mature under the influence of gonadotropins?

Before any line of investigation is undertaken to resolve this puzzle, it should be taken into consideration that any suggested mechanism for LH-induced oocyte maturation should result in a drop in cAMP levels in the oocyte (Schultz et al., 1983; Vivarelli et al., 1983).

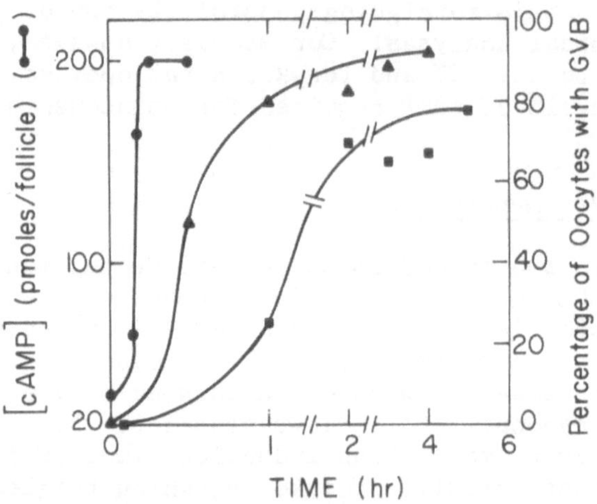

Fig. 3: Effect of forskolin on cAMP accumulation and oocyte maturation in rat follicles. Cyclic AMP determinations (●-●) were performed by the competitive protein binding assay on isolated follicles incubated for the indicated times in the presence of 100 μM forskolin. To establish the minimal effective exposure-time for forskolin-induced GVB in follicle-enclosed oocytes (▲-▲) isolated follicles were exposed to 10 μM of forskolin, rinsed at the indicated times and reincubated in forskolin-free-medium for 20 h. Cumulus-oocyte complexes were recovered and oocytes examined for the presence of GV by Nomarski Interference Contrast microscopy. The time-course of forskolin-induced GVB in follicle-enclosed oocytes (■-■) was established following incubation of the isolated follicles in the presence of 10 μM forskolin. At the indicated times cumulus oocyte complexes were recovered and the presence of GV in the oocyte was examined.

If, as appears from the first part of this review, maintenance of meiotic arrest is dependent upon communication of an inhibitory signal, then uncoupling between the oocyte and the cumulus cells could provide the conditions for the oocyte to resume meiosis. This hypothesis appeared very intriguing since it seems to correspond with the actual events in vivo. Gilula et al. (1978) had demonstrated that following hCG administration the maturing oocyte no longer communicates with the surrounding cumulus cells. In addition, we have shown that follicle-enclosed oocytes induced to mature in vitro by LH, are uncoupled from the cumulus cells and that uncoupling in this system is also induced by dibutyryl cAMP and MIX (Dekel et al., 1981).

Based on the fact that LH terminates communication in the cumulus-oocyte complex and that this action is mimicked by cAMP, we proposed the following hypothesis for LH-induced oocyte maturation. Cyclic AMP generated by the follicular cells, but not by the oocyte, is transferred via junctional communications with the cumulus cells to the oocyte to keep it meiotically arrested. As a result of LH action, which terminates communication in the cumulus-oocyte complex, the transfer of cAMP is stopped, inhibition is relieved and the oocyte is allowed to resume meiosis.

Although it is clearly evident that both meiosis resumption and breakdown of communication are subsequent to the preovulatory LH surge, some difficulties regarding the temporal sequence of these two events appeared to be present. If termination of communication is the signal for oocyte maturation it should precede meiosis resumption. However, our findings (Dekel et al., 1981), and those of others (Moor et al., 1980; Eppig, 1982), seem to suggest that reinitiation of meiosis is the earlier event detected and that it is followed by communication breakdown. The discrepency in time obtained in our study (Dekel et al., 1981), in which electrical coupling was used to analyze communication, could be easily explained since this technique actually measures the absolute lack of detectable channels. But, as both Moor et al. (1980) and Eppig (1981) seemed to measure the alternations in the actual flow prior to complete uncoupling their findings appeared to undermine our suggested theory.

Both Moor et al. (1980) and Eppig (1981) studies are based on the assumption that the amount of either choline or uridine transferred to cumulus-enclosed oocytes is a function of the extent of cell coupling since cumulus-free oocytes cannot incorporate these markers. However, both these investigators ignored the possibility that besides its effect on the extent of communication, hormonal treatment can also influence the uptake of these markers by the cumulus cells. Uptake variations of the marker in the donor (cumulus) cells would probably be followed by changes in its transfer to the recipient cell (the oocyte) not necessarily reflecting uncoupling changes. Testing this possibility Salustri and Siracusa (1983) recently demonstrated that gonadotropin treatment does stimulate uridine uptake by the cumulus cells. These investigators therefore expressed coupling as the amount of uridine transferred to cumulus-enclosed oocytes as a fraction of total cumulus uptake. Their results demonstrate a good temporal correlation between the resumption of meiosis and the onset of uncoupling. The possibility that oocyte maturation is the outcome of breakdown of communication is now open for further investigations.

CONCLUSIONS

Based on the information provided by the studies described in the present review the following conclusions can be withdrawn:

1. Cyclic AMP within the oocyte acts to physiologically maintain meiotic arrest. Alternatively, maturation is associated with a drop in cAMP levels within the oocyte.

2. The inhibitory signal for oocyte maturation is provided by the cumulus cells.

3. LH-induced oocyte maturation is a cAMP-mediated response.

4. The temporal correlation between reinitiation of meiosis and onset of uncoupling suggests that termination of communication can be the signal for oocyte maturation.

REFERENCES

Amsterdam, A., Josephs, R., Lieberman, M.E., and Lindner, H.R., 1976, Organization of intermembrane particles in freeze-cleaved gap junctions of rat Graafian follicles: Optical diffraction analysis. J. Cell Sci., 21:93-105.

Anderson, E., and Albertini, D.F., 1976, Gap junctions between the oocyte and the companion follicle cells in the mammalian ovary. J. Cell Biol., 71:680-686.

Ayalon, D., Tsafriri, A., Lindner, H.R., Cordova, R., and Harell, A., 1972, Serum gonadotrophin levels in pro-estrous rats in relation to the resumption of meiosis by the oocytes. J. Reprod. Fert. 31:51-58.

Biggers, J.D., 1972, Metabolism of the oocyte. in: "Oogenesis", J.D. Biggers and A.W. Schuetz, eds., University Park Press, Baltimore, pp. 241-251.

Cho, W.K., Stern, S., and Biggers, J.D., 1974, Inhibitory effect of dibutyryl cAMP on mouse oocyte maturation in vitro. Exp. Zool., 187:383-386.

Dekel, N., and Beers, W.H., 1978, Rat ooyte maturation in vitro: Relief of cyclic AMP inhibition by gonadotropins. Proc. Natl. Acad. Sci. USA 75:4369-4373.

Dekel, N., Hillensjö, T., and Kraicer, P.F., 1979, Maturational effects of gonadotropins on the cumulus-oocyte complex of the rat. Biol. Reprod., 20:191-197.

Dekel, N., and Beers, W.H., 1980, Development of the rat oocyte in vitro: Inhibition and induction of maturation in presence or absence of the cumulus oophorus. Devel. Biol., 75:247-254.

Dekel, N., Lawrence, T.S., Gilula, N.B., and Beers, W.H., 1981, Modulation of cell-to-cell communication in the cumulus-oocyte complex and the regulation of oocyte maturation by LH. Devel. Biol., 86:356-362.

Dekel, N., and Sherizly, I., 1983, Induction of maturation in rat follicle-enclosed oocytes by forskolin. FEBS Lett., 151:153-155.

Dekel, N., Aberdam, E. and Sherizly, I., 1983, Spontaneous maturation in vitro of cumulus-enclosed rat oocyte is inhibited by forskolin. Biol. Reprod. Vol. 28, Suppl. 1, p. 86.

Donahue, R.P., 1972, The relation of oocyte maturation to ovulation in mammals. in: "Oogenesis", J.D. Biggers and A.W. Schuetz, eds., University Park Press, Baltimore, Butterworths, London, pp. 413-438.

Edwards, R.G., 1965, Maturation in vitro of mouse, sheep, cow, pig, rhesus monkey and human ovarian oocytes. Nature, 208:349-351.

Eppig, J.J., 1977, Mouse oocyte development in vitro with various culture systems. Devel. Biol., 60:371-388.

Eppig, J.J., 1982, The relationship between cumulus cell-oocyte coupling, oocyte meiotic maturation, and cumulus expansion. Devel. Biol., 89:268-272.

Foote, W.D., and Thibault, C., 1969, Recherches expérimentales sur la maturation in vitro des ovocytes de truie et de veau. Ann. Biol. Anim. Biochem. Biophys., 9:329-349.

Gilula, N.B., Epstein, M.C., and Beers, W.H., 1978, Cell-to-cell communication and ovulation. A study of the cumulus-oocyte complex. J. Cell Biol., 78:58-75.

Hillensjö, T., Ekholm, C. and Ahrén, K., 1978, Role of cAMP in oocyte maturation and glycolysis in the preovulatory rat follicle. Acta Endocr. Copenh. 87:377-388.

Lawrence, T.S., Beers, W.H., and Gilula, N.B., 1978, Transmission of hormonal stimulation by cell-to-cell communication. Nature, 272:501-506.

Lindner, H.R., Tsafriri, A., Lieberman, M.E., Zor, U., Koch, Y., Bauminger, S., and Barnea, A., 1974, Gonadotrophin action on cultured Graafian follicles: induction of maturation division of the mammalian oocyte and differentiation of the luteal cell. Recent Prog. Horm. Res. 30:79-138.

Magnusson, C. and Hillensjö, T., 1977, Inhibition of maturation and metabolism in rat oocytes by cyclic AMP. J. Ex. Zool., 201:139-147.

Maller, J.L., and Krebs, E.G., 1980, Regulation of oocyte maturation. Cur. Top. Cell Regul., 16:271-311.

Moor, R.M., Smith, M.W., and Dawson, R.M.C., 1980, Measurement of intercellular coupling between oocytes and cumulus cells using intracellular markers. Exp. Cell Res., 126:15-29.

Paladino, G., 1890, Il ponte intercellulare tra l'uovo ovarico e la cellula follicolare e la formazion della zona pellucida. Anat. Anz., 15:254-259.

Pincus, G., and Enzmann, E.V., 1935, The comparative behaviour of mammalian eggs in vivo and in vitro. I. The activation of ovarian eggs. J. Exp. Med. 62:665-675.

Salustri, A., and Siracusa, G., 1983, Metabolic coupling, cumulus expansion and meoitic resumption in mouse cumuli oophori cultured in vitro in presence of FSH or dcAMP, or stimulated in vivo by hCG. J. Reprod. Fert., 68:335-341.

Schorderet-Slatkine, S., and Baulieu, E.E., 1982, Forskolin increases cAMP and inhibits progesterone induced meiosis reinitiation in xenopus laevis oocytes. Endocrinology, 111:1385-1387.

Schultz, R.M., Montgomery, R.R., Ward-Bailey, P.F., and Eppig, J.J., 1983, Regulation of oocyte maturation in the mouse: Possible roles of intercellular communication, cAMP and testosterone. Devel. Biol., 95:294-304.

Seamon, K. and Daly, W.J., 1981, Forskolin: A unique diterpene activator of cyclic AMP-generating systems. J. Cyc. Nucl. Res. 7:201-224.

Tsafriri, A. and Channing, C.P., 1975, An inhibitory influence of granulosa cells and follicular fluid upon porcine oocyte meiosis in vitro. Endocrinology 96:922-927.

Tsafriri, A., 1978, Oocyte maturation in mammals. in: "The Vertebrate Ovary", pp. 409-442, R.E. Jones, ed., Plenum Press, N.Y.

Vivarelli, E., Conti, M., De Felici, M. and Siracusa, G., 1983, Meiotic resumption and intracellular cAMP levels in mouse oocytes treated with compounds which act on cAMP metabolism. Cell Differentiation 12:271-276.

MECHANISMS INVOLVED IN FOLLICULAR RUPTURE IN THE RAT

Reuven Reich and Alex Tsafriri

Department of Hormone Research
The Weizmann Institute of Science
Rehovot, 76100, Israel

INTRODUCTION

Ovulation in mammals can be subdivided into at least three functional components: ovum maturation, luteinization of granulosa cells and follicular rupture. Although all three processes are initiated by the preovulatory surge of LH, it seems that different mechanisms mediate LH action on these processes.

The process of follicular rupture, frequently related to as "ovulation", has been the subject of much interest recently. Several reviews have been published on this aspect of ovarian function (Rondell, 1970a, 1974; Lipner, 1973; Espey, 1978, 1980; Marsh and LeMaire, 1974; Parr, 1975; Wallach et al., 1980). An increase in intrafollicular pressure to bursting point has for long been assumed to be the cause of follicular rupture. The increased pressure has been ascribed to hyperemia (Pearson, 1944), contraction of smooth muscle and the secretion of osmotically active substances and proteoglycans into the follicular antrum (Zachariae and Jensen, 1958). This hypothesis was accepted until the 1960's when it was shown by direct measurements that the intrafollicular pressure does not increase before ovulation (Blandau and Rumery, 1963; Espey and Lipner, 1963; Rondell, 1964). Recently, the demonstration of proteolytic activities in the follicle led to the concept of enzymatic weakening of the follicular wall. Thus, the observed increase in follicular volume, which is not accompanied by increase in intrafollicular pressure, is related to the decrease in the tensile strength of follicular wall resulting from proteolytic activity.

Microscopical examination of the wall of ovulatory follicles revealed dissolution of the connective tissue matrix and of collagen fibers in the tunica albuginea and theca externa. Hence, it seems likely that enzymatic digestion is involved in follicular rupture. Many enzymes have been identified in follicular tissues or fluid including proteolytic enzymes (Reichert, 1962; Espey and Rondell, 1967), hyaluronidase (Zachariae and Jensen, 1958), acid phosphatases and esterases (Banon et al., 1964), collagenase-like activity (Espey, 1975; Espey and Coons, 1976; Morales et al., 1978, 1983; Fukumoto et al., 1981; Fujii et al., 1981) and plasminogen activator (Beers, 1975; Beers et al., 1975; Strickland and Beers, 1976). It was shown that injection of proteolytic enzymes into the follicular antrum resulted in follicular rupture (Espey and Lipner, 1965) and application of enzyme solutions to follicular wall resulted in ovulatory changes (Espey, 1967b; Espey and Rondell, 1967; Rondell, 1970b).

In order to establish a physiological role of an enzyme in follicular rupture, several requirements should be met. Among these: it should be produced in the follicle; its activity in the follicle should be regulated by the ovulation-inducing hormone; it should be capable of weakening the follicular wall; and inhibitors of its action should prevent ovulation. Here our recent studies on the involvement of collagenolysis, plasminogen activator and of lipoxygenase products of arachidonic acid in follicular rupture, and hence in ovulation, will be reviewed.

COLLAGENOLYSIS AND FOLLICULAR RUPTURE

In view of the observed changes in follicular collagen it appears that collagen degrading enzymes play a major role in follicular rupture. Nevertheless, experiments to extract follicular collagenase and to demonstrate its ability to degrade follicular wall were not successful (Espey and Stacy, 1970), nor has a correlation between collagenase activity and ovulatory changes been demonstrated as yet. This failure should probably be attributed to the following characteristics of mammalian collagenase: (i) it is secreted as an inactive zymogen; (ii) it is firmly bound to its natural substrate - the ovarian thecal collagen; (iii) it is kept inactivated by serum and follicular fluid inhibitors and activated by protease activators (Espey, 1978). In this regard follicular proteases, including plasmin, may have an important role in ovulation (Birkedal-Hansen et al., 1975; Horwitz et al., 1976).

We labelled ovarian collagen by injecting L-(5-^{3}H) proline peritoneally into immature (26 day old) rats (see Fig. 1). Part of the injected ^{3}H-Pro is first incorporated into the collagen and is then enzymatically converted into labelled-Hyp. The presence of the latter is unique to collagen. Ovarian or follicular collagen was

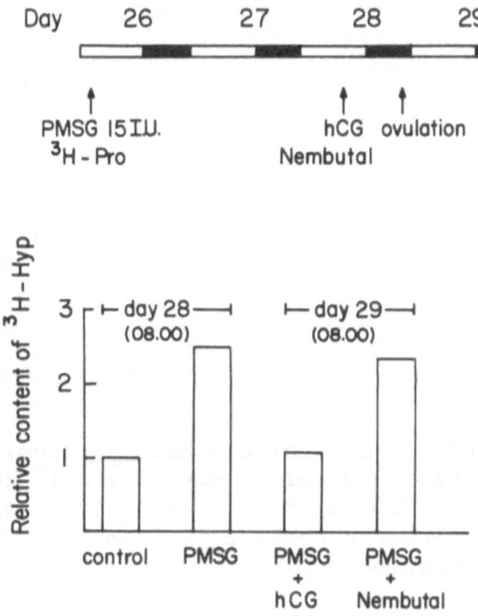

Fig. 1. Labeling of ovarian collagen by ^{3}H-proline in immature rats. Upper panel indicates the treatment schedule of rats and lower panel ^{3}H-hydroxyproline (^{3}H-Hyp) content of the ovaries on days 28 and 29. Animals which received PMSG + hCG, ovulated at night of day 28, and those treated with Nembutal did not ovulate. (From Reich et al., in preparation.)

extracted as described by Morales et al (1978). The extract was either (i) directly hydrolized in acid (HCl 6N, 105°C, 18 h) or (ii) first endogenous collagenase was activated by trypsin, plasmin or p-amino-phenyl-mercuric acetate (APMA) and tested after 48 h incubation and separation and only afterwards acid hydrolized as in (i). The labeled Hyp was separated from the acid hydrolyzate of the collagenous fraction by HPLC on an ion exchange column (Beckman type AA 15) using citrate buffer (0.2 M, pH 2.8 and 2% in n-propanol). Specific activity was calculated as cpm/Hyp μmole and cpm/leucine μmole equivalents. Hyp was determined colorimetrically according to Woessner (1961) and total amino acids by fluorometric measurement (Bleecker and Romeo, 1982).

Administration of PMSG (15 I.U.) to immature rats enhanced incorporation of labeled Hyp into the ovary (2.5-fold) as compared to

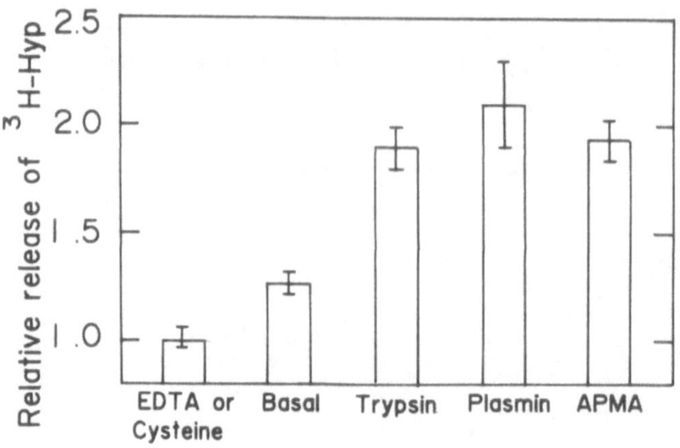

Fig. 2. Activation of ovarian collagenase in vitro. Endogenous collagenase extracted alone with the collagen was activated by trypsin (0.01 mg/ml), plasmin (0.01 mg/ml) and p-amino-phenyl mercuric acetate (1.5 mM). (From Reich et al., in preparation.)

untreated immature rats. Following ovulation, the fraction of labeled ovarian Hyp was reduced by 60% evidencing degradation of collagen. Prevention of the preovulatory surge of gonadotropins, and hence ovulation, by Nembutal abolished this reduction in labeled ovarian Hyp. (Fig. 1). Furthermore, known activators of collagenase, i.e. trypsin (0.01 mg/ml) plasmin (0.01 mg/ml) and p-amino-phenyl-mercuric acetate (APMA, 1.5 mM), induced collagenolytic activity in ovarian collagen extracts in vitro (Fig. 2). This in vitro activity was inhibited by cysteine (0.01M) and EDTA (0.02M), known inhibitors of metalo-proteinases including collagenase. These results suggest that the decomposition of collagen was most likely due to an ovarian collagenase extracted along with the collagen fraction. This suggestion is corroborated by a pharmacological approach: intra bursal administration of cysteine, an inhibitor of collagenase (0.025-0.12 mmole), prevented ovulation in a dose-dependent manner when injected on the day of proestrus (Fig. 3). Histological examination of the ovaries did not reveal any morphological deleterious changes in the periovulatory Graafian follicles by the amino acid. Cysteine not only inhibited ovulation but also prevented breakdown of ovarian collagen; these two effects of cysteine were dose-related (Fig. 4). Similar results were obtained by a microbial metalo-protease inhibitor, talopeptine, which inhibited ovulation in vitro from hamster ovaries (Ichikawa et al., 1983).

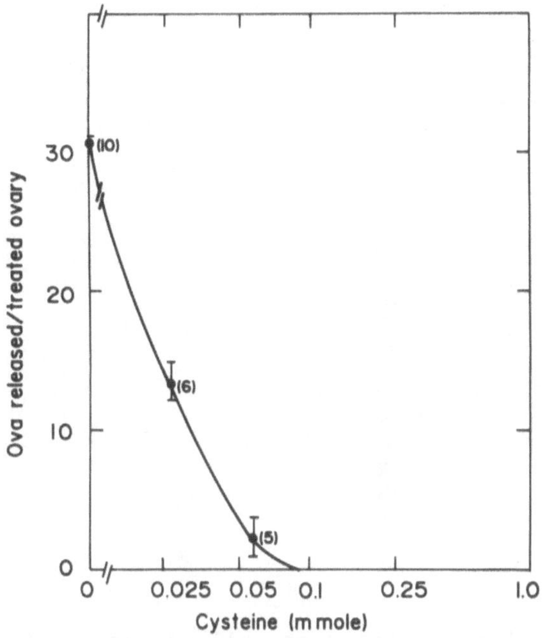

Fig. 3. Effect of cysteine on ovulation. The amino acid was injected into one of the ovarian bursae and hCG (4 I.U.) intraperitoneally 52 h following PMSG (15 I.U.) administration. The contralateral ovary served as control (0). (From Reich et al., in preparation.)

ROLE OF PLASMINOGEN ACTIVATOR (PA) IN FOLLICULAR RUPTURE

Previous studies demonstrated an enhancement of PA production by rat granulosa cells by gonadotropins (Beers, 1975; Beers et al., 1975; Strickland and Beers, 1976; 1979). It was suggested that the product of PA action, plasmin, is involved in the activation of latent follicular collagenase and thus in follicular rupture (Espey, 1980). In our studies, we did observe activation of ovarian collagenolysis *in vitro* by exogenous plasmin (Fig. 2).

One major difficulty for the suggested role of plasminogen activator in follicular rupture was the observation that FSH (NIH-FSH-S11 or rat FSH-B1) was more potent, on a mass basis, in inducing PA in granulosa cells than LH (NIH-LH-S19 or rat LH-I-4; Strickland and Beers, 1976). By contrast, *in vivo* studies revealed that while both LH and FSH are capable of inducing ovulation in the rat, only LH may be regarded as the physiological ovulation induc-

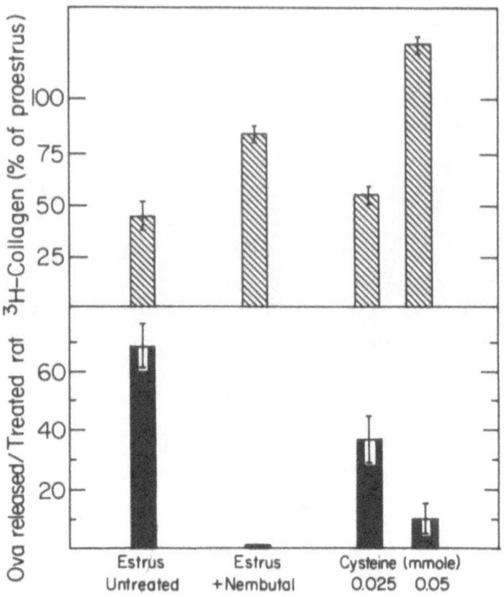

Fig. 4. The effect of cysteine on collagen degradation and ovulation. The rats were treated as in Fig. 1. On day 28, the rats were injected, in addition to hCG, with the indicated dose of cysteine. On day 29, the content of ^{3}H-Hyp in the ovaries, and number of ova in the oviducts were determined (from Reich et al., in preparation).

ing hormone (Schwartz et al., 1973; Tsafriri et al., 1976). Therefore, we re-examined the activity of LH and FSH on production of PA by rat Graafian follicles in culture. It is assumed that the follicular wall, rather than the isolated granulosa cells, is the tissue involved in follicular rupture. PA activity was determined by the iodinated fibrin plate assay (Soreq and Miskin, 1981) by measuring the fibrinolytic activity of plasmin, which was converted by PA from plasminogen included in the assay mixture.

Graafian follicles were explanted at various times on the day of proestrus and the PA content of the follicles was determined. Considering the fact that the preovulatory surge of gonadotropins is initiated in our colony only after 15:00 (Ayalon et al., 1972), no increase in PA activity was observed in ovaries collected prior to the surge (Fig. 5). By contrast, at 20:00 h (about 5 h after the beginning of the surge) almost maximal production of PA was observed. The elevation of PA production on the day of proestrus is

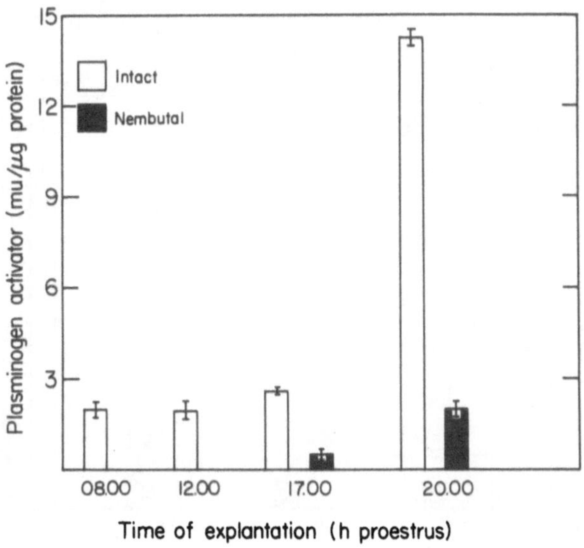

Fig. 5. Plasminogen activator content of ovarian folllicles on day of proestrus. Follicles were dissected at the indicated time and assayed for plasminogen activator (PA) content. Nembutal was injected to the indicated groups at 14.00 h. (From Reich, Miskin and Tsafriri, in preparation.)

gonadotropin-dependent since administration of Nembutal blocked the rise of PA activity on the evening of the day of proestrus (Fig. 5). We compared the relative potency of LH (NIH-LH-S21; biopotency equal to 2.5 NIH-LH-S1 U/mg; FSH activity < 0.5% by weight) and FSH (NIH-FSH-S14; biopotency equal to 9 NIH-FSH-S1 U/mg; LH activity equal to 0.01 NIH-LH-S1 by OAAD bioassay) on follicular secretion of PA in vitro. In the explanted proestrus rat follicles, LH was almost 5 times more potent, on a mass basis, than FSH in increasing PA activity (Fig. 6). Our results suggest, therefore, that while in isolated granulosa cells FSH is more potent than LH in increasing PA activity (Beers, 1975; Beers et al., 1975; 1976; Strickland and Beers, 1979), in the whole follicle, LH is more potent. However, when follicular rupture is considered, we assume that the response of the entire follicle wall is relevant.

In addition to the documentation of PA presence and secretion in the follicle, a pharmacological approach was used to relate this activity to the process of ovulation. Benzamidine (0.05-0.25 mmole) and ε-amino caproic acid (0.05-0.25 mmole), two selective inhibitors of serine proteases, including plasminogen activator and plasmin, were injected locally into one of the bursal cavities of proestrus rats. Both inhibitors prevented ovulation in a dose dependent manner in the treated ovary without causing morphological

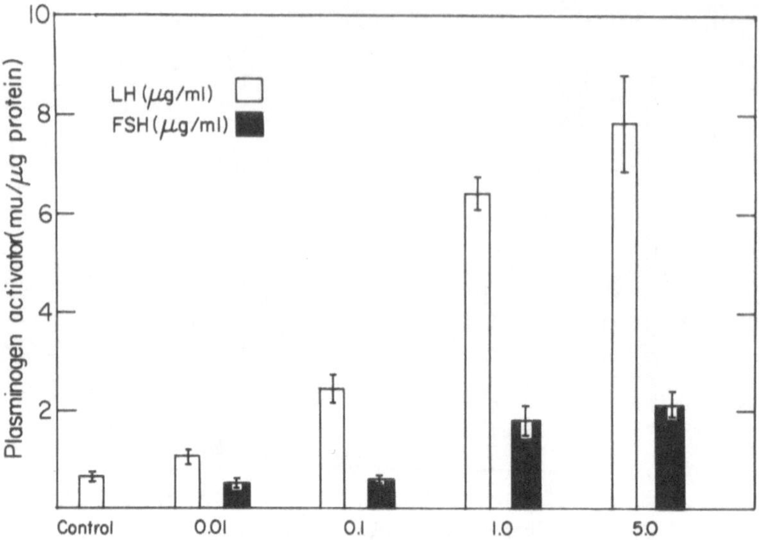

Fig. 6. Plasminogen activator production by ovarian follicles *in vitro*. The follicles were explanted on the morning of the day of proestrus and cultured for 6 h and then assayed for their PA content. (From Reich, Miskin and Tsafriri, in preparation.)

changes discernible by histological examination or affecting the ovulation of the control side (Fig. 7 describes the effect of benzamidine; similar dose response was obtained with ε-amino caproic acid). Similarly, several inhibitors of serine proteases inhibited *in vitro* ovulation of hamster ovaries (Ichikawa et al., 1983). Even though follicular rupture occurs 9-12 h after hCG stimulation, administration of inhibitors of serine proteases prior to 1.5 h after hCG blocked ovulation in rats (> 65%) but had limited effect (< 30%) after 3 h. This result implies that the activity of serine proteases is required only during the first 3 h after hCG stimulation.

INVOLVEMENT OF METABOLITES OF ARACHIDONIC ACID IN OVULATION

Most of the ovulatory processes, i.e. activation of adenylate cyclase, ovum maturation, steroidogenesis and luteinization, evoked by LH in the preovulatory follicle are reinforced by local prostaglandin (PG) synthesis. Nevertheless, they will proceed even when PG synthesis is inhibited by drugs. The exception is follicular rupture, which is prevented by administration of aspirin and indomethacin (Armstrong and Grinwich, 1972; Orczyk and Behrman, 1972; Tsafriri et al., 1972; 1973) or PG antibody (Armstrong et al.,

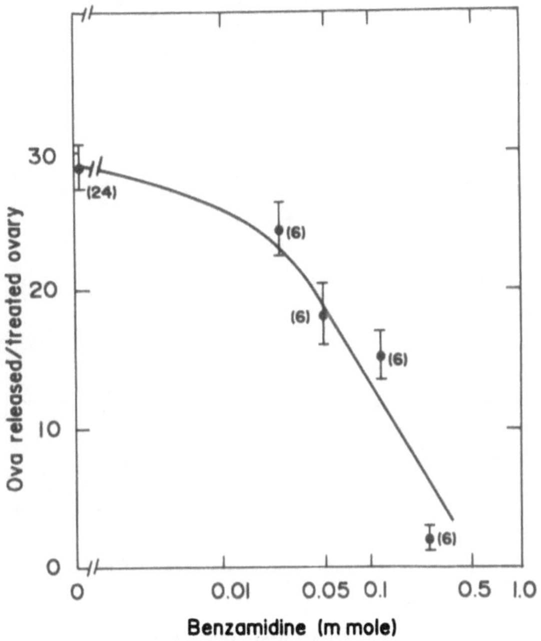

Fig. 7. Effect of benzamidine on ovulation. The drug was injected into one of the ovarian bursae and hCG (4 I.U.) intraperitoneally 52 h following PMSG (15 I.U.) administration. The contralateral ovary served as control (0). (From Reich, Miskin and Tsafriri, in preparation.)

1974). Thus cyclooxygenase products of arachidonic acid have a physiological role on follicular rupture (reviewed by Zor and Lamprecht, 1974; Patrono, 1983). It was suggested, therefore, that ovulation may be considered as an inflammatory process (Espey, 1980) and the involvement of prostaglandins can be viewed in this context. The recent recognition of the potential importance of the lipoxygenase pathway of the arachidonic acid (AA) cascade in the process of inflammation and the availability of specific inhibitors of lipoxygenase such as nordihydroguaiaretic acid (NDGA) (Panaganamala et al., 1977), 5,8,11, eicosatriynoic acid (5,8,11 ETYA) (Hammarstrom, 1977), and 3-amino-1-(3-trifluromethyl phenyl)-2-pyrazoline hydrochloride (BW755c) (Casey et al., 1983), prompted us to test the possible involvement of the lipoxygenase pathway in follicular rupture.

Unilateral administration of these drugs into the ovarian bursa at 18.00 h ($\pm$ 15 min) of the day of proestrus, resulted in the reduction of the number of ovulated ova in a dose dependent manner,

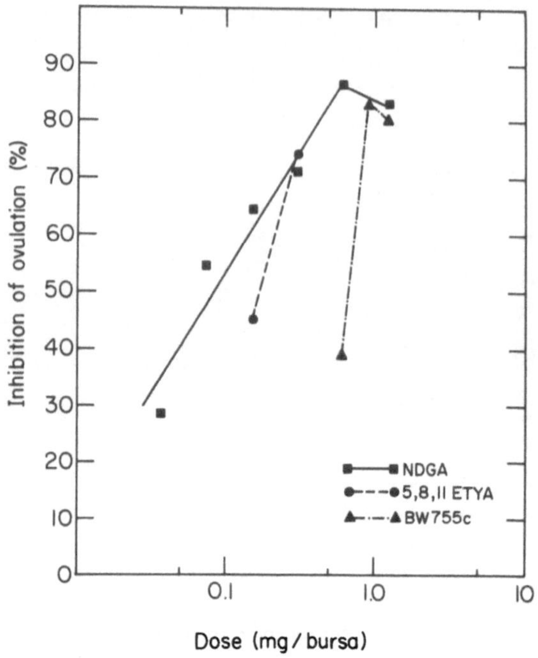

Fig. 8. Effect of inhibitors of lipoxygenase pathway on ovulation. The drugs were injected at 18.00 on the day of proestrus into the ovarian bursa. The contralateral ovary served as control. (Data from Reich, Kohen, Naor and Tsafriri, submitted for publication.)

but they did not affect the ovulation from the contralateral ovary (Fig. 8). NDGA and 5,8,11 ETYA were found to be more effective in preventing ovulation than BW755c. NDGA was the most potent since it completely blocked ovulation in 17/38 rats receiving a dose higher than 0.15 mg/bursa. Unilateral administration of NDGA (0.3 mg) into the bursal cavity inhibited only partially (N.S.) the LH-induced rise in ovarian prostaglandin E (E_1 + E_2; PGE) content measured at midnight of the proestrus, 6 h after administration of NDGA and about 8 h after the gonadotropin surge. By contrast, administration of indomethacin (0.3 mg) abolished completely the rise in PGE at the same time (Fig. 9). It should be noted, that the partial reduction in ovarian PGE content by NDGA was exerted on both treated and untreated ovaries, indicating that this partial reduction cannot be responsible for the block of ovulation. The results of this pharmacological approach suggest involvement of products of the lipoxygenase cascade in the process of follicular rupture. Since lipoxygenase products of AA were described mainly

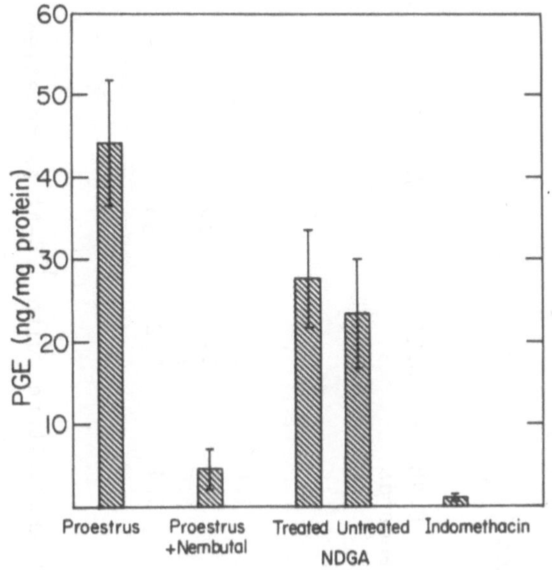

Fig. 9. Prostaglandin content of ovaries on the day of proestrus. All ovaries were dissected at 24.00 h. Other details in the text. (Data from Reich et al., submitted for publication.)

in the immune system, it was important to check whether the ovary converts AA to hydroxyeicosatetranoic acids (HETE's) via the lipoxygenase pathway. This was tested by following metabolism of ^{14}C-arachidonic acid by preovulatory follicles according to the procedures described by Jakschik et al. (1982). Following incubation of 30 min, the follicles were homogenized and extracted.

The extracts were chromatographed in a solvent system of n-hexane, ethyl-acetate, acetic acid (50:30:1). The radioactive bands were then visualized by radioautography (curix RP2-AGFA-GEVAERT film) and monitored on a densitometer (Beckman DU-8 spectrophotometer). In this solvent system, PGF, PGE and TBX_2 standards remain at the origin while 5-HETE, 11-HETE, 12-HETE and AA standards migrate with Rf values of 0.36, 0.47, 0.51 and 0.75 respectively. Follicular tissue from proestrus rats converted ^{14}C-AA into metabolites of the cyclooxygenase and the lipoxygenase pathways (Table 1). Autoradiography of the TLC plates revealed at least 6 different bands in the autoradiogram. Band I, near the origin, most likely represents prostanoids PGE, PGF and TBX_2. Band II co-migrated with synthetic 5-HETE, band III with 11-HETE, band V 12-HETE

Table 1: Conversion of ^{14}C-arachidonic acid by preovulatory follicles in vitro. The data are expressed as percentage of total radioactivity as measured by optical density on the radioautogramme bands. (Data from Reich, Kohen, Naor and Tsafriri, submitted.)

Treatment	I	II	III	IV	V	VI
	R_f values					
	Origin	0.36	0.46	0.48	0.51	0.72
	Comigrating standards					
	Prostanoids	5-HETE	11-HETE	?	12-HETE	AA
None[a]	12	0.4	0.5	1.6	2.2	65
hCG[b]	32.7	1.0	7.0	5.2	5.1	35
hCG+I (6μM)[c]	23	1.0	4.2	6.5	6.1	49
hCG+NDGA (20μM)[c]	30.1	0.2	6.9	5.1	3.2	36

a. Follicles explanted from rats on the morning of proestrus and cultured with ^{14}C-AA as detailed in Materials and Methods section.
b. Follicles explanted 6 h after administration of hCG (10 IU/rat) on 08.00 of the day of proestrus and cultured as in a.
c. Follicles as in b, but cultured in the presence of the indicated dose of indomethacin (I) or NDGA.

and band VI was AA as revealed by authentic standards. Treatment with hCG enhanced follicular arachidonic acid conversion into all the metabolites as compared to untreated proestrus follicular tissue. Addition of indomethacin (6 μM) to the reaction mixture reduced bands I and III. Inclusion of 20 μM NDGA in the reacting mixture reduced bands II and V (Table 1). Omission of Ca^{++} from the reaction mixture reduced band II substantially (data not shown).

Two of the visualized bands, II and V seem to be products of lipoxygenase; 5-HETE comigrated with the first one and 12-HETE with the second. They were not affected by indomethacin, but NDGA decreased their formation by 80% and 40% respectively. Omission of Ca^{++} reduced band II supporting the suggestion that this band represents 5-HETE. While these identifications need further confirmation by complementary methods, the available data seem sufficient to suggest lipoxygenase activity in the preovulatory follicle. Of special interest is the 2,5-fold increase in these bands after treatment with hCG. The cellular site of lipoxygenase activity remains to be determined. This could be within any of follicle cell-types, granulosa or theca, or of blood cells such as mast or basophil cells which accumulate and degranulate around the time of ovulation (Zachariae et al, 1958; Zachariae and Jensen, 1958; Jones et al., 1980).

This is the first indication of the involvement of lipoxygenase and its products in the process of follicular rupture, but the mechanism(s) by which their effect is exerted remains obscure. These may include activation of collagenase or effects on follicular microvasculature such as increase in capillary permeability or constriction, changes which were observed in periovulatory follicles.

CONCLUDING REMARKS

By a combination of in vivo and in vitro studies we have been able to demonstrate an increase in ovarian collagenolysis dependent upon the preovulatory surge of gonadotropins and related to follicular rupture; ovulation was prevented by an inhibitor of metaloproteinases. An inactive collagenase was extracted along with ovarian collagen and it was activated in vitro chemically by APMA or enzymatically by trypsin or plasmin. Evidence for the involvement of plasminogen activator in follicular rupture has been presented (Beers, 1975; Beers et al., 1975; Strickland and Beers, 1976; 1979). Nevertheless, when PA activity of rat granulosa cell cultures was tested, there was a discrepancy between the potency of the gonadotropins, LH and FSH, in enhancing production and ovulation (see above). Now, by testing PA activity of whole preovulatory follicles, LH was more effective than FSH, on a weight basis, in enhancing PA activity. Furthermore, inhibitors of serine proteases prevented ovulation. Collectively, the previous studies by others and our data presented here, demonstrate the involvement of serine proteases, most probably plasmin and of metalo-proteases, most probably collagenase, in follicular rupture.

Lipoxygenase products also seem to be involved in follicular rupture. This suggestion is based on our following observations: specific inhibitors of lipoxygenase prevented ovulation; preovulatory follicles converted in vitro arachidonic acid into lipoxygenase products and this conversion was enhanced by hCG. Further studies are needed in order to define the cellular and molecular mechanisms by which lypoxygenase products are involved in ovulation.

ACKNOWLEDGEMENTS

We thank our colleagues Dr. Fortune Kohen, Dr. Z. Naor and Dr. Ruth Miskin for permission to quote unpublished studies; Mrs. R. Slager and Mrs. A. Tsafriri for excellent technical assistance; Mrs. M. Kopelowitz for diligent secretarial help; Dr. S. Hammarström of the Karolinska Institutet for kindly providing us with 5,8,11-ETYA; and the National Pituitary Agency, NIAMD, for providing the gonadotropins. The work was supported by the Ford Foundation and the Rockefeller Foundation.

REFERENCES

Armstrong, D.T., Grinwich, D.L., Moon, Y.S., and Zamecnik, J., 1974, Inhibition of ovulation in rabbits by intrafollicular injection of indomethacin and PGF_2 antiserum. Life Sci. 14:129.

Armstrong, D.T., and Grinwich, D.L., 1972, Blockade of spontaneous and LH-induced ovulation in rats by indomethacin, an inhibitor of prostaglandin biosynthesis, Prostaglandins, 1:21.

Ayalon, D., Tsafriri, A., Lindner, H.R., Cordova, T., and Harell, A., 1972, Serum gonadotrophin levels in pro-oestrous rats in relation to the resumption of meiosis by the oocytes, J. Reprod. Fert. 31:51.

Banon, P., Brandes, D. and Frost, J.K., 1964, Lysosomal enzymes in the rat ovary and endometrium during the estrous cycle, Acta. Cytol. 8:416.

Beers, W.H., 1975, Follicular plasminogen and plasminogen activator and the effect of plasmin on follicular wall, Cell 6:379.

Beers, W.H., Strickland, S., and Reich, E., 1975, Ovarian plasminogen activator: Relationship to ovulation and hormonal regulation, Cell 6:387.

Birkedal-Hansen, H., Cobb, C.M., Taylor, R.E. and Fullmer, H.M., 1975, Trypsin activation of latent collagenase from several mammalian sources, Scand. J. Dent. Res. 83:302.

Blandau, R.J. and Rumery, R.E., 1963, Measurements of intrafollicular pressure in ovulatory and preovulatory follicles of rat, Fertil. Steril. 14:330.

Bleecker, A.B. and Romeo, J.T., 1982, Automatic fluorometric amino acid analysis: The determination of non-protein cyclic imino acids, Anal. Biochem. 121:295.

Casey, F.B., Appleby, B.J., and Buck, D.C., 1983, Selective inhibition of lipoxygenase pathway of arachidonic acid by the SRS-A antagonist FPL 55712. Prostaglandins 25:1.

Espey, L.L., 1967, Ultrastructure of the apex of the rabbit's Graafian follicle during ovulatory process, Endocrinology 81:267.

Espey, L.L., 1974, Ovarian proteolytic enzymes and ovulation. Biol. Reprod. 10:216.

Espey, L.L., 1975, Evaluation of proteolytic activity in mammalian ovulation, in: "Proteases and Biological Control" E. Reich, D.B. Rifkin and E. Shaw, eds., Cold Spring Harbor Laboratory, Cold Spring Harbor, N.Y., pp. 767-776.

Espey, L.L., 1978, Ovulation, in: "The Vertebrate Ovary", R.E. Jones, ed., Plenum Press, pp. 503-532.

Espey, L.L., 1980, Ovulation as an inflammatory reaction - a hypothesis. Biol. Reprod. 22:73.

Espey, L.L. and Lipner, H., 1963, Measurements of intrafollicular pressures in the rabbit ovary. Amer. J. Physiol. 205:1067.

Espey, L.L. and Lipner, H., 1965, Enzyme-induced rupture of rabbit Graafian follicle, Amer. J. Physiol. 208:208.

Espey, L.L. and Rondell, P., 1967, Estimation of mammalian collagenolytic activity with a synthetic substrate, J. Appl. Physiol. 23:457.

Espey, L.L. and Stacy, S., 1970, Failure of an ovarian collagenolytic extract to decompose the connective tissue in the mature sow Graafian follicle, Fed. Proc. 29:833.

Espey, L.L. and Coons, P.J., 1976, Factors which influence ovulatory degradation of rabbit ovarian follicles, Biol. Reprod. 14:233.

Fujii, M., Tojo, H. and Kogo, K., 1981, Detection and properties of collagenase in ovarian follicle wall of domestic fowl, Int. J. Biochem. 13:1043.

Fukumoto, M., Yajima, Y., Okamura, H. and Midoribawa, O., 1981, Collagenolitic enzyme activity in human ovary: On ovulatory enzyme system, Fertil. Steril., 36:746.

Hammarström, S., 1977, Selective inhibition of platelet n-8 lipoxygenase by 5,8,11-eicosatriynoic acid. Biochim. Biophys. Acta, 484:517.

Horwitz, A.L., Kelman, J.A. and Crystal, R.G., 1976, Activation of alveolar macrophage collagenase by a natural protease secreted by the same cell, Nature (London) 264:772.

Ichikawa, S., Morioka, H., Ohta, M., Oda, K. and Murao, S., 1983, Effect of various proteinase inhibitors on ovulation of explanted hamster-ovaries. J. Reprod. Fert. 68:407.

Jakschik, B.A., Harper, T. and Murphy, R.C., 1982, The 5-lipoxygenase and leukotriene forming enzymes, Methods in Enzym. 86:30-37.

Jones, R.E., Duvall, D. and Guillette, L.J., 1980, Rat ovarian mast cells: distribution and cyclic changes. Anat. Rec. 197:489.

Lipner, H., 1973, Mechanism of mammalian ovulation, in: "Handbook of Physiology, Endocrinology" Vol. II, Part 1, R. Greep, ed., American Physiological Soc., Washington, D.C., pp. 409-437.

Marsh, J.M. and LeMaire, W.J., 1974, The role of c-AMP and prostaglandins in the action of luteinizing hormone, in: "Gonadotropins and Gonadal Function", N.R. Moudgal, ed., AP, N.Y., pp. 376-380.

Morales, T.I., Woessner, J.F., Howell, D.S., March, J.M., and LeMaire, W., 1978, A microassay for the direct demonstration of collagenolytic activity in Graafian follicles of the rat, Biochim. Biophys. Acta. 524:428.

Morales, T.I., Woessner, J.F., Marsh, J.M. and LeMaire, W.J., 1983, Collagen collagenase and collagenolytic activity in rat Graafian follicles during follicular growth and ovulation, Biochim. Biophys. Acta 756:119.

Orczyk, G.P., and Behrman, H.R., 1972, Ovulation blockade by aspirin or indomethacin - in vivo evidence for a role of prostaglandin in gonadotropin secretion. Prostaglandins, 1:3.

Panaganamala, R.V., Miller, J.S., Gueba, E.T., Harma, H.M., and Cornwell, D.G., 1977, Differential inhibitory effects of vitamin E and other antioxidant on prostaglandin synthetase, platelet aggregation and lipoxidase. Prostaglandins, 14:261.

Parr, E.L., 1975, Rupture of ovarian follicles at ovulation, J. Reprod. Fertil. Suppl. 22:1.

Patrono, C., 1983, Arachidonic acid metabolism in the ovary: Biochemistry methodology and physiology. in: "Comprehensive Endocrinology - The Ovary", G.B. Serra, ed., N.Y., pp. 45-56.

Pearson, O.P., 1944, Reproduction in the shrew, Ann. J. Anat. 75:39.

Reich, R., Kohen, F., Naor, Z., and Tsafriri, A., Possible involvement of lipoxygenase products of arachidonic acid pathway in ovulation. Prostaglandins (submitted).

Reichert, L.E., 1962, Endocrine influences on rat ovarian proteinase activity, Endocrinology 70:657.

Rondell, P., 1970a, Biophysical aspects of ovulation, Biol. Reprod. (Suppl.) 2:64.

Rondell, P., 1970b, Follicular processes in ovulation, Fed. Proc. 29:1875.

Rondell, P., 1974, Role of steroid synthesis in the process of ovulation. Biol. Reprod. 10:199.

Schwartz, N.B., Krone, K., Talley, W.L., and Ely, C.A., 1973, Administration of antiserum to ovine FSH in the female rat;

Failure to influence immediate events of cycle. Endocrinology 92:1165.

Soreq, H. and Miskin, R., 1981, Plasminogen activator in the rodent brain, Brain Res. 216:361.

Strickland, S. and Beers, W.H., 1976, Studies on the role of plasminogen activation in ovulation, J. Biol. Chem. 251:5694.

Strickland, S. and Beers, W.H., 1979, Studies of the enzymatic basis and hormonal control of ovulation. in: "Ovarian Follicular Development and Function", A.R. Midgley and W.A. Sadler, eds., Raven Press, New York, pp. 143-153.

Tsafriri, A., Lindner, H.R., Zor, U. and Lamprecht, S.A., 1972, In vitro induction of meiotic division in follicle-enclosed rat oocytes by LH, cyclic AMP and Prostaglandin E_2. J. Reprod. Fertil. 31:39.

Tsafriri, A., Lieberman, M.E., Barnea, A., Bauminger, S. and Lindner, H.R., 1973, Induction by luteinizing hormone of ovum maturation and of steroidogenesis in isolated Graafian follicles of the rat: Role of RNA and of protein synthesis, Endocrinology 93:1378.

Tsafriri, A., Lieberman, M.E., Koch, Y., Bauminger, S., Chobsieng, P., Zor, U., and Lindner, H.R., 1976, Capacity of immunologically purified FSH to stimulate cAMP accumulation and steroidogenesis in Graafian follicles and to induce ovum maturation and ovulation in the rat. Endocrinology, 98:655.

Wallach, E.E., Bronson, R.A., Hamada, Y., Karen, H. and Wright, M.S., 1980, The physiology of ovulation, in: "Endocrine Physiopathology of the Ovary", Rozzini, Reeves and Pinola, eds., Elsevier/North Holland Biomedical Press, pp. 153-163.

Woessner, J.F., 1961, The determination of hydroxyproline in tissue and protein samples containing small proportions of this imino acid, Arch. of Biochem and Biophys. 93:440.

Zachariae, F., 1958, Studies on the mechanism of ovulation, Permeability of the blood-liquor barrier, Acta Endocrinol. (Copenhagen) 27:339-342.

Zachariae, F., and Jensen, C.E., 1958, Studies on the mechanism of ovulation: Histochemical and physico-chemical investigations on genuine follicular fluids, Acta Endocrinol. (Copenhagen) 27:343.

Zor, U., and Lamprecht, S.A., 1977, Mechanism of prostaglandin action in endocrine glands, in: "Biochemical Actions of Hormones", vol. 4, G. Litwack, ed., Academic Press, pp. 85-133.

THE ROLE OF CELL-CELL COMMUNICATION IN NEUROPEPTIDE-STIMULATED AND DOPAMINE-INHIBITED PROLACTIN RELEASE *

Carl Denef, Myriam Baes, Carla Schramme and Luc Swennen

Laboratory of Cell Pharmacology
School of Medicine, University of Leuven
Campus Gasthuisberg, B-3000 Leuven, Belgium

The anterior pituitary is composed of different cell types producing different protein or peptide hormones. Although at first look these different cells are scattered throughout the gland, a more careful examination clearly shows that the topographical arrangement of the different cells is not random (1). Certain cell types are more abundant in certain areas than in others. Moreover, one cell type may display a selective topographical affinity for another. More than 10 years ago Nakane mentioned in his paper on immunocytochemical studies of the anterior pituitary cell types of the adult male rat that gonadotrophs and lactotrophs are frequently found in close association with each other (2). Many of these lactotrophsare cup-shaped, embracing and sometimes completely surrounding a gonadotroph. It has also been mentioned that gonadotrophs may have some affinity for somatotrophs (3). Nakane as well as others also found that corticotrophs (2,4,5) and thyrotrophs (6) are in close juxtaposition with somatotrophs. Horvath *et al.* (7) reported that gonadotrophs and lactotrophs form between each other specialized junctional complexes of the "macula adhaerens diminuta" type, described by Overton (8). The length of attachment of these adherence junctions varies between 50 and 300 nm, the intercellular gap measuring approximately 150 Å. It has also been demonstrated that not all lactotrophs have affinity for a gonadotroph. Nogami and Yoshimura distinguished 4 morphologically distinct subtypes in adult male rat pituitary (9) : 1) oval or polygonal cells with only small spherical granules (130-200 nm diam.); 2) oval or polygonal cells with medium-sized spherical and polymorphic granules (250-300 nm); 3) polygonal cells with only large polymorphic granules

*Supported by grants from "Geconcerteerde Onderzoeksakties", I.W.O.N.L., F.G.W.O. and "Koninging Elisabcth Stichting".

(300-700 nm diam.) in the cytoplasm and small granules in the Golgi region; 4) cup-shaped cells with usually spherical (300 nm diam.) and a few polymorphic granules (300-700 nm diam.). Type 3 is the commonly accepted lactotroph in the female rat but it is not predominant in the male. The most frequently found lactotrophs in the male are the type 2 and the cup-shaped cells and these are the cells which have a special affinity for gonadotrophs (9,10). According to Sato (10) polygonal cells appear to gather around an enlarged gonadotroph and extend cytoplasmic processes to the gonadotroph to envelop it. The latter are the cup-shaped cells and some of them can completely surround a gonadotroph. Cup-shaped cells, while intermingled with oval and polygonal cells, accumulate in the marginal layer of the gland, particularly in the vicinity of the sex zone (10), in which there is a high proportional number of gonadotrophs (2). However, these different cell types are also found to be scattered throughout the gland and sometimes in clusters (9,10).

The functional significance of the topographical affinity of lactotrophs to gonadotrophs is not known. However, since there are dramatic developmental changes, sex differences and alterations during the estrous cycle in the proportional number of the different lactotroph cell types and in their affinity for the gonadotrophs (10), an intimate functional interrelationship seems plausible. Cup-shaped cells do not seem to occur before puberty whereas in adult life they are more numerous in the male than in the female rat. During the estrous cycle the number and/or immunostainability of cup-shaped cells increase during proestrous and significantly fall during estrous.

Since techniques have been developed to separate the different pituitary cell types into highly enriched populations (for review, see 11), a direct experimental approach to study the functional significance of the above morphological data has become possible. Using superfused reaggregate pituitary cell cultures (12,13) of a mixture of lactotrophs and gonadotrophs, we have recently demonstrated that gonadotrophs can activate the secretory activity of the lactotrophs, most likely through the release of (a) paracrine humoral factor(s) (14,15). We here report our progress in this area.

I. Interaction between Gonadotrophs and Lactotrophs during Exposure to Neuropeptides

LHRH : In superfused reaggregate cell cultures derived from dispersed anterior pituitary cells from 14-day-old rats, LHRH was found capable of stimulating PRL release from concentrations as low as 10^{-11} M (15). The onset of the PRL response was rapid and comparable to that of the LH response (< 2 min). However, when LHRH was withdrawn from the superfusion medium, there was a 4-6 min delay before the secretion rate of PRL decreased whereas LH release was turned off immediately (16). LHRH was more potent in stimulating PRL release than thyrotropin releasing hormone (TRH) (16) and vasoactive intestinal peptide (VIP) (12). Upon withdrawal of TRH, there was no residual stimulation of PRL release. The PRL response to a prolonged superfusion with LHRH was biphasic (16). After an initial sustained peak response during about 20 min, the secretion rate declined to considerably lower levels but started rising again after about 1 h. Interestingly, the latter response pattern paralleled that of LHRH-stimulated LH release.

In aggregates prepared from adult rat pituitary the PRL response to LHRH was weak and seen only after a longer time in culture (15). As the proportional number of gonadotrophs in adult rat pituitary is 3-4 times lower, and that of large gonadotrophs about 7 times lower than in the pituitary of 14-day-old female rats (17), we hypothesized that LHRH is capable of stimulating PRL release only in the presence of a critical number of gonadotrophs and that this is brought about by signal transmission from gonadotrophs to lactotrophs.

The latter hypothesis was supported by the following findings : 1) The PRL response to LHRH was not seen in reaggregate tissue cultures of pituitary cell subpopulations, obtained by unit gravity sedimentation, in which there were lactotrophs but very little (< 1 %) and only small gonadotrophs (15). 2) LHRH readily stimulated PRL release in subpopulations containing lactotrophs and a higher number of gonadotrophs (15). At each concentration of LHRH used (0.01-10 nM) the magnitude of stimulation was dependent on the proportional number and size of the gonadotrophs present. 3) When a lactotroph-enriched/gonadotroph-deprived population was reaggregated with a highly-enriched population of large gonadotrophs (70-75 % gonadotrophs) LHRH also stimulated PRL release (15). In the latter case, a proportional number of about 3 % large gonadotrophs in the coculture was sufficient to induce a more than half-maximal response. 4) Whereas the PRL response to LHRH was weak in aggregates from the total pituitary cell population of adult rats it was high in a gonadotroph-enriched subpopulation (15).

Stimulus-transfer from gonadotrophs to lactotrophs appeared to be quite selective. Whereas LHRH readily stimulated PRL release in pituitary reaggregates, provided there was a critical number of gonadotrophs present, the decapeptide failed to stimulate TSH release (data not shown). However, as shown in Fig. 1 LHRH slightly stimulated GH release but only at relatively high concentrations (10 nM). There is also no evidence that gonadotrophs and lactotrophs are readily excitable by other cell types. TRH was not capable of stimulating LH release in aggregates prepared from a population consisting of 75 % gonadotrophs and 12 % thyrotrophs (15). As shown in Fig. 2 Growth hormone releasing factor (GH-RF) failed to stimulate

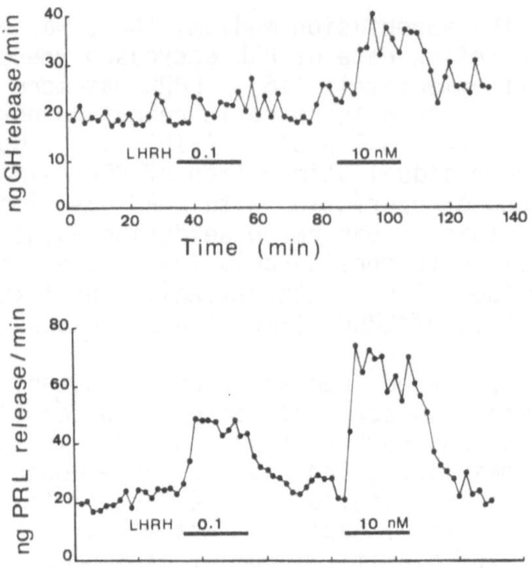

Fig. 1 : Stimulation of PRL and GH release in superfused anterior pituitary reaggregate cell cultures by LHRH. Methods as described in reference 15.

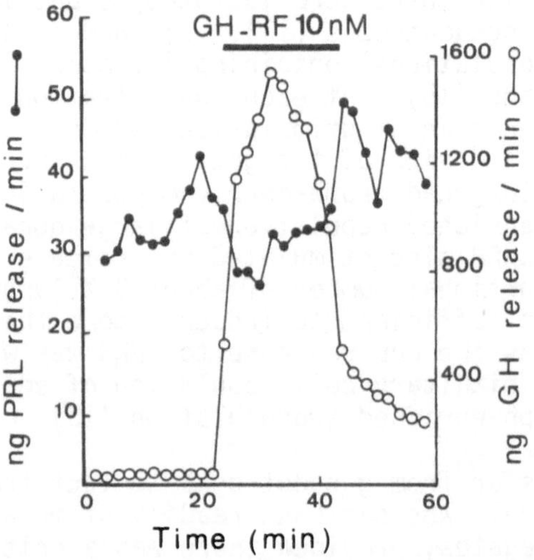

Fig. 2 : Failure of GH-RF to stimulate PRL release in superfused reaggregate cell cultures of a lactotroph/somatotroph-enriched pituitary cell population from 14-day-old female rats (∼ 30 % of each lactotrophs and somatotrophs). The enriched population was prepared by unit gravity sedimentation and taken from combined gradient fraction 2 and 3 as described in reference 15.

PRL release in a population consisting predominantly of lactotrophs and somatotrophs.

TRH : We could not find evidence for a stimulus transfer from lactotrophs to gonadotrophs when lactotrophs were stimulated by TRH (15). In gonadotroph-lactotroph cocultures in which LHRH stimulated PRL release, TRH failed to stimulate LH release at concentrations up to 100 times higher than those effective on PRL release.

VIP : It is well known that VIP stimulates PRL release at concentrations between 10^{-9} - 10^{-6} M. Similar concentrations were also effective in our reaggregate cell cultures (12). As shown in Fig. 3A VIP (10^{-9}-10^{-7}M) dose-dependently stimulated PRL release in the lactotroph-enriched/gonadotroph-deprived subpopulation from 14-day-old female pituitaries. However, quite surprising responses to VIP were seen when the peptide was superfused over reaggregates consisting of a mixture of the above population and the highly enriched population of large gonadotrophs. At a concentration of 10^{-9} M, VIP slightly inhibited PRL release and this was followed by a rebound secretion upon withdrawal of the peptide. VIP had almost no effect on PRL release at 10^{-8} M, except for a rebound secretion when it was withdrawn. Only at 10^{-7} M a clearcut stimulation was seen. These data strongly suggest that gonadotrophs can also engage in an inhibitory interaction with lactotrophs. The latter interpretation was supported by the data presented in Fig. 3B where it is shown that VIP dose-dependently inhibits spontaneous LH release from the gonadotroph-rich population.

Angiotensin II (AII) : It has been recently shown that AII is capable of stimulating PRL release by a direct action on the pituitary In both monolayer cultures (18) and superfused reaggregate cell cultures (19) AII was effective from concentrations as low as 10^{-10}M. In order to find out whether the effect was elicited directly on the PRL-cells, AII was tested in various pituitary cell subpopulations including lactotroph-enriched/gonadotroph-poor populations. To our surprise the latter populations displayed the weakest response to AII (unpublished observations). However, as shown in Fig. 4, the response to AII was significantly enhanced when the latter population was mixed with a small number of large gonadotrophs. A final proportional number as low as 1 % of these large gonadotrophs was effective. This potentiating effect, however, faded when the number of gonadotrophs in the coculture was raised to 15 %, again suggesting that gonadotrophs are capable of transmitting not only stimulatory but also inhibitory signals.

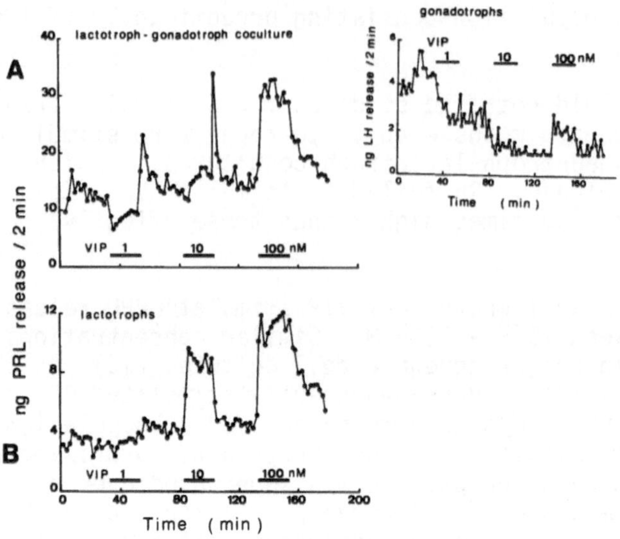

Fig. 3 : A. Influence of coculturing a highly-enriched population of large gonadotrophs with a lactotroph-enriched/gonadotroph-deprived population on VIP-stimulated PRL release. Cell separation and co-aggregation of the two populations (gradient fraction 2 and fraction 6-9 from 14-day-old female rats as described in reference 15). The approximate number of large gonadotrophs from fraction 6-9 in the coculture was 15 %.
B. Effect of VIP on spontaneous LH release from superfused reaggregate cell cultures of the gonadotroph-rich fraction 6-9.

2. Interaction between Gonadotrophs and Lactotrophs during and after Exposure to Dopamine (DA)

The interaction between gonadotrophs and lactotrophs is not abolished when PRL release is inhibited for 90 % by tonic exposure to 10 nM DA. LHRH was found equally potent in stimulating DA-inhibited PRL release as spontaneous PRL release, concentrations as low as 10^{-11} M already being effective (15). Even in the presence of DA, LHRH was more potent than TRH in stimulating PRL release (16).

The extent of inhibition induced by 10 nM DA, however, was not affected when the gonadotrophs were not stimulated. This is clearly shown in Fig. 5 which compares the inhibition by a 10 min pulse of 10 nM DA in a lactotroph-enriched/gonadotroph-deprived population with that seen in a coculture of the latter population with a gonadotroph-rich population. However, a remarkable finding was that resumption of PRL release upon withdrawal of DA was considerably slower in the coculture. In fact, we have recently shown

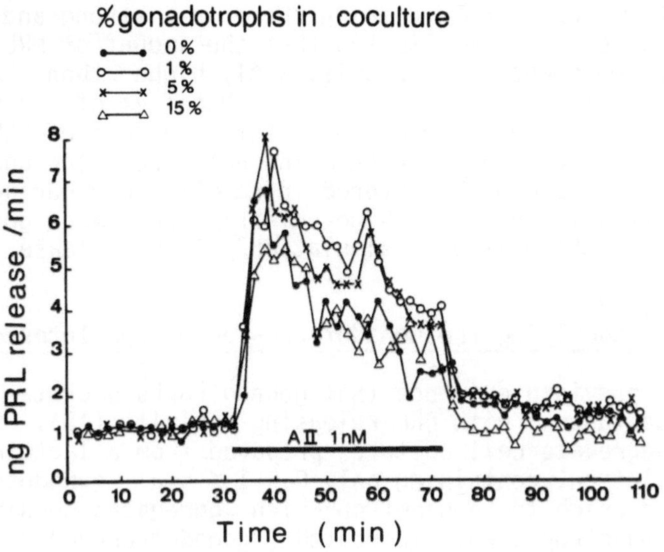

Fig. 4 : Influence of coculturing a highly enriched population of large gonadotrophs with a lactotroph-enriched gonadotroph-deprived population on angiotensin II (AII)-stimulated PRL release. The same populations as in Fig. 3 were used.

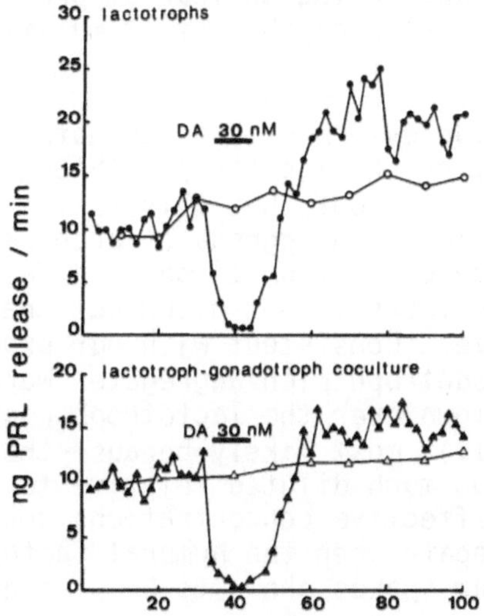

Fig. 5 : PRL release during a 10 min pulse and subsequent to withdrawal of 10 nM DA in reaggregate cell cultures of lactotroph-enriched/gonadotroph-deprived pituitary cell population from 14-day-old females and in a coculture of the latter population with a gonadotroph-rich population. The same populations as in Fig. 3 were used. The final number of large gonadotrophs in the coculture was approx. 7.5 %.

that after short-term exposure to DA there is a strong and prolonged rebound secretion of PRL and that the amount of PRL secreted during this rebound phase was significantly higher than the amount inhibited during the time DA was present (Denef *et al.*, submitted). Several lines of evidence suggested that this excess of PRL secretion is a stimulated type of release and not merely the consequence of spontaneous release of PRL stored intracellularly during the period of DA-inhibition. Fig. 5 now clearly shows that gonadotrophs attenuate the post-DA "stimulation" of PRL release.

3. Mechanisms Underlying the Gonadotroph-Lactotroph Interactions

We have provided evidence that gonadotrophs secrete a substance (or substances) with PRL-releasing activity (15). Superfusion of reaggregate cell cultures prepared from a lactotroph-enriched population, containing only 0.5-1 % small gonadotrophs, with medium in which the gonadotroph-rich aggregates consisting of 75 % large gonadotrophs were incubated ("gonadotroph-conditioned medium"), provoked a 40-120 % rise of PRL (15,16). The gonadotroph-rich aggregates released this substance spontaneously and quite rapidly and LHRH augmented this release. However, after 1 h of incubation a steady state condition appeared to develop, the mechanism and significance being unclear at present. "Gonadotroph-conditioned medium" was also capable of stimulating PRL release inhibited by 10 nM DA.

These data provide evidence that gonadotrophs can activate the secretory activity of the lactotrophs through the release of a paracrine factor. Direct proof that this factor also mediates the LHRH-stimulated PRL release in aggregates prepared from the total population of pituitary cells from 14-day-old females or in lactotroph-gonadotroph cocultures is not given but the findings are at least highly suggestive. Consistent with our proposal is another finding that when gonadotroph-rich aggregates were superfused and the eluate directly flown over the lactotroph aggregates, there was no PRL response (15), most likely because the presumptive paracrine substance was too much diluted relative to its stimulatory potency. Presumably effective concentrations could rapidly be obtained inside an aggregate when the humoral factor is released in the small intercellular spaces shown to be present in the reaggregate cell cultures (12).

Although the chemical nature of the substance could not be determined yet, we have excluded the involvement of LH, FSH and the small amount of PRL secreted in the "gonadotroph-conditioned medium" (15). The involvement of LHRH could also be excluded as the "gonadotroph-conditioned medium" stimulated PRL release in the presence of an LHRH-antagonist (15). Possible candidates are peptides. TRH (20), VIP (21,22), neurotensin (23-25), substance P (23,24), calcitonin (26), angiotensin II (18,19) and under certain conditions also opioid peptides (27) have PRL-releasing activity in pituitary *in vitro* preparations. All these peptides have been identified by immunocytochemical techniques in cells of the intact anterior pituitary (28-38). TRH (28), substance P (35), opioid material (36,37), and angiotensin (38) have been detected in gonadotrophs.

In our reaggregate cell culture system, however, neurotensin and substance P failed to stimulate PRL release but angiotensin II did (19). Furthermore, acid extracts of gonadotroph-rich aggregates have PRL-releasing potency and contain radioimmunoassayable angiotensin I but little angiotensin II (unpublished data). Angiotensin I stimulates PRL release in our system but not when conversion to angiotensin II is blocked by the dipeptidylcarboxypeptidase inhibitor captopril (Schramme and Denef, in preparation). Work is in progress to determine whether or not angiotensin is the paracrine factor responsible for the stimulation of PRL release by LHRH.

As shown in the present paper, gonadotrophs also appear to be capable of transmitting inhibitory signals to the lactotrophs. So far, we have not tested whether or not a paracrine mechanism is also involved in this phenomenon.

REFERENCES

1. B. L. Baker, Functional cytology of the hypophyseal pars distalis and intermedia, in : "Handbook of Physiology", sect. 7, vol. 4, pt. 1. The Pituitary Gland and its Neuroendocrine Control, E. Knobil, and W. H. Sawyer, eds., American Physiological Society, Washington DC, p. 45 (1974).
2. P. K. Nakane, Classification of pituitary cell types with immunoenzyme histochemistry, J. Histochem. Cytochem. 18:9 (1970).
3. K. Kovacs, and E. Horvath, The Pituitary, in : "Principles and Practice of Surgical Pathology", S. G. Silverberg, ed., John Wiley & Sons, p. 1393 (1983).
4. E. R. Siperstein, and K. J. Miller, Endocrinology 86:451 (1970).
5. M. A. Nagata, S. E. Mizunaga, and F. Yoshimura, Endocrinol. Japon. 27:13 (1980).
6. F. Yoshimura, and H. Nogami, Endocrinol. Japon. 27:43 (1980).
7. E. Horvath, K. Kovacs, and C. Ezrin, Functional contact between lactotrophs and gonadotrophs in rat pituitary, IRCS Med. Sci. 5:511 (1977).
8. J. Overton, Development of cell junctions of the adhaerens type, Curr. Top. Dev. Biol. 10:1 (1975).
9. H. Nogami, and F. Yoshimura, Fine structural criteria of prolactin cells identified immunocytochemically in the male rat, Anat. Rec. 202:261 (1982).

10. S. Sato, Postnatal development, sexual difference and variation during the sexual cycle of prolactin cells in rats : The special reference to the topographic affinity to a gonadotroph, Endocrinol. Japon. 27:573 (1980).
11. C. Denef, L. Swennen, and M. Andries, Separated anterior pituitary cells and their response to hypophysiotropic hormones, Int. Rev. Cytol. 76:225 (1982).
12. B. Vanderschueren, C. Denef, and J.-J. Cassiman, Ultrastructural and functional characteristics of rat pituitary cell aggregates, Endocrinology 110:513 (1982)
13. C. Denef, M. Baes, B. Vanderschueren, and J.-J. Cassiman, Aggregate cell cultures as a tool for studying cell-to-cell communication in rat anterior pituitary, Les Colloques de l'INSERM, INSERM 110:451 (1982).
14. C. Denef, LHRH stimulates prolactin release from rat pituitary lactotrophs cocultured with a highly purified population of gonadotrophs, Ann. Endocrinol. (Paris) 42:65 (1981).
15. C. Denef, and M. Andries, Evidence for paracrine interaction between gonadotrophs and lactotrophs in pituitary cell aggregates, Endocrinology 112:813 (1983).
16. C. Denef, Functional interrelationships between pituitary cells, in : "Proceedings of the 3rd European Workshop on Pituitary Adenomas", Blackwell Scientific, London, in press (1984).
17. C. Denef, Functional heterogeneity of separated dispersed gonadotropic cells, in : "Synthesis and Release of Adenohypophyseal Hormones", M. Jutisz, and K. W. McKerns, eds., Plenum Publishing Corporation, p. 659 (1980).
18. G. Aguilera, C. L. Hyde, and K. J. Catt, Angiotensin II receptors and prolactin release in pituitary lactotrophs, Endocrinology 111:1045 (1982).
19. C. Schramme, and C. Denef, Stimulation of prolactin release by angiotensin II in superfused rat anterior pituitary cell aggregates, Neuroendocrinology 36:483 (1983).
20. C. Y. Bowers, H. C. Friesen, P. Hwang, H. J. Guyda, and K. Folkers, Prolactin and thyrotropin release in man by synthetic pyroglutamyl-histidyl-prolinamide, Biochem. Biophys. Res. Commun. 45:1033 (1971).
21. Y. Kato, Y. Iwasaki, J. Iwasaki, H. Abe, N. Yanaihara, and H. Imura, Prolactin release by vasoactive intestinal peptide in rats, Endocrinology 103:554 (1978).
22. M. Ruberg, W. H. Rotsztejn, S. Arancibia, J. Besson, and A. Enjalbert, Stimulation of prolactin release by vasoactive intestinal peptide (VIP), Eur. J. Pharmacol. 51:319 (1978).
23. E. Vijayan, and S. M. McCann, *In vivo* and *in vitro* effects of substance P and neurotensin on gonadotropin and prolactin release, Endocrinology 105:64 (1980).
24. E. Vijayan, and S. M. McCann, Effect of substance P and neurotensin on growth hormone and thyrotropin release *in vivo* and *in vitro*, Life Sci. 26:321 (1980).

25. A. Enjalbert, S. Aracibia, M. Priam, M. T. Bluet-Pajot, and C. Kordon, Neurotensin stimulation of prolactin secretion *in vitro*, Neuroendocrinology 34:95 (1982).
26. Y. Iwasaki, K. Chihara, J. Iwasaki, H. Abe, and T. Fujita, Effect of calcitonin on prolactin release in rats, Life Sci. 25:1243 (1979).
27. A. Enjalbert, M. Ruberg, S. Arancibia, M. Priam, and C. Kordon, Endogenous opiates block dopamine inhibition of prolactin secretion *in vitro*, Nature 280:595 (1979).
28. G. V. Childs (Moriarty), D. E. Cole, M. Kubek, R. B. Tobin, and J. F. Wilber, Endogenous thyrotropin releasing hormone in the anterior pituitary : sites of activity as identified by immunocytochemical staining, J. Histochem. Cytochem. 26:901 (1978).
29. G. Morel, J. Besson, G. Rosselin, and P.M. Dubois, Ultrastructural evidence for endogenous vasoactive intestinal peptide-like immunoreactivity in the pituitary gland, Neuroendocrinology 34:85 (1982).
30. G. Uhl, M. J. Kuhar, and S. H. Snyder, Neurotensin : immunohistochemical localization in rat central nervous system, Proc. Natl. Acad. Sci. USA 74:4059 (1977).
31. M. Goedert, S. L. Lightman, J. I. Nagy, P. D. Marley, and P. C. Emson, Neurotensin in the anterior pituitary gland, Nature 298:163 (1982).
32. W. R. Watkins, and R. Y. Moore, Immunoreactive calcitonin in the rat anterior pituitary gland and its localization in thyrotrophs, Am. J. Anat. 158:445 (1980).
33. W. Vale, C. Rivier, L. Yang, S. Minick, and R. Guillemin, Effects of purified hypothalamic corticotropin-releasing factor and other substances on the secretion of adrenocorticotropin and endorphin-like immunoreactivities *in vitro*, Endocrinology 103:1910 (1978).
34. L. R. DePalatis, R. P. Fiorindo, and R. H. Ho, Substance P immunoreactivity in the anterior pituitary gland of the guinea pig, Endocrinology 110:282 (1982).
35. G. Morel, J. A. Chayvialle, B. Kerdelhué, and P. M. Dubois, Ultrastructural evidence for endogenous substance P-like immunoreactivity in the rat pituitary gland. Neuroendocrinology 35:86 (1982).
36. G. Tramu, and J. Leonardelli, Immunohistochemical localization of enkephalines in median eminence and adenohypophysis, Brain Res. 168:457 (1979).
37. K. M. Braas, J. F. Wilber, and G. V. Childs, Opiocortin peptide storage sites in gonadotrophs and corticotrophs in the rat pituitary. J. Cell. Biol. 87:173 (abstract) (1980).
38. M. K. Steele, M. S. Brownfield, and W. F. Ganong (1982) Immunocytochemical localization of angiotensin immunoreactivity in gonadotrophs and lactotrophs of the rat anterior pituitary gland, Neuroendocrinology 35:155 (1982).

ACKNOWLEDGEMENTS

The excellent technical assistance of R. Dewals, A. De Wolf, D. Manet and M.J. Vanderheyden and secretarial work of M. Bareau is gratefully acknowledged. The authors are grateful to the U.S. National Hormone and Pituitary Program and the National Institute of Arthritis, Diabetes and Digestive and Kidney Diseases for providing rat PRL, LH, GH and TSH RIA kits.

MODULATION OF PROLACTIN SECRETION AT THE PITUITARY LEVEL : INVOLVEMENT OF ADENYLATE CYCLASE

Alain Enjalbert, Joël Bockaert*, Jacques Epelbaum, Emmanuel Moyse and Claude Kordon

Unité 159 de Neuroendocrinologie INSERM, 75014 Paris and *Centre CNRS-INSERM de Pharmacologie-Endocrinologie 34000 Montpellier (France).

The original concept of adenohypophyseal regulation postulated that exteroceptive and interoceptive inputs were integrated at the hypothalamic level and relayed to the pituitary in the form of simple messages. The hypophysis was thus considered a passive responder to such messages which increased or reduced hormonal secretion. It appears now that the situation is more complex in particular for prolactin secretion.

A large number of substances have been shown to directly affect prolactin cells (Fig. 1), either as prolactin inhibiting factors (PIF), such as dopamine (Mac Leod, 1969), but also gamma-aminobutyric acid (GABA) (Schally et al., 1977 ; Enjalbert et al., 1979d), and histidyl proline diketopiperazine (DKP), a degradation product of TRH (Bauer et al., 1978 ; Enjalbert et al., 1979a), or as prolactin releasing factor (PRF), such as TRH (Tashjian et al., 1971 ; Gourdji et al., 1972), vasoactive intestinal peptide (VIP) (Ruberg et al., 1978 ; Gourdji et al., 1979 ; Enjalbert et al., 1980), neurotensin (Vijayan and McCann, 1980 ; Enjalbert et al., 1982a), or bombesin (Westendorf and Schonbrunn, 1982).

In addition to these multiple inhibiting and stimulating factors, a new type of hypothalamic factors has also been identified : prolactin modulating factors (PMF) (Enjalbert and Kordon, 1982). These factors also act at the pituitary level without affecting the spontaneous release of prolactin by themselves, but by interfering with stimulatory or inhibitory inputs caused by other factors.

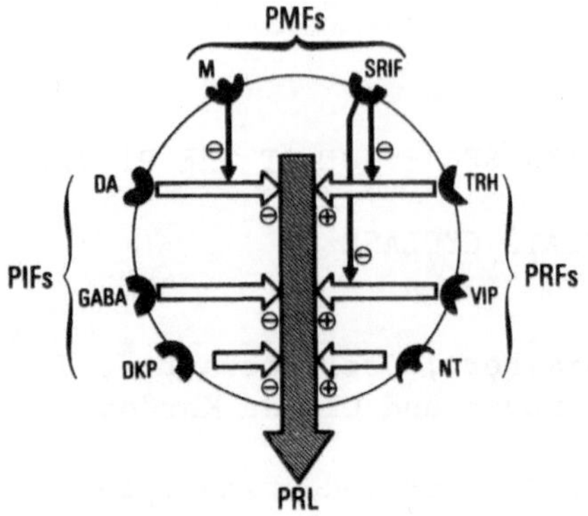

Fig. 1. Summary of the various interactions occuring at the level of the prolactin cell (from Enjalbert, 1982).

Opiates are thus able to block the dopamine inhibition of prolactin secretion without affecting the spontaneous prolactin release (Enjalbert et al., 1979b, c ; Cheung, 1982). This effect of opiates seems to occur only after short-term incubations, and to disappear after longer exposure (Cheung, 1982). This phenomenon could explain why other authors using long incubation time (Login and Mac Leod, 1979) did not find any effect of morphine or morphinomimetic peptides. This interaction of opiates with dopamine inhibition directly at the pituitary level has also been demonstrated in vivo. After destruction of the mediobasal hypothalamus, a perfusion of dopamine reduces plasma prolactin levels. Under these conditions, met-enkephalin or morphine elevates these levels of prolactin. This effect can only be accounted for by a direct effect at the pituitary level since the hypothalamus has been destroyed (Wuttke and Duker, 1983).

This effect of opiates is limited to dopamine inhibition since neither prolactin inhibition by GABA nor stimulation by TRH or VIP is affected by opiates (Enjalbert and Kordon, 1982).

On the other hand, somatostatin blocks the stimulation of prolactin secretion induced by TRH or VIP (Enjalbert et al., 1982b) (furthermore, a reciprocal interaction occurs on somatotrophs, since

TRH or VIP, which have no effect on the spontaneous growth hormone release, can counteract the inhibition of somatostatin on growth hormone release) (Tapia-Arancibia et al., 1980 ; Enjalbert et al., 1982b).

Prolactin secretion is thus controlled by multiple hypothalamic factors. The hypophyseal cell thus appears as the last level of integration of information coming from the central nervous system.

INTEGRATION OF INFORMATION BY LACTOTROPHS

How does the prolactin cell respond to the two concomitant signals ? Under certain conditions, additivity of the effects can be observed. For example, TRH and VIP stimulate prolactin release in an additive manner from both normal (Fig. 2) and tumoral (GH_3) cells (Enjalbert et al., 1980 ; Gourdji et al., 1979). Effects of neurotensin and TRH or VIP are also additive (Enjalbert et al.,

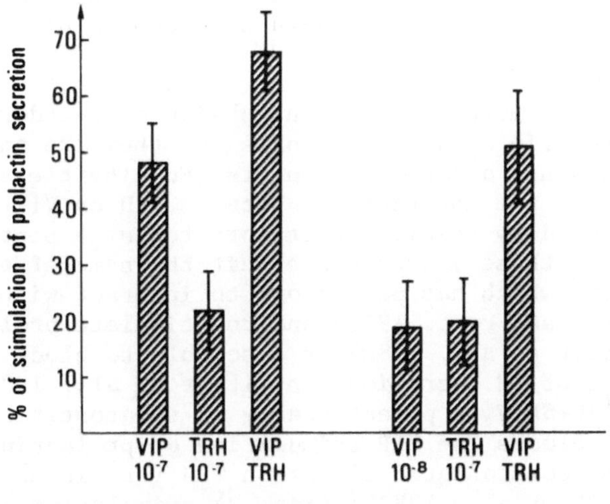

Fig. 2. Additive effects of VIP and TRH on in vitro prolactin release. Stimulation by VIP + TRH was significantly higher ($p < 0.05$) than when each peptide was added alone (from Enjalbert et al., 1980).

1982a). These results demonstrate that these peptides act through independent specific receptors, specific of each peptide. Similarly, when dopamine and VIP are both added to the incubation medium of anterior pituitaries, the resulting effect is the algebrical sum of the effects (Arancibia et al., 1981).

On the contrary, modulatory effects are non-additive. These modulations could theoretically be accounted for by three distinct mechanisms. They could involve :

1) Direct competition of the modulatory peptide for the specific binding site of the PIF or PRF.

2) Modulation of the number or the affinity of the specific receptor for PIF or PRF by the modulatory peptide (through its own specific receptor).

3) Interaction of the modulatory peptide with intracellular mechanisms coupled with PIF or PRF receptors.

In the case of the dopamine-opiate interaction as well as of the reciprocal interaction of somatostatin with TRH or VIP, the first hypothesis can be discarded as demonstrated by binding studies. Opiates do not displace ^{3}H-dihydroergocriptine (Caron et al., 1978) or ^{3}H-spiroperidol (Cronin and Weiner, 1979 ; Enjalbert and Kordon, 1982) binding to pituitary membrane preparation. On the other hand, the ineffectiveness of VIP and TRH in displacing ^{125}I-[Tyr_1]-SRIF binding to anterior pituitary membranes even at very high concentrations (Enjalbert et al., 1982b) indicates that the three peptides must be recognized by independent receptors on the pituitary cells.

The effects of morphine, met-enkephalin or β-endorphin seem to involve a specific opiate receptor since they are antagonized by naloxone and other opiate antagonists (Enjalbert et al., 1979c). On the other hand, the interactions between TRH or VIP and SRIF seem to be mediated by specific receptors for each peptide, since known agonists of these substances elicit the same effects. For example, secretin which has been shown to interact with VIP receptors (Taylor and Pert, 1979) and to stimulate prolactin release (Enjalbert et al., 1980) is also able to block the somatostatin inhibition of GH secretion (Enjalbert et al., 1982b). [D-Trp^{8}, D-Cys^{14}]-SRIF, a potent analog of somatostatin on GH secretion, also blocks the VIP stimulation of prolactin release. Furthermore, the somatostatin effect on TRH (Drouin et al., 1976) or VIP (Enjalbert et al., 1982b) (Fig. 3) stimulation of prolactin release appears non competitive, since SRIF reduces the maximal effect but not the apparent affinity of the two PRF.

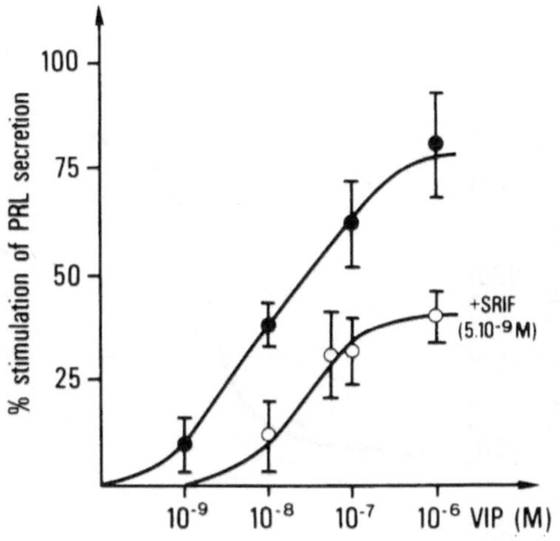

Fig. 3. Non competitive inhibition by somatostatin of VIP stimulation of prolactin secretion (from Enjalbert et al., 1982).

If the modulations cannot be accounted for by a direct competition on the same receptor, a modulation of the specific receptors for PIF or PRF by modulatory peptide (through its own specific receptors) cannot be discarded. In fact, such interaction between TRH receptors and somatostatin receptors has been described on GH_4C_1 cells (Schonbrunn and Tashjian, 1980). TRH, without competing with somatostatin binding, increased the number of somatostatin binding sites after short-term incubation and subsequently decreased somatostatin binding sites after longer exposure. Such interactions between receptors could account for the peptide interactions demonstrated on hormone release.

The alternate hypothesis is that these interactions occur at the level of the transducing mechanism involved after the initial step of binding or PRF (s) or PIF (s) to their specific receptors.

COUPLING OF PITUITARY RECEPTORS WITH ADENYLATE CYCLASE

Although the coupling mechanism of PIF, PRF and PMF receptors are still not completely understood, adenylate cyclase seems to be involved in the mechanism of action of at least three neurohormones.

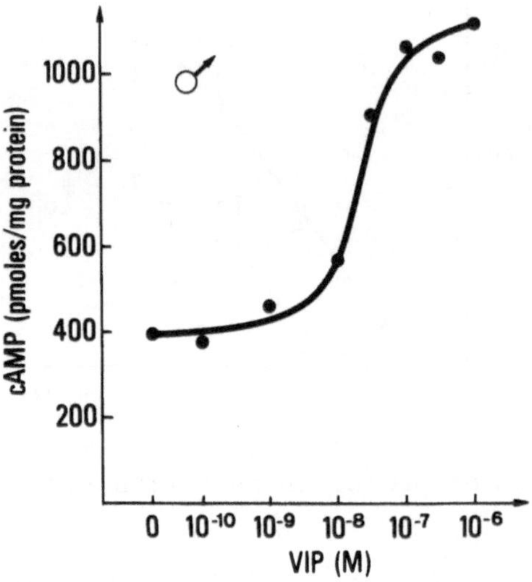

Fig. 4. Stimulation by VIP of basal adenylate cyclase of male anterior pituitary homogenates.

1) VIP

It seems clear that, as in other structures, adenohypophyseal receptors for VIP are positively coupled with adenylate cyclase. A direct stimulation of adenylate cyclase activity has been described on rat adenohypophyseal membranes (Robberecht et al., 1979) (Fig. 4), as well as on human prolactinoma (Bataille et al., 1979). This last result demonstrates that this effect on cyclic AMP production occurs, at least in part, in lactotroph cells. This has been confirmed on a rat tumor cell line (GH_3 B_6) in which VIP concomitantly increases prolactin release and cyclic AMP accumulation (Gourdji et al., 1979).

2) Dopamine

The dopamine receptor involved in prolactin secretion has been characterized as a D_2 receptor (Caron et al., 1978 ; Cronin and Weiner, 1979). This receptor type has been initially described as unrelated to adenylate cyclase in contrast to the D_1 dopamine receptor which activates the enzyme (Kebabian and Calme, 1979). However, recently in the intermediate pituitary lobe, D_2 dopamine receptor has been shown to inhibit adenylate cyclase activity (Munemura et al., 1980 ; Meunier and Labrie, 1982 ; Frey et al., 1982). In the anterior pituitary lobe, after a series of contradictory reports, two groups have demonstrated an inhibition of adenylate cyclase activity by dopamine in rat (Giannattasio et al., 1981 ; Onalli et al., 1981) or in human prolactinema (De Camilli et al., 1979). However, the involvement in prolactin secretion of the dopamine receptor negatively coupled with adenylate cyclase has been questioned. For example, ergot alkaloids, which are more potent than dopamine for inhibiting prolactin secretion has been shown weaker than the amine for inhibiting the enzyme (Onalli et al., 1981). For these reasons, these authors proposed that the dopamine receptor inhibiting pituitary adenylate cyclase were distinct from the classical D_2 receptors.

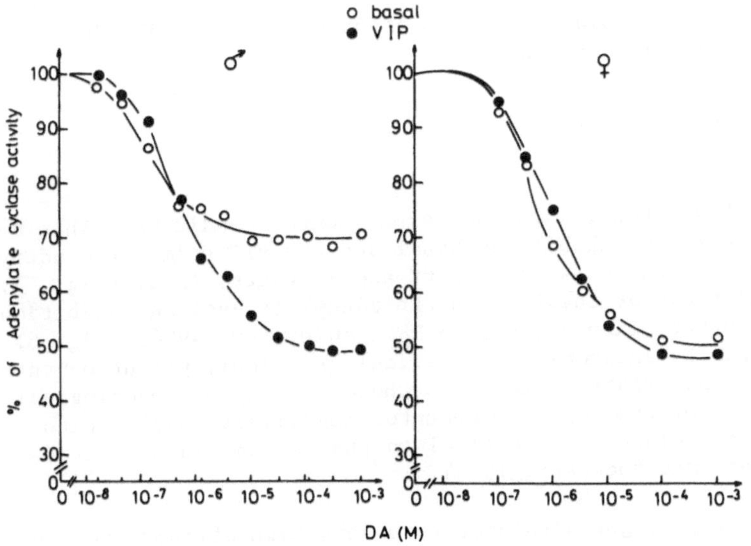

Fig. 5. Inhibition by dopamine of basal and VIP-stimulated adenylate cyclases of male and female anterior pituitary homogenates.

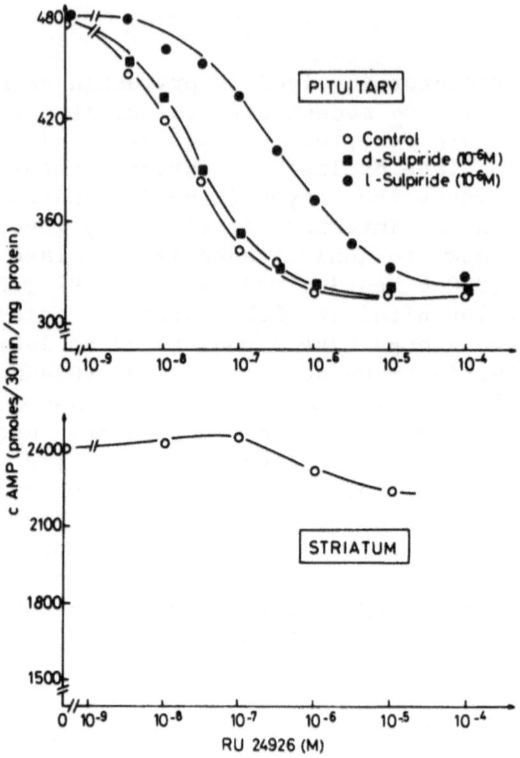

Fig. 6. Effect of RU 24926, a specific D_2 agonist, on basal adenylate cyclases of anterior pituitary and striatum homogenates.

We have shown, under our experimental conditions, that dopamine is able to inhibit the basal and the VIP-stimulated adenylate cyclase in both sexes (Enjalbert and Bockaert, 1983) (Fig. 5). The dopamine receptor involved in the adenylate cyclase inhibition is a D_2 receptor since a specific D_2 agonist (RU 24926) (Fig. 6) and a specific D_2 antagonist (sulpiride) are highly potent on anterior pituitary adenylate cyclase. Furthermore, the pharmacological properties of the dopamine receptor negatively coupled with adenylate cyclase are identical to that of D_2 binding sites (Enjalbert and Bockaert, 1983).

Finally, ergot alkaloids have very high affinity for the dopamine receptor negatively coupled with adenylate cyclase. We have demonstrated that the use of short incubation times leads to an underestimation of the apparent affinity (from 1 to 100 nM in the case of α-DMEC) (Enjalbert and Bockaert, 1983). In fact, due to their high affinity, these compounds slowly interact with dopamine receptors. For instance, Caron et al. (1978) reported that equilibrium of ^{3}H-DHEC binding to anterior pituitary membranes is reached only after 30 min at 25°C.

The fact that the binding of various agonists on pituitary D_2 receptors has been shown to be GTP-sensitive is constant with a coupling of these receptors with adenylate cyclase (Sibley and Creese, 1979 ; De Lean et al., 1982 ; Sibley et al., 1982). On the other hand, these D_2 receptors negatively coupled with an adenylate cyclase are the dopamine receptors involved in prolactin secretion since the pharmacological specificity characterized for the two biological responses are identical. In fact, increasing intracellular cyclic AMP by pharmacological agents results in an increase in prolactin release and synthesis (Ojeda et al., 1974 ; Hill et al., 1976 ; Tam and Dannies, 1981 ; Maurer, 1982). Conversely, dopamine agonists have been shown to decrease cyclic AMP production in anterior pituitary cells (Schettini et al., 1983) or in enriched lactotroph preparations (Barnes et al., 1978 ; Swennen and Denef, 1982). Finally, the toxin from Bordetella Pertussis, which suppresses hormone-induced adenylate cyclase inhibition in several system, is able to block the dopamine inhibition of prolactin secretion (Cronin et al., 1982).

In the case of stimulation of adenylate cyclase, activation of the nucleotide binding protein (N_S) is the rate limiting step. This activation is probably the result of a Mg^{++} GTP-dependent dissociation of the two subunits which compose N_S (NORTHRUP et al., 1982). Stimulating hormones increase N_S activation by increasing its affinity for Mg^{++} (Iyengar and Birnbaumer, 1983). In the case of anterior pituitary adenylate cyclase, it appears that GTP requirements for N_S and N_i (nucleotide binding protein involved in negative coupling) are different. Inhibition of adenylate cyclase requires much higher concentrations of GTP and dopamine seems to suppress the GTP-dependent adenyl-cyclase activation rather than to directly inhibit the enzyme. This adenylate cyclase inhibition by dopamine seems to be the result of a decrease of Mg^{++} affinity without any change in the maximal velocity of the system.

3) <u>Somatostatin</u>

In the case of somatostatin, there are also some data suggesting that cyclic AMP could be involved in the effect on GH secretion (Borgeat et al., 1974 ; Rouleau and Barden, 1981). However, other studies suggest that somatostatin exerts its inhibitory effect independently of cyclic nucleotide metabolism, by preventing cytoplasmic Ca^{++} rise (Bicknell et al., 1977 ; Kraicer and Chow, 1982).

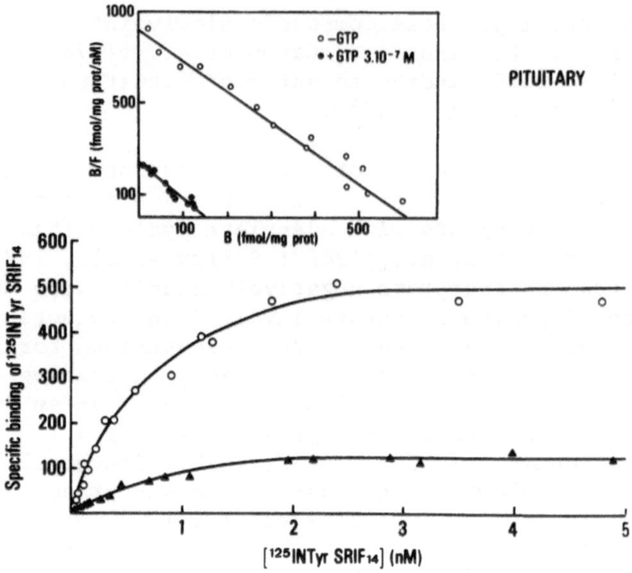

Fig. 7. Effect of GTP on specific binding on [^{125} I]-NTyr-somatostatin to adenohypophyseal membranes.

Using [^{125} I]-NTyr-somatostatin as a ligand, we have demonstrated the presence of a single population of high affinity binding sites on adenohypophyseal membranes. In the presence of 3.10^{-7}M GTP, specific binding was reduced (Fig. 7). The apparent affinity of the remaining binding sites is not significantly affected by the guanine nucleotide (Enjalbert et al., 1983). GTP and GDP are also able to reduce binding capacity of adenohypophyseal membranes in a dose-dependent manner whereas ATP, ADP, AMP, GMP or cGMP are ineffective (Enjalbert et al., 1983). It thus seems that guanine nucleotides induce a transformation of somatostatin binding sites to a lower affinity state that cannot be detected under our experimental conditions (ligand concentration up to 4nM). Kinetic experiments confirm this phenomenon since GTP increases the dissociation rate without affecting the association rate. The sensitivity of the [^{125} I]-NTyr-somatostatin binding sites to guanine nucleotides strongly suggests a coupling with a GTP-binding protein which could be linked to an adenylate cyclase.

It has been reported that on adenohypophyseal preparation, somatostatin decreases both basal and prostaglandin stimulated adenylate cyclase activity (Borgeat et al., 1977 ; Rouleau and Barden, 1981) (Fig. 8). However, all these experiments have been performed on whole anterior pituitary preparations and somatostatin can affect GH but also TSH and prolactin secretion.

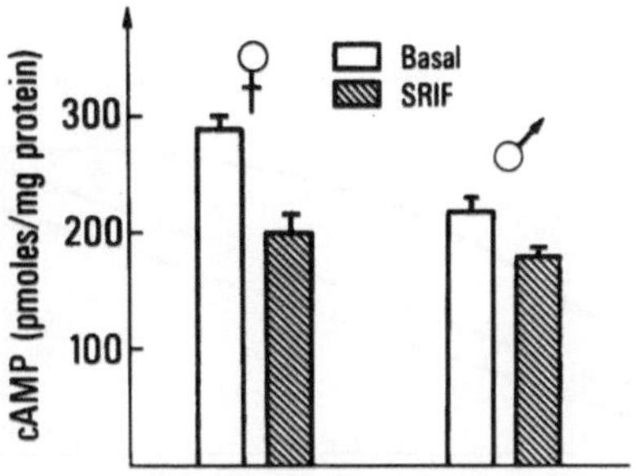

Fig. 8. Inhibition by somatostatin (10^{-7}M) of basal adenylate cyclase of male and female anterior pituitary homogenates.

Nevertheless, the single population of high affinity binding sites observed on whole pituitary membranes (Enjalbert et al., 1982c), as well as the complete disappearance of these sites in the presence of guanine nucleotides (Enjalbert et al., 1983) suggest that similar somatostatin receptors could be present on different cell types and that their coupling mechanism could be identical. In this respect, we have demonstrated the presence of such specific binding not only on membranes of human acromegalic tumors but also of prolactinomas (Fig. 9) with similar apparent affinity. The only difference between the two populations is the density of binding sites which is higher in GH secreting tumors.

CONCLUSION

Three receptors located on prolactin cells appear coupled with adenylate cyclase, one positively (VIP) and two negatively (dopamine, somatostatin).

The inverse effect of VIP and dopamine on cyclic AMP production can account for the resulting effect observed in the presence of both neurohormones on prolactin secretion. In the case of modulation of prolactin secretion, one of the mechanism involved could be an interaction at the level of the coupling mechanism of

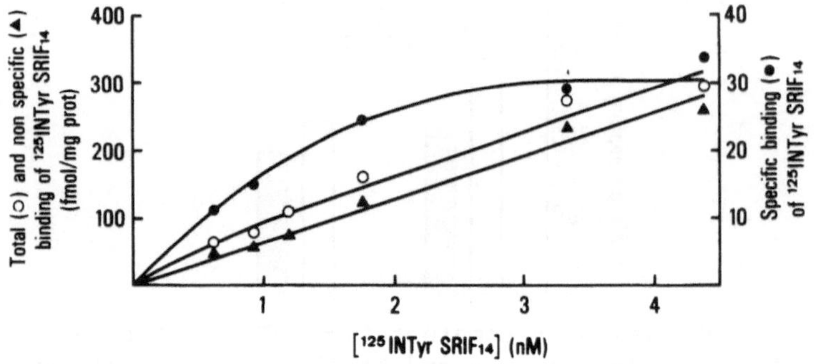

Fig. 9. Binding of [^{125} I]-NTyr-somatostatin to human prolactinoma membranes in the presence of increasing concentrations of ligand.

the receptor with adenylate cyclase. We have seen that VIP is a potent stimulator of adenylate cyclase and that somatostatin receptors are negatively coupled with the enzyme. The antagonism of both peptides on prolactin and growth hormone secretion could thus take place at the level of cyclic AMP production. This could also be the case for modulation of dopamine inhibition of prolactin secretion by opiates since interactions between dopamine and opiates on adenylate cyclase activity have been described in the central nervous system. (Motomatsu et al., 1977 ; Tang and Lotzias, 1978).

In conclusion, it appears that the release of prolactin is controlled by more than one specific releasing and/or inhibiting factor. Direct interactions at the level of the lactotrophs could represent an additional mechanism in the hypothalamic control of prolactin secretion. This capacity of integration resembles to that of neurones. In fact, some endocrine cells, including lactotrophs, have been shown to be excitable. Integration of the information thus seems to be a common property of these two types of cells and could involve similar mechanisms. The prolactin cells thus appear as a good model to study neurotransmitter receptors and their transduction mechanisms.

Arancibia, S., Enjalbert, A., Ruberg, M., Priam, M., Bluet-Pajot, M. T., and Kordon, C., 1981, Activité PRF (prolactin releasing factor) du VIP (vasoactive intestinal peptide) in vitro, J. Physiol. (Paris),77:979.

Barnes, G. D., Brown, B. L., Gard, T. G., Atkinson, D., and Ekins, R. P., 1978, Effect of TRH and dopamine on cyclic AMP levels in enriched mammotroph and tyrotroph cells, Mol. Cell. Endocr., 12:275.

Bataille, D., Peillon, F., Besson, J., and Rosselin, G., 1979, Vasoactive intestinal peptide (VIP) : Récepteurs spécifiques et activation de l'adénylate cyclase dans une tumeur hypophysaire humaine à prolactine, C. R. Acad. Sci. (Paris), 288:1315.

Bauer, K., Graf, K. J., Faivre-Bauman, A., Beier, S., Tixier-Vidal, A., and Kleinkauf, M., 1978, Inhibition of prolactin secretion by histidyl-proline-diketopiperazine. Nature, 274:174.

Bicknell, R. J., Young, P. W., Schofield, J. G., and Albano, J., 1977, Mechanism of action of somatostatin : Growth hormone release, [^{45}Ca] calcium ion efflux and cyclic nucleotides metabolism of bovine anterior-pituitary slices in the presence of prostaglandin E_2 and L-methyl-3-isobutyl-xanthine, Biochem. Soc. Trans., 5:219.

Borgeat, P., Labrie, F., Drouin, J., Belanger, A., Immer, I., Seetany, K., Nelson, V., Grotz, M., Schally, A. V., Coy, D. H., and Coy, E. J., 1974, Inhibition of adenosine 3', 5' monophosphate accumulation in anterior pituitary gland in vitro by growth hormone release inhibiting hormone, Biochem. Biophys. Res. Commun., 56:1052.

Caron, M. G., Beaulieu, M., Raymond, V., Gagné, B., Drouin, J., Lefkowitz, R., and Labrie, F., 1978, Dopaminergic receptors in the anterior pituitary gland, J. Biol. Chem., 253:2244.

Cheung, C. Y., 1982, Beta-endorphin modulates the dopamine inhibition of prolactin secretion at the anterior pituitary, in : 12th Neuroscience Meeting, Abstract N°18.1.

Cronin, M. J., Myers, G. A., Dabney, L. G., and Hewlett, E. L., 1982, Pertussis toxin uncouples dopamine receptor-mediated inhibition of prolactin release, in : 64th Annual Meeting of the Endocrine Society.

Cronin, M. J., and Weiner, R. I., 1979, [^{3}H]-spiroperidol (spiperone) binding to a putative dopamine receptor in sheep and steer pituitary and stalk median eminence, Endocrinology, 104:307.

De Camilli, P., Macconi, D., and Spada, A., 1979, Dopamine inhibits adenylate cyclase in human prolactin secreting pituitary adenomas, Nature, 278:252.

De Lean, A., Kilpatrick, B. F., and Caron, M. G., 1982, Guanine nucleotides regulate both dopaminergic agonist and antagonist binding in porcine anterior pituitary, Endocrinology,

110:1064.

Drouin, J., De Lean, A., Rainville, D., Lachance, R., and Labrie, F., 1976, Characteristics of the interaction between thyrotropin releasing hormone and somatostatin for thyrotropin and prolactin release, Endocrinology, 98:514.

Enjalbert, A., 1982, Multiplicité des facteurs qui influencent la sécrétion de prolactine au niveau hypophysaire, in : " Prolactine, Neurotransmission et Fertilité ", Masson, Paris.

Enjalbert, A., Arancibia, S., Priam, M., Bluet-Pajot, M. T., and Kordon, C., 1982a, Neurotensin stimulation of prolactin secretion in vitro, Neuroendocrinology,34:95.

Enjalbert, A., Arancibia, S., Ruberg, M., Priam, M., Bluet-Pajot, M. T., Rotsztejn, W. H., and Kordon, C., 1980, Stimulation of in vitro prolactin release by vasoactive intestinal peptide, Neuroendocrinology, 31:200.

Enjalbert, A., and Bockaert, J., 1983, Pharmacological characterization of the D_2-dopamine receptor negatively coupled with adenylate cyclase in rat anterior pituitary, Mol. Pharmacol. 23:576.

Enjalbert, A., Epelbaum, J., Arancibia, S., Tapia-Arancibia, L., Bluet-Pajot, M. T., and Kordon, C., 1982b, Reciprocal interactions of SRIF with TRH and VIP on prolactin and growth hormone secretion in vitro, Endocrinology, 111:42.

Enjalbert, A., and Kordon, C., 1982, Neuropeptides and modulation of adenohypophyseal secretions, in : " Multihormonal Regulations in Neuroendocrine Cells ", Vol. 110, INSERM, Paris.

Enjalbert, A., Rasolonjanahary, R., Moyse, E., Kordon, C., and Epelbaum, J., 1983, Guanine nucleotide sensitivity of [^{125}I]-iodo-NTyr-somatostatin binding in rat adenohypophysis and cerebral cortex, Endocrinology, 113:822.

Enjalbert, A., Ruberg, M., Arancibia, S., Priam, M., Bauer, K., and Kordon, C., 1979a, Inhibition of in vitro prolactin secretion by histidyl-proline-diketopiperazine, a degradation product of TRH, Eur. J. Pharmacol., 58:97.

Enjalbert, A., Ruberg, M., Fiore, L., Arancibia, S., Priam, M., and Kordon, C., 1979b, Effect of morphine on the dopamine inhibition of pituitary prolactin release in vitro, Eur. J. Pharmacol., 53:211.

Enjalbert, A., Ruberg, M., Arancibia, S., Priam, M., and Kordon, C., 1979c, Endogenous opiates block dopamine inhibition of prolactin secretion in vitro, Nature, 280:595.

Enjalbert, A., Ruberg, M., Fiore, L., Arancibia, S., Priam, M., and Kordon, C., 1979d, Independent inhibition of prolactin secretion by dopamine and γ-amino-butyric acid in vitro, Endocrinology, 105:823.

Enjalbert, A., Tapia-Arancibia, L., Rieutort, M., Brazeau, P., Kordon, C., and Epelbaum, J., 1982c, Somatostatin receptors on rat anterior pituitary membranes, Endocrinology, 110:1634

Frey, E. A., Cote, T. E., Grewe, C. W., and Kebabian, J. W., 1982, ^{3}H-spiroperidol identifies a D_2 dopamine receptor inhibiting adenylate cyclase activity in the intermediate lobe of the rat pituitary gland, Endocrinology, 110:1897.

Giachetti, A., Borghi, C., Nicosia, S., and Said, S. I., 1979, Vasoactive intestinal peptide (VIP) activates rat pituitary adenylate cyclase, Fed. Proc., 38:1129.

Giannattasio, G., De Ferrari, M. E., and Spada, A., 1981, Dopamine-inhibited adenylate cyclase in female rat adenohypophysis, Life Sci., 28:1605.

Gourdji, D., Bataille, D., Vauclin, N., Grouselle, D., Rosselin, G., and Tixier-Vidal, A., 1979, Vasoactive intestinal peptide (VIP) stimulates prolactin (PRL) release and cAMP production in a rat pituitary cell line (GH_3/B_6). Additive effects of VIP and TRH on PRL release, FEBS Lett., 104:165.

Gourdji, D., Kerdelhué, B., and Tixier-Vidal, A., 1972, Ultrastructure d'un clone de cellules hypophysaires sécrétant de la prolactine (clone GH_3). Modification induite par l'hormone de libération de l'hormone thyréotrope (TRF), C. R. Acad. Sci. (Paris), 274:437.

Hill, M. K., Mac Leod, R. M., and Orcutt, P., 1976, Dibutyryl cyclic AMP, adenosine and guanosine blockade of the dopamine, ergocryptine and apomorphine inhibition of prolactin release in vitro, Endocrinology, 99:1612.

Iyengar, R., and Birnbaumer, L., 1982, Hormone receptor modulates the regulatory component of adenylate cyclase by reducing its requirement for Mg^{++} and enhancing its extens of activation by guanine nucleotides, Proc. Natl. Acad. Sci. (USA), 79:5179.

Kebabian, J. W., and Cagne, C. B., 1979, Multiple receptors for dopamine, Nature, 277:93.

Kraicer, J., and Chow, A. E. H., 1982, Release of growth hormone from purified somatotrophs. Use of perifusion system to elucidate interrelations among Ca^{++} adenosine, 3', 5'-monophosphate, and somatostatin, Endocrinology, 111:1173.

Login, I. S., and Mac Leod, R. M., 1979, Failure of opiates to reverse dopamine inhibition of prolactin secretion in vitro, Eur. J. Pharmacol., 60:253.

Mac Leod, R. M., 1969, Influence of norepinephrine and catecholamines depleting agents on the synthesis and release of prolactin and growth hormone, Endocrinology, 85:916.

Maurer, R. A., 1982, Adenosine 3', 5'-monophosphate derivates increase prolactin synthesis and prolactin messenger ribonucleic acid levels in ergocriptine-treated pituitary cells, Endocrinology, 110:1957.

Meunier, H., and Labrie, F., 1982, The dopamine receptor in the intermediate lobe of the rat pituitary gland is negatively coupled to adenylate cyclase, Life Sci., 30:963.

Motomatsu, T., Lis, M., Seidan, N., and Chretien, M., 1977, Inhibition by beta-endorphin of dopamine sensitive adenylate cyclase in rat striatum, Biochem. Biophys. Res. Commun., 77: 442.

Munemura, M., Cote, T. E., Tsuruta, K., Eskay, R. L., and Kebabian, J. W., 1980, The dopamine receptor in the intermediate lobe of the rat pituitary gland : pharmacological characteristization, Endocrinology, 107:1676.

Northrup, J. K., Smigel, M. D., and Gilman, A. G., 1982, The guanine nucleotide activating site of the regulatory component of adenylate cyclase. Identification by ligand binding, J. Biol. Chem., 257:11416.

Ojeda, S. R., Harms, P. G., and McCann, S. M., 1974, Possible role of cyclic AMP and prostaglandin E_1 in the dopaminergic control of prolactin release, Endocrinology, 95:1694.

Onalli, P., Schwartz, J. P., and Costa, E., 1981, Dopaminergic modulation of adenylate cyclase stimulation by vasoactive intestinal peptide in anterior pituitary, Proc. Natl. Acad. Sci. (USA), 78:6531.

Robberecht, P., Deschodt-Lanckman, M., Camus, J. C., De Neef, P., Lambert, N., and Christophe, J., 1979, VIP activation of rat anterior pituitary adenylate cyclase, FEBS Lett., 103:229.

Rouleau D., and Barden, N., 1981, Inhibition of anterior pituitary prostaglandin-stimulated adenyl cyclase activity by somatostatin, Can. J. Biochem., 59:307.

Ruberg, M., Rotsztejn, W. H., Arancibia, S., Besson, J., and Enjalbert, A., 1978, Stimulation of prolactin release by vasoactive intestinal peptide (VIP), Eur. J. Pharmacol., 51:319.

Schally, A. V., Redding, T. W., Arimura, A., Dupont, A., and Linthicum, G. L., 1977, Isolation of gamma-amino butyric acid from pig hypothalami and demonstration of its prolactin release-inhibiting (PIF) activity in vivo and in vitro, Endocrinology, 100:681.

Schettini, G., Cronin, M. J., and Mac Leod, R. M., 1983, Adenosine 3', 5'-monophosphate (cAMP) and calcium-calmodulin interrelation in the control of prolactin secretion : evidence for dopamine inhibition of cAMP accumulation and prolactin release after calcium mobilization, Endocrinology, 112:1801.

Schonbrunn, A., and Tashjian, A. H., 1982, Modulation of somatostatin receptors by thyrotropin releasing hormone in a clonal pituitary strain, J. Biol. Chem., 288:190.

Sibley, D. R., and Creese, I., 1979, Guanine-nucleotides regulate anterior pituitary dopamine receptors, Eur. J. Pharmacol., 55:341.

Sibley, D. R., De Lean, A., and Creese, I., 1982, Anterior pituitary dopamine receptors. Demonstration of interconvertible high and low affinity states of the D_2 dopamine receptor, J. Biol. Chem., 257:6351.

Swennen, L., and Denef, C., 1982, Physiological concentrations of dopamine decrease adenosine 3', 5'-monophosphate levels in cultured rat anterior pituitary cells and enriched populations of lactotrophs : evidence for a causal relationships to inhibition of prolactin release, Endocrinology, 111:398.

Tam, S. W., and Dannies, P. S., The role of adenosine 3', 5'-monophosphate in dopaminergic inhibition of prolactin release in anterior pituitary cells, Endocrinology, 109:403.

Tang, L. C., and Cotzias, G. C., 1978, Morphine sulfate stimulates adenylate cyclase in mouse caudate nuclei, Proc. Natl. Acad. Sci. (USA), 75:1546.

Tapia-Arancibia, L., Arancibia, S., Bluet-Pajot, M. T., Enjalbert, A., Epelbaum, J., Priam, M., and Kordon, C., 1980, Effect of vasoactive intestinal peptide (VIP) on somatostatin inhibition of pituitary growth hormone secretion in vitro, Eur. J. Pharmacol., 63:235.

Tashjian, A. H., Barousky, N. J., and Jensen, D. K., 1971, Thyrotropin-releasing hormone : direct evidence for stimulation of prolactin production by pituitary cells in culture, Biochem. Biophys. Res. Commun., 43:516.

Taylor, D. P., and Pert, C. B., 1979, Vasoactive intestinal polypeptide : specific binding to rat brain membranes, Proc. Natl. Acad. Sci. (USA), 76:660.

Vijayan, E., and McCann, S. M., 1980, In vivo and in vitro effects of substance P and neurotensin on gonadotropin and prolactin release, Endocrinology, 105:64.

Westendorf, J. M., and Schonbrunn, A., 1982, Bombesin stimulates prolactin and growth hormone release by pituitary cells in culture, Endocrinology, 110:352.

Wuttke, W., and Düker, E., 1983, Control of pituitary prolactin release, in : " Integrative Neurohumoral Mechanisms ", Endröczi, E. et al. Eds., Elsevier Science Publisher, Amsterdam.

HORMONAL REGULATION OF CASEIN GENE EXPRESSION IN NORMAL AND TRANSFORMED MAMMARY CELLS

Jeffrey M. Rosen, William K. Jones and Li-Yuan Yu-Lee

Department of Cell Biology
Baylor College of Medicine
Houston, TX 77030

INTRODUCTION

The mammary gland provides an excellent model system in which to study the mechanisms by which both steroid and peptide hormones regulate gene expression. Both glucocorticoids and prolactin are required for maximal expression of the milk protein genes, while progesterone antagonizes the inductive effects of these lactogenic hormones. As a necessary prerequisite for elucidating the mechanism of action of these hormones, we have isolated a series of recombinant cDNA and genomic DNA clones encoding three members of the casein multigene family and a fourth, abundant rat milk protein, the whey acidic protein. Complete nucleic acid sequences have been determined for all four of these milk protein mRNAs and for portions of the large and complex, split genes encoding these mRNAs. Comparison of these sequences has revealed three regions of unusual conservation among the rapidly diverging members of the casein gene family. These include the 5' noncoding regions of the mRNAs, the major sites of casein phosphorylation and calcium binding, and the signal peptide sequences. The 5' noncoding region and the signal peptide sequence each appear to be encoded by a separate exon, while the site of phosphorylation is generated by an RNA splicing event. Analysis of the 5' flanking regions of the casein genes revealed several structural features which may represent potential progesterone and glucocorticoid receptor binding sites. All 3 casein genes contain a 16-nucleotide consensus sequence which constitutes part of a palindrome and is homologous with a chicken ovalbumin gene 5' sequence involved in progesterone receptor binding and induction of ovalbumin gene expression. Preferential binding of the chicken progesterone receptor and a 5' flanking DNA fragment of the mammalian γ-casein gene has been demonstrated. Casein genes also contain short nucleotide sequences which share 90% homology with viral transcriptional enhancer core elements. These results will be briefly illustrated in the following presentation.

RESULTS

Hormonal Regulation of Milk Protein Gene Expression

Individual recombinant DNA clones for each of the four abundant rat milk proteins have been used to study the regulation of milk protein gene expression during normal mammary development,[1] in explant cultures in the presence of hormones,[1] and in hormone-dependent mammary tumors.[2] In general the levels of the three casein mRNAs appear to be coordinately regulated during mammary development and during induction by hormones in culture. This is consistent with the observations that the α-, β- and γ-caseins are members of a small multigene family,[3] which is present as a gene cluster[4] on a single mouse chromosome.[5] Some differences were observed, however, in the ratio of the levels of three casein mRNAs in the mammary glands of virgin and lactating rats and in the presence and absence of prolactin in explant cultures. This may reflect differences in the stabilities of the three casein mRNAs observed in the presence and absence of prolactin.[6,7]

The multihormonal regulation of milk protein gene expression is illustrated in Fig. 1. The use of mammary explant cultures derived from midpregnant rats under serum-free, chemically-defined conditions has allowed us to assess the relative importance of both peptide and steroid hormones in the induction of the milk protein mRNAs.[1] Both prolactin and hydrocortisone (in the presence of insulin) are required for the maximal induction of all four milk protein mRNAs.[1] However, a differential effect of hydrocortisone and prolactin was observed on the induction of the whey acidic protein (WAP) and casein mRNAs.[1] Thus, a 68-fold induction of WAP mRNA was observed after 72 hrs of culture with insulin and hydrocortisone as compared to insulin alone, while γ-casein mRNA levels remained unchanged. Following the addition of prolactin for the final 24 hrs of culture WAP mRNA levels further increased 3-fold, while γ-casein mRNA levels were elevated 450-fold. Smaller inductive effects were observed following prolactin addition on the levels of the other two casein mRNAs.[1] This differential response is consistent with the independent origin of the WAP gene and its location on a different chromosome from the members of the casein gene family.[5]

While hydrocortisone potentiates milk protein gene expression, progesterone is known to antagonize milk protein synthesis during pregnancy.[8]

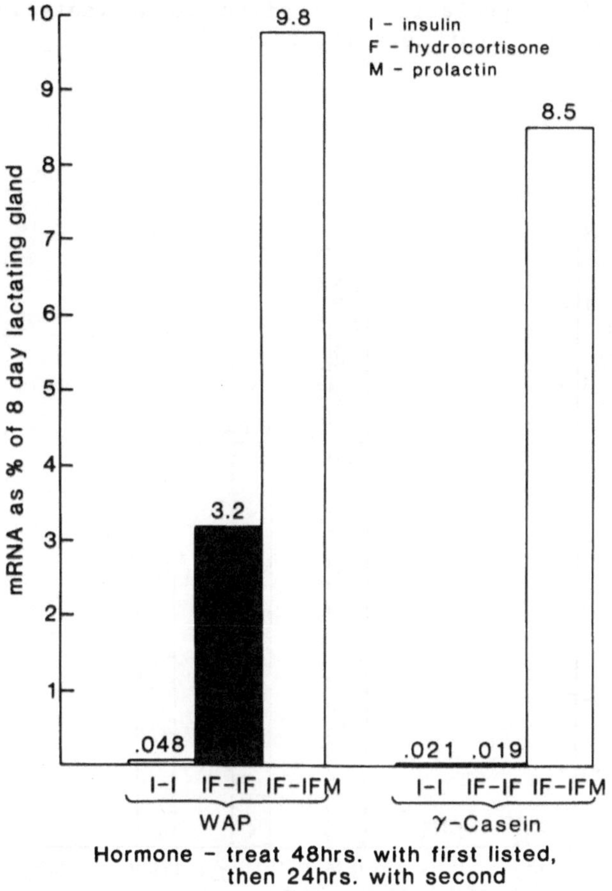

Fig. 1. Hormonal regulation of WAP and casein mRNA levels. Details of this experiments are provided in Hobbs et al., 1982.[1] I=insulin, F=hydrocortisone, M=prolactin.

In both in vivo and in vitro experiments it has been demonstrated that when progesterone is administered prior to, or simultaneously with prolactin, the induction of milk protein synthesis is inhibited.[8,9] Progesterone administration at the end of parturition will delay the onset of lactation.[10] In explant cultures increasing concentrations of progesterone block the prolactin- and hydrocortisone-mediated induction of the α- and β-casein mRNAs (Fig. 2). Approximately, a 50% inhibition is observed when equivalent concentrations of progesterone and glucocorticoids are added to the explant cultures. Interestingly, if progesterone is added 4 hrs after prolactin, or given to a lactating rat, no inhibition of casein synthesis is observed.

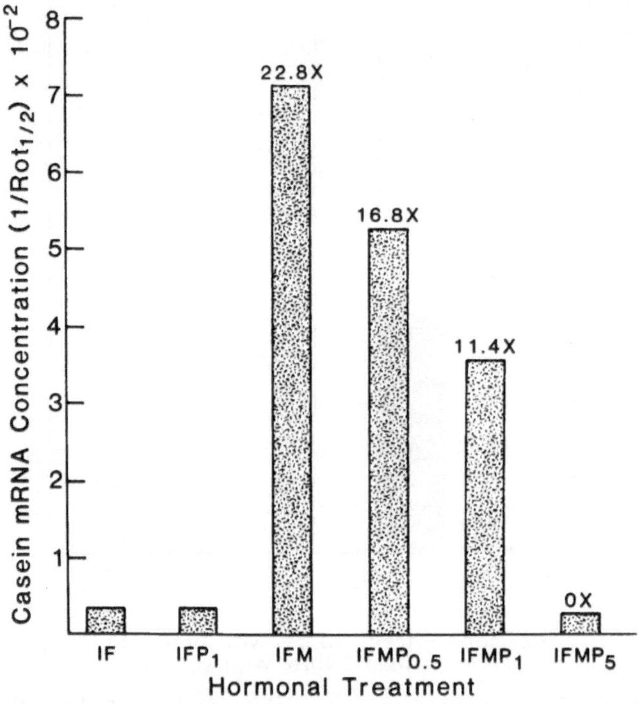

Fig. 2. Progesterone-mediated inhibition of prolactin-induced casein mRNA accumulation. Experimental details are provided in Rosen et al., 1978.[8] P=progesterone. Subscripts indicate the hormonal concentration in μg/ml.

The detailed mechanistic implications of these experiments are unclear at present. However, it appears that progesterone exerts its antagonistic effect by a dual mechanism involving both competition for the binding of glucocorticoids to their receptors, as well as by the direct action of the progesterone-receptor complex on specific gene expression.[8] Support for the second mechanism is provided by the analysis of <u>in vitro</u> binding studies of the chicken progesterone receptor to 5'-flanking regions of the rat casein genes discussed later in this chapter.

Casein Gene Structure

In order to elucidate the mechanism by which steroid and peptide hormones regulate milk protein gene expression, we have isolated and characterized approximately 100 kb of genomic DNA encompassing the α-, β- and γ-casein and the WAP genes. In addition, the complete nucleic acid sequences of the four milk protein mRNAs encoded by these genes has been determined. This permitted the location of the 5' ends of the α- and γ-casein and WAP genes and the analysis of flanking DNA sequences for conserved regions presumably important for hormonal regulation.

Comparison of the mRNA sequences for the calcium-sensitive rat caseins revealed three specific areas showing a high degree of homology among the three casein mRNAs, the sequences encoding the signal peptides, the 5' non-coding regions, and the phosphorylation sites.[3] All of the calcium-sensitive caseins examined to date have a highly conserved 15 amino acid signal peptide sequence, presumably of importance for the efficient secretion of casein. Analysis of the rate of divergence of these conserved sequences has suggested that the casein genes diverged 270-440 million years ago. This supports the hypothesis that the casein gene family arose by gene duplication at about the time of the appearance of the primitive mammals, about 300 million years ago, well before the mammalian radiation which occurred approximately 75 million years ago. The conservation of the 5' non-coding regions of the casein mRNAs may be related in part to functions such as ribosome binding and the initiation of translation. It may also be related to the post-transcriptional regulation by hormones of casein mRNA accumulation. A major effect of prolactin on casein gene expression appears to be mediated by selectively regulating casein mRNA stability. Of interest in this regard is the observation that sequences within the 5' non-coding region of α-casein mRNA capable of stably base-pairing with other regions at the 3' end of the mRNA are conserved in both the guinea pig and bovine α_{s1}-casein mRNAs.[11] A potentially stable stem-loop structure has also been observed in the 5' non-coding region of β-casein mRNA. Thus, regions of secondary structure within the casein mRNAs may be important determinants in regulating their selective stabilization in the presence of hormones.

Support for the concept of functional domains within casein comes from the analysis of the structure of the large and complex casein genes. As illustrated in Fig. 3, the caseins are encoded by large, complex split genes.[12] The γ-casein gene is approximately 15 kb long and is, therefore, 17.4 times larger than the mature γ-casein mRNA. The coding regions of the γ-casein gene are split into at least nine small segments, interspersed with long intervening sequences.

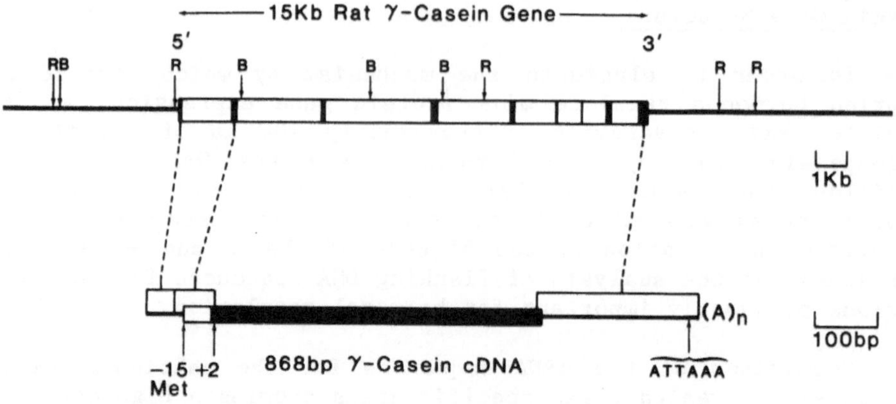

Fig. 3. Strucuture of the rat γ-casein gene.[12] Solid regions indicate exons, and open regions introns within the gene. Flanking sequences are depicted by the solid line. The mRNA sequence is shown below with the dashed lines depicting the positions of the exons. The solid bar is the region encoding the mature protein, the open region the signal peptide, and the solid lines indicate the 5' and 3' non-coding regions of the mRNA, respectively.

The first exon is 44 nucleotides long and encodes the majority of the 5' non-coding region of the mRNA, while the second exon is 62 nucleotides long and encodes the entire signal peptide sequence and the first two amino acids of the mature γ-casein. An identical arrangement for the first two exons has also been observed in the α-casein gene with the splice junctions occurring at the same positions. Thus, both the highly conserved 5' non-coding region and the signal peptide sequence are encoded by a separate exon. This supports both hypotheses that these may be important functional domains that were "recruited" during the evolution of the primordial casein gene, and that the members of the casein gene family have arisen by a process of intergenic duplication of a primordial gene.

Examination of the third region of conservation within the calcium-sensitive caseins, the phosphorylation sties, indicates that most sites contain a variable number of serine residues followed by two glutamic acid residues, e.g., ser-ser-ser-glu-glu. Comparison of the nucleic acid sequences of all of the phosphorylation sites in the rat casein which conform to this sequence indicates that there are two types of serine codon, AGX and TCX, which can each accept silent mutations, but cannot be interconverted without a transition form in which the codon no longer codes for a serine residue. Thus, if there is a selection pressure to retain serine residues, the distribution of the types of serine codons should be retained. In general, the distribution of serine codons has been retained in all the phosphorylation sites analyzed to date in rat, mouse, guinea pig and bovine caseins. Also of interest is the observation that the sequence coding for the two glutamic acid residues, GAGGAA, is identical in all the phosphorylation sites. The conservation of the nucleotide sequences of the phosphorylation sites, at least within the α- and γ-casein mRNAs, supports the suggestion that the caseins have arisen by a series of internal duplications. According to this hypothesis the primordial casein gene may have evolved by intragenic duplication of a sequence coding for a phosphorylation site. This is difficult to establish by analyzing only the cDNA sequence, but recent studies of the rat β-casein gene support this hypothesis. One exon contains the major phosphorylation site for β-casein ending with an intron between the two glutamic acid codons (Fig. 4).

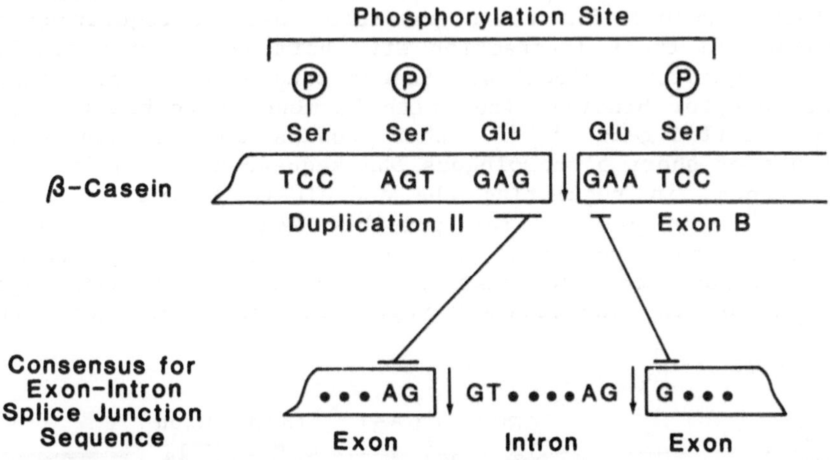

Fig. 4. Exon structure of the conserved β-casein phosphorylation site. The vertical arrows indicate the positions of splice junctions.

The reason for the conservation of the positions of the glutamic acid codons is apparent if one compares these codons to the consensus sequence derived for intron-exon splice junctions.[13] Thus, the GAG at the 5' junction is required because of the conserved AG at the 5' splice junction, and the GAA in the second glutamic codon is the 3' codon because of the conserved G at the 3' junction. If the positions of these two codons were reversed, the consensus sequence at the 5' junction would be lost and aberrant splicing would occur. Thus, there may be significant pressure to retain this particular codon arrangement for efficient splicing of the casein mRNAs. In the absence of this splicing event, a functional recognition sequence for the casein kinase would not be generated preventing both the phosphorylation and efficient calcium binding of the caseins. Analysis of the 5' sequences of both the rat and bovine α- and β-casein mRNAs, therefore, supports the hypothesis that the casein gene family has arisen by a process of intergenic duplication of a primordial site of calcium binding and phosphorylation. Thus, the evolution of the casein gene family appears to have involved processes of intragenic and intergenic duplication, recruitment of 5' non-coding and signal peptide domains and possibly 3' hydrophobic and non-coding domains. In addition, the rat and mouse casein mRNAs have undergone the insertion of an apparent transposable element which is composed of a series of 18 base pair repeats.[3]

Possible Regulatory Elements Involved in the Hormonal Regulation of the Rat Casein Gene Family

DNA sequences in the 5' flanking regions of several genes have been examined for their possible role in regulating gene expression via their interaction with hormone receptor complexes or other regulatory molecules. Recent studies have correlated 5' hormone receptor binding sites with hormone inducible transcription of specific genes.[14-19] Other studies have demonstrated the importance of short 5' homologous DNA sequences, specific to each set of genes, in regulating the coordinate expression of gene families.[20] In looking for possible regulatory elements, we searched for both potential hormone receptor binding sites and other homologous sequences that existed in the 5' flanking regions of members of the coordinately regulated rat casein gene family (Fig. 5).

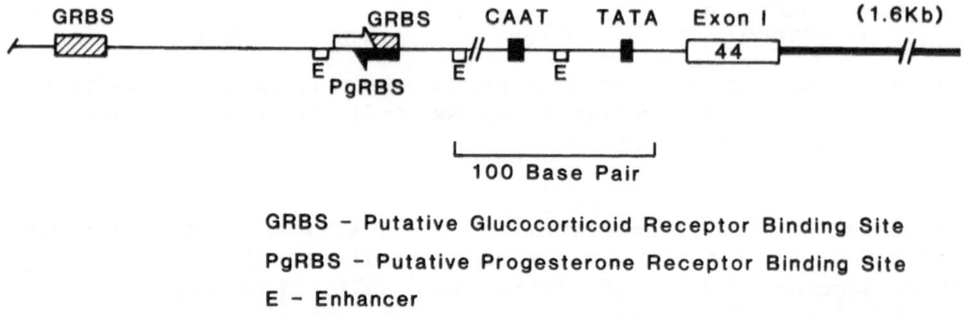

Fig. 5 Putative steroid hormone receptor binding sites and enhancer sequences at the 5' end of the rat γ-casein gene.

The α- and γ-casein (and the WAP) genes share the same unusual TATA signal, TTTAAAT, while only the γ-casein gene appears to contain a weak CAAT sequence as previously described.[12] The transition of an A to a C, T or G in the second position of the TATA sequence has been demonstrated to reduce the efficiency of this promoter sequence.[21] Further upstream in the γ-casein gene 5' flanking region is a 33-nucleotide palindrome sequence (head-to-head arrows) which shares homology with a sequence at the 5' end of the chicken ovalbumin gene. This sequence has been shown to be involved in progesterone receptor binding by DNase I footprinting[19,22] as well as in progesterone-mediated induction of ovalbumin gene expression by gene transfection experiments.[16] Only one half (about 20 nucleotides) of the γ-casein palindrome shares extensive homology with the putative ovalbumin progesterone receptor binding site (PgRBS), while the other half exhibits a greater sequence divergence. These two sequences form an imperfect palindrome and may represent putative PgRBS in the γ-casein gene flanking region.

Since all three casein genes are regulated by progesterone, we searched for possible progesterone receptor binding sites in the other casein genes.[23] Two overlapping sequences spanning 36 nucleotides in the α-casein flanking region were found to share sequence homology with the putative γ-casein gene PgRBS. These shared sequences are in contrast to a lack of homology observed in the remainder of the flanking DNA sequences between the two genes. A 31-nucleotide sequence located in the 5' region of the β-casein gene also shows extensive homology with the putative PgRBS in the γ-casein gene. All of the casein sequences seem to share a 16-nucleotide consensus sequence, 5'-TATGCAATATGTTTT$^{A}_{T}$-3'. This 16-nucleotide sequence may be involved in the coordinate regulation by progesterone of casein gene expression, analogous to the regulation of other gene families by their respective, short 5' homologous sequence elements.[20] Direct DNA binding studies have demonstrated that there is preferential binding of the chicken progesterone receptor A subunit to a γ-casein flanking DNA fragment containing the putative rat PgRBS.[23] Preferential binding of avian progesterone receptor to the γ-casein DNA is comparable to that demonstrated with a similarly-sized ovalbumin DNA fragment.[23]

Multiple glucocorticoid receptor binding sites have been shown to be present in several glucocorticoid-responsive genes by direct DNA binding studies *in vitro*[17,18] as well as by gene transfection studies *in vivo*.[14,15] As depicted in Fig. 5, about 170 bp upstream from the γ-casein palindrome structure is a 25-nucleotide sequence which shares homology with a sequence in the long terminal repeat (LTR) region of the mouse mammary tumor virus (MMTV). This sequence has been demonstrated to be a glucocorticoid receptor binding site (GRBS), and is contained within the LTR region required for glucocorticoid regulation as determined by gene transfection experiments.[14,15] A second region exhibiting a considerable homology with the MMTV LTR GRBS is the complementary strand of half of the γ-casein palindrome. Interestingly, a putative GRBS in the α-casein gene flanking region also overlaps the putative PgRBS. The 16-nucleotide casein consensus sequence which may be associated with progesterone receptor binding is also homologous with part of the MMTV LTR GRBS. Whether the two steroid hormone receptor complexes bind the same DNA sequence or not in vivo is unknown. The dual binding sites may explain the antagonistic effects of glucocorticoids (stimulatory) versus progesterone (inhibitory) on casein gene expression during pregnancy. The antagonism may be due to the competition between the two hormone-receptor complexes for an overlapping DNA binding site as well as the competition of the two steroid hormones for binding sites on the same receptor molecule.

Aside from potential steroid hormone receptor binding sites, both casein genes also contain short nucleotide sequences which share 90% homology with viral enhancer core elements (E).[23,24] Enhancer elements can act in either orientation, as well as upstream or downstream of a promoter and over considerable distances, in stimulating eukaryotic gene transcription. Interestingly, these enhancer sequences flank the putative γ-casein PgRBS sequence and may act as entry sites for regulatory molecules such as the progesterone receptor complex or other DNA binding proteins. Alternatively, the binding of the progesterone-receptor complex may alter the activity of enhancers, as first proposed by Parker[25] for the glucocorticoid activation of the MMTV LTR enhancer. Again, the proximity of enhancer-like sequences to steroid hormone receptor binding sites may indicate a coordinate role of these putative regulatory elements on casein gene expression.

Perhaps the most interesting observation is that the putative steroid hormone receptor binding sites represent the only observed regions of flanking DNA sequence homology between the α- and γ-casein genes, in sharp contrast to the complete lack of conservation in the rest of the flanking sequences. The putative PgRBS sequences are palindromes and part of the PgRBS sequences overlap the putative GRBS. This unique arrangement of sequences found in both the γ- and α-casein flanking region may underlie a simple mechanism of antagonism between progesterone and glucocorticoid action on casein gene expression. How prolactin fits into this scheme is unknown. It is noted that no other conserved sequences, which may represent potential prolactin relay or second messenger binding sites, have been detected. The relationships of these observed sequence homologies and conservation to hormonal control of gene expression remains to be established. Whether the enhancer-like sequences found in close association with either the 5' promoter elements and/or the putative steroid hormone receptor binding sites, have any effect on gene transcription in vivo is also unknown. However, it is possible that the family of rat casein genes is controlled in a coordinate fashion by a unique set of DNA sequences which interact with regulatory molecules such as hormone receptors or other proteins. We are presently conducting gene transfection experiments to test the function of these putative regulatory sequences on casein gene expression.

ACKNOWLEDGEMENT

This research was supported by NIH grant CA16303. The excellent technical assistance of Elizabeth Richter and Craig Couch, as well as the typing expertise of Patricia Kettlewell, is greatly appreciated.

REFERENCES

1. A.A. Hobbs, D.A. Richards, D. Kessler, and J.M. Rosen, J. Biol. Chem. 257:3598 (1982).
2. M.L. Johnson, J. Levy, S.C. Supowit, L.-Y. Yu-Lee, and J.M. Rosen, J. Biol. Chem. 258:10805 (1983).
3. A.A. Hobbs and J.M. Rosen, Nucl. Acids Res. 10:8079 (1983).
4. V.S. Matyukov and A.P. Urnyshev, Genetika 16:884 (1980).
5. P. Gupta, J.M. Rosen, P. D'Eustachio, and F.H. Ruddle, J. Cell Biol. 93:199 (1982).
6. W.A. Guyette, R.J. Matusik, and J.M. Rosen, Cell 17:1013 (1979).
7. J.R. Rodgers and J.M. Rosen, unpublished observations.
8. J.M. Rosen, D.L., O'Neal, J.E. McHugh, and J.P.Comstock, Biochemistry 17:290 (1978).
9. R.J. Matusik and J.M. Rosen, J. Biol. Chem. 253:2343 (1978).
10. R.T. Chatterton, Jr.,W.T. King, D.A. Ward, and J.L. Chien, Endocrinology 96:861 (1975).
11. T.L. Brown and J.M. Rosen, unpublished observations.
12. L.-Y. Yu-Lee and J.M. Rosen, J. Biol. Chem. 258:10794 (1983).
13. R. Breathnach and P. Chambon, Ann. Rev. Biochem. 50:349 (1981).
14. V.L. Chandler, B.A. Maler, and K.R. Yamamoto, Cell 33:489 (1983).
15. N. Hynes, A.J.J. van Ooyen, N. Kennedy, P. Herrlich, H. Ponta, and B. Groner, Proc. Natl. Acad. Sci. USA 80:3637 (1983).
16. D.C. Dean, B.J. Knoll, M.E. Riser, and B.W. O'Malley, Nature 305:551 (1983).
17. M. Pfahl, D. McGinnis, M. Hendricks, B. Groner, and N. Hynes, Science 222:1341 (1983).
18. C. Scheidereit, S. Geisse, H.M. Westphal, and M. Beato, Nature 304:749 (1983).

19. J.G. Compton, W.T. Schrader, and B.W. O'Malley, Proc. Natl. Acad. Sci. USA 80:16 (1983).
20. E.H. Davidson, H.T. Jacobs, and R.J. Britten, Nature 301:468 (1983).
21. M. Concino, R.A. Goldman, M.H. Caruthers, and R. Weinmann, J. Biol. Chem. 258:8493 (1983).
22. J.G. Compton, W.T. Schrader, and B.W. O'Malley, submitted for publication.
23. L.-Y. Yu-Lee, W.K. Jones, J.G. Compton, W.T. Schrader, and J.M. Rosen, submitted for publication.
24. N. Rosenthal, M. Kress, P. Gruss, and G. Khoury, Science 222:749 (1983).
25. M. Parker, Nature 304:687 (1983).

IN VIVO REGULATION BY ESTRADIOL OF THE MESSENGER RNAs ENCODING LH AND FSH SUBUNITS AND THE SECRETION OF GONADOTROPINS

Raymond Counis, Maithé Corbani and Marian Jutisz

Laboratoire des Hormones Polypeptidiques, CNRS
91190 Gif sur Yvette, France

1. Introduction

Gonadotropins are glycoproteins composed of two dissimilar, non-covalently linked α- and β-subunits. Within a given species, the amino acid sequences of the α-subunits of LH and FSH are identical, while those of the hormone specific β-subunits differ (Pierce and Parsons, 1981).

Using the translation of rat, ovine and bovine pituitary poly(A^+)mRNAs in a cell-free system, we and others have recently shown that gonadotropin subunits (α, LHβ, FSHβ) are synthesized as precursors encoded by separate messengers (for bibliography see Jutisz et al., 1983). Recently, cDNAs for the α-subunit of rat (Godine et al., 1982) and bovine (Nilson et al., 1983) pituitary glycoprotein hormones and rat LHβ (Chin et al., 1983) have been cloned and sequenced. Further, evidence has been obtained that gonadectomy in female rats (Counis et al., 1982a,b,c), in male sheep (Alexander and Miller, 1982) and in ewes (Landefeld et al., 1983) results in the enhancement of precursors to α, LHβ and FSHβ encoded by specific mRNAs. These results suggest that gonadal steroids can regulate the level of specific mRNAs. Indeed, treatment of gonadectomized animals with 17β-estradiol (E_2) reverses the effect of gonadectomy (Alexander and Miller, 1982 ; Counis et al., 1983a,b ; Landefeld et al., 1983).

As a continuation of our study on the regulation of the expression of specific genes coding for gonadotropin subunits, we have prepared mRNAs from anterior pituitaries of male and female rats at different times following gonadectomy. Using the cell-free translation of these mRNAs, we have studied the time-dependent post-operative increase of the precursors to gonadotropin subunits α, LHβ and FSHβ. In parallel, we have determined, by radioimmunoassay, LH release in the same rats. Furthermore, using synthetic oligodeoxynucleotides (15-16 bases) corresponding to partial sequences of α, LHβ and FSHβ as probes, we have demonstrated that the number of copies of specific mRNAs was higher in gonadectomized as compared to normal rats. This observation confirmed our hypothesis that estradiol negatively regulates the synthesis of gonadotropin subunits via changes in specific mRNA levels.

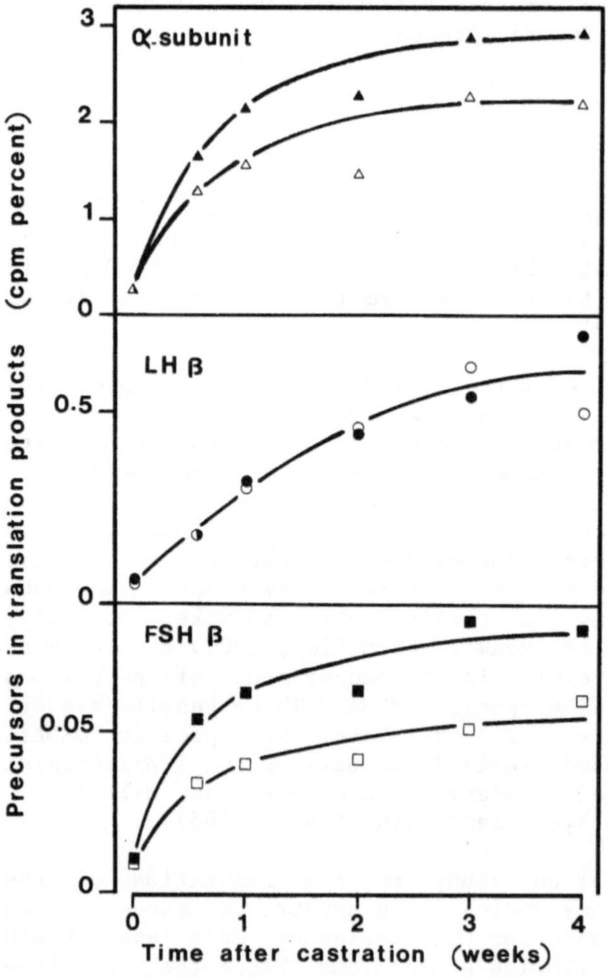

Figure 1. Time-course of the gonadectomy-induced increase in gonadotropin subunit precursor levels (α, LHβ,FSHβ) in the cell free translation media using pituitary mRNAs derived from gonadectomized adult male (solid symbols) and female (open symbols) rats, sacrificed at appropriate post-operative delays. Messenger RNAs were translated in the presence of ^{35}[S] Met and ^{35}[S] Cys and the precursors to subunits were isolated by immunoprecipitation and SDS-PAGE. Precursor levels are expressed as cpm per cent of total radioactive proteins. See the text for details.

2. Gonadectomy-induced increase in translational potency of mRNAs encoding gonadotropin subunits is a time-dependent process.

Figure 1 shows the time-course of the gonadectomy-induced increase in gonadotropin subunit precursor (α, LHβ and FSHβ) levels in the cell-free translation media using pituitary mRNAs derived from gonadectomized adult male and female rats, sacrificed at appropriate post-operative delays (Corbani et al., 1984). Messenger RNAs were extracted in parallel from pituitary glands in each group and translated in the presence of ^{35}S-labeled methionine and cysteine. Precursors were isolated from the translation media by immunoprecipitation with specific sequential antisera and electrophoresis on SDS-polyacrylamide slab gels (SDS-PAGE). Bands corresponding to precursors were excised and counted after solubilization. Precursor levels are expressed as cpm per cent of total radioactive proteins. In both, gonadectomized male and female rats, the rate of synthesis of the α precursor increased rapidly until 7 days after surgery and more slowly afterwards, until about 21 days, when a plateau was reached. The maximal increase was slightly greater in the male than in the female (about 25 % higher). In the case of LHβ, precursor synthesis increased after castration somewhat slower than for α-precursor and reached a plateau after 3 weeks. No significant difference was detected in either the kinetics or the relative values between males and females. Increase in FSHβ-precursor was comparable to that of α-precursor. However, due to the low values of radioactivity incorporated into FSHβ-precursor, the difference between males and females was difficult to determine.

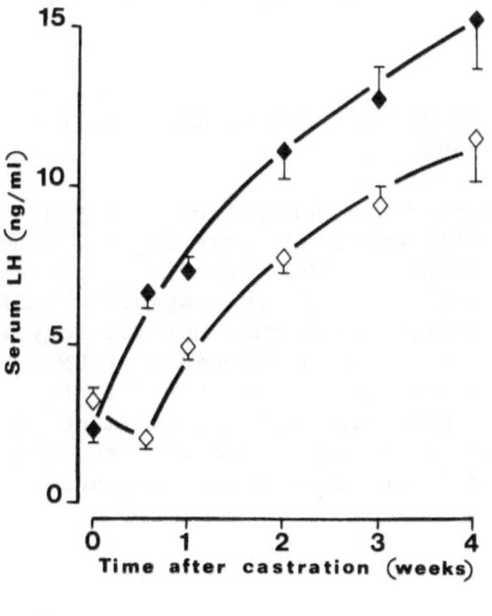

Figure 2. Time-course of the gonadectomy-induced increase in serum LH in gonadectomized adult male (solid symbols) and female (open symbols) rats, sacrificed at appropriate post-operative delays.

3. Does the post-gonadectomy increase in the rate of synthesis of the precursors correlate with the simultaneous enhancement in LH release ?

Figure 2 shows the time-course of the gonadectomy-induced, well known increase in serum LH. LH levels increased rapidly in the male from about 2 ng/ml in normal rats to more than 15 ng/ml 28 days after surgery. In the female, LH levels decreased until the 4th day (from 3.2 to 2 ng/ml) and then increased to about 12 ng/ml 28 days after ovariectomy. In addition, LH levels were always somewhat higher in the male than in the female.

Comparing the time dependence of the post-gonadectomy increase in LH release and in LH subunit precursor synthesis, some similarities and divergencies can be observed. In the male rats, the time-course of LH release paralleled the post-operative pattern of the synthesis of LH subunit precursors during the first 7 days, while in the female, the release of LH was somewhat delayed as compared to the synthesis of LH precursors. Subsequently, serum LH continued to increase in both males and females, even after 28 days (data not shown), the rate of synthesis of precursors to LH subunits slowed down starting from about 7 days post-castration and plateaued 14 days later. Thus, after gonadectomy when an increase in the translational capacity of mRNAs encoding LH subunits as well as in the release of LH was observed, no evidence was provided for a direct, closely dependent relationship between the two. Though some interconnections might exist between the two phenomena, it is evident that the synthesis and release of gonadotropins are relayed via different mechanisms, which implies they are regulated in different manners. However, it is clear that gonadectomy affects synthesis as well as release of gonadotropins, by consistently stimulating both processes.

4. Gonadectomy increases the amount of each of the specific mRNAs encoding α, LHβ and FSHβ.

In order to investigate whether the control of the synthesis of gonadotropin subunits by estradiol occurs by lowering the number of copies of the specific mRNAs coding for the subunit precursors or by decreasing the messenger activity of the specific mRNAs present, we used the cDNA hybridization technique. Our strategy was first to chemically synthesize oligodeoxynucleotides (ODNs) of 15-16 bases with a nucleotide sequence complementary to a portion of each specific mRNA. Considering that some regions of amino acid sequences in α, LHβ and FSHβ from different species are highly conserved (Pierce and Parsons, 1981), we deduced the sequences of ODNs to be synthesized.

LHα : amino acid sequence	...	^{33}MET -	GLY -	CYS -	CYS -	PHE^{37} ...
mRNA (all possible codons)	...	$^{5'}$<u>AUG</u> -	GGC -	UGC -	UGC -	UUC$^{3'}$ ...
			U	U	U	U
			A			
			G			
Complementary ODNs	...d	TAC -	CCG -	ACG -	ACG -	AAG$^{5'}$ ...
			A	A	A	A
			T			
			C			
hCGα - cDNA (Fiddes and Goodman, 1979)	...d	TAC -	CCG -	ACG -	ACG -	AAG$^{5'}$ ...
Rat LHα - cDNA (Godine et al., 1982)	...d	TAC -	CCG -	ACA* -	ACG -	AAG$^{5'}$ ...
15-mer ODN synthesized :	$_{3'}$d	TAC -	CCG -	ACA -	ACG -	AAG$^{5'OH}$

Figure 3. Deduction of the specific sequence of a 15-mer oligodeoxynucleotide complementary to mRNA of rat α subunit, taking as a model the cDNA of hCGα. The amino acid sequence 29-33 in hCGα was selected.

In order to circumvent any ambiguity due to variations in the codons used for some amino acid residues in the chosen pentapeptide sequences, we took as a model the sequence of cDNAs coding for hCGα and hCGβ as determined by Fiddes and Goodman (1979, 1980).

Figure 3 shows the way of deducing the sequence of a specific oligodeoxynucleotide probe corresponding to residues 29-33 in the amino acid sequence of hCGα. This sequence is conserved in all known pituitary glycoprotein α subunits from different species. (Pierce and Parsons, 1981). Due to the degeneracy of genetic code, excepting for methionine which possesses only one codon, all other amino acid residues of this sequence have at least 2 or even 4 codons as in the case of glycine. Among all possible complementary ODNs, we first selected the sequence contained in cDNA corresponding to hCGα (Fiddes and Goodman, 1979). Meanwhile, before starting synthesis of the chosen 15-mer ODN, we have been aware of work in which the nucleotide sequence of cloned cDNA corresponding to rat pre-α subunit was published (Godine et al., 1982). This latter sequence shows that in this particular region, a G in the cDNA corresponding to hCGα is replaced by an A in the rat pre-α cDNA (see Fig. 3). Consequently, this latter 15 oligomer ODN was finally selected and synthesized.

Very similar strategies were used to deduce and synthesize a 16-base oligomer corresponding to LHβ and a 15-base oligomer corresponding to FSHβ.

The three synthetic ODNs were 5'-end labeled with ^{32}P and their hybridization to specific messengers was tested. Rat and ovine pituitary poly(A^+) and poly(A^-) RNAs were first separated by agarose gel electrophoresis, transferred on a solid support (gene screen, NEN) and then hybridized with the ^{32}P-labeled ODNs.

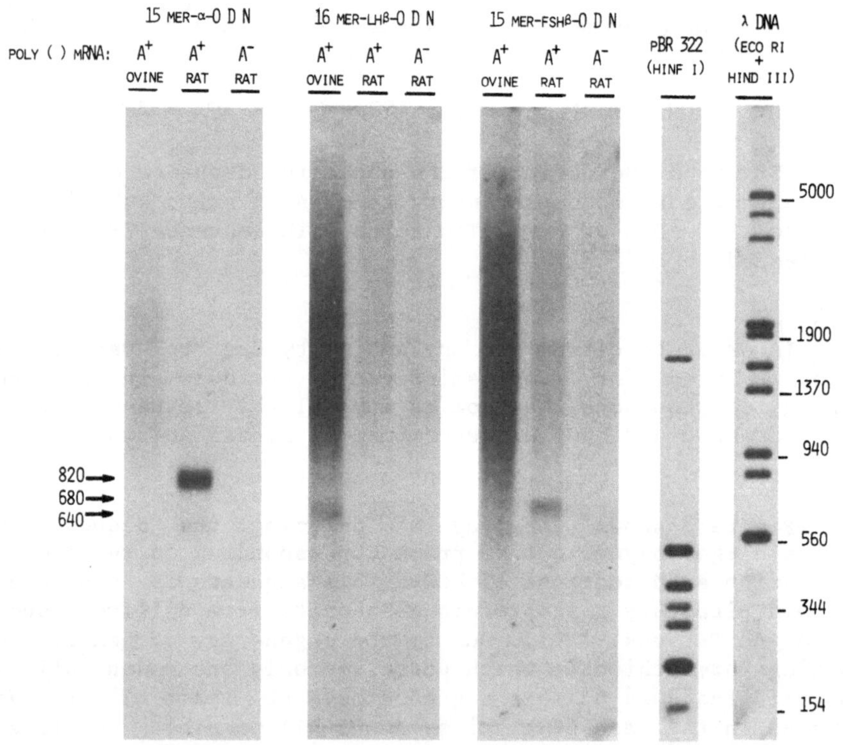

Figure 4. Autoradiograph after transfer of rat and ovine pituitary poly (A^+) and poly (A^-) RNAs and hybridization with ^{32}P-labeled oligodeoxynucleotides specific to a part of the sequence of mRNAs encoding α, LHβ and FSHβ. Glyoxal-denatured RNAs were first separated by agarose gel electrophoresis then transferred on a solid support (gene screen, NEN) for hybridization. On the right are reference DNAs with their nucleotide numbers.

Figure 4 presents an autoradiograph of the filters after hybridization and subsequent washing. It shows that : 1) the oligomers hybridized only to poly(A^+)RNAs ; 2) the 15-mer ODNs corresponding to α as well as to FSHβ only hybridized with a single mRNA sequence of rat pituitary origin; their positions indicate that they contain approximately 820 and 680 bases, respectively ; 3) the 16-mer ODN corresponding to LHβ hybridized only to an ovine mRNA of about 640 nucleotides.

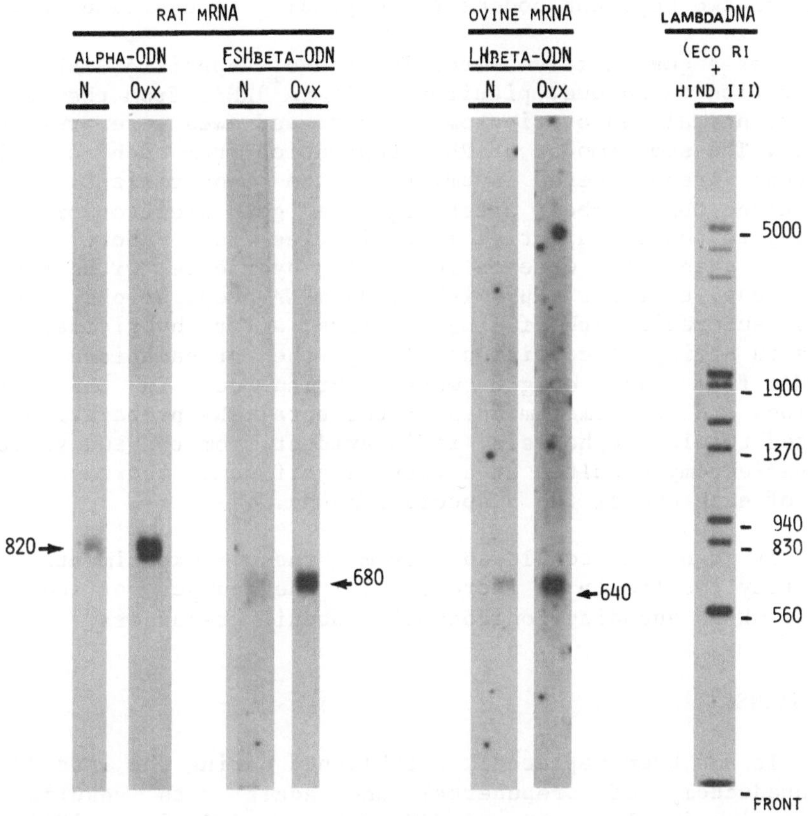

Figure 5. Autoradiograph of the filters after transfer of pituitary poly (A^+) RNAs derived from normal (N) and ovariectomized (ovx) adult rats and ewes and hybridization with ^{32}P-labeled oligodeoxynucleotides. Oligomers were specific to a part of the sequence on mRNAs encoding α, LHβ and FSHβ. RNAs were extracted in parallel from the pituitary tissue of normal and castrated animals. Messenger RNAs were glyoxal-denatured, separated by agarose gel electrophoresis and transferred to a solid support (gene screen, NEN) for hybridization. On the right are reference DNAs with their nucleotide numbers.

These results demonstrate that the hybridization of oligomers is highly specific ; only one or two mismatches in a 15 to 16-base oligomer sequence might be sufficient to prevent hybridization, or to render the hybrid unstable (Wallace et al., 1979 ; Wallace et al., 1981). Furthermore, it appears that even in the case of the highly conserved amino acid sequences of the pituitary glycoproteins, the gene contains cryptic mutations. The best example of such a mutation is in the region of 29-33 residues in hCGα. Although this amino acid sequence is exactly the same in hCGα as in rat α (33-37 residues), a mutation occured in the DNA in one of the two adjacent codons corresponding to cysteine residues.

For a quantitative determination of specific mRNAs using hybridization technique, pituitary poly (A^+)RNAs from the same series of normal and ovariectomized rats and ewes were prepared in parallel. The same amount of RNA preparation from each normal and castrated group were submitted to hybridization with ^{32}P-labelled ODN probes after agarose gel electrophoresis. According to their respective specificities (see above) the ODN probes for α and FSHβ were allowed to hybridize with rat mRNA preparations, that for LHβ, with ovine mRNA preparations. Figure 5 shows an autoradiograph of the filters after hybridization and washing in stringent conditions. Though the preparations of poly (A^+)mRNAs from each origin were carried out in the same conditions and the same amounts of the total RNA preparations were submitted to electrophoresis, it is evident from the autoradiograph that ovariectomy resulted in a very significant increase in the amount of each one of the 3 specific mRNAs.

It can be concluded from these experiments, that ovariectomy results in an increase in the number of copies of specific mRNAs encoding gonadotropin subunit precursors.

CONCLUSIONS

It has been repeatedly established during the last 20 years that gonadectomy of prepubertal and adult rats results in a dramatic rise in plasma LH and FSH (McCann and Ramirez, 1964 ; see also the review by Schally et al., 1972a). It has been also reported that serum LH concentrations increase more rapidly following orchidectomy than following ovariectomy (Gay and Midgley, 1969 ; Yamamoto et al., 1970). Although it was shown many years ago that estradiol exerts both positive and negative feedback on the release of LH (reviewed by Everett, 1964 ; Davidson, 1969), the mechanism of estrogen action as well as the sites of the estrogen effect are still controversial. Most of the evidence obtained _in vivo_ suggests that the negative feedback of estrogen on LH secretion occurs principally on the hypothalamus rather than the pituitary gland (Lisk and Newlon, 1963). However, in vitro, studies using either isolated rat pituitaries (Schally et al., 1972b) or rat pituitary cells in culture (Debeljuk et al., 1978) demonstrate that a part of the negative feedback on LH and FSH secretion is exerted directly at the hypophysis.

Recent studies from our laboratory (Counis et al., 1983a, b) showed that a single s.c. injection of 25 µg 17β-estradiol (but not of progesterone injected alone or in combination with E_2) into ovariectomized rats, dramatically reduced, 48h after administration, the synthesis of all three gonadotropin subunit precursors, α, LHβ and FSHβ, produced in cell-free conditions by pituitary mRNAs. Inhibition of the translational capacity of the mRNAs encoding the precursors was nearly 80 %. Similar data on the inhibition of the synthesis of FSHβ (Alexander and Miller, 1982) and α (Landefeld et al., 1983) subunits with estradiol in castrated sheep have been reported. These results strongly suggest that the synthesis of α, LHβ and FSHβ precursors is negatively controlled by E_2 and that specific mRNAs coding for all three subunits are regulated by this steroid. Preliminary data obtained more recently in our laboratory (unpublished results) indicate that other gonadal steroids also participate in this regulation and that some of them have selective effects.

These studies of the time-course (during a 4 week period) of the gonadectomy-induced increase in gonadotropin subunit precursor levels as well as serum levels of LH show that, 1) the rate of synthesis of the precursors increased rapidly up to 7 days after surgery, then slower until reaching a plateau at about 21 days ; 2) LH levels increased at about a constant rate during the four weeks after surgery and even afterwards ; 3) although, no direct correlation seems to exist between the two phenomena, it is evident that both are dependent on gonadal steroids, which affect through different routes, but consistently, the synthesis of gonadotropin subunits and the release of gonadotropins.

Besides gonadal steroids, the secretion of gonadotropins is regulated by numerous factors and mainly by the hypothalamic GnRH. It is well known that gonadectomy in both male and female rats results in a significant elevation of circulating GnRH (Wheaton and McCann, 1976). Further, the number of pituitary GnRH receptors also increases in gonadectomized rats (Frager et al., 1981; Clayton and Catt, 1981 ; Aubert et al., 1983). The increase in GnRH and in its pituitary receptors certainly contribute to the elevation in serum LH, but also probably to the stimulation of gonadotropin synthesis (Khar et al., 1978).

In conclusion, estradiol and other gonadal steroids, affect both the synthesis and the release of pituitary gonadotropins, where their regulatory role appears essential. In the case of the synthesis of gonadotropins, estradiol negatively regulates the expression of specific genes encoding all three subunit precursors. However it is not known at present whether estradiol is involved or not in the cellular processing of gonadotropins. In gonadectomized rats of both sexes, a simultaneous dramatic increase in gonadotropin subunit synthesis as well as in LH release can be observed, the two processes being regulated in different ways. Their patterns, which present some similarities in the early stages after surgery, diverge later. Finally, our results clearly demonstrate that ovariectomy results, probably among several effects, in an increase in the number of copies of specific mRNAs encoding gonadotropin subunit precursors. The resulting increase in the synthesis of LH and FSH subunit precursors, together with their subsequent processing into authentic hormones, is certainly an essential factor for the chronic increase in their post-castration release.

SUMMARY

Using the translation of rat and ovine pituitary poly(A^+) mRNAs in a cell-free system, we previously showed that gonadotropin subunits (α, LHβ, FSHβ) are synthesized as precursors encoded by separate messengers. Further, evidence has been obtained that gonadectomy increases the rate of synthesis of subunits by 10 to 15 fold, thus suggesting the involvement of steroids in this process. We recently demonstrated that this effect of gonadectomy was significant as soon as 4 days after surgery. The rate of synthesis of the precursors increased rapidly up to 7 days, then more slowly until reaching a plateau at 21 days. Radioimmunoassay of circulating LH following gonadectomy showed the hormone increased at about a constant rate during the first 4 weeks after castration. Although no direct correlation seems to exist between the two processes, it is evident that both are dependent on gonadal steroids, which affect through different routes, but consistently the synthesis of gonadotropin subunits and the release of LH. Supplementation of gonadectomized rats with estradiol rapidly reversed the stimulatory effect of gonadectomy almost to the levels observed in normal rats. In order to check whether estradiol regulates the expression of subunit genes by lowering the number of copies of the specific mRNAs, oligodeoxynucleotides (15-16 bases) corresponding to partial sequences of the α, LHβ and FSHβ genes were synthesized. These oligomers hybridized with corresponding mRNA sequences with a high specificity and were species specific. Using these oligomers as probes, we have demonstrated that the gonadectomy effects result from an increase in the intracellular pool of each of the specific mRNAs, thus suggesting a probable role for gonadal steroids at genomic level.

ACKNOWLEDGEMENTS

We wish to thank the National Hormone and Pituitary Program (NIADDK) and Dr A. Parlow for rat LH RIA kit, Dr J.G. Pierce for his gift of antisera to RCMX bovine LH subunits, Drs A. Bérault and M. Théoleyre for their help in performing RIA and Mr M. Poissonnier for his help in preparing antisera to RCXM ovine α, LHβ and FSHβ. The valuable technical assistance of Mme G. Ribot is acknowledged. M.C. is a recipient of a Fondation pour la Recherche Medicale fellowship. This work was supported by a grant from Fondation de Recherche en Hormonologie.

REFERENCES

Alexander, D.C., and Miller, W.L., 1982, Regulation of ovine follicle-stimulating hormone β-chain mRNA by 17β-estradiol in vivo and in vitro . J. Biol. Chem. , 257 : 2282-2286.

Aubert, M.L., Conne, B.S., Winniger, B.P., Lang, U., and Sizonenko, P.C., 1983, Hormonal regulations of pituitary GnRH binding sites, in "Multihormonal Regulations in Neuroendocrine Cells", A. Tixier-Vidal and P. Richard, eds., pp.319-346, INSERM, Paris (INSERM Symposium no 110, Colmar, France, 1-4 september 1982).

Chin, W.W., Godine, J.E., Klein, D.R., Chang, A.S., Lee, K.T., and Habener, J.F., 1983, Nucleotide sequence of the cDNA encoding the precursor of the β subunit of rat lutropin, Proc. Natl. Acad. Sci. USA, 80 : 4649-4653.

Clayton, R.N., and Catt, K.H., 1981, Regulation of pituitary gonadotropin-releasing hormone receptors by gonadal hormones. Endocrinology , 108 : 887-895.

Corbani, M., Counis, R., Starzec, A., and Jutisz, M., 1984, Effect of gonadectomy on pituitary levels of mRNA encoding gonadotropin subunits and secretion of luteinizing hormone. Mol. Cell. Endocrinol. , (in press).

Counis, R., Corbani, M., Poissonnier, M., and Jutisz, M., 1982a, Characterization of the precursors of α and β subunits of follitropin following cell-free translation of rat and ovine pituitary mRNAs, Biochem. Biophys. Res. Chem. 107 : 998-1005.

Counis, R., Corbani, M., Ribot, G., and Jutisz, M.,1982b, Cell-free synthesis of rat lutropin subunits, in "Hormonally active Brain Peptides : Structure and Function", K.W. McKerns and V. Pantic, eds., pp. 567-579, Plenum Press, New York.

Counis, R., Corbani, M., and Jutisz, M., 1982c, Studies on cell-free biosynthesis of lutropin (LH) and characterization of its subunit precursors, in : "Pituitary Hormones and Related Peptides", M. Motta, M. Zanisi and F. Piva, eds., pp. 49-61, Academic Press, London and New York.

Counis, R., Corbani, M., and Jutisz, M., 1983a, Régulation de la biosynthèse des gonadotropines hypophysaires, in "Multihormonal Regulations in Neuroendocrine Cells", A. Tixier-Vidal and P. Richard, eds., pp. 509-523, INSERM, Paris (INSERM Symposium no 110, Colmar, France, 1-4 September 1982).

Counis, R., Corbani, M., and Jutisz, M., 1983b, Estradiol regulates mRNAs encoding precursors to rat lutropin (LH) and follitropin (FSH) subunits, Biochem. Biophys. Res. Commun., 114 : 65-72.

Davidson, J.M., 1969, Feedback control of gonadotropin secretion, in : "Frontiers in neuroendocrinology", W.F. Ganong and L. Martini, eds., pp. 343-388, Oxford University Press, New York.

Debeljuk, L., Khar, A., and Jutisz, M., 1978, Effects of gonadal steroids and cycloheximide on the release of gonadotrophins by rat pituitary cells in culture, J. End., 77 : 409-415.

Everett, J.W., 1964, Central neural control of reproductive functions of the adenohypophysis, Physiol. Rev., 44 : 373-431.

Fiddes, J.C., and Goodman, H.M., 1979, Isolation, cloning and sequence analysis of the cDNA for the α-subunit of human chorionic gonadotropin, Nature, 281 : 351-356.

Fiddes, J.C., and Goodman, H.M., 1980, The cDNA for the β-subunit of human chorionic gonadotropin suggests evolution of a gene by readthrough into the 3'-untranslated region, Nature, 286 : 684-687.

Frager, M.S., Pieper, D.R., Tonetta, A., Duncan, J.A., and Marshall, J.C., 1981, Pituitary gonadotropin-releasing hormone receptors : Effects of castration, steroid replacement, and the role of gonadotropin-releasing hormone in modulating receptors in the rat. J. Clin. Invest., 67 : 615-623.

Gay, V.L., and Midgley, A.R., 1969, Response of the adult rat to orchidectomy and ovariectomy as determined by LH radioimmunoassay Endocrinology, 84 : 1359-1364.

Godine, J.E., Chin, W.W., and Habener, J.F., 1982, α subunit of rat pituitary glycoprotein hormones. Primary structure of the precursor determined from the nucleotide sequence of cloned cDNAs, J. Biol. Chem., 257 : 8368-8371.

Jutisz, M., Counis, R., and Corbani, M., 1983, Biosynthesis of pituitary gonadotropins and its regulation by gonadoliberin (GnRH) and estradiol, in "Regulation of target cell responsiveness", K.W. McKerns, ed., Plenum Press, New York, (in press).

Khar, A., Debeljuk, L., and Jutisz, M., 1978, Biosynthesis of gonadotropins by rat pituitary cells in culture and in pituitary homogenates : Effect of gonadotropin-releasing hormone, Mol. Cell. Endocrinol. , 12 : 53-65.

Landefeld, T.D., Kepa, J, and Karsch, F.J., 1983, Regulation of α subunit synthesis by gonadal steroid feedback in the sheep

Lisk, R.D., and Newlon, M.,1963, Estradiol: evidence for its direct effect on hypothalamic neurons , Science , 139 : 223-224.

McCann, S.M., and Ramirez, V.D., 1964, The neuroendocrine regulation of hypophyseal luteinizing hormone secretion. Rec. Progr. Hormone Res. , 20 : 131-181.

Nilson, J.H., Thomason, A.R., Cserbak, M.T., Moncman, C.L., and Woychik, R.P., 1983, Nucleotide sequence of cDNA for the common α subunit of the bovine pituitary glycoprotein hormones, J. Biol. Chem. , 258 : 4679-4682.

Pierce, J.G., and Parsons, T.F., 1981, Glycoprotein hormones : structure and function, Ann. Rev. Biochem. 50 : 465-495.

Schally, A.V., Kastin, A.J., and Arimura, A., 1972a, FSH-releasing hormone and LH-releasing hormone, Vitamins and Hormones , 30 : 83-164.

Schally, A.V., Redding, T.W., Matsuo, H., and Arimura, A., 1972b, Stimulation of FSH and LH release in vitro by natural and synthetic LH and FSH releasing hormone, Endocrinology 90 : 1561-1568.

Wallace, R.B., Shaffer, J., Murphy, R.F., Bonner, J., Hirose, T., and Itakura, K., 1979, Hybridization of synthetic oligodeoxynucleotides to ϕX 174 DNA : The effect of single base pair mismatch, Nucleic Acids Res. , 6 : 3543-3557.

Wallace, R.B., Johnson, M.J., Hirose, T., Miyake, T., Kawashima, E.H., and Itakura, K., 1981, The use of synthetic oligo nucleotides as hybridization probes. II. Hybridization of oligonucleotides of mixed sequence to rabbit β-globin DNA, Nucleic Acids Res. , 9 : 879-894.

Wheaton, J.E., and McCann, S.M., 1976, Luteinizing hormone-releasing hormone in peripheral plasma and hypothalamus of normal and ovariectomized rats, Neuroendocrinology 20 : 296-310.

Yamamoto, M., Diebel, N.D., and Bogdanove, E.M., 1970, Analysis of initial and delayed effects of orchidectomy and ovariectomy on pituitary and serum LH levels in adult and immature rats, Endocrinology , 86 : 1102-1111.

FOLLICLE STIMULATING HORMONE REGULATION OF PHOSPHODIESTERASE AND CELL RESPONSE

M. Conti, R. Geremia, M.V. Toscano
and M. Stefanini

Institute of Histology and General Embryology
University of Rome, Rome, Italy

INTRODUCTION

In the last decade a large body of work has focused on the mechanisms of action of protein hormones. Properties of receptors, receptor-hormone interaction, activation of adenylate cyclase, and initiation of the cAMP-dependent cascade have been described in many systems in great detail. Conversely, little attention has been devoted to the termination of the hormonal stimulus, and little is known about the mechanisms that govern this process. There is now abundant evidence that hormone binding to the receptor is not always completely reversible (1-3), and in some instances a stable hormone-receptor complex is internalized in the cell (4-8). Therefore dissociation of the hormone from its receptor can no longer be considered the primary cause of the cessation of the hormonal stimulation. In addition to stimulating the function of their targets, it has also become clear that hormones induce profound changes in the response of the cells (9) so that repeated exposure to the same hormone leads to an attenuated response (refractoriness). The boundary between the mechanisms of regulation of cell response and cessation of the primary stimulation is not clearly defined, and it is possible that both are aspects of a common phenomenon.

In those systems in which the signal evoked by the formation of the hormone-receptor complex is translated into an elevation of intracellular cyclic nucleotides, the most obvious cause of the attenuation of the hormonal effect is a decrease in the intracellular concentration of these second messenger molecules. Since it has been generally recognized that "desensitization" of the adenylate cyclase is a common event that follows an agonist stimulation (9-10), it is probable that cessation of cyclic nucleotide synthesis plays an important role in the return of the cyclic nucleotide levels to basal values. Equally important, however, appear to be those mechanisms that reduce cyclic nucleotides levels by degradation and by escape outside the cell. Escape of cyclic nucleotides from the cell is a common finding in hormone responsive systems, but it is not known how relevant this is to cellular regulation. In the intracellular environment, phosphodiesterase is the only known enzyme that inactivate cyclic nucleotides by degradation. Only recently has it become clear that hormones are able to regulate phosphodiesterases (11-12), and therefore they control cell function by regulating cyclic nucleotide degradation.

In this chapter, the FSH regulation of phosphodiesterase in Sertoli and granulosa cells will be briefly reviewed, and more recent studies on the correlation of changes of phosphodiesterase activity with changes in cell responsiveness will be reported.

FSH REGULATION OF PHOSPHODIESTERASE IN THE SERTOLI CELL

Incubation of cultures of immature Sertoli cells with FSH produces an elevation of intracellular cAMP and a host of effects that include the stimulation of synthesis and secretion of protein and the activation of steroid metabolism (13). Among the described modifications of Sertoli cell function are marked effects of gonadotropin on phosphodiesterase (14-16). FSH has a biphasic effect on phosphodiesterase activity of the Sertoli cell, as shown in Fig.1. During the first 30 min of hormone treatment, FSH produces a decrease in the phosphodiesterase activity measured in total cell homogenate. These early FSH inhibitory effects on phosphodiesterase are similar to those reported by Fakunding et al. (17) and might represent a mechanism of potentiation of the hormone action. Thus, elevation of intracellular cAMP in the Sertoli cell is caused by stimulation of cAMP synthesis through activation of the adenylate cyclase and by inhibition of cAMP catabolism through inhibition of phosphodiesterase. The inhibition of phosphodiesterase is followed by a delayed but marked stimulation of the enzyme activity (Fig. 1). This stimulation of phosphodiesterase requires ongoing protein and RNA synthesis since both cycloheximide and actinomycin D

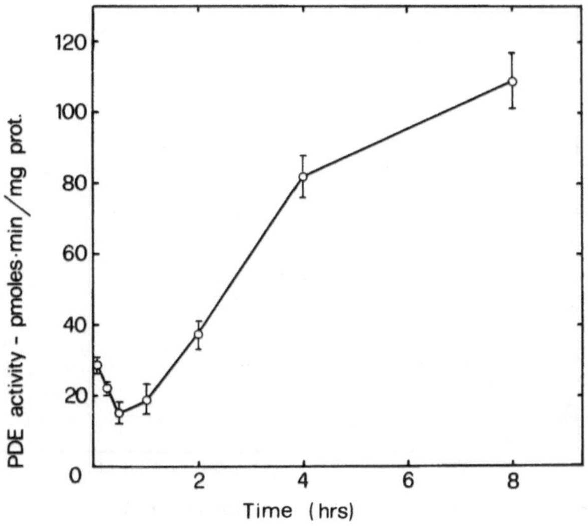

Fig.1 FSH regulation of Sertoli cell phosphodiesterase activity
Ovine FSH-S14 was added to Sertoli cell culture at 0 time and incubation prolonged for the indicated times. PDE activity was measured in the cell homogenate using 1 µM cAMP as substrate.

have been shown to completely abolish hormonal stimulation (14-16). If phosphodiesterase activity is measured with cGMP as substrate, the hormonal stimulation is no longer detected (14,16).

The mechanism by which FSH regulates the phosphodiesterase activity of the Sertoli cell probably requires the mediatory role of cAMP. In fact, it has been shown that activation of the phosphodiesterase temporally follows the peak of intracellular cAMP, and MIX potentiates the FSH effect (16). When intracellular cAMP levels are raised by incubating the cells with the analog dibutyryl cAMP, a marked stimulation of phosphodiesterase is observed. There is also a strong positive correlation between the FSH-dependent cAMP accumulation and the induction of phosphodiesterase activity (Fig. 2). In addition, β-adrenergic agonists and cholera-toxin, which are known to elevate the intracellular cAMP of the Sertoli cell (13,18), also produce a stimulation of phosphodiesterase (15,16). Thus, it appears that the phosphodiesterase activity is markedly elevated as a consequence of sustained cAMP levels. This is also consistent with the finding that removal of the stimulatory agents

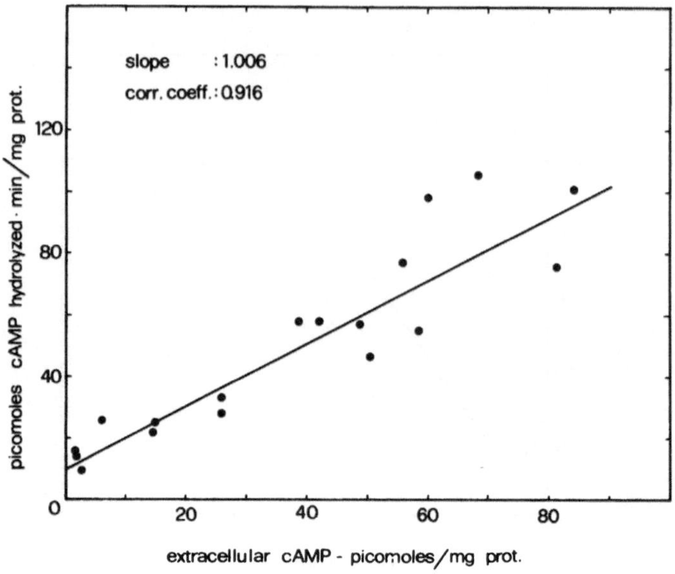

Fig.2 Correlation between FSH dependent stimulation of phosphodiesterase and cAMP accumulation

Sertoli cells were incubated with graded FSH doses for 24 hrs, after which medium was used for cAMP-RIA while PDE activity was measured in the cell homogenate with 1 μM cAMP as substrate.

leads to a reversal of the phosphodiesterase stimulation (16).

Like many other cells and organs, Sertoli cells possess multiple forms of phosphodiesterase; in most mammalian cells, three different forms have been isolated (12). The first form, called cGMP phosphodiesterase, hydrolyses cGMP with high affinity, and its activity is stimulated by Ca^{++} and calmodulin. The second form, present only in rod outer segments and liver and lung cells, is a cyclic nucleotide phosphodiesterase whose activity is stimulated by cGMP and is called cGMP binding phosphodiesterase. The third form is insensitive to Ca^{++} and calmodulin and usually hydrolyses cAMP with higher affinity than cGMP and is called "low K_m" cAMP phosphodiesterase. Sertoli cell soluble extract apparently possesses only two of the three forms mentioned (16); these forms have characteristics similar to the cGMP phosphodiesterase and to the low K_m phosphodiesterase (Table 1). When the phosphodiesterase activity of cells treated with FSH for 24 hrs and the activity of untreated

Table 1. Characteristics of the forms of phosphodiesterase present in the soluble extract of Sertoli and granulosa cells.

	Sertoli cells		Granulosa cells	
	cGMP PDE (Peak1)	cAMP PDE (Peak2)	cGMP PDE (Peak1)	cAMP PDE (Peak2)
K_m cGMP	3.5 μM	-	1.5 μM	-
K_m cAMP	23 μM	1.8 μM	6.7 μM	2.0 μM
	-	-	60 μM	-
Kinetics cAMP	linear	linear	non linear two sites	linear
Kinetics cGMP	linear	-	linear	-
Calmodulin stim.	yes	no	yes	no
FSH stimulation	no	yes	yes	yes

cells are compared by DEAE-cellulose chromatography, it appears that FSH treatment stimulates selectively the activity of the second form without affecting the cGMP phosphodiesterase (16). In agreement with these findings, dbcAMP, shown to stimulate total Sertoli cell phosphodiesterase, also stimulates only the low K_m phosphodiesterase. The latter finding is similar to early reports that cAMP analogs and phosphodiesterase inhibitors stimulate the phosphodiesterase activity in hepatoma and glioma cell lines (19,20).

The stimulatory effects of FSH on phosphodiesterase are not only observed in vitro. Marked stimulation of testicular phosphodiesterase follows prolonged FSH treatment of immature male rats (21). Such stimulation is detected in the seminiferous tubules, but FSH has no effect on the phosphodiesterase activity of the interstitium. It is likely that the increased phosphodiesterase activity observed in the seminiferous tubules is due to an FSH stimulation of the Sertoli cell, since FSH treatment stimulates phosphodiesterase activity of the seminiferous tubules depleted of germ cells by irradiation in utero (data not shown). Confirming the observations in vitro, the enzyme affected by the FSH treatment is a high affinity, low K_m cAMP phosphodiesterase (21).

FSH REGULATION OF GRANULOSA CELL PHOSPHODIESTERASE

Since granulosa cells of the ovarian follicle share many similarities with Sertoli cells, it has been studied whether FSH, which regulates the metabolism and differentiation of these cells, acts on phosphodiesterase in a manner similar to that observed in the Sertoli cell. FSH treatment of granulosa cells from immature, hypophysectomized diethylstilbestrol treated animals has an effect similar to that observed in the Sertoli cell; although an initial decrease is not detected, after a time lag of 1 hr hormone treatment produces a marked stimulation of phosphodiesterase reaching an apparent plateau in 6-48 hrs (22). Again, dbcAMP has an effect similar to FSH, and MIX potentiates the gonadotropin stimulation. In agreement with other reports on the lack of hCG effect on the preantral granulosa cells, hCG does not stimulate phosphodiesterase (22). The FSH effect on granulosa cell phosphodiesterase is also dose-dependent, and inhibitors of protein synthesis block the hormonal stimulation (22).

The forms of phosphodiesterase present in the granulosa cell have also been characterized by ion exchange chromatography, and they appear to be similar to those present in the Sertoli cell extract (22). As shown in Table 1, a high affinity cGMP-calcium-calmodulin-dependent enzyme (peak 1) is present together with a low K_m phosphodiesterase (peak 2). Again, FSH treatment for 48 hrs produces a marked stimulation of the low K_m phosphodiesterase. However, unlike that observed in Sertoli cells, the activity of the first peak appears to be elevated when assayed with Ca^{++} and calmodulin. It can be speculated that FSH either renders this enzyme more sensitive to Ca^{++}-calmodulin stimulation or induces the appearance of a new form of phosphodiesterase with the characteristics of a high affinity, cAMP-Ca^{++}-calmodulin-dependent enzyme. The latter hypothesis is of particular interest since only recently such an enzyme has been isolated in tissues such as the testis and the spleen (12). Experiments so far performed to reevaluate the FSH effect on the Sertoli cell have given a negative result, and it is not clear why stimulation of this form is undetectable in the cells of the male gonad.

INVOLVEMENT OF PHOSPHODIESTERASE IN THE REGULATION OF CELL RESPONSE

Once established that gonadotropin regulates the phosphodiesterase activity of its target cells, the question to be answered is whether this regulation has any physiological importance in the process of the termination of hormonal stimulus or in the refractoriness of the target cell (reduced cAMP response measured in the intact cell). The consistent finding that FSH affects the activity of a phosphodiesterase form that hydrolyses cAMP with high affinity is by itself suggestive that marked changes in cAMP turnover are to be expected after hormonal stimulation.

Sertoli cells, like most other target cells, enter a refractory state after FSH treatment, and a second hormonal treatment is no longer effective in stimulating intracellular cAMP accumulation (23). Previous studies have shown that receptor down-regulation (24) and adenylate cyclase desensitization (24,25) accompany the loss of responsiveness of the intact cell. Studies undertaken to characterize this refractory state have indicated that indeed a correlation can be established between the altered Sertoli cell response and the FSH regulation of phosphodiesterase (25). First, the time course of the onset of refractoriness is compatible with the time course of the stimulation of phosphodiesterase (25). Using 500 ng/ml FSH, refractoriness becomes evident after two hours and reaches a maximum in 4-8 hrs. Similarly, phosphodiesterase stimulation is not detected until 2 hrs after the addition of hormone, and it approaches a maximum in 4-8 hrs. Second, a comparison of the ability of different stimulatory agents to induce Sertoli cell refractoriness and to stimulate phosphodiesterase shows that in no instance can refractoriness be induced without a concomitant stimulation of the phosphodiesterase activity (Table 2). Conversely, there is evidence that refractoriness is apparently not always associated with desensitization of adenylate cyclase (Table 2, see also below). Third, refractoriness of the Sertoli cell in terms of cAMP accumulation can be markedly reduced by inhibitors of phosphodiesterases (Fig. 3). In fact, cells apparently rendered insensitive to hormone, once incubated in the presence of 1 mM MIX, recover the ability to respond to FSH. The effect of xanthine is dose dependent, and half maximal stimulation is obtained at 200-300 μM MIX (data not shown). The less potent xanthine, theophylline, is equally effective in restoring the hormonal stimulation of the FSH-dependent cAMP accumulation (25).

Table 2. Comparison of the effect of different treatments on the phosphodiesterase (PDE) and adenylate cyclase (AC) activity and the intact cell cAMP response of the Sertoli cell.

Treatment	PDE stimulation	AC desensitization	cAMP refractoriness
FSH	+	+	+
Isoproterenol	+	+	+
MIX	±	-	±
Choleratoxin	+	ND	+
dbcAMP	+	±	+

ND: not determined

Another set of experiments carried out in different conditions is also suggestive of phosphodiesterase involvement in cell refractoriness. As previously mentioned, inhibitors of protein synthesis block the FSH-dependent stimulation of phosphodiesterase (14-16). In agreement with this finding, cycloheximide partially prevents the onset of the FSH-dependent refractoriness (25). It is speculated that when the increase of the phosphodiesterase activity is prevented, the onset of cell refractoriness is also prevented. Since adenylate cyclase desensitization is not affected by inhibition of protein synthesis (25), the partial refractoriness present in cells treated with FSH+cycloheximide is apparently due to adenylate cyclase desensitization.

The above mentioned studies indicate that the decreased cAMP accumulation in the refractory Sertoli cell is caused by a decreased cAMP synthesis consequent to adenylate cyclase desensitization and to an increased cAMP catabolism caused by the stimulation of the high affinity phosphodiesterase. On a quantitative basis, phosphodiesterase appears to contribute to refractoriness as much as the adenylate cyclase desensitization, at least at the doses of FSH employed to induce refractoriness. Phosphodiesterase stimulation might be even more determinant in the induction of refractoriness at very low doses of gonadotropin. It has been observed, in fact, that at nanogram doses of FSH, refractoriness of the cell is associated with stimulation of phosphodiesterase but not with desensitization of the adenylate cyclase (25).

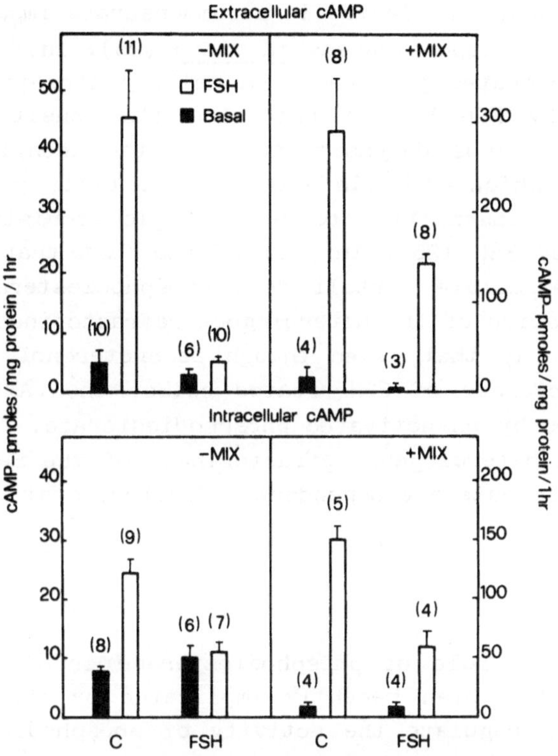

Fig.3 Effect of MIX on the response of the refractory Sertoli cell
Cells were preincubated for 4 hrs with 500 ng/ml FSH. At the end of this preincubation cells were rinsed and restimulated for 1 hr with 10 μg/ml FSH in the absence or presence of 1 mM MIX. At the end of the second incubation, intracellular and extracellular cAMP were measured by RIA (25). Each bar represents the mean ± se (N).

A further detailed evaluation of the properties of the Sertoli cell and its regulation suggest another phenomenon probably caused by the FSH-dependent regulation of phosphodiesterase. Sertoli cells not only respond to FSH, but also possess a receptor-cyclase system sensitive to β-adrenergic agonists (18). Thus, these cells respond to β-adrenergic agents such as isoproterenol with an increase in cAMP production and in protein and steroid secretion. It has also been reported that refractoriness induced by FSH pretreatment causes an impaired response of the cell to both FSH and isoproterenol (23,25). This heterologous refractoriness of the intact cell, however, is not reflected in a commensurate impairment of the adenylate cyclase responsiveness in vitro (25). In fact, adenylate cyclase of homogenates prepared from cells pretreated with FSH is not activated by FSH but it maintains its sensitivity to isoproterenol (homologous desensitization of the adenylate cyclase). In a similar fashion, adenylate cyclase of cells pretreated with isoproterenol is insensitive to B-adrenergic agonists, but it can be stimulated by FSH (25). In view of the fact that both FSH and isoproterenol stimulate Sertoli cell phosphodiesterase, the most probable explanation of the heterologous refractoriness observed in the intact cell is that, even though isoproterenol can stimulate the adenylate cyclase of FSH-treated cells, the cAMP produced is rapidly degraded by an activated phosphodiesterase. Thus it can be speculated that heterologous refractoriness of the Sertoli cell is a "pure" phosphodiesterase-dependent refractory state.

CONCLUSIONS

The mediatory role of phosphodiesterase in the mechanism of hormone action has been recently implicated by the finding that several hormones regulate the activity of phosphodiesterases. The gonadotropin FSH appears to have marked effect on the phosphodiesterases of cells of the male and female gonads. Thus, gonadotropin not only regulates cAMP synthesis by activating the adenylate cyclase, but it can also regulate cAMP catabolism by modulating the activity of phosphodiesterase. FSH has been shown to suppress cAMP response of the Sertoli cell by activating a high affinity cAMP phosphodiesterase. The process of refractoriness induced by gonadotropin then appears to be a complex phenomenon composed of regulations that operate at different levels of the hormone dependent cascade. In the Sertoli cell, these include: 1) regulation of receptor number (down-regulation); 2) desensitization of the adenylate cyclase; 3) stimulation of phosphodiesterase; and 4) stimulation of the synthesis of a protein kinase inhibitor (26).

ACKNOWLEDGMENT

This work was supported by CNR finalized project M.P.R. Grant N. 82.02317.56 and by Ministero Pubblica Istruzione, 1st and 2nd University of Rome.

REFERENCES

1. Kahn, C.R., and Baird, K., The fate of insulin bound to adipocytes. Evidence for compartmentalization and processing, J. Biol. Chem. 253:4900 (1978).
2. Linsley, P.S., Blifeld, C., Wrann, M., and Fox, C.F., Direct linkage of epidermal growth factor to its receptor, Nature 278:745 (1979).
3. van der Gugten, A.A., Waters, J., Murthy, G.S., and Friesen, H.G., Studies on the irreversible nature of prolactin binding to receptors, Endocrinology 106:402 (1980).
4. Carpenter, G., and Cohen, S., ^{125}I-Labeled human epidermal growth factor. Binding, internalization, and degradation in human fibroblasts, J. Cell Biol. 71:159 (1976).
5. Goldfine, I.D., Smith, G.J., Wong, K.Y., and Jones, A.L., Cellular uptake and nuclear binding of insulin in human cultured lymphocytes: evidence for potential intracellular sites of insulin action, Proc. Natl. Acad. Sci. USA 74:1368 (1977).
6. Conn, P.M., Conti, M., Harwood, J.P., Dufau, M.L., and Catt, K.J., Internalization of gonadotropin receptors complexes in ovarian luteal cells, Nature 274:598 (1978).
7. Amsterdam, A., Berkowitz, A., Nimrod, A., and Kohen, F., Aggregation of luteinizing hormone receptors in granulosa cells: a possible mechanism of desensitization to the hormone, Proc. Natl. Acad. Sci. USA 77:3440 (1980).
8. Pastan, I.H., and Willingham, M.C., Journey to the center of the cell: role of the receptosome, Science 214:504 (1981).
9. Catt, K.J., Harwood, J.P., Aguilera, G., and Dufau, M.L., Hormonal regulation of peptide receptors and target cell responses, Nature 280:109 (1979).
10. Caron, H.G., Limbird, L.E., and Lefkowitz, R.J., Biochemical characterization of the β-adrenergic receptor for the frog erytrocyte, Mol. Cell. Biochem. 28:45 (1979).
11. Thompson, J.W., and Strada, S.J., Hormonal regulation of cyclic nucleotide phosphodiesterase, in: "Receptors And Hormone Action", L. Birnbaumer, B.W. O'Malley eds., p. 553, Academic Press, New York (1978).
12. Beavo, J.A., Hansen, R.S., Harrison, S.A., Hurwitz, R.L., Martins, T.J., and Mumby, M.C., Identification and properties of cyclic nucleotide phosphodiesterases, Mol. Cell. Endocrinol. 28:387 (1982).
13. Dorrington, J.H., and Armstrong, D.T., Effect of FSH on gonadal function, Rec. Prog. Horm. Res. 35:301 (1979).

14. Conti, M., Geremia, R., Adamo, S., and Stefanini M., Regulation of Sertoli cell cyclic adenosine 3':5' monophosphate phosphodiesterase activity by follicle stimulating hormone and dibutyryl cyclic AMP, Biochem. Biophys. Res. Commun. 98:1044 (1981).
15. Verhoeven, J., Cailleau, J., and de Moor, P., Hormonal control of phosphodiesterase activity in cultured rat Sertoli cells, Mol. Cell. Endocrinol. 24:41 (1981).
16. Conti, M., Toscano, M.V., Petrelli, L., Geremia, R., and Stefanini, M., Regulation by Follicle-Stimulating Hormone and dibutyryl Adenosine 3':5'-monophosphate of a phosphodiesterase isoenzyme of the Sertoli cell, Endocrinology 110:1189 (1982).
17. Fakunding, J.L., Tindall, D.J., Dedman, J.R., Mena, C.R., and Means, A.R., Biochemical actions of follicle-stimulating hormone in the Sertoli cell of the rat testis, Endocrinology 98:392 (1976).
18. Verhoeven,G., Dierickx,P. and de Moor,P., Stimulation effect of neurotransmitters on the aromatization of testosterone by Sertoli cell-enriched cultures, Mol.Cell.Endocrinol. 13:241(1979).
19. Uzunov, P., Shein, H.M., and Weiss, B., Cyclic AMP phosphodiesterase in cloned astrocytoma cells: norepinephrine induces a specific enzyme form, Science 180:304 (1973).
20. Ross, P.S., Manganiello, V.C., and Vaughan, M., Regulation of cyclic nucleotide phosphodiesterases in cultured hepatoma cells by dexamethasone and N^6,O^2-dibutyryl adenosine 3':5'-monophosphate, J. Biol. Chem. 252:1448 (1977).
21. Conti, M., Toscano, M.V., Geremia, R., and Stefanini, M., Follicle-stimulating hormone regulates in vivo testicular phosphodieasterase, Mol. Cell. Endocrinol. 29:79 (1983).
22. Conti, M., Kasson, B.G., and Hsueh, A.J.W., Hormonal regulation of 3',5'-adenosine monophosphate phosphodiesterases in cultured rat granulosa cells, submitted for publication.
23. Verhoeven, G., Cailleau, J. and de Moor, P., Desensitization of cultured rat Sertoli cells by Follicle-Stimulating Hormone and by L-isoproterenol, Mol. Cell. Endocrinol. 20:113 (1980).
24. O'Shaughnessy, P.J., FSH receptor autoregulation and cyclic AMP production in the immature rat testis, Biol. Reprod. 23:810 (1980).
25. Conti, M., Toscano, M.V., Petrelli, L., Geremia, R., and Stefanini, M., Involvement of phosphodiesterase in the refractoriness of the Sertoli cell, Endocrinology 113 (1983) in press.
26. Tash, J.S., Welsh, M.J., and Means, A.R., Regulation of protein kinase inhibitor by Follicle-Stimulating Hormone in Sertoli cells in vitro. Endocrinology 108:427 (1981).

REGULATION OF STEROIDOGENIC ACTIVITIES IN LEYDIG CELLS BY LH AND AN LHRH AGONIST

Focko F.G. Rommerts, Rinkje Molenaar, Axel P.N. Themmen and Henk J. van der Molen

Department of Biochemistry (Division of Chemical Endocrinology), Medical Faculty, Erasmus University Rotterdam, The Netherlands

INTRODUCTION

Regulation of steroidogenesis in Leydig cells is the result of interactions between stimulatory and inhibitory processes regulated by protein hormones, peptides and steroid hormones. Investigations of isolated intact Leydig cells can assist in the elucidation of the individual regulating systems, provided that specific steps of the complete process can be measured, inhibited or activated. The mechanism of action of LH on Leydig cells has been studied for many years and much information has been obtained about the initial events. It is now generally accepted that LH stimulation of steroid production involves a concomitant increase in cAMP-dependent protein kinase and phosphorylation of various specific proteins. It is not clear yet if, and which phosphoproteins are important for stimulation of steroid production. Direct activation of mitochondrial cholesterol side-chain cleavage activity (CSCC) by phosphoproteins appears to be unlikely and there are indications that some specific rapidly turning over proteins regulate the CSCC enzyme. The ultimate regulation of CSCC activity by LH depends probably on a sequence of reactions which involves activation of membrane receptors, increased concentrations of second messengers, protein phosphorylation and synthesis of specific proteins. Recently, it has been shown that LHRH and analogues may directly regulate steroid production in gonadal cells and various preliminary observations indicate that the mechanism of action of gonadotrophic hormones and releasing hormones may be different (Hsueh et al., 1981). From a comparison of the effects of LH and LHRH on metabolic activities of Leydig cells, common important regulatory pathways for regulation of steroid production can be discerned. In addition, other regulatory systems may modulate the effects of LH.

Methods and materials used for isolation and incubation of Leydig cells as well as analytical methods have been described elsewhere (Bakker et al., 1981; Rommerts et al., 1982; Molenaar et al., 1983). Further details are given in the tables and figures.

SITES FOR REGULATION OF STEROID PRODUCTION

Testosterone is quantitatively and physiologically the most important steroid secreted by the testis. The production of testosterone can be regulated at three different levels: 1. availability of intracellular cholesterol, 2. conversion of cholesterol to pregnenolone, 3. conversion of pregnenolone to testosterone. Different investigators employing isolated interstitial cells have shown that LH stimulates pregnenolone and testosterone production in a similar fashion and it has been generally accepted that the rate-limiting step for the control of steroid production is at the level of CSCC and that LH acts as the primary regulatory hormone (Eik-Nes, 1975). Recent findings obtained with cells from rats 24 h after <u>in vivo</u> treatment with LH, oestrogens or LHRH analogues have shown that the rate of pregnenolone production and testosterone production may be different and that enzyme activities involved in pregnenolone metabolism may be inhibited by these hormones (Rommerts & Brinkmann, 1981). Moreover, the presence of substantial amounts of 17 -hydroxyprogesterone and progesterone in testis tissue indicates that the capacity of pregnenolone metabolism <u>in vivo</u> does not always exceed the production rate of pregnenolone (Cigorraga et al., 1980). Thus, depending on the relative activities of pregnenolone production and metabolism, the conversion of pregnenolone may become rate-<u>limiting</u> for the production of testosterone, whereas the CSCC activity is always the rate-<u>determining</u> step for production of steroids. The availability of cholesterol via uptake of lipoproteins can be regulated in steroidogenic cells, but in Leydig cells this appears not to be a rate-limiting step under normal conditions (Gwynne & Strauss, 1982). The relative activities of CSCC and pregnenolone metabolism will depend on the age and endocrine status of the animal, but also on experimental conditions, such as the use of isolated tissue, cells, homogenates or incubation conditions. We have recently shown that the LH-dependent testosterone production by isolated Leydig cells from adult rats depends on the cell preparation method and that not more than 5-10% viable Leydig cells are recovered (Molenaar et al., 1983).

It is not clear if the CSCC activity or pregnenolone metabolism is predominantly affected by the isolation procedure and we have therefore estimated these two activities in various cell preparations. The pregnenolone conversion rate in Leydig cells from mature rats selected by preincubation and attachment to plastic was equal to the pregnenolone production rate in control cells and in cells stimulated with LH. However, when the activity of CSCC was stimulated with 22R-hydroxycholesterol as substrate, testosterone production was also increased, but the proportion of pregnenolone which was converted to testosterone was much smaller (Table 1). These selected collagenase-dispersed Leydig cells still contain a certain amount of damaged cells (Molenaar et al., 1983). The presence of such cells in isolated cell preparations may create an apparent overcapacity for pregnenolone metabolism which can obscure inhibiting effects of hormones on this pathway. Specific enzyme activities in homogenates or intact cells rather than endogenous steroid productions must therefore be measured for detection of hormone-induced leasions in this pathway. The rate of conversion of progesterone in isolated Leydig cells from mature rats decreased to 50% of the original activities after incubation for 24 h. However, no significant effects of LHRHa, LH or combinations of these hormones on this activity could be shown in this period. Preliminary experiments showed major effects of LHRH and LH at the level of the CSCC activity. In further experiments we have therefore measured pregnenolone production in the presence of inhibitors of pregnenolone metabolism as the most accurate and direct parameter of CSCC activity.

Table 1. PRODUCTION OF PREGNENOLONE* AND TESTOSTERONE BY ISOLATED LEYDIG CELLS

condition	pregnenolone* (P)	testosterone (T)	$\frac{T}{P}$ x100%
	(ng/h per 10^6 Leydig cells)		
control	59 ± 13	49 ± 13	81
LH (100 ng/ml)	634 ± 116	432 ± 64	71
22R-hydroxy-cholesterol (30 μM)	5541 ± 1170	1088 ± 202**	21

* Pregnenolone production was measured in the presence of inhibitors of pregnenolone metabolism.
Mean results ± S.E.M. (4 different cell preparations).
**Significantly different from P production ($p < 0.01$).

REGULATION OF CHOLESTEROL SIDE-CHAIN CLEAVAGE ACTIVITY

Isolated interstitial cells from 21-23 day old rats were incubated in plastic dishes for 1 h at 32°C in culture medium containing 1% foetal calf serum. In this period viable interstitial cells, but not erythrocytes, germinal cells and damaged cells, attach to the surface. The absence of effects of NADPH on steroid production indicates the absence of damaged cells (Molenaar et al., 1983). After this period fresh medium containing hormones etc. was added and cells were further incubated. Pregnenolone production was measured in the final 1-2 h. The dose-response curve for LH action on steroidogenesis shows that the first significant stimulation can be shown with 0.05 ng LH/ml and that steroid production is fully stimulated (more than 30-fold) with 1 ng LH/ml (Fig. 1).

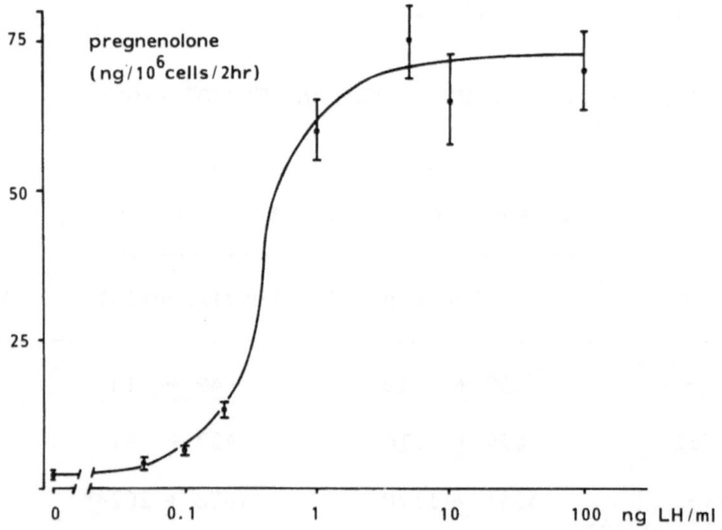

Fig. 1. Dose-response curve for action of LH (NIH-LH S20) on pregnenolone production by isolated Leydig cells obtained from 21 day-old rats. Cells were preincubated for 1-2 h.
Mean results ± S.E.M. of 10 different observations (3 different cell preparations) are shown.

Short-term and long-term effects of LHRH agonist (LHRHa) were investigated with a maximally stimulating dose of the LHRH agonist (Hoe-766; 50 ng/ml), according to Sharpe & Cooper (1982) (Fig. 2). Initially LHRHa stimulated steroid production nine-fold and this effect of LHRHa, but not that of LH, was abolished when the LHRH antagonist ORG-30093D (0.5 µg/ml) was present. The maximally LH-stimulated steroid production could not be further stimulated when LHRH was present (results not shown). Steroid production in cells incubated for 48 h without hormones could still be stimulated by LH, but not by LHRHa. No significant effect on the maximally LH-stimulated steroid production could be shown when cells were incubated for 48 h either in the presence of LH or LHRH. However, the LH-stimulated steroid production was significantly decreased when cells had been cultured for 48 h with LH together with LHRH. This inhibitory effect of LHRH was abolished when ORG-30093D was present during the 48 h incubation period (Fig. 2).

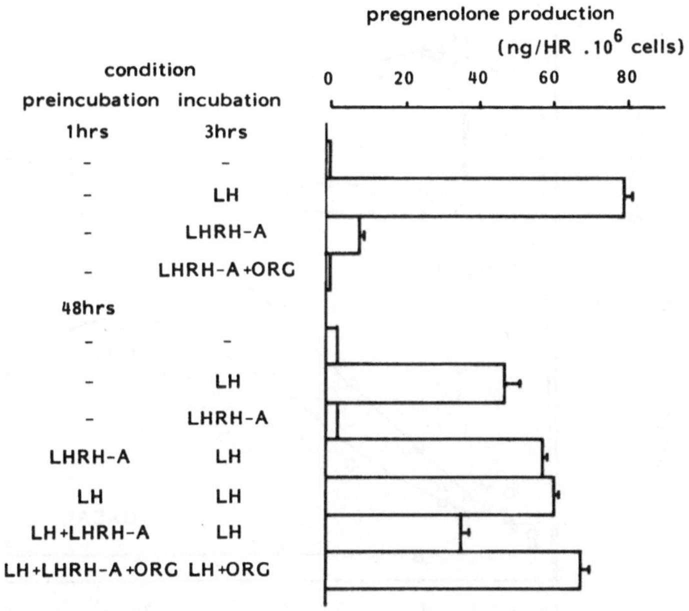

Fig. 2. Short-term and long-term effects of LH (100 ng/ml), LHRH agonist Hoe-766 (50 ng/ml) and LHRH antagonist ORG-30093 (0.5 µg/ml) and combinations on pregnenolone production by isolated Leydig cells from 21 day-old rats. Cells were incubated at 32°C in culture medium containing 1% foetal calf serum and the indicated additions. Mean results ± S.D. of 10 observations are shown.

Steroid production in isolated Leydig cells can be stimulated by LH within several minutes (Rommerts et al., 1982). Effects of LHRH, however, have only been observed after several hours (Sharpe & Cooper, 1982). This difference in kinetics of LH and LHRH action may reflect that the mechanism of action of these hormones is not the same and kinetic studies with LH and LHRH were therefore carried out. Cells were incubated with or without hormones for 3 h and steroid concentrations in the incubation media were measured each 10 min. The results in Fig. 3 show that stimulation of steroid production by 100 ng/LH starts a few minutes after addition of LH and that full stimulation is obtained within approximately 30 min. The first significant effects of LHRH could be detected after approximately 20 min, whereas for the maximum effect 3 h were required. The results show that also more than 3 h are required to reach a steady state stimulation of steroid production with 0.1 ng LH/ml. Stimulatory effects of low

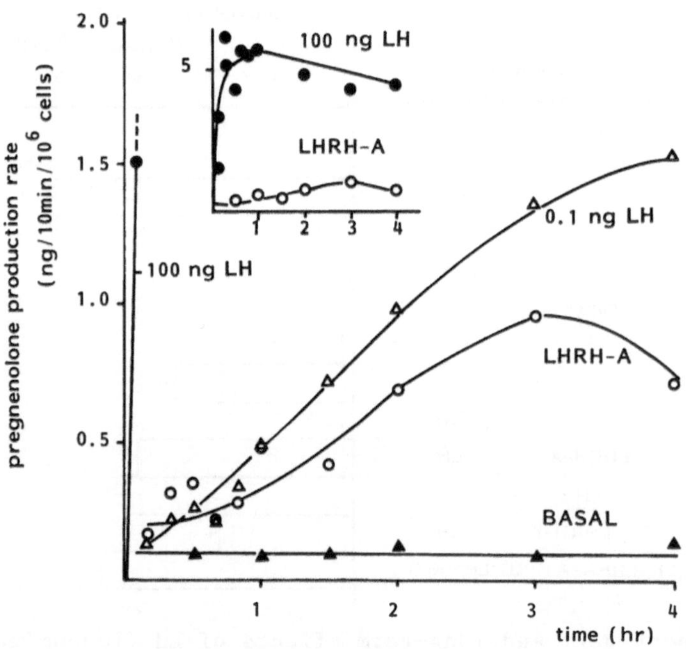

Fig. 3. Kinetics of LH and LHRH agonist action on pregnenolone production by isolated Leydig cells. Pregnenolone production per 10 min was calculated from the concentrations of pregnenolone in culture media from cells incubated during different periods.
Mean results of triplicate determinations are shown.

concentrations of LH may therefore be underestimated when relatively short incubation periods are used. As a consequence the dose-response relationship of LH action on steroid production becomes dependent on the duration of the incubation period. The results also indicate that the mechanism of action of high and low concentrations of LH may be different and that the mechanism of action of LHRHa and the low dose of LH appear similar in this respect. Moreover, comparisons between the effects of LH and LHRH analogues must at least include experiments with concentrations of LH and LHRHa which stimulate steroid production in a similar fashion.

It is generally accepted that LH stimulates steroid production via cAMP as second messenger and that phosphoproteins are somehow involved in the ultimate regulation of the CSCC activity. The effect of LHRHa on cellular cAMP levels in Leydig cells sometimes incubated in the presence of 1-methyl-3-isobutyl-xanthine (MIX) was therefore compared with that of LH. In the presence of 100 ng LH/ml cAMP levels were approximately 6-fold increased, but no significant effects could be shown when 0.2 ng LH/ml or 50 ng/ml LHRHa were used (Table 2). Pregnenolone production stimulated by 0.2 ng LH/ml, however, is further stimulated by addition of MIX, which indicates an involvement of

Table 2

EFFECTS OF MIX ON HORMONE STIMULATED cAMP-LEVELS AND PREGNENOLONE PRODUCTION

ADDITIONS	PREGNENOLONE (ng/hr.10^6cells)		cAMP (pmol/10^6cells)	
	-	MIX 200 μM	-	MIX 200 μM
-	0.5 ± 0.1	1.9 ± 0.5	7.3/7.9	6.4 ± 2.1
100 ng/ml LH	25.6 ± 1.1	25.2 ± 4.6	25.1/23.2	37.4 ± 9.1
0.2 ng/ml LH	5.9 ± 1.6	27.6 ± 4.0	7.7/9.8	7.1 ± 1.8
LHRHa	4.2 ± 1.2	5.9 ± 2.7	9.5/11.6	7.4 ± 1.4

Means ± S.D. (n=4)

cAMP action with this dose of LH. LHRH action was not affected by MIX, which argues against an important role of cAMP. The results in Table 2 show also that small and almost undetectable changes in cAMP can cause complete stimulation of steroid production. Measurements of cAMP are thus inadequate for discerning the mechanism of action of hormone concentrations, which do not overstimulate the cell. In order to compare with more sensitive techniques the effects of LH and LHRHa, we have measured endogenous protein phosphorylation in intact cells as a parameter for intracellular cAMP action on phosphokinase activity. The patterns of ^{32}P-labelled phosphoproteins after separation of cellular proteins on SDS gels showed that the intensity of the 17000 Da and 33000 Da phosphoproteins was increased after incubations of cells with 100 ng LH/ml, confirming earlier observations (Bakker et al, 1982). The highest increase was observed for the phosphorylation of the 17000 Da protein. The effect of 0.2 ng LH/ml on protein phosphorylation was much less, although effects of LH could still be detected for both proteins (Fig. 4). It appears that the resolution of the one-dimensional

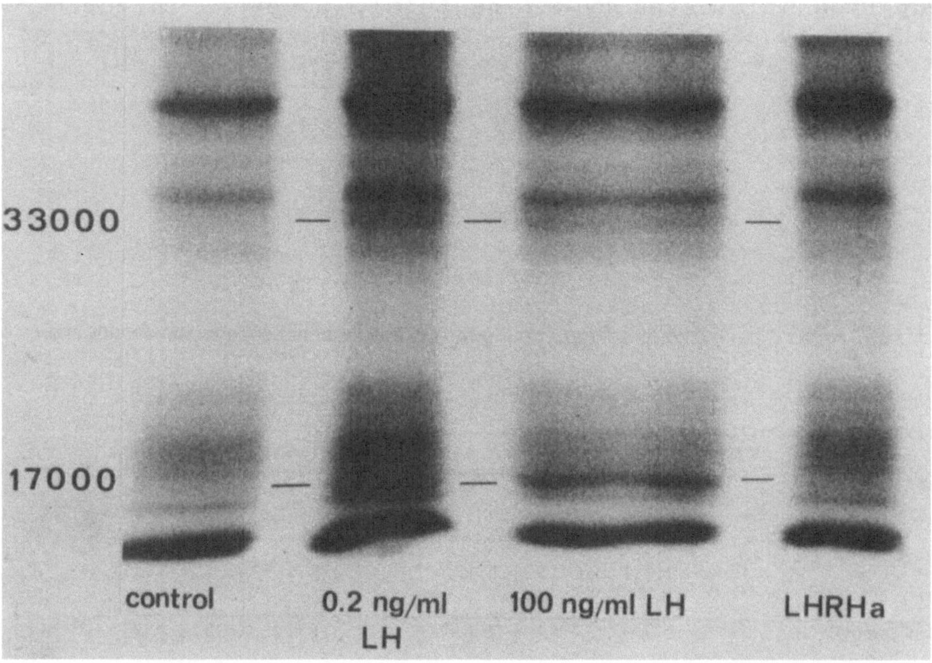

Fig. 4. Effect of LH 0.2 ng/ml and 100 ng/ml and LHRHa (50 ng/ml) on protein phosphorylation in isolated Leydig cells from 21 day-old rats. Cells were incubated wth ^{32}P-phosphate and extracted proteins were analyzed on SDS-polyacrylamide-gel-electrophoresis.

separation system is a major limitation for the detection of the other LH-dependent phosphoproteins. When LHRHa was employed to stimulate steroid production, no changes in protein phosphorylation could be shown. Apparently LHRH acts differently from LH (not via cAMP?) and it could be possible that the LH-dependent phosphoproteins are not a prerequisite for stimulation of CSCC activity. It may also be possible that LH stimulates protein phosphorylation partly via non-cAMP-mediated mechanisms. This hypothesis is supported by results that were obtained during investigations with tumour Leydig cells in culture (Bakker et al., 1983a). When comparing the actions of LH and dcAMP, a discrepancy between the effects of both compounds on protein phosphorylation and steroid production was observed (Fig. 5). The effect of LH on

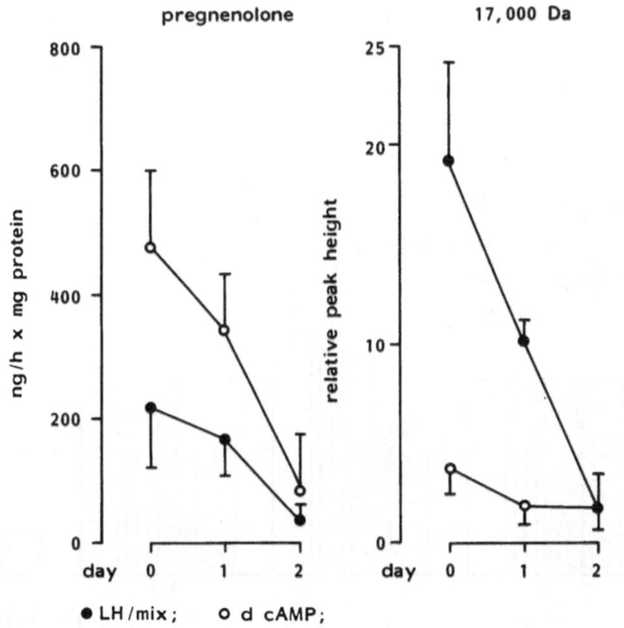

Fig. 5. Pregnenolone production and protein phosphorylation in cultured tumour Leydig cells incubated at 32°C and stimulated with LH (100 ng/ml) and 1-methyl-3-isobutyl-xanthine (MIX; 0.25 mM) or dibutyryl cyclic AMP (dcAMP 0.5 mM). Pregnenolone was measured by radioimmunoassay in the incubation media. Effects on protein phosphorylation of the 17000 Da protein were measured from densitograms of autoradiograms as shown in Figure 4. Mean results ± S.D. of three different cell preparations are shown.

phosphorylation of the 17000 Da protein was much greater than that of dcAMP, whereas stimulation of steroid production by LH was much less than with dcAMP. This discrepancy was not observed with 5 other hormone-dependent phosphoproteins. Effects of dcAMP and LH on these phosphoproteins changed in parallel during the culture period. There are indications that not the 17000 Da protein, but (one of) the other phosphoproteins are involved in the regulation of the CSCC activity (Bakker et al., 1983b).

It is well-known that in general calcium plays an important role in the transduction of hormonal signals (Campbell, 1983). Calcium appears to be involved in regulation of steroid production in Leydig cells (Hall et al., 1981). In this respect we have investigated the calcium dependency of LH and LHRHa effects on Leydig cells. Increasing concentrations of the calcium ionophore A23187 caused a progressive inhibition of the effect of high concentrations of LH on steroid production (Fig. 6). However, the production of pregnenolone in the presence of 25-hydroxy-

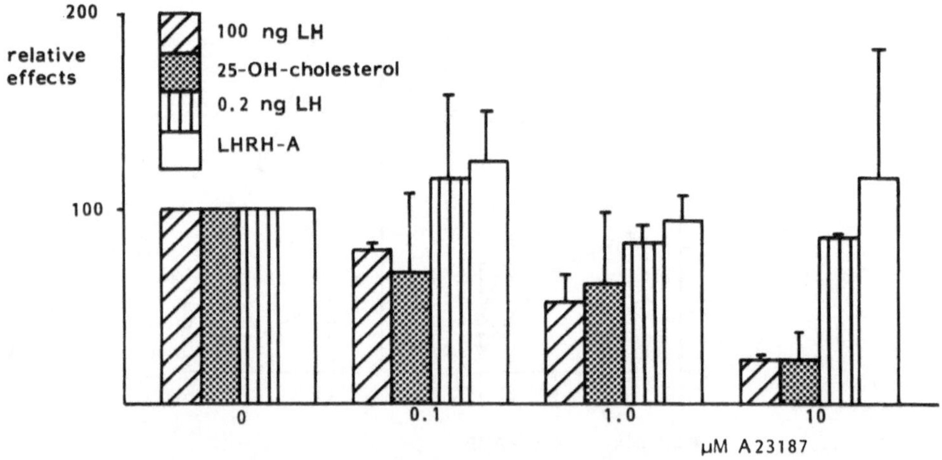

Fig. 6. Effect of various concentrations of calcium ionophore A23187 on steroid production by Leydig cells from 21 day-old rats. Steroid production was stimulated by LH (0.2 or 100 ng/ml), LHRH agonist (50 ng/ml) or 25-hydroxycholesterol (30 μM). Cells were incubated for 2 h in the presence of ionophore. For estimation of steroid production fresh medium, containing ionophore, hormones and inhibitors of pregnenolone metabolism, was added. Mean results ± S.D., n = 4.

cholesterol, which is independent of LH action, was also inhibited by the ionophore. This indicates that 1-10 uM ionophore acts aspecifically, which makes it difficult to draw definite conclusions about the mechanisms of hormone stimulation. On the other hand, no effects of any ionophore concentration on the action of LHRH or low concentrations of LH could be demonstrated. These results may suggest that these LH or LHRHa actions are not affected by increased intracellular calcium levels. For expression of LH and LHRHa action extracellular calcium is required. The results in Fig. 7 show that at low concentrations of extracellular calcium the maximal steroidogenic response triggered by LH or LHRHa is reduced and that the effects of LH and LHRHa at the various calcium concentrations are inhibited in a similar fashion. In this respect LH and LHRHa action have the same requirements for calcium.

The different effects of low and high concentrations of LH on protein phosphorylation and kinetics of steroid production as well as the discrepancies between dcAMP- and LH-stimulated phosphorylation of the 17000 Da protein and steroid production may indicate

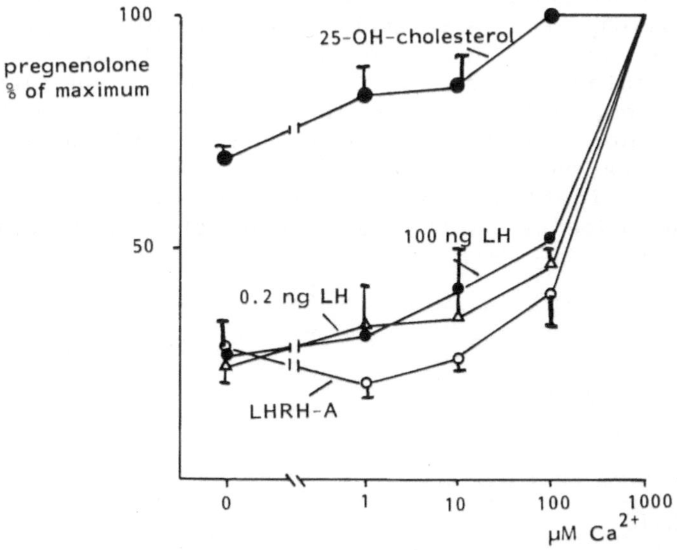

Fig. 7. Effect of various extracellular calcium concentrations on steroid production stimulated by LH (100 or 0.2 ng/ml) or LHRHa (50 ng/ml). For incubation conditions see Fig. 6. Mean results ± S.D. of 4 observations are shown.

that, depending on the concentration, LH action on Leydig cells may require other mediators in addition to cAMP. LHRH action may depend more on other mediators than on cAMP. Calcium may be an important candidate for this alternative mediator in Leydig cells, but we have not yet been able to obtain support for this possibility.

Specific stimulatory or inhibitory effects of LHRH analogues on steroid production have also been shown for Leydig cells in vivo (Sharpe et al, 1982). Moreover, activities which can interfere with binding of LHRH to Leydig cells are present in the testis and can be produced by the Sertoli cells (Sharpe et al., 1981; Bhasin et al., 1983). It has been shown recently, that in addition to LHRH or LHRH-like molecules, other peptides, such as the neuropeptide vasopressin, can also regulate Leydig cell function (Adashi & Hsueh, 1981). Similar effects of LHRH analogues have been shown in ovarian cells (Hsueh & Jones, 1981). In addition, peptides may also play a role within the cell in the regulation of mitochondrial CSCC in adrenals (Pedersen & Brownie, 1983). The physiological importance of these peptide effects for gonadal function can at the present time not be evaluated. However, there is no doubt that peptides play a very important role in the regulation of the nervous system. Connections between peptide effects on gonadal cells and neuronal cells could indicate that the regulation of these different cell functions may have common basic principles. These connections between regulation of brain function and steroidogenesis have recently been extended to the regulation of haematopietic and germ-cell systems (Golub, 1982). In addition, we have recently been able to show that Leydig cells and testicular macrophages may be functionally connected, because, depending on the stage of development, an overlap in enzyme activities, cell surface antigens and phagocytosis could be demonstrated (Molenaar et al., 1983). Investigations of protein and peptide action on functional properties of different cells may help in the elucidation of the basic mechanisms of action of peptides and proteins in the regulation of (testicular) cell function.

ACKNOWLEDGEMENTS

We thank Miss W. Bakhuizen for typing the manuscript. Dr. A.V. Shally and Organon for supply of ORG-30093, Hoechst Company for supply of the LHRH agonist (HOE-766) and the National Pituitary Agencya, NIAMDD for supply of LH.

REFERENCES

Adashi, E.Y., and Hsueh, A.J.W., 1981, Direct inhibition of testicular androgen biosynthesis by arginine-vasopressin: mediation through pressor-selective testicular recognition sites, Endocrinology, 109:1793.

Bakker, G.H., Hoogerbrugge, J.W., Rommerts, F.F.G., and van der Molen, H.J., 1981, Lutropin-dependent protein phosphorylation and steroidogenesis in rat tumour Leydig cells, Biochem. J., 198:339.

Bakker, G.H., Hoogerbrugge, J.W., Rommerts, F.F.G., and van der Molen, H.J., 1982, Lutropin increases phosphorylation of a 33000-dalton ribosomal protein in rat tumour Leydig cells, Biochem. J., 204:809.

Bakker, G.H., Hoogerbrugge, J.W., Rommerts, F.F.G., and van der Molen, H.J., 1983a, LH-dependent steroid production and protein phosphorylation in culture of rat tumour Leydig cells, Molec. Cell. Endocr., in press.

Bakker, G.H., Hoogerbrugge, J.W., Rommerts, F.F.G., and van der Molen, H.J., 1983b, Subcellular localization of LH-dependent phosphoproteins and their possible role in regulation of steroidogenesis in rat tumour Leydig cells, FEBS Lett., in press.

Bhasin, S., Heber, D., Peterson, M., and Swerdloff, R., 1983, Partial isolation and characterization of testicular GnRH-like factors, Endocrinology, 112:1144.

Campbell, A.K., 1983, "Intracellular calcium, its universal role as regulator", John Wiley & Sons Ltd., New York.

Cigorraga, S.B., Sorrell, S., Bator, J., Catt, K.J., and Dufau, M.L., 1980, Estrogen dependence of a gonadotropin-induced steroidogenic lesion in rat testicular Leydig cells, J. Clin. Invest., 65:699.

Eik-Nes, K.B., 1975, Biosynthesis and secretion of testicular steroid, in: "Handbook of Physiology", section 7: Endocrinology, vol. V, R.O. Greep and E.B. Astwood, eds, American Physiological Society, Washington D.C., p. 95-115.

Golub, E.S., 1982, Connections between the nervous, haematopoietic and germ-cell systems, Nature, 299:483.

Gwynne, J.T., and Straus, J.F. III, 1982, The role of lipoproteins in steroidogenesis and cholesterol metabolism in steroidogenic glands, Endocr. Rev., 3:299.

Hall, F., Osawa, S., and Mrotek, J., 1981, Influence of calmodulin on steroid synthesis in Leydig cells from rat testis, Endocrinology, 109:1677.

Hsueh, A.J.W., and Jones, P.B.C., 1981, Extra-pituitary actions of gonadotropin-releasing hormone, Endocr. Rev., 2:437.

Molenaar, R., Rommerts, F.F.G., and van der Molen, H.J., 1983, The steroidogenic activity of isolated Leydig cells from mature rats depends on the isolation procedure, Int. J. Androl., 6:261.

Molenaar, R., Rommerts, F.F.G., and van der Molen, H.J., 1983, Characteristics of Leydig cells and macrophages from developing testicular interstitial cells, in: Proc. 8th Testis Workshop, Bethesda.

Pedersen, A.D., and Brownie, A.C., 1983, Cholesterol side-chain cleavage in the rat adrenal cortex: Isolation of a cycloheximide-sensitive activator peptide, Proc. Natl. Acad. Sci. USA, 80:1882.

Rommerts, F.F.G., and Brinkmann, A.O., 1981, Modulation of steroidogenic activities in testis Leydig cells, Molec. Cell. Endocr., 21:15.

Rommerts, F.F.G., van Roemburg, M.J.A., Lindh, L.M., Hegge, J.A.J., and van der Molen, H.J., 1982, The effects of short-term culture and perifusion on LH-dependent steroidogenesis in isolated rat Leydig cells, J. Reprod. Fert., 65:289.

Sharpe, R.M., Fraser, H.M., Cooper, I., and Rommerts, F.F.G., 1981, Sertoli-Leydig cell communication via an LHRH-like factor, Nature, 290:785.

Sharpe, R.M., Cooper, I., 1982, Stimulatory effect of LHRH and its agonists on Leydig cell steroidogenesis in vitro, Molec. Cell. Endocr., 26:141.

Sharpe, R.M., Doogan, D.C., and Cooper, I., 1982, Stimulation of Leydig cell testosterone secretion in vitro and in vivo in hypophysectomized rats by an agonist of luteinizing hormone releasing hormone, Biochem. Biophys. Res. Commun., 106: 1210.

MOLECULAR HETEROGENEITY OF LUTEINIZING HORMONE-RELEASING HORMONE

Robert P. Millar and Judy A. King

Department of Chemical Pathology
University of Cape Town Medical School
Observatory 7925, South Africa

INTRODUCTION

Following the structural elucidation of luteinizing hormone-releasing hormone (LH-RH) by Schally and associates, it became generally accepted that the decapeptide was a unique molecular form. This belief arose from:

(a) A number of studies purporting to have shown non-ribosomal biosynthesis of LH-RH and thereby excluding the possibility of ribosomally biosynthesised prohormonal forms.

(b) The assumption that LH-RH was confined to the CNS and thus unlikely to be present in other tissues in a modified form.

(c) Immunological and low resolution chromatographic studies demonstrating that LH-RH in the hypothalamus of nonmammalian vertebrates was identical to the mammalian peptide. This conclusion of a lack of interspecific differences in LH-RH structure in vertebrates was supported by the demonstration that synthetic mammalian LH-RH was biologically active in a wide range of mammalian species and in nonmammalian vertebrates (1).

A number of factors argued against this view of a universal conservation of LH-RH structure:

(a) The LH-RH structure, comprising exclusively L-amino acids, α-amino peptide linkages and a cyclised N-terminal Glu and C-terminal amide, is characteristic of ribosomally synthesised peptides; in contrast, the presence of D-amino acids and unusual peptide linkages (γ glutamyl in glutathione and β alanyl in carnosine) characterises prokaryote and eukaryote peptides synthesised by nonribosomal mechanisms.

(b) The related neurohypophysial peptide, vasopressin, had been convincingly shown to be synthesised ribosomally with the production of a prohormone. Moreover, the neurohypophysial peptides exhibit structural heterogeneity in vertebrates which is consistent with single nucleotide base changes in the triplet codons (2).

(c) Accepting that LH-RH is synthesised ribosomally, it appeared highly likely that different LH-RH molecular forms would have arisen in vertebrates during over 400 million years of evolution, as is the case with the neurohypophysial hormones (2).

Research over the past six years has now firmly established that there is considerable diversity in the structure of LH-RH and related molecular forms. Higher molecular weight prohormonal forms have been convincingly demonstrated, while structural variations in vertebrate hypothalamic LH-RH have been shown in several species from all the major classes. These structural differences have been confirmed by the isolation and structural analysis of LH-RH from a single species of bird, amphibian and teleost (see Fig. 1). Furthermore, LH-RH-like peptides differing structurally from the mammalian hypothalamic peptide have been found in mammalian tissues such as the pineal, testis and ovary.

In this chapter our current knowledge of LH-RH molecular heterogeneity will be briefly reviewed and the functional and evolutionary implications discussed.

PROHORMONAL LH-RH

The existence of higher molecular weight immunoreactive forms of LH-RH in hypothalamic extracts suggested that these might constitute prohormonal species. In both rat and sheep hypothalami (3-5) we have detected LH-RH immunoreactive peptides of molecular weights of $\geqslant$ 5K, 3K and 2K in addition to decapeptide LH-RH. Since the 5K peptide eluted in the void volume of a Sephadex G-25 column it is possible that it comprised even higher molecular weight forms. Extensive studies provided evidence for the prohormonal nature of these peptides. The peptides were specifically retained on immunoaffinity columns using an appropriate antiserum directed towards the "middle" of the LH-RH sequence; they were not dissociated by rigorous treatment with 8M urea and 6M guanidinium hydrochloride and did not bind or degrade ^{125}I-LH-RH (3-5). Physiological manipulations which altered hypothalamic LH-RH content also changed the occurrence of the putative prohormonal forms, and in tissues lacking LH-RH no immunoreactive higher molecular weight material was detected (4,5). Specific chemical modifications of each of the amino acids comprising the LH-RH sequence resulted in a similar loss of immunoreactivity of both LH-RH and the ≥5K prohormonal form when quantitating with appropriate antisera requiring the particular residues for binding (4,5). Similarly, proteolytic cleavage of LH-RH and the prohormones with a range of enzymes yielded appropriate losses of immunoreactivity with the different antisera (3-5). The presence of relatively higher proportions of the prohormonal forms in hypothalamic regions containing LH-RH cell bodies (localised by immunocytochemistry) than in the stalk median eminence, supported the classical concept of neuronal peptide processing for LH-RH biosynthesis (4,5). The prohormonal forms were also more prevalent in the microsomal fraction than in purified synaptosomes which contained exclusively fully-processed decapeptide LH-RH (5). HPLC separation of the synaptosomal extract confirmed that only decapeptide LH-RH is present in contrast to the presence of both somatostatin-28 and somatostatin-14 in these extracts (6).

Other studies addressed the question as to the location of the LH-RH sequence within the prohormonal peptide. The interaction of the ≥5K LH-RH putative prohormonal species with seven region- and/or conformation-specific LH-RH antisera clearly demonstrated that the molecule is modified at both the N- and C-termini (4,5). This indication of both N- and C-terminal extensions to the LH-RH sequence were confirmed by demonstrating that aminopeptidase and carboxypeptidase digestions led to increases in immunoreactivity (4,5). The 5K LH-RH species was partially converted by hypothalamic peptidases into an immunoreactive peptide eluting in the position of LH-RH. Progressive trypsin digestion released a 2-3K immunoreactive species followed by complete conversion to a single form migrating in the position of LH-RH on Sephadex G-25 (3-5). It is apparent, therefore, that there are both N- and C-terminal extensions to LH-RH in the putative prohormonal LH-RH and that trypsin-sensitive cleavage sites (basic amino acids) are interposed between the LH-RH sequence and these extensions. This arrangement is common to many prohormones which are processed by trypsin-like cleavages at pairs of basic amino acids followed rapidly by removal of the exposed basic residues by carboxypeptidase-B-like activity. We previously proposed (5) that prohormonal LH-RH is also characterised by Gln in position 1 of the LH-RH sequence which is spontaneously (or enzymically) cyclised after cleavage of the N-terminal extension to give rise to $pGlu^1$. In addition, the amide ($Gly^{10}.NH_2$) was presumed to arise from the amino group of an additional Gly preceding the basic residues. This now seems a very likely possibility as structural analysis of prohormonal forms of eleven propeptides with C-terminus amides has revealed that all have this additional Gly, and recent studies on a pituitary amidating enzyme using synthetic peptide substrates have demonstrated an absolute requirement for Gly in this oxidative transamidation (7).

Recent studies have demonstrated 26K and 1.8K higher molecular weight immunoreactive forms of LH-RH in extracts of rat hypothalamus, cortex and placenta (8). The primary LH-RH translation product of rat hypothalamic mRNA in reticulocyte lysate was recently shown to be a 28K peptide (9). Allowing for the cleavage of a signal/leader sequence this is comparable to the 26K peptide reported above. The 26K peptide was recognised almost exclusively by an N-terminus-directed antibody, suggesting it is C-terminally extended. Unfortunately, the authenticity of the 26K species is uncertain as dissociating conditions were not used. It is also uncertain as to whether both N- and C-extensions were present as a middle-directed antiserum which would recognise such forms was not employed.

Although all the above studies provide a persuasive argument for the existence of prohormonal LH-RH, final proof resides in the isolation and sequence analysis of putative prohormones and a demonstration of their conversion to LH-RH by the tissues concerned. The demonstration of incorporation of ^{3}H-tyrosine into LH-RH by human placental trophoblast (10) indicates the potential of this tissue for these biosynthetic and processing studies.

An alternative approach to establishing the structure of prohormonal LH-RH is by recombinant DNA technology. Several laboratories have initiated programmes aimed at elucidating the sequence of LH-RH mRNA. We have recently detected clones in cDNA and genomic libraries which hydridise with labelled synthetic oligomers (17-mers) coding for both N- and C-terminal sequences of LH-RH. The successful cloning of LH-RH cDNA holds the promise of exciting studies on the endocrine regulation of expression of the LH-RH gene.

LH-RH IN MAMMALIAN EXTRAHYPOTHALAMIC TISSUES

Extrahypothalamic Brain LH-RH

Although the presence of immunoreactive LH-RH in extrahypothalamic brain regions is well-documented, few studies have investigated the molecular nature of the peptide/s. Studies in our laboratory demonstrated that the sheep pineal gland has an LH-RH which is identical to the hypothalamic peptide in its interaction with different region-specific antisera and which cannot be distinguished using gel filtration chromatography, cation exchange chromatography, or higher resolution HPLC (11-13). A second form of LH-RH was clearly structurally distinct from the hypothalamic hormone (11-13). This LH-RH species is of similar size to LH-RH as it co-migrates with the decapeptide on Sephadex G-25 but is less positively charged and elutes earlier on cation exchange chromatography. The peptide has similar properties to chicken hypothalamic LH-RH (Gln^8-LH-RH; see later) in co-eluting on cation exchange chromatography and reverse phase HPLC. Interactions with N- and C-terminally-directed antisera and resistance to degradation by aminopeptidase and carboxypeptidase A confirm that $pGlu^1$ and $Gly^{10}.NH_2$ are present in the molecule (11,12). This pineal species of LH-RH has intrinsic LH-releasing activity but decreases the LH response to synthetic LH-RH suggesting that it may be a weak agonist (11). The presence of an LH-RH species in the pineal which is similar to hypothalamic LH-RH of a lower vertebrate is reminiscent of reports on the presence of vasotocin in the mammalian pineal (14). The possibility that this peptide performs a neurotransmitter role in the CNS is currently being investigated.

Gonadal and Placental LH-RH

LH-RH has direct effects on the gonads of laboratory animals, and high affinity binding sites for LH-RH analogues have been demonstrated in testicular Leydig cells and in ovarian granulosa cells (see review 15). Testicular extracts were reported to displace ^{125}I-LH-RH in radioreceptor assays (16). Immunoreactive LH-RH species from acetic acid-extracted and immunoaffinity-purified rat testicular material (17) have been characterised by region-specific antisera and by gel filtration and HPLC. The molecular species of approximately 100K, 32K, 5K and 1K were all found to interact strongly with a C-terminally-directed antiserum and poorly with middle- and N-terminal-directed antisera suggesting they contain the C-terminal sequence of hypothalamic LH-RH. Only the lower molecular weight forms displaced ^{125}I-LH-RH from rat pituitary LH-RH receptors. A recent report of a similar study on rat testis extracts also suggests that the testicular material shares C-terminal sequences in common with LH-RH and displaces ^{125}I-LH-RH in the radioreceptor assay (18). Somewhat different results were obtained in another study on rat testicular LH-RH which showed that the high molecular weight form could be dissociated to molecules of the same size as LH-RH which reacted more poorly with C-terminally-directed antisera than with an antiserum specific for the N- and C-terminus and one recognising the middle region of the molecule (19).

Immunoreactive LH-RH has been described in the placenta, which has immunological, chromatographic and biological properties identical to the hypothalamic decapeptide

(10,20,21). Higher molecular weight forms have also been detected in this tissue (8). In porcine follicular fluid we have recently detected three LH-RH immunoreactive peptides in the molecular range 30K to 50K. Immunoreactivity of these peptides increased after trypsin digestion.

Immunoreactive LH-RH in Other Tissues

LH-RH in milk extracts appears to be identical to the hypothalamic peptide (22). Immunoreactive LH-RH reported in pancreas (23) and rat submandibular gland (this laboratory) has not been characterised.

INTERSPECIFIC STRUCTURAL HETEROGENEITY IN VERTEBRATE LH-RHs

Birds

Some early studies suggested an identity (24) of bird hypothalamic LH-RH with mammalian LH-RH (mLH-RH), but others indicated that there were structural differences (25-27). Chicken and pigeon hypothalamic LH-RHs had a similar molecular size to the mammalian peptide but were less positively charged and differed immunologically (26,28). Antisera directed towards the middle region of mLH-RH and those recognising the C-terminal three amino acids gave lower quantitation and nonparallel radioimmunoassay displacement curves. Antisera requiring the extreme N- and C-termini and tolerant of certain amino acid substitutions in the middle region of the molecule gave high quantitation and parallel displacement curves (26,28). Examination of overlapping sequence requirements of these antisera indicated that the alteration in chicken hypothalamic LH-RH (cLH-RH) resided in the position of Arg^8 (Fig. 1). The difference was investigated in more detail by noting the interaction with the different antisera after selectively modifying the molecule at each amino acid residue in turn by specific chemical and enzymic treatment (29). These data clearly showed that cLH-RH differed at Arg^8. The difference in isoelectric points of cLH-RH and mLH-RH was compatible with a neutral amino acid substitution for Arg^8 of mLH-RH. On the basis of evolutionary probability of amino acid interchange for Arg, Gln was a likely candidate. The putative cLH-RH (Gln^8-LHRH) was synthesised and shown to have identical immunological, chromatographic and biological properties to natural cLH-RH (29). Other LH-RH analogues with substitutions of Ser, Trp, Leu, Met, Ile, Phe, His, Asn, Glu, Cit, Orn and Lys in the eight position had properties different from that of natural cLH-RH.

Mammalian	pGlu-His-Trp-Ser-Tyr-Gly-Leu-Arg-Pro-Gly.NH_2
Chicken	——————————— Leu-Gln ————
Lizard	——————————— Trp-Leu ———— ?
Frog	——————————— Leu-Arg ————
Salmon	——————————— Trp-Leu ————

Fig. 1. Structure of Vertebrate Hypothalamic LH-RHs

In concurrent studies, 17 µg of cLH-RH was purified from 250,000 chicken hypothalami using a combination of affinity chromatography, cation exchange HPLC and reverse phase HPLC. Amino acid analysis of an acid hydrolysate showed an absence of Arg and the presence of an additional Glu, compatible with the proposed structure (30,31). Partial sequence analysis was consistent with the location of Gln as a replacement for Arg in the eight position (30). Other workers have subsequently confirmed the structure of cLH-RH as Gln^8-LH-RH (32). Recently, we have fully sequenced the material and confirmed the structure (J. Spiess, J.A. King and R.P. Millar, in preparation). Whether the Gln^8-LH-RH structure is conserved in all bird species remains to be determined.

Reptiles

LH-RH immunoreactive material in extracts of lizard and tortoise hypothalami exhibited immunological and chromatographic (cation exchange) properties different from those of mLH-RH and similar to those of cLH-RH and teleost LH-RH (26,28). The data pointed to alterations in the vicinity of Leu^7. Since LH-RH in reptile species is also less positively charged than mLH-RH, as in cLH-RH, it appears that Arg^8 is also not present in reptile LH-RH. Recent immunological and reverse phase HPLC studies in our laboratory indicate that the major form of lizard brain LH-RH is clearly different from both mLH-RH and cLH-RH. The peptide is more hydrophobic than these forms and co-elutes in three reverse phase HPLC systems with salmon brain LH-RH (Trp^7, Leu^8-LH-RH; see below).

Amphibians

Anuran (frogs and toads) hypothalamic LH-RH has identical physicochemical properties to that of mLH-RH (see review 33). HPLC purification of frog brain LH-RH revealed a single species with an amino acid composition identical to that of mLH-RH (34). Immunological and HPLC studies have revealed that frog retina extracts have the mammalian type of peptide in addition to a more hydrophobic species which has HPLC properties similar to fish brain LH-RH and which is thought to differ from mLH-RH at Arg^8 (35). This additional species of LH-RH is the major form found in the frog sympathetic ganglion and adrenal gland (35).

Fish

Fish (teleost, elasmobranch and cyclostome) brain LH-RHs were found to differ from mLH-RH in the vicinity of Leu^7 and were less positively charged suggesting the absence of Arg^8 (26,28). Purification and sequence analysis of salmon brain LH-RH (sLH-RH) revealed the structure Trp^7,Leu^8-LH-RH (36) (Fig. 1). Our own work on hake (Merluccius capensis) pituitary and hypothalamic LH-RH indicates that it has identical immunological and HPLC properties to sLH-RH. The absorbance (280 nm) of purified hake pituitary LH-RH confirmed the presence of two Trp residues.

In both our studies and those of Barnett and co-workers (37) additional less hydrophobic species of LH-RH were detected in teleost brain. It is possible that these represent different decapeptide LH-RHs, LH-RH precursors, or degradation products of teleost LH-RH.

INTERSPECIFIC GONADOTROPIN-RELEASING ACTIVITIES OF VERTEBRATE LH-RHs

Synthetic ovine and porcine LH-RH have high biological activity in a wide variety of domestic and laboratory mammals (1,38) and also in feral mammalian species (39) including rock hyrax, impala, Soay sheep and hyaena (unpublished), suggesting that the LH-RH structure is conserved throughout the class Mammalia. Lys substitution for Arg^8 in LH-RH retains substantial biological activity (40). It is possible, therefore, that this substitution has occurred in LH-RH of some mammalian species especially as Arg is replaced by Lys in vasopressin of certain mammals (2).

cLH-RH has low gonadotropin-releasing activity using sheep (40,41) and rat (26,42) pituitary cells in vitro, and in the rat in vivo (42). Neutral and acidic amino acid substitutions for Arg^8, in general, have low LH-releasing activity in the mammalian system (43, unpublished). Synthetic sLH-RH has low LH-releasing activity in rat pituitary cells (36). Thus, the mammalian pituitary is highly discriminating with regard to substitutions for Arg^8. The receptor may be somewhat less selective for substitutions for Leu^7 since Ile^7 and Ser^7 analogues retain some activity (43).

Table 1. Interspecific Gonadotropin-Releasing Activity of Vertebrate LH-RHs

LH-RH Type	Mammal	Reptile	Bird	Amphibian	Fish
Mammalian	++++	0 or +	++++	++++	++++
Chicken	+	0	++++	++++	++++
Salmon	+	?	++++	?	++++

0, no activity +, slight activity ++++, full activity compared with homologous peptide

In birds, cLH-RH and mLH-RH are equipotent in releasing LH and FSH from chicken pituitary cells in vitro, with low ED_{50}s of 10^{-9} M (41). They are also equipotent in vivo in quail (B.K. Follett, personal communication). The two peptides have identical affinities for chicken pituitary receptors (41). Analogues of cLH-RH with substitutions of Ile, Ser, Met, Phe, Trp, Leu, His and Lys for Gln^8 all have substantial biological activity in releasing LH from chicken pituitary cells. The acidic amino acid substitution of Glu^8 (and also Asn^8) had reduced biological activity. Thus, unlike the mammalian pituitary LH-RH receptor, the chicken receptor is "promiscuous" with regard to its requirements for the amino acid in the eight position.

In our laboratory, an LH-RH analogue with alterations in both positions seven and eight (Gln^7,Leu^8-LH-RH) had a potency of approximately 4% relative to that of the natural peptide. However, sLH-RH (Trp^7,Leu^8-LH-RH) was at least as active as cLH-RH. There is consequently some uncertainty regarding the importance of the amino acid in position seven of LH-RH for biological activity in birds and further studies are needed to clarify this.

In turtles and snakes, mLH-RH, cLH-RH and superactive analogues of the peptides are inactive (44,45). In contrast, another study reported some ability of mLH-RH to stimulate the reproductive system in turtles (46).

Amongst amphibians, mLH-RH (i.e. frog LH-RH) stimulates gonadotropic hormone secretion, steroidogenesis and spawning in anurans (45,47). cLH-RH is equipotent with mLH-RH in stimulating gonadotropin secretion from frogs in vivo (45). The doses required to achieve these effects are considerably higher than those required to induce gonadotropin release in rats, despite the fact that the natural hypothalamic hormone in frogs has the structure of mLH-RH. A lower affinity of mLH-RH for frog pituitary receptors and/or more rapid degradation of mLH-RH may account for this relatively poor activity. We have observed very rapid degradation of mLH-RH by Xenopus laevis plasma. The sensitivity of frog pituitaries to LH-RH in vitro (P. Licht, personal communication) suggests that the receptor binding affinity is high.

mLH-RH and its analogues have relatively poor gonadotropin-releasing activity in fish (33, 48-51). The structural characterisation of salmon brain LH-RH as Trp^7,Leu^8-LH-RH (sLH-RH) (36) suggested that this might be due to inter-class specificity of LH-RH. However, we have recently found that mLH-RH and sLH-RH are equally effective in stimulating plasma testosterone and 17-ß-estradiol in the cichlid (Tilapia sparrmanii) in vivo. All three peptides (mLH-RH, cLH-RH and sLH-RH) are equipotent in stimulating gonadotropin secretion in goldfish in vivo (R.E. Peter, personal communication).

These differences in gonadotropin-releasing activity of synthetic vertebrate LH-RHs in different vertebrates in vivo and in vitro are summarised schematically in Table 1.

STRUCTURE/ACTIVITY RELATIONS OF LH-RH IN VERTEBRATES

cLH-RH and sLH-RH have low gonadotropin-releasing activity in mammals as do a wide range of position eight-substituted analogues. Of the naturally occurring L-amino acids, only Lys substitution for Arg^8 retains substantial biological activity (40) in accordance with the postulate that His^2, Tyr^5 and Arg^8 in mLH-RH form a combined unit of hydrogen bonding important in stabilising the molecule for biological activity (52). By monitoring the fluorescence of Trp^3 when titrating LH-RH through the pH range 4-11 the degree of stabilisation can be monitored. In the analogues with poor biological activity (including cLH-RH), a significant feature was the extended titration range (>1.74 pH units) for His^2 compared with <1.74 for the Arg^8 and Lys^8 peptides (40). This is indicative of a heterogeneous population of His residues in the inactive analogues due to the presence of a series of different conformers. Thus, the mammalian receptor appears to have evolved a stringent requirement for a privileged conformer.

In the bird these structural requirements clearly do not pertain as LH-RH analogues with a wide range of amino acid substitutions (except Glu and Asn) have high LH- and FSH-releasing activity. Thus, if the structural conformation model is true we must infer that, unlike the mammalian LH-RH receptor, the bird receptor is less discriminating and binds a number of LH-RH conformers of the structurally unstabilised analogues.

Although the data for activity of the substituted analogues in fish and amphibians are less extensive, in these vertebrate classes too, there appears to be a lack of discrimination of the receptor for the amino acid in the eight position of LH-RH. On the other hand, the pituitary LH-RH receptor in reptiles may have more stringent requirements as the analogues tested to date are lacking in, or have low, biological activity.

These comparative differences in receptor requirement may be of value in elucidating the mechanisms of LH-RH-receptor interactions and the stimulation of gonadotropin release. In this regard it may be significant that the frog and chicken pituitary do not exhibit the desensitization phenomenon characteristic of the mammalian pituitary. The reasons for the more stringent LH-RH structure requirements of the mammalian receptor are not clear but may be a consequence of a need to discriminate between related LH-RH molecular forms performing other biological functions. The effects of synthetic mLH-RH on the CNS and gonads in mammals may merely reflect overlap interaction with receptors normally bound by different specific forms functioning in vivo.

CONCLUSIONS

It is now abundantly clear that there is considerable molecular heterogeneity in LH-RH and structurally related molecules. A number of putative prohormonal forms have been described, some of which may even have specific biological activity in their own right or contain sequences with biological activity. Within the vertebrates there are at least three distinct structural forms of decapeptide LH-RH in the brain, while still other different immunologically-related peptides are present in other tissues. All of the structural differences in variants of decapeptide LH-RH are in amino acids in positions seven and eight. The structure of three forms of LH-RH (Arg^8-LH-RH in mammalian hypothalamus and frog brain, Gln^8-LH-RH in chicken hypothalamus and Trp^7Leu^8-LH-RH in salmon brain) have been established by isolation and structural analysis. Lizard LH-RH has similar properties to sLH-RH. It should be emphasized that these structures are not necessarily representative of the entire vertebrate class as it is feasible that some interspecific variation might have occurred in the course of evolution, especially in fish genera which have experienced some 400 million years of independent evolution.

The elucidation of the structure of LH-RH in some of the lower vertebrates held the hope that administration of synthetic homologous (endogenous) LH-RH might result in a greater specific activity. This is apparently not the case for the bird, frog and some teleosts where it appears that the pituitary receptor is "promiscuous" in its acceptance of many amino acid substitutions in the eight position. Only in reptiles are the heterologous LH-RHs from other species apparently relatively inactive and there remains a possibility that reptile species are highly specific for their own endogenous LH-RH. This may also pertain to certain fish species which have experienced separate evolution over an extended period.

In mammals the high specificity of the pituitary receptor for Arg^8 of LH-RH may reflect a need to discriminate between different, but related, molecular forms of LH-RH serving other functions such as in the CNS and in the gonads. The demonstration of different forms of LH-RH in the pineal and gonads of mammals, together with the indication of different LH-RH structural requirements for Leydig cell receptors, support this speculative notion. In teleosts and in frogs more than one form of LH-RH has been demonstrated and in the latter species the tissue distribution varies.

LH-RH may originally have evolved as a neurotransmitter/ modulator possibly regulating reproductive behaviour. Subsequent gene duplications allowed the evolution of other molecular forms which were co-opted as regulators of functions in other tissues such as the pituitary and gonad. An early evolution of LH-RH as a regulator of reproductive behaviour is suggested by the structural elucidation of the yeast alpha-mating factor which has remarkable structural homology with mLH-RH (53). This homology is, however, less convincing when the structure is compared to cLH-RH and sLH-RH.

ACKNOWLEDGEMENTS

We gratefully acknowledge generous gifts of research materials and collaboration from the following: A. Arimura, K. Bauer, S. Blahser, D. Coy, W. Day, B. Follett, E. Griffiths, P. Licht, T. Nett, G. Niswender, L. Reichert, J. Rivier, R. Roeske, J. Sandow, W. Vale, Y. Yabe and N. Yanaihara. This work was financed by grants from the University of Cape Town and the Medical Research Council.

REFERENCES

1. A.V. Schally, Aspects of hypothalamic regulation of the pituitary gland, Science 202:18 (1978).
2. R. Acher, Recent discoveries in the evolution of proteins, Angewandte Chemie International Edition 13:186 (1974).
3. R.P. Millar, C. Aehnelt, and G. Rossier, Higher molecular weight immunoreactive species of luteinizing hormone releasing hormone : possible precursors of the hormone, Biochem. Biophys. Res. Commun. 74:720 (1977).
4. R.P. Millar, P. Denniss, C. Tobler, J.C. King, A.V. Schally, and A. Arimura, Presumptive prohormonal forms of hypothalamic peptide hormones, in "Cell biology of hypothalamic neurosecretion", J.D. Vincent, and C. Kordon, eds., Centre National de la Recherche Scientifique 280, Bordeaux, pp. 487 (1978).
5. R.P. Millar, I. Wegener, and A.V. Schally, Putative prohormone of luteinizing hormone-releasing hormone, in "Neuropeptides: biochemical and physiological studies", R.P. Millar, ed., Churchill-Livingstone, New York, pp. 111 (1981).
6. C.F. Kewley, R.P. Millar, M.C. Berman, and A.V. Schally, Depolarization- and ionophore-induced release of octacosa somatostatin from stalk median eminence synaptosomes, Science 213:913 (1981).
7. A.F. Bradbury, M.D.A. Finnie, and D.G. Smyth, Mechanism of C-terminal amide formation by pituitary enzymes, Nature 298:686 (1982).
8. J.P. Gautron, E. Pattou, and C. Kordon, Occurrence of higher molecular forms of LHRH in fractionated extracts from rat hypothalamus, cortex and placenta, Mol. Cell. Endocrinol. 24:1 (1981).
9. A. Curtis, and G. Fink, A high molecular weight precursor of luteinizing hormone-releasing hormone from rat hypothalamus, Endocrinology 112:390 (1983).
10. L. Tan, and P. Rousseau, The chemical identity of the immunoreactive LHRH-like peptide biosynthesized in the human placenta, Biochem. Biophys. Res. Commun. 109:1061 (1982).
11. R.P. Millar, and C. Tobler, Structural and functional differences in pineal and hypothalamic luteinizing hormone-releasing hormone, in "Neuropeptides : biochemical and physiological studies", R.P. Millar, ed., Churchill-Livingstone, New York, pp. 263 (1981).
12. R.P. Millar, P. Denniss, C. Tobler, and R.B. Symington, Immunological, biochemical and functional differences in pineal and hypothalamic luteinizing hormone-releasing hormone, in "Pineal function", C.D. Matthews, and R.F. Seamark, eds., Elsevier/North-Holland Biomedical Press, Amsterdam, pp. 151 (1981).

13. J.A. King, and R.P. Millar, Decapeptide luteinizing hormone-releasing hormone in ovine pineal gland, J. Endocr. 91:405 (1981).
14. S. Pavel, The mechanism of action of vasotocin in the mammalian brain, in "The pineal gland of vertebrates including man. Progress in brain research vol. 52", J. Ariens Kappers, and P. Pevet, eds., Elsevier/North-Holland Biomedical Press, Amsterdam, pp. 445 (1979).
15. R.P. Millar, J.A. King, I. Wegener, C. Tobler, C. Dutlow, R.W. Roeske, W.A. Day, J.E. Rivier, W.W. Vale, and P. Licht, Molecular evolution of vertebrate luteinizing hormone-releasing hormone, in " Neuronal Communications", B. Meyer, and S. Kramer, eds., Balkema Press, Cape Town, (1983) in press.
16. R.M. Sharpe, H.M. Fraser, I. Cooper, and F.F.G. Rommerts, Sertoli-Leydig cell communication via an LHRH-like factor, Nature 290:785 (1981).
17. C.M. Dutlow, and R.P. Millar, Rat testis immunoreactive LH-RH differs structurally from hypothalamic LH-RH, Biochem. Biophys. Res. Commun. 101:486 (1981).
18. S. Bhasin, D. Heber, M. Peterson, and R. Swerdloff, Partial isolation and characterization of testicular GnRH-like factors, Endocrinology 112:1144 (1983).
19. C. Turkelson, T. Kenjo, and A. Arimura, Effects of an LHRH agonist in rat Leydig cell culture and purification of a testicular LHRH-like substance, 65th Annual Meeting of the Endocrine Society, abstract no. 373 (1983).
20. G.S. Khodr, and T.M. Siler-Khodr, Placental luteinizing hormone-releasing factor and its synthesis, Science 207:315 (1980).
21. J.N. Lee, M. Seppala, and T. Chard, Characterization of placental luteinizing hormone-releasing factor-like material, Acta Endocrinol. 96:394 (1981).
22. T. Amarant, M. Fridkin, and Y. Koch, Luteinizing hormone-releasing hormone and thyrotropin-releasing hormone in human and bovine milk, Eur. J. Biochem. 127:647 (1982).
23. M. Seppala, and T. Wahlstrom, Identification of luteinizing hormone-releasing factor and alpha-subunit of glycoprotein hormones in human pancreatic islets, Life Sci. 27:395 (1980).
24. S.L. Jeffcoate, P.J. Sharp, H.M. Fraser, D.T. Holland, and A. Gunn, Immunochemical and chromatographic similarity of rat, rabbit, chicken and synthetic luteinizing hormone releasing hormones, J. Endocr. 62:85 (1974).
25. M. Hattori, K. Wakabayashi, and M. Nozaki, Difference of Japanese quail LH-RF from mammalian LH-RF revealed by biological and immunochemical studies, Gen. Comp. Endocrinol. 41:217 (1980).

26. J.A. King, and R.P. Millar, Heterogeneity of vertebrate luteinizing hormone-releasing hormone, Science 206:67 (1979).
27. K. Miyamoto, Y. Hasegawa, T. Minegishi, M. Nomura, Y. Takahashi, M. Igarashi, K. Kangawa, and H. Matsuo, Isolation and characterisation of chicken hypothalamic luteinizing hormone-releasing hormone, Biochem. Biophys. Res. Commun. 107:820 (1982).
28. J.A. King, and R.P. Millar, Comparative aspects of luteinizing hormone-releasing hormone structure and function in vertebrate phylogeny, Endocrinology 106:707 (1980).
29. J.A. King, and R.P. Millar, Structure of chicken hypothalamic luteinizing hormone-releasing hormone. I. Structural determination on partially purified material, J. Biol. Chem. 257:10722 (1982).
30. J.A. King, and R.P. Millar, Structure of chicken hypothalamic luteinizing hormone-releasing hormone. II. Isolation and characterization, J. Biol. Chem. 257:10729 (1982).
31. J.A. King, and R.P. Millar, Structure of avian hypothalamic gonadotrophin-releasing hormone, S. Afr. J. Sci. 78:124 (1982).
32. K. Miyamoto, Y. Hasegawa, M. Igarashi, N. Chino, S. Sakakibara, K. Kangawa, and H. Matsuo, Evidence that chicken hypothalamic luteinizing hormone-releasing hormone is [Gln^8]LH-RH, Life Sci. 32:1341 (1983).
33. J.A. King, and R.P. Millar, Phylogeny of vertebrate luteinizing hormone-releasing hormone and somatostatin, in "Neuropeptides : biochemical and physiological studies", R.P. Millar, ed., Churchill-Livingstone, New York, pp. 217 (1981).
34. J. Rivier, C. Rivier, D. Branton, R. Millar, J. Spiess, and W. Vale, HPLC purification of ovine CRF, rat extrahypothalamic brain somatostatin and frog brain GnRH, in " Peptides : synthesis-structure-function", Proc. Seventh American Peptide Symposium, D.H. Rich, and E. Gross, eds., Pierce Chemical Company, Illinois, pp. 771 (1981).
35. L.E. Eiden, E. Loumaye, N. Sherwood, and R.L. Eskay, Two chemically and immunologically distinct forms of luteinizing hormone-releasing hormone are differentially expressed in frog neural tissues, Peptides 3:323 (1982).
36. N. Sherwood, L. Eiden, M. Brownstein, J. Spiess, J. Rivier, and W. Vale, Characterization of a teleost gonadotropin-releasing hormone, Proc. Natl. Acad. Sci. 80:2794 (1983).

37. F.H. Barnett, J. Sohn, S. Reichlin, and I.M.D. Jackson, Three luteinizing hormone-releasing hormone-like substances in a teleost fish brain : none identical with the mammalian LH-RH decapeptide, Biochem. Biophys. Res. Commun. 105:209 (1982).
38. R. Guillemin, Peptides in the brain : the new endocrinology of the neuron, Science 202:390 (1978).
39. R.P. Millar, and C. Aehnelt, Application of ovine luteinizing hormone (LH) radioimmunoassay in the quantitation of LH in different mammalian species, Endocrinology 101:760 (1977).
40. R.C.deL. Milton, J.A. King, M.N. Badminton, C.J. Tobler, G.G. Lindsey, M. Fridkin, and R.P. Millar, Comparative structure-activity studies on mammalian [Arg^8]LH-RH and chicken [Gln^8]LH-RH by fluorimetric titration, Biochem. Biophys. Res. Commun. 111:1082 (1983).
41. R.P. Millar, and J.A. King, Synthesis, luteinizing hormone releasing activity, and receptor binding of chicken hypothalamic luteinizing hormone-releasing hormone, Endocrinology (in press).
42. N. Yanaihara, C. Yanaihara, T. Hashimoto, Y. Kenmochi, T. Kaneko, H. Oka, S. Saito, A.V. Schally, and A. Arimura, Syntheses and LH- and FSH-RH activities of LH-RH analogs substituted at position 8, Biochem. Biophys. Res. Commun. 49:1280 (1972).
43. J. Sandow, W. Konig, R. Geiger, R. Uhmann, and W. von Rechenberg, Structure-activity relationships in the LH-RH molecule, in "Control of ovulation", D.B. Crighton, N.B. Haynes, G.R. Foxcroft, and G.E. Lamming, eds., Butterworths, London, pp. 49 (1978).
44. P. Licht, Evolutionary and functional aspects of pituitary gonadotropins in the green turtle, Chelonia mydas, Amer. Zool. 20:561 (1980).
45. P. Licht, R. Millar, J.A. King, B.R. McCreery, M.T. Mendonca, A. Bona-Gallo, and B. Lofts, Effects of chicken and mammalian gonadotropin-releasing hormones (GnRH) on in vivo pituitary gonadotropin release in amphibians and reptiles, Gen. Comp. Endocrinol. (in press).
46. I.P. Callard, and V. Lance, The control of reptilian follicular cycles, in "Reproduction and evolution", J.H. Calaby, and C.H. Tyndale-Biscoe, eds, Australian Acad. Sci., Canberra City, pp. 199 (1977).
47. B.R. McCreery, P. Licht, R. Barnes, J.E. Rivier, and W.W. Vale, Actions of agonistic and antagonistic analogs of gonadotropin releasing hormone (Gn-RH) in the bullfrog Rana catesbeiana, Gen. Comp. Endocrinol. 46:511 (1982).
48. J.N. Ball, Hypothalamic control of the pars distalis in fishes, amphibians, and reptiles, Gen. Comp. Endocrinol. 44:135 (1981).

49. L.W. Crim, D.M. Evans, D.H. Coy, and A.V. Schally, Control of gonadotropic hormone release in trout : influence of synthetic LH-RH and LH-RH analogues in vivo and in vitro, Life Sci. 28:129 (1981).
50. E.M. Donaldson, G.A. Hunter, and H.M. Dye, Induced ovulation in coho salmon (Oncorhynchus kisutch). II Preliminary study of the use of LH-RH and two high potency LH-RH analogues, Aquaculture 26:129 (1981).
51. R.E. Peter, Serum gonadotropin levels in mature male goldfish in response to luteinizing hormone-releasing hormone (LH-RH) and des-Gly^{10}-[D-Ala^{6}]-LH-RH ethylamide, Can. J. Zool. 58:1100 (1980).
52. M. Shinitzky, E. Hazum, and M. Fridkin, Structure-activity relationships of luliberin substituted at position 8, Biochim. Biophys. Acta 453:553 (1976).
53. J.M. Stewart, and K. Channabasavaiah, Evolutionary aspects of some neuropeptides, Fed. Proc. 38:2302 (1979).

THE BIOLOGICAL ACTIONS OF 'TESTICULAR LHRH'

Richard M. Sharpe and Irene Cooper

MRC Reproductive Biology Unit
37 Chalmers Street
Edinburgh, Scotland

INTRODUCTION

Although it is now established that LHRH and its agonistic analogues can exert direct effects on the gonads of several mammalian and non-mammalian species (Hsueh & Jones, 1981; Sharpe & Harmer, 1983), the physiological significance of these actions has not been resolved. In the rat testis, LHRH has direct effects only on the Leydig cells and these effects are believed to reflect the actions of an LHRH-like peptide which is secreted within the testis by the Sertoli cells (Sharpe et al. 1982a; Bhasin et al. 1983; Nagendranath et al. 1983; Sharpe & Harmar, 1983). In view of the critical dependence of normal Sertoli cell function on testosterone produced by the Leydig cells, such a line of communication has obvious physiological significance (see also Sharpe, 1983, 1984). Unfortunately, purification of 'testicular LHRH' has made poor progress (Bhasin et al. 1983; Sharpe & Harmar, 1983), so that the only line of investigation that has been possible is to explore the effects of synthetic LHRH and its analogues on the testis, and from the results obtained to infer the likely actions of the endogenous peptide. This paper summarizes our recent findings in this area which have been obtained using two different approaches: 1) by examining the effects of an LHRH agonist on Leydig cell function *in vitro* and *in vivo*, and 2) by examining the effects of an LHRH antagonist on Leydig cell function *in vivo*, as this compound should block any actions of endogenous 'testicular LHRH'.

EFFECTS OF LHRH AGONIST ON LEYDIG CELL FUNCTION IN VITRO

Short-term (5h) incubation of dispersed Leydig cells *in vitro* with increasing concentrations of an LHRH agonist ((D-Ser-*t*-bu^6, *des*-Gly-NH$_2$^{10}) LHRH ethylamide; Hoechst) results in dose-dependent stimulation of testosterone secretion (Fig.1), an effect which can be magnified by depriving the donor animals of LH, either by prior treatment with an LHRH antiserum (Sharpe & Fraser, 1983; Fig.1) or by hypophysectomy (Bourne et al. 1982; Sharpe et al. 1982b). These stimulatory effects of LHRH agonist on testosterone secretion are, equally evident in the presence of LH, hCG or dibutyryl cyclic AMP (Hunter et al. 1982; Sharpe & Cooper, 1982). However, during longer term (12h+) incubations with LHRH agonist, inhibitory rather than stimulatory effects on steroidogenesis become evident (Hunter et al. 1982; Browning et al. 1983).

EFFECTS OF LHRH AGONIST ON LEYDIG CELL FUNCTION IN VIVO

Initially, studies *in vivo* on the effects of LHRH agonist were done using hypophysectomized rats as this ruled out any pituitary-mediated effects of the peptide on the testis.

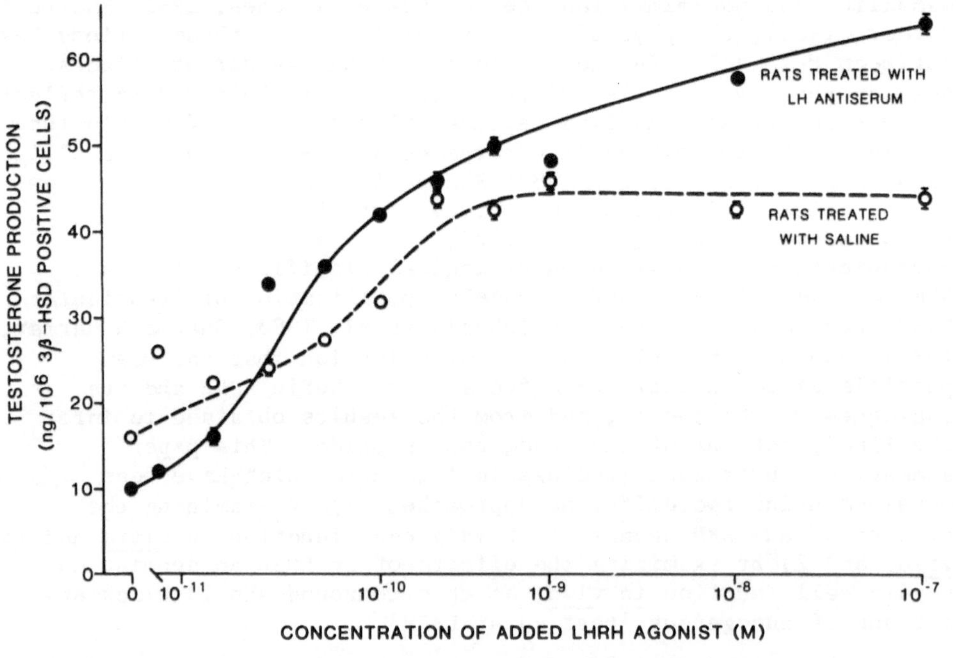

Fig.1 Dose-dependent stimulation of testosterone secretion *in vitro* by an LHRH agonist, using Leydig cells isolated from the testes of adult rats treated 20h previously with saline or an antiserum to oLH (mean ± S.D., N=3 per point).

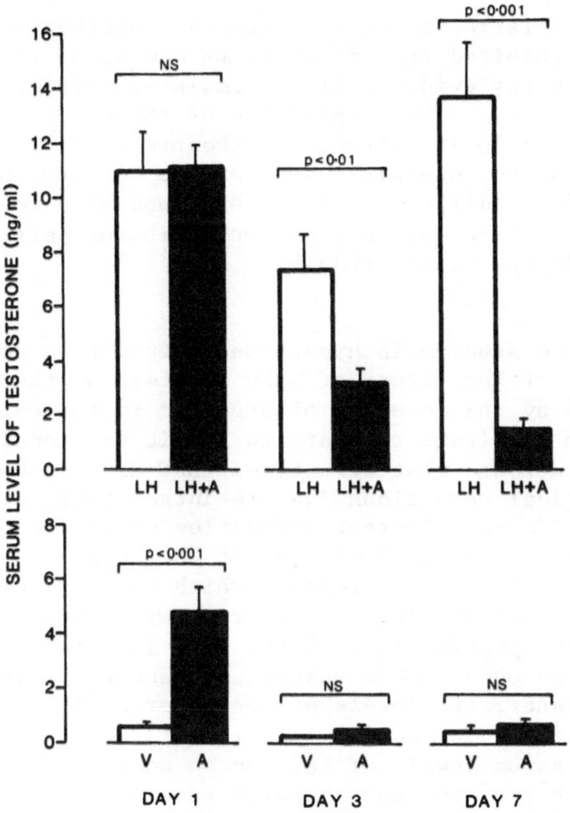

Fig.2 Effect of repeated daily injection of 55-day-old hypophysectomized male rats with vehicle (V), 100 ng LHRH agonist (A), 20 ug oLH-S24 (LH) or 20 ug LH + 100 ng LHRH agonist (LH+A) on the serum levels of testosterone 2h after injection on days 1,3 and 7 of treatment (Mean $\pm$ S.D., N=7).

Such studies have demonstrated unequivocally that, in the short term, LHRH agonists are capable of stimulating testicular testosterone secretion to the extent that peripheral and intratesticular levels of this steroid are returned to within or above the normal range for intact rats (Sharpe et al. 1982b, 1983a). A typical experiment is illustrated in Fig.2. Thus, a single subcutaneous injection of 100 ng LHRH agonist alone resulted 2h later in 'normal' peripheral levels of testosterone (Mean 4.8 ng/ml), although continued daily treatment with this dose of peptide resulted by day 3 in complete loss of this stimulatory response (Fig.2, bottom). In similar rats in which testosterone secretion was stimulated by daily injection of LH concomitant administration of LHRH agonist together with the LH progressively inhibited the effect of LH and at no time during the 7 days was there any evidence of a stimulatory effect of the LHRH agonist (Fig.2, top). This opposition of the effects of LHRH agonist on its own to its effects in the presence of high levels of LH is now thought to explain many of the 'discrepancies' in results obtained by different research groups with respect to whether LHRH has direct stimulatory or inhibitory effects on the Leydig cells (Sharpe et al. 1983a).

Because such studies in hypophysectomized rats demonstrated that the nature of the effect of LHRH agonists on the testis was determined both by the duration of exposure to the peptide and by the degree of concomitant exposure to LH, it was considered essential to elucidate what effects of LHRH agonist were obtained under physiological conditions i.e. in intact rats, as this would presumably provide the clearest indication of what effect endogenous 'testicular LHRH' exerted on the Leydig cells. To circumvent the problem of LH release which would result from peripheral injection of intact adult rats with LHRH agonist, small quantities of the peptide (0.1-10 ng) were injected intratesticularly under ether anaesthesia and at times ranging from ½ to 24h later, the levels of testosterone in peripheral serum and testicular interstitial fluid (IF) were measured and related to the serum levels of LH. As an additional in-built control for each rat, the LHRH agonist was injected only into the right testis whilst the left testis was injected with vehicle alone. Then, by comparing the levels of testosterone in IF from right and left testes it was possible to assess the local steroidogenic effect of LHRH agonist. Detailed studies using this technique demonstrated that intratesticular injection of adult rats with 1 ng LHRH agonist or less did not result in any detectable increase in peripheral LH levels and, as would be predicted from this finding, such treatment did not alter the levels of testosterone in IF from the left (control) testis (see Sharpe et al. 1983b; 1984 and Fig. 3).

Results from a typical experiment in which adult rats were injected intratesticularly with 1 ng LHRH agonist, are illustrated in Fig.3. This treatment resulted in a large unilateral increase in the IF levels of testosterone in each of the 12 rats receiving the LHRH agonist and, compared with overall control animals (i.e. injected bilaterally intratesticularly with vehicle), there was a significant increase in the peripheral serum levels of testosterone. The obvious conclusion from such an experiment is that the increase in peripheral levels of testosterone is solely a

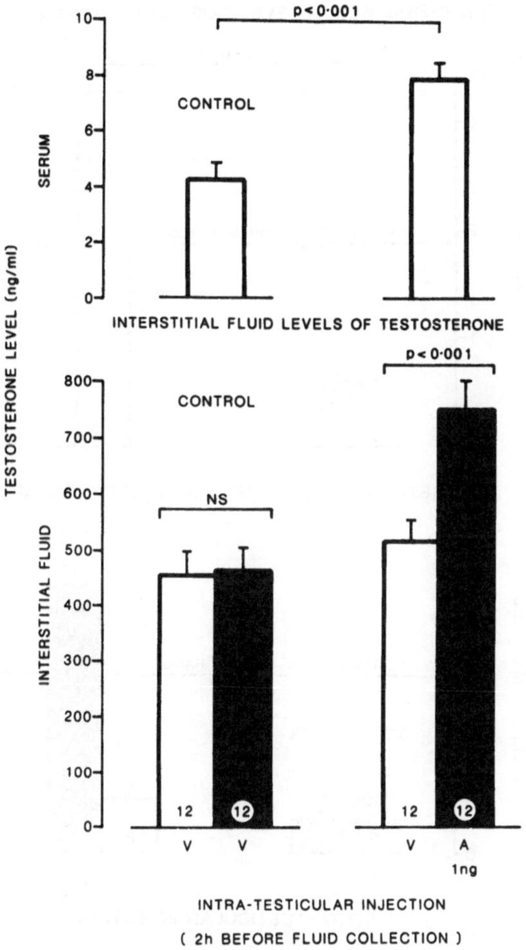

Fig.3 Direct stimulation of testicular testosterone secretion in intact adult rats by intratesticular injection of an LHRH agonist. Rats were injected in the left (open columns) or right (closed columns) testis with either vehicle (V) or 1 ng LHRH agonist (A), and 2h later the levels of testosterone in peripheral serum (top) and in testicular interstitial fluid (bottom) were measured. Values are the mean ± S.D. for the number of animals shown in parentheses.

consequence of the unilateral intratesticular increase in testosterone levels induced by the LHRH agonist, but to remove any possible doubt as to the lack of involvement of LH in this effect the experiment was repeated in rats which had been treated 20h

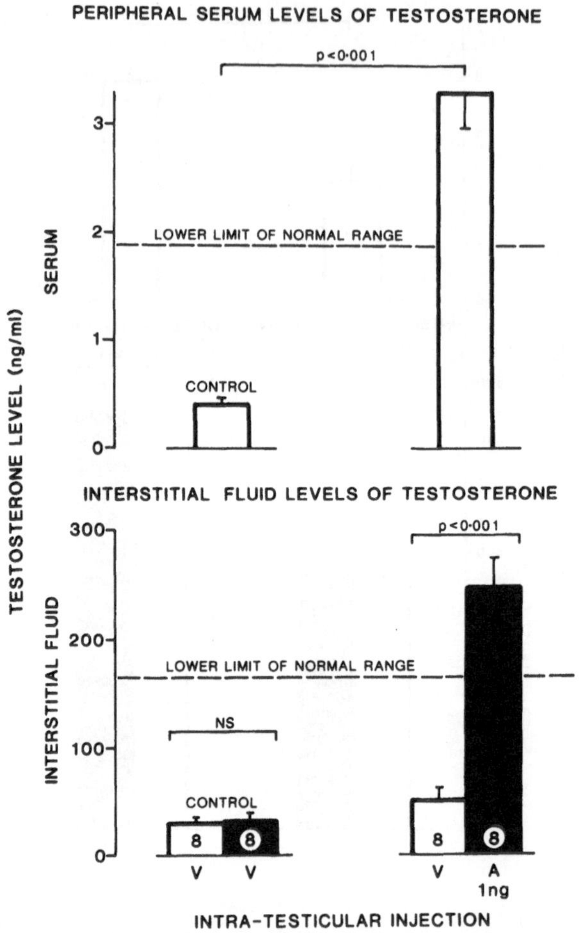

Fig. 4 Direct stimulation of testicular testosterone secretion by LHRH agonist in intact adult rats treated 20h previously with 1 ml antiserum to oLH. Other details are as given in the legend to Fig. 3.

previously with a potent antiserum to oLH (Sharpe & Fraser, 1983). This treatment reduced the concentration of testosterone in testicular IF and peripheral serum (Fig.4) to levels found in hypophysectomized rats. Unilateral intratesticular injection of such rats with 1 ng LHRH agonist returned the IF levels of testosterone in the treated testis to within the normal range for rats of this age, whilst levels of testosterone in IF from the contralateral control testis remained at the hypophysectomized

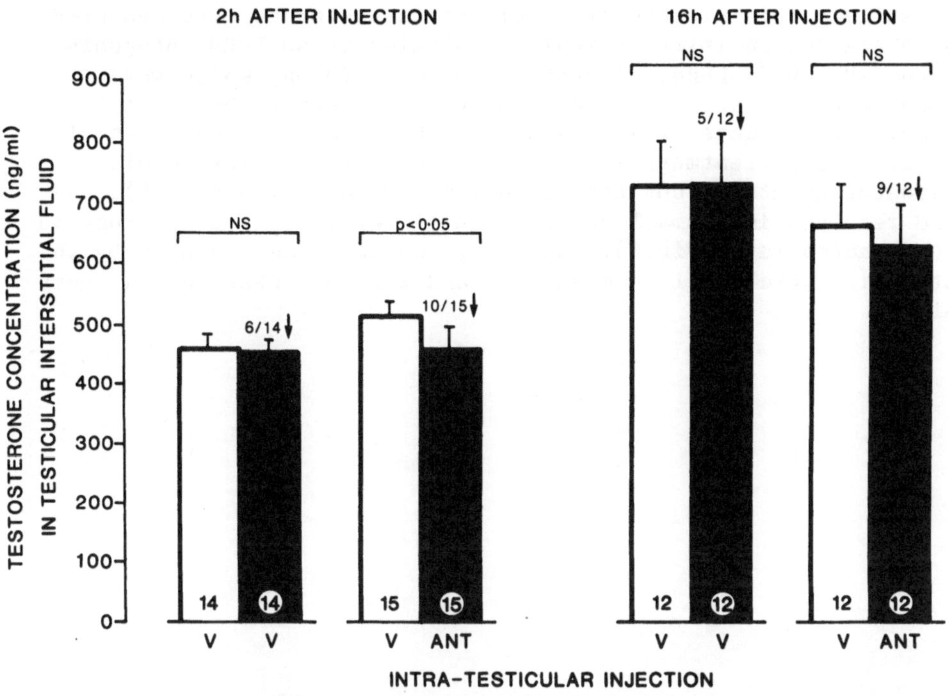

Fig.5 Effect of a single unilateral intratesticular injection of 10 ug LHRH antagonist on the levels of testosterone in testicular interstitial fluid 2 or 16h later. Mean (± S.E.M) values are shown for left (open columns) and right (closed columns) testes for the number of animals indicated at the foot of each column. V=vehicle injected testes. The number of animals in which IF testosterone levels were lower in the right than in the left testis is also indicated.

level (Fig.4). In the same animals, the peripheral serum levels of testosterone were returned to within the normal range, and the only conclusion possible is that the latter increase was a consequence of the direct unilateral stimulation of testosterone secretion by the LHRH agonist.

EFFECTS OF AN LHRH ANTAGONIST ON LEYDIG CELL FUNCTION IN VIVO

The preceding studies have shown that 'testicular LHRH' has the potential to alter the intratesticular levels of testosterone by acting on Leydig cell steroidogenesis. However, such studies tell us nothing about the extent to which this potential is utilized *in vivo* in the normal adult testis. Therefore, to investigate this problem IF levels of testosterone were measured in rats given an intratesticular injection of an LHRH antagonist (D-$Phe^{2,6}$, Phe^{3}) LHRH; Hoechst) at a dose (10 ug) which was known to be in excess of that required to prevent the local stimulatory effects of 1 ng injected LHRH agonist (Sharpe et al. 1983b). This treatment marginally reduced the IF levels of testosterone at 2h, but not at 16h, after injection (Fig.5), and also resulted in a small decrease in IF levels of testosterone in hCG-injected rats (Fig.6). However, the decreases induced by the antagonist were small in magnitude and were not observed in every animal.

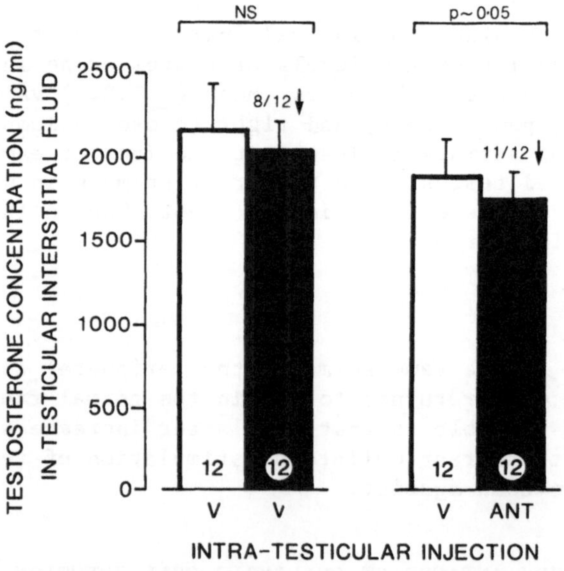

Fig.6 Effect of a single unilateral intratesticular injection of 10 ug LHRH antagonist on the levels of testosterone in testicular interstitial fluid in hCG-injected rats. Animals were injected subcutaneously with 100 IU hCG at the same time as administration of the intratesticular treatments and killed 16h later. Other details are as shown in the legend to Fig.5.

DISCUSSION

The aim of the present series of experiments was first, to identify the likely biological effects of 'testicular LHRH' on the Leydig cell and, second, to evaluate the physiological importance of these effects. The results obtained have been clearcut in showing that testosterone secretion, and thus the intratesticular levels of testosterone, is altered considerably by local exposure of the Leydig cells to LHRH agonist, and this effect is demonstrable in intact rats exposed to physiological levels of LH-stimulation. However, when the actions of endogenous 'testicular LHRH' were blocked by intratesticular administration of an LHRH antagonist, little if any change in the intratesticular levels of testosterone was observed. The straightforward interpretation of these findings would therefore be that 'testicular LHRH' has either no role or, at best, a trivial role to play in the short-term regulation of the intratesticular levels of testosterone. If this is true, then it does seem rather surprising that the mechanisms exist to enable 'LHRH' to play such a potentially major role (see also Sharpe, 1984), to the extent that LHRH-stimulation of the Leydig cell can, in the short-term, maintain normal levels of testosterone (Fig.4). Moreover, the fact that 'LHRH-like' material has been extracted from the testis (see Introduction), surely argues that it plays some local role.

There are several possible explanations for the apparent lack of effect of LHRH antagonist on the IF levels of testosterone. Chief amongst these is the possibility that 'testicular LHRH' is not secreted continuously, but is produced only under certain specific circumstances e.g. when intratesticular levels of testosterone fall below the 'danger' level necessary for the full support of spermatogenesis; such conditions might occur in the interval between successive episodes of LH release. Alternatively, it is possible that 'testicular LHRH' is only produced by Sertoli cells at a specific stage(s) of the spermatogenic cycle and that its action is therefore restricted to the immediate vicinity of tubules at this stage (Sharpe, 1984). If either of these possibilities is correct, then it would be predicted that effects of treatment with an LHRH antagonist would either be restricted to a certain proportion of the rats or that there would be relatively little overall effect on the IF levels of testosterone. As these predictions match the present observations, definitive conclusions as to the physiological importance of 'testicular LHRH' in the adult rat must wait at least until further possibilities such as these have been explored.

ACKNOWLEDGEMENTS

We are grateful to Dr. Jurgen Sandow and Hoechst for provision of the LHRH analogues.

REFERENCES

Bhasin, S., Heber, D., Peterson, M., and Swerdloff, R., 1983, Partial isolation and characterization of testicular GnRH-like factors, Endocrinology, 112: 1144.

Bourne, G.A., Regiani, S., Payne, A.H., and Marshall, J.C., 1980, Testicular GnRH receptors-characterization and localization on interstitial tissue. J. Clin. Endocr. Metab., 51: 407.

Browning, J.Y., D'Agata, R., Steinberger, A., Grotjan, H.E. Jr., and Steinberger, E., 1983, Biphasic effect of GnRH and its agonist analog (HOE 766) on in vitro testosterone production by purified rat Leydig cells, Endocrinology, 113: 985.

Hsueh, A.J.W., and Jones, P.B.C., 1981, Extrapituitary actions of gonadotropin-releasing hormone, Endocr. Rev., 2: 437.

Hunter, M.G., Sullivan, M.H.F., Dix, C.J., Aldred, L.F., and Cooke, B.A., 1982, Stimulation and inhibition by LHRH analogues of cultured rat Leydig cell function and lack of effect on mouse Leydig cells. Molec. Cell. Endocr., 27: 31.

Nagendranath, N., Jose, T.M., and Juneja, H.S., 1983, Bioassayable gonadotropin releasing hormone-like activity in the spent nutrient medium of rat Sertoli cells in primary cultures, Horm. Metab. Res., 15: 99.

Sharpe, R.M., 1983, Local control of testicular function, Qu. J. Exp. Physiol., 68: 265.

Sharpe, R.M., 1984, Intratesticular factors controlling testicular function. Biol. Reprod., (In press).

Sharpe, R.M., and Cooper, I., 1982, Stimulatory effect of LHRH and its agonists on Leydig cell steroidogenesis in vitro, Molec. Cell. Endocr., 26: 141.

Sharpe, R.M., Doogan, D.G., and Cooper, I., 1982b, Stimulation of Leydig cell testosterone secretion in vitro and in vivo in hypophysectomized rats by an agonist of luteinizing hormone releasing hormone, Biochem. biophys. Res. Commun., 106: 1210.

Sharpe, R.M., Doogan, D.G., and Cooper, I., 1983a, Factors determining whether the direct effect of an LHRH agonist on Leydig cell function in vivo are stimulatory or inhibitory, Molec. Cell. Endocr., 32: 57.

Sharpe, R.M., Doogan, D.G., and Cooper, I., 1983b, Direct effects of an LHRH agonist on intratesticular levels of testosterone and interstitial fluid formation in intact male rats, Endocrinology, 113: 1306.

Sharpe, R.M., and Fraser, H.M., 1983, The role of LH in regulation of Leydig cell responsiveness to an LHRH agonist, Molec. Cell. Endocr., 33: 131.

Sharpe, R.M., Fraser, H.M., Cooper, I., and Rommerts, F.F.G., 1982a, The secretion, measurement and function of a testicular LHRH-like factor, Ann. N.Y. Acad. Sci., 383: 272.

Sharpe, R.M., and Harmar, A.J., 1983, The nature and biological actions of 'testicular LHRH', In: Hormones and Cell Regulation, vol. 7, (Eds. J.E. Dumont, J. Nunez and R.M. Denton), pp. 217-230, Elsevier Biomedical Press, Amsterdam.

LUTEINIZING HORMONE-RELEASING HORMONE INDEPENDENTLY STIMULATES CYTODIFFERENTIATION OF GRANULOSA CELLS

J.H. Dorrington, H.L. McKeracher, A. Chan and R.E. Gore-Langton

Banting and Best Department of Medical Research
University of Toronto, and Department of Physiology
University of Western Ontario, London, Canada

INTRODUCTION

Luteinizing hormone-releasing hormone (LHRH) and the potent LHRH agonists are known to inhibit various hormone-regulated reproductive processes in the female rat. These inhibitory effects include inhibition of ovarian follicular maturation (Johnson *et al.*, 1976) and ovulation (Baumann *et al.*, 1980), delay of implantation (Lin and Yoshinaga, 1976), termination of pregnancy in its early stages (Corbin and Beattie, 1975) and delay of parturition (Bercu *et al.*, 1980). These actions of LHRH *in vivo* are associated with decreases in the circulating levels of estrogen and progesterone, and may therefore account, at least in part, for the observed inhibitory effects. Several mechanisms have been proposed to explain the inhibitory effects observed *in vivo*; exogenous LHRH may directly desensitize the pituitary causing reduced gonadotrophin secretion, an effect which would require long-term treatment. Alternatively, gonadal cells may be desensitized by the excessive gonadotrophin secretion produced by the acute stimulation of the pituitary by LHRH. LHRH and the potent agonists also directly inhibit the actions of FSH and LH on the stimulation of progesterone or estrogen secretion by rat granulosa and luteal cells. These actions appear to be mediated through the specific high-affinity receptors which are present on granulosa cells (Jones and Hsueh., 1981; Pieper *et al.*, 1981) and luteal cells (Pieper *et al.*, 1981; Clayton *et al.*, 1979). Knecht and Catt (1981) have suggested that the mechanism of direct inhibition of granulosa cell functions may be due to the inhibition of the FSH-induced decrease in cyclic nucleotide phosphodiesterase and the FSH-induced increase in adenylate cyclase activity.

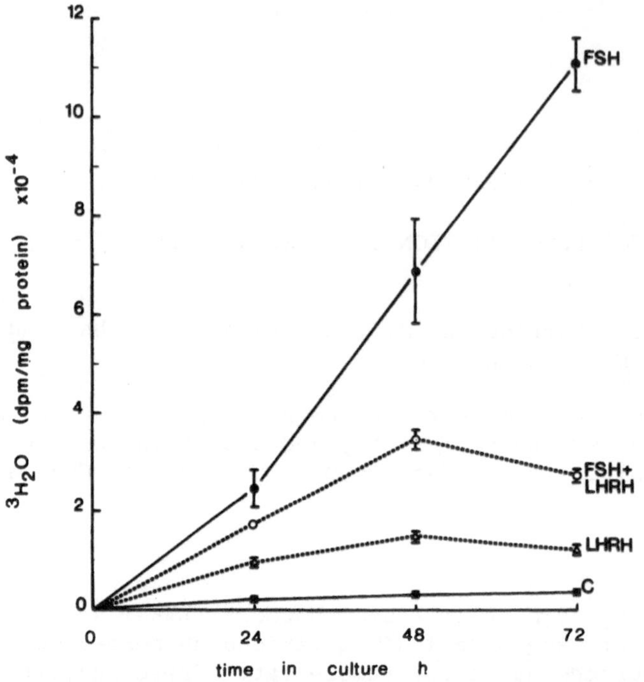

Figure 1. Effect of LHRH on aromatase activity in granulosa cell cultures. Granulosa cells were cultured for periods of 24, 48, or 72 h in the presence or absence of 500 ng/ml NIH-FSH-S14 and/or 10^{-7} M LHRH. Aromatase activity was assessed at each time point by incubating the cells for 2 h with 0.25 μCi [1β-^{3}H]testosterone (0.25 μM) and measuring the amount of ^3H_2O released. Each value is a mean ± SE (n=4). From Dorrington *et al*. 1983.

Since LHRH influenced steroidogenesis *in vivo* we have examined the effects of LHRH agonist [D-Ser(Bu^t)^6, des-Gly-NH_2^{10}]LHRH ethylamide (LHRH-A) on the activity of three key steroidogenic enzymes; aromatase, cholesterol side-chain cleavage and 3β-hydroxysteroid dehydrogenase, and on the activity of cAMP-binding proteins of granulosa cells, and compared these effects with those elicited by FSH. All experiments were carried out using cultures of granulosa cells isolated from immature rats which had been treated daily from day 20 to 23 of age with diethylstilbestrol in 0.1 ml sesame oil by subcutaneous injection (Gore-Langton and Dorrington, 1981). The cells were cultured in Falcon tissue culture plates using Eagle's Minimum Essential Medium with supplements and antibiotics and maintained at 37°C in a humidified atmosphere of 95% air and 5% CO_2. The hormonal treatments were made shortly after plating and after each daily medium change.

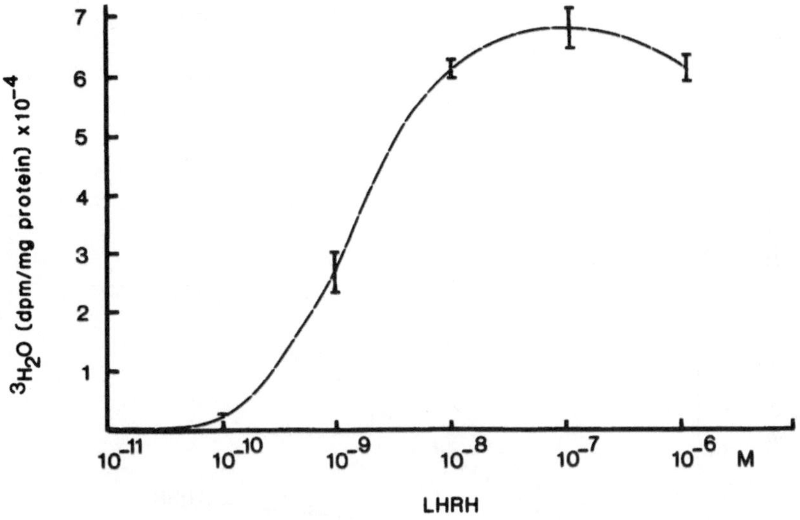

Figure 2. Dose response curve for the action of LHRH alone on aromatase activity in granulosa cell cultures. The cells were cultured in the presence of LHRH agonist (10^{-10}M to 10^{-6}M) for 48 h. The aromatase activity was assessed by measuring the amount of ^3H_2O released from 0.25 µCi [1β-^{3}H]testosterone, 0.25 µM, during a 2 h incubation. Each value is a mean ± SE (n=4). From Dorrington _et al_. 1983.

EFFECT OF LHRH-A ON STEROIDOGENIC ENZYMES

1. Aromatase

The aromatase activity of cell cultures was assessed using a radiometric assay which measures the stereospecific release of ^{3}H from [1β-^{3}H]testosterone to give ^3H_2O (Gore-Langton and Dorrington, 1981). Treatment of cells with LHRH-A alone caused a significantly greater aromatase activity during the first 24 h of culture and this remained elevated at 48 h and 72 h. The degree of stimulation with LHRH-A was however considerably less than that acheived in the presence of FSH. LHRH-A added simultaneously with FSH at the beginning of culture effectively inhibited FSH-induced aromatase activity at each time point (Figure 1). The stimulation of aromatase activity by LHRH-A was dose-dependent with an ED_{50} of 3.8 x 10^{-9} M and a maximal effect produced by 10^{-8} M (Figure 2). By comparing cells treated with FSH and LHRH-A for the entire 72 h culture period with cells in which the LHRH-A component was removed after 24 h of culture, we showed that the inhibitory effect of LHRH-A was irreversible (Dorrington _et al_. 1983).

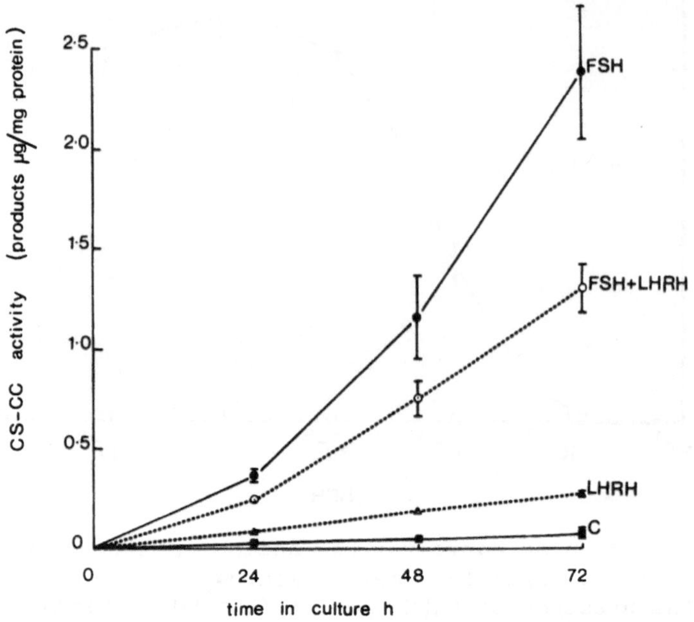

Figure 3. Effect of LHRH on cholesterol side-chain cleavage (CS-CC) activity. Granulosa cells were cultured in the presence or absence of 10^{-7}M LHRH agonist and/or 500 ng/ml NIH-FSH-S14. Medium was collected at 24, 48 and 72 h of culture. The total secreted products were measured as pregnenolone, progesterone and 20α-hydroxypregn-4-en-3-one individually determined by RIA. Each value is a mean ± SE (n=4).

Table 1. Comparison of secreted and cellular levels of cholesterol side-chain cleavage products.

Treatment	Sum of products* Secreted 0-72h		Cell Extract	
	ngs	Fold Stimulation	ngs	Fold Stimulation
Control	18	1	7	1
FSH	2434	137	550	83
LHRH-A	365	21	139	21
FSH + LHRH-A	1023	57	193	29

*See Legend for figure 3. The data is expressed as total products synthesized during 72 h culture.

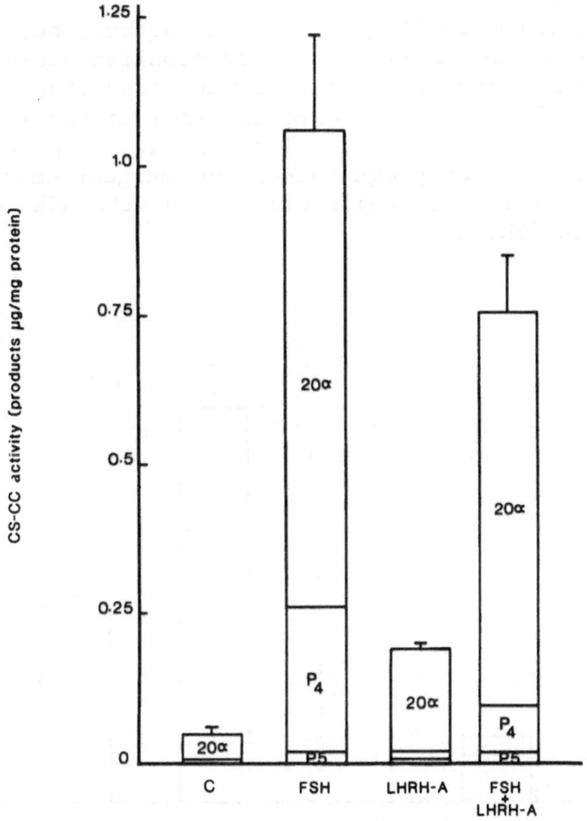

Figure 4. Composition of the steroid products secreted by granulosa cells during a 48 h culture period in the presence of FSH and LHRH (10^{-7}M). P_5 denotes pregnenolone, P_4: progesterone, and 20α: 20α-hydroxypregn-4-en-3-one.

2. Cholesterol side-chain cleavage

The effects of LHRH-A acting either independently or in combination with FSH were then examined on the key steroidogenic steps involved in the synthesis of progesterone. The first step involves the conversion of cholesterol to pregnenolone by the cholesterol side-chain cleavage (CS-CC) system. The subsequent metabolism of pregnenolone to progesterone results from the action of Δ^5-3β-hydroxysteroid dehydrogenase and Δ^5-Δ^4-isomerase. Cholesterol side-chain cleavage activity was assessed by measuring the total secreted products synthesised from endogenous cholesterol, by individual radioimmunoassays. Untreated cells had a low level of CS-CC activity and synthesised 20α-hydroxypregn-4-en-3-one as the major product (Fig.3, 4). Cultures treated with LHRH-A alone had small but significantly elevated levels of CS-CC activity, the major product also being 20α-hydroxypregn-4-en-3-one. FSH greatly increased CS-CC activity in granulosa cells after 24,48, and 72 h in culture, but this activity was suppressed when LHRH-A was added simultaneously. It was apparent that pregnenolone was rapidly metabolised since 20α-hydroxypregn-4-en-3-one and progesterone were secreted in far higher concentrations than pregnenolone (Fig. 4). The relative proportions of progesterone and 20α-hydroxypregn-4-en-3-one suggest enhanced metabolism of progesterone in cells stimulated with LHRH alone or in combination with FSH.

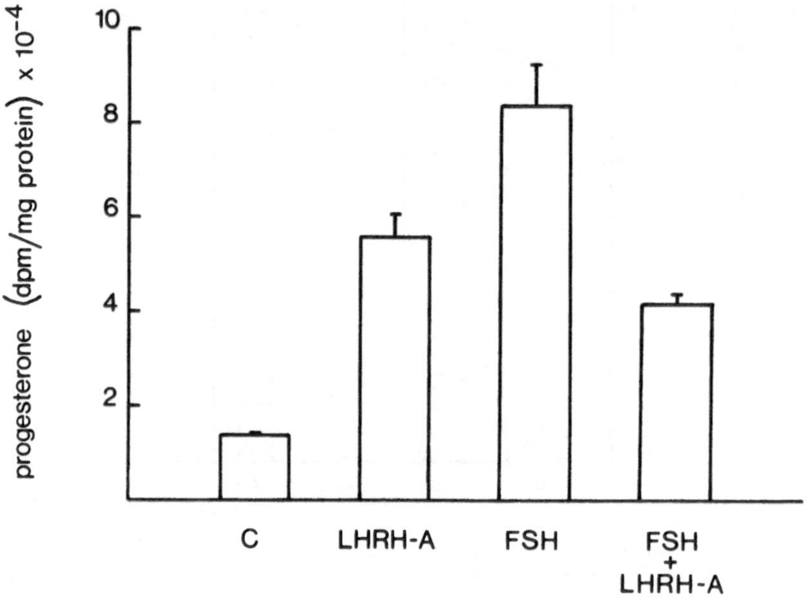

Figure 5. Δ^5-3β-Hydroxysteroid dehydrogenase activity in rat granulosa cells cultured with LHRH agonist (10^{-7}M) and/or FSH for 72 h. The activity was measured in a cell-free system under optimal conditions using [^{3}H]pregnenolone as the substrate. [^{3}H]Progesterone was the only product obtained after a 20 min incubation and this was purified by TLC. From Dorrington et al. 1983.

3. 3β-Hydroxysteroid dehydrogenase activity

The activity of 3β-hydroxysteroid dehydrogenase was determined by measuring the rate of conversion of ^{3}H-pregnenolone to ^{3}H-progesterone in cell-free preparations under optimal conditions (Dorrington and Armstrong, 1979). Pretreatment of cultures with LHRH-A alone for 72 h increased the activity 4-fold whereas FSH alone produced a 6-fold increase. The combined treatment with LHRH-A and FSH resulted in an increase in 3β-hydroxysteroid dehydrogenase activity but this was less than that elicited by either FSH or LHRH alone.

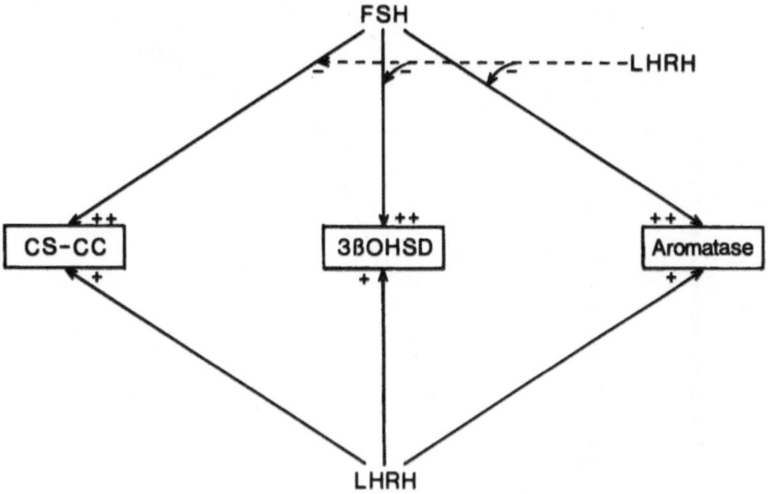

Figure 6. Summary of the interactions between FSH and LHRH on steroidogenic enzymes. —Denotes inhibitory actions and + indicates stimulatory actions.

From the experiments described above one can conclude that FSH acts directly on undifferentiated granulosa cells previously primed with DES to induce the appearance of the domain of proteins required for the synthesis of steroids. These steroids are required for the co-ordination of events within the follicle and for communication between the ovary and the hypothalamus-pituitary and the uterus, to synchronize the events which occur during the normal cycle. The ability of LHRH to inhibit these essential functions of FSH provide the biochemical basis for the antigonadal actions of this peptide, since the normal process of follicular development is interrupted.

To determine if LHRH exclusively inhibits the expression of steroidogenic enzymes we examined its effects on the activity of other intracellular proteins induced by FSH namely cAMP binding proteins.

EFFECTS OF FSH AND LHRH ON cAMP BINDING ACTIVITY

Richards and Rolfes (1980) showed that FSH stimulated the cAMP-binding activity of granulosa cells isolated from immature hypophysectomized rats. We have established conditions under which these effects of FSH could be demonstrated *in vitro* in order to study in more detail those factors which could modulate the action of FSH. Granulosa cells freshly isolated from DES-primed immature rats contained cAMP binding activity in the 20,000g supernatant fraction but this tended to decrease with increasing time in culture in

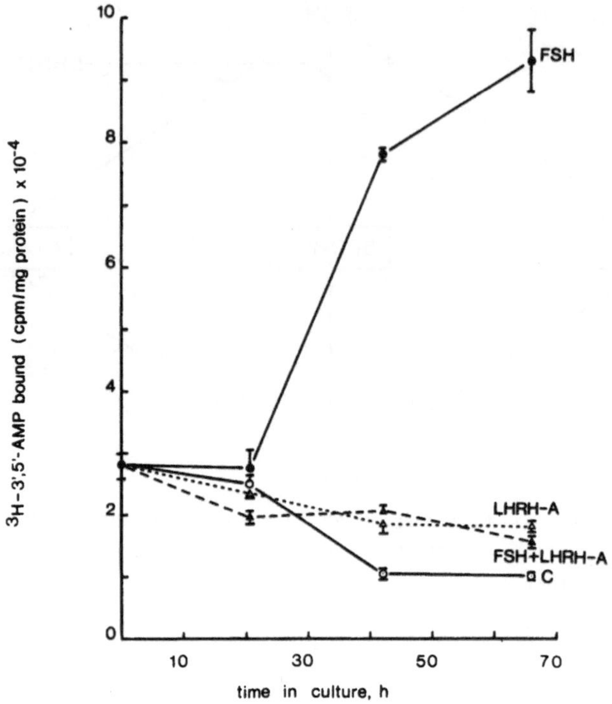

Figure 7. Specific binding of [^{3}H]cAMP to the 20,000g supernatant fraction from granulosa cells cultured for 66 h with 500ng NIH-FSH-S14/ml and/or 10^{-7}M LHRH-A. Supernatants were incubated with 0.12μM [^{3}H]cAMP with and without 100-fold excess of unlabelled cAMP to estimate the specifically bound [^{3}H]cAMP. The methods used were the same as those described by Richards and Rolfes (1980). Each value is the mean ± SE (n=4).

medium alone (Figure 7). When the cells were cultured in the presence of FSH there was little change in the amount of cAMP binding activity for the first 20 h. A large increase in binding capacity occurred on the second day of culture and this increase continued for 66 h after plating when the experiment was terminated (Fig. 7). This parameter was also slightly stimulated by the addition of LHRH-A alone. LHRH-A suppressed the FSH-stimulated increase in cAMP binding activity after 42 h and 66 h of culture.

In order to determine the molecular weights of the proteins in the 20,000g supernatant fraction which bound cAMP the granulosa cell preparation was labelled with the photoreactive probe [^{3}H]8-N_3 cAMP and the proteins separated by one dimensional SDS-gel electrophoresis. The autoradiographs revealed two major proteins with molecular weights of 48,000 and 54,000 which specifically bound [^{3}H]8-N_3 cAMP in preparations from control cells (lane 1). After

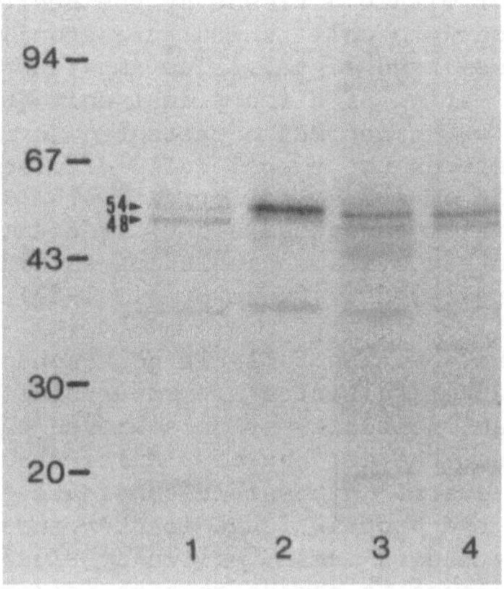

Figure 8. Autoradiograph of a one-dimensional SDS-gel following the electrophoresis of 20,000g supernatant fractions labelled with the photoreactive probe, [^{3}H]8-N_3 cAMP. Labelled proteins from control granulosa cells maintained in culture for 66 h are shown in lane 1, from FSH- treated cells in lane 2, LHRH (10^{-7}M)-treated cells in lane 3, and FSH and LHRH-treated cells in lane 4. The molecular weights (x 10^{-3}) were obtained from standard proteins run on the same gel.

treatment of the cells with FSH for 66 h there was an increase in the amount of binding to the 54,000 molecular weight protein with little change in the 48,000 molecular weight component (lane 2). The small increase in cAMP binding activity after treatment with LHRH alone, demonstrated in figure 7 could also be attributed to an increase in the binding to the 54,000 molecular weight protein (lane 3). LHRH suppressed the FSH-induced increase in cAMP binding activity by interfering with the ability of FSH to increase the binding capacity of the higher molecular weight protein (lane 4).

DISCUSSION

In developing tissues, such as the follicle, cells interact in a number of ways in order to support morphogenesis and cytodifferentiation. Cell-cell interaction can exist between cells of the same type and between cell types of different embryonic origins. Cells can interact by acquiring specific proteins on their cell surface which then serve as recognition sites for other neighbouring cells and allow the progression of the developmental program. Communication can occur within a tissue by the secretion and transport of specific products to cells which have acquired the ability to respond to the transmitted signal. The importance of cell-cell interaction in the formation of a functional unit is exemplified by the dominant follicle which becomes competent to ovulate as a result of the interactions between the thecal cells of mesenchymal origin and the granulosa cells of epithelial origin. The influence of the mesenchyme on epithelial morphogenesis and differentiation has been studied in detail in other systems, including the mammary gland, uterus and prostate (reviewed by Cunha et al. 1983).

Once selected, the dominant follicle continues to grow in an environment in which other follicles are undergoing atresia. The eminence of the dominant follicle may be achieved by the secretion of factor(s) which cause the atrophy of similar structures in the same or contralateral ovary. A possible candidate for one of these inhibitory factors is the protein found in the venous drainage of the preovulatory ovary and in human follicular fluid, which suppresses follicular response to gonadotrophins (diZerega et al. 1982, 1983).

It is our working hypothesis that the dominant follicle acquires autocrine and paracrine mechanisms for local regulation in order to complete its developmental program. We know that steroids are important local regulators; testosterone synthesised in the thecal cells acts as a substrate for aromatization and as a hormone to influence FSH-induced steroidogenesis in the granulosa cells. Estrogen produced by granulosa cells is an "autocrine" regulator since it causes proliferation of granulosa cells and modulates FSH action.

The possibility that proteins synthesised by the follicle may also play a role in local regulation was suggested by the observation that insulin (and insulin-like growth factors) could augment the action of FSH on aromatase activity in human granulosa cells (Garzo and Dorrington, 1983). The concentration of insulin required, however, was higher than that found in human plasma suggesting that if these effects are important physiologically then other insulin-like factors may be involved. Insulin interacts with a low affinity with the somatomedin C receptor raising the possibility that somatomedin C or a similar "growth factor" may be important physiologically. The identification of inhibitory and stimulatory factors produced by the follicle is clearly essential to determine the maintenance of fertility and the underlying causes of infertility.

The study of LHRH actions has been particularly useful since it has provided us with an example of a small peptide which can alter ovarian function. It is unlikely that LHRH itself plays a physiological role outside the hypothalamic-pituitary axis, since the concentration found in human plasma is low (8 x 10^{-12}M) (Elkind-Hirsch et al. 1982) compared with the amount required to produce a response in granulosa cells (Fig. 2). Nevertheless, pharmacological doses of LHRH and its potent analogues can stimulate the principle enzymatic steps in the synthesis of estrogen and progesterone by rat granulosa cells. We have shown that the activities of aromatase, cholesterol side-chain cleavage enzyme, and Δ^5-3β hydroxysteroid dehydrogenase are directly and independently stimulated by LHRH agonist, even though the extent of the stimulation is in each case, less than that obtained with FSH. In addition to steroidogenic enzymes, LHRH alone can influence cAMP binding proteins (Dorrington et al. 1983), secretion of plasminogen activator (Wang, 1983) and the resumption of meiosis in the oocyte and ovulation (Ekholm et al. 1981). LHRH alone can stimulate cAMP accumulation, albeit to a small extent, and it may be this ability which enables it to mimic the actions of FSH on the rat follicle (Dorrington et al. 1983).

We have confirmed that LHRH agonist can partially inhibit estrogen and progesterone secretion by inhibiting the action of FSH on steroidogenic enzymes (Hsueh and Jones, 1981), and have shown that the inhibitory action can also be extended to other FSH end-responses eg. cAMP binding proteins. The mechanism by which LHRH inhibits FSH-stimulated end-responses also seems to involve changes in cAMP level (Massicotte et al. 1980; Dorrington et al. 1983). Knecht and Catt (1981) and Knecht et al. (1983) have suggested that the inhibitory effects of LHRH on FSH actions are attributable to a reduction in cyclic AMP accumulation by influencing cyclic nucleotide phosphodiesterase and adenylate cyclase activity.

The work on LHRH has re-emphasized two important concepts: Firstly, factors which increase cAMP levels can mimic the actions of FSH, supporting the role of cAMP as an intracellular mediator of the events which occur during the cytodifferentiation of granulosa cells. Secondly, follicular development can be arrested by factors which interfere with the ability of FSH to increase cAMP. The question of whether the follicle synthesises LHRH-like peptides remains; nevertheless, the concepts which have evolved from the study of the antigonadal actions of LHRH have stimulated a new interest in the role of peptides in the control of follicular maturation.

REFERENCES

Baumann, R., Kuhl, H., Taubert, H.-D. and Sandow, J., 1980, Contraception, 21: 191.
Bercu, B.B., Hyashi, A., Poth, M., Alexandrova, M., Soloff, M.S., and Donahoe, P.K., 1980, Endocrinology, 107: 504.
Clayton, R.N., Harwood, J.P., and Catt, K.J., 1979, Nature, 282: 90.
Corbin, A., and Beattie, C.W., 1975, Endocr. Res. Commun. 2: 445.

Cunha, G.R., Chung, L.W.K., Shannon, J.M., Taguchi, O., and Fujii, H., 1983, Rec. Progr. Hormone, Res., 39: 559.
DiZerega, G.S., Goebelsmann, U., and Nakamura, R.M., 1982, J. Clin. Endocrinol. Metab., 54: 1901.
DiZerega, G.S., Marrs, R.P., Campeau, J.D., and Kling, O.R., 1983, J. Clin. Endocrinol. Metab., 56: 35.
Dorrington, J.H., and Armstrong, D.T., 1979, Rec. Progr. Hormone Res., 35: 301.
Dorrington, J.H., McKeracher, H.L., Chan, A.K., and Gore-Langton, R. J. Steroid Biochem., 19: 17.
Ekholm, C., Hillensjo, T., and Isaksson, O., 1981, Endocrinology, 108: 2022.
Elkind-Hirsch, K., Ravnikar, V., Schiff, I., Tulchinsky, D., and Ryan, K.J., 1982, J. Clin. Endocr. Metab., 54: 602.
Garzo, G., Dorrington, J.H., 1983, Am. J. Obs. Gyn. in press.
Gore-Langton, R.E., and Dorrington, J.H., 1981, Mol. Cell Endocr., 22: 135.
Hsueh, A.J.W., and Jones, P.B.C., 1981, Endocr. Rev., 2: 437.
Johnson, E.S., Gendrich, R.L., and White, W.F., 1976, Fertil. Steril., 27: 853.
Jones, P.B.C., and Hsueh, A.J.W., 1981, J. Biol. Chem. 256: 1248.
Knecht, M., and Catt, K.J., 1981, Science, 214: 1346.
Knecht, M., Ranta, T., Naor, Z., and Catt, K.J., 1983, in: "Factors regulating ovarian function", G.S. Greenwald, and P.F. Terranova, ed., Raven Press, New York.
Lin, Y.C., and Yoshinaga, K., 1976, Program 58th Annual Meeting Endocrine Soc. San Francisco, p. 143.
Massicotte, J., Veilleux, R., Lavoie, M., and Labrie, F., 1980, Biochem. Biophys. Res. Commun., 94: 1362.
Pieper, P.R., Richards, J.S., and Marshall, J.C., 1981, Endocrinology, 108: 1148.
Richards, J.S., and Rolfes, A.I., 1980, J. Biol. Chem. 255: 5481.
Wang, C., 1983, Endocrinology, 112: 1130.

ACTION OF LHRH ANALOGUES ON RAT LEYDIG CELLS IN VITRO: EFFECTS ON CYCLIC AMP, Ca^{2+}, CHOLESTEROL SIDE CHAIN CLEAVAGE AND CELL SIZE

Brian A. Cooke, Mark H.F. Sullivan and Louise F. Aldred

Department of Biochemistry and Chemistry
Royal Free Hospital School of Medicine
(University of London)
Rowland Hill Street
London NW3 2FP

INTRODUCTION

Previous studies from this laboratory (Hunter et al., 1982) demonstrated that LHRH analogues bind specifically to purified rat but not mouse Leydig cells. During short term (less than 24 h) these analogues stimulate steroidogenesis in the rat Leydig cells (Hunter et al., 1982; Sharpe & Cooper, 1982; Sharpe et al., 1982) but long term (in excess of 24 h) effects are inhibitory on LH-stimulated steroidogenesis (Hunter et al., 1982; Massicotte et al., 1981). Further studies have now been carried out to determine the effects and roles of cyclic AMP, Ca^{2+} in LHRH agonist action during stimulation of steroidogenesis (Sullivan & Cooke 1984 a,b) and to determine the effects of LHRH agonist on cholesterol side chain cleavage, enzyme activity (Sullivan & Cooke, 1984c) and size of the Leydig cells (Aldred & Cooke, unpublished).

METHODS AND MATERIALS

Rat Leydig cells were prepared and purified as described previously (Hunter et al, 1982; Aldred and Cooke, 1982). All preparative procedures were carried out in media containing 2.0 - 2.5 mM Ca^{2+}. Media depleted in Ca^{2+} were prepared by adding 2.8 mM EGTA to complex the calcium.

Purified rat Leydig cells were plated out in Costar culture

wells (10^5 cells/well unless otherwise stated) and the media (Dulbecco's Modified Eagles Medium) (Gibco Europe) added. LHRH agonist (ICI 118630) (dissolved in media) and LH (LH-NIH-S 20; 2.3 i.u. NIH-SI/mg) (dissolved in media) were added as stated in the text. The calcium ionophore A23187 (Sigma Chemical Co., London) was dissolved in dimethylsulphoxide at 100 times the final concentration and 10 µl/ml medium was added. The same amount of dimethylsulphoxide was added to the controls. 1-methylisobutylxanthine (MIX) (Sigma Chemical Co., London) was dissolved in media at the final concentration stated in the text. Hydroxy cholesterol or pregnenolone (in ethanol, 10 µl/ml media, were added as appropriate after 2 hours in culture, unless stated otherwise in the text. The cells were then incubated at 32°C. After 4 hours, incubations were stopped with $HClO_4$ (final concentration 0.5 M) and frozen at -20°C until neutralised with K_3PO_4 (final concentration 0.23 M) and assayed for testosterone (Verjans et al., 1973) and cyclic AMP (Steiner et al., 1972, as modified by Harper and Brooker, 1975). ICI 118630 (< Glu-His-Trp-Ser-Tyr-D-Ser(Bu^t)-Leu-Arg-Pro-AzaGly-NH_2) was a gift from ICI PLC. All data are total (intracellular plus extracellular) levels of testosterone and cyclic AMP; unless stated otherwise. Initial levels were not subtracted.

To measure intra- and extracellular cyclic AMP and testosterone levels, the medium was removed from the cells, acidified with $HClO_4$ as above and frozen. 150µl of $HClO_4$ was added to the cells, and this was followed by freezing. Before assay, the cellular extract was neutralized with 300 µl K_3PO_4; the medium was treated as above.

RESULTS

Effects of LHRH Agonist

(i) Cyclic AMP Production: An investigation of the initial 2 hours of incubation of rat testis Leydig cells showed (Fig. 1) that intracellular and extracellular cyclic AMP levels are unaffected by LHRH agonist in the presence of the phosphodiesterase inhibitor, MIX. A significant increase in extracellular testosterone production was detected after 40 minutes incubation and the major increase occurred in the period from 120 minutes to 240 minutes incubation (Fig. 2).

Comparison of LHRH agonist and low concentrations of LH (Fig. 3) in the absence of MIX showed that 0.050 ng/ml LH was equipotent with 10^{-7} M LHRH agonist in stimulating testosterone production during a 4 hour incubation. In the presence of MIX, the effect of LH were greatly potentiated, however, no potentiation of the LHRH agonist effect on testosterone production was found. In the absence and presence of MIX cyclic AMP levels were increased by LH but not by LHRH agonist.

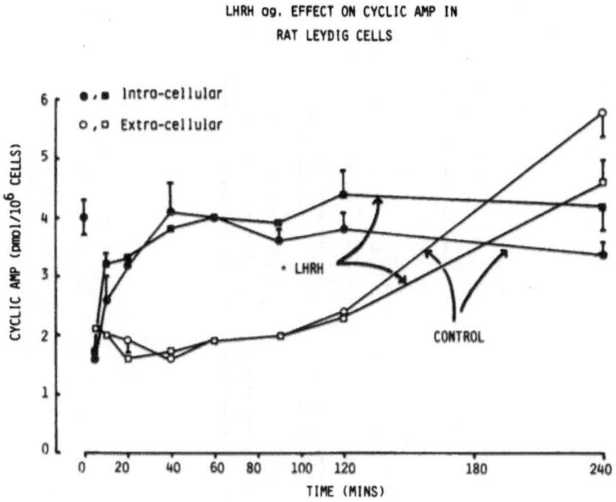

Figure 1

(Data from Sullivan & Cooke 1984 a).

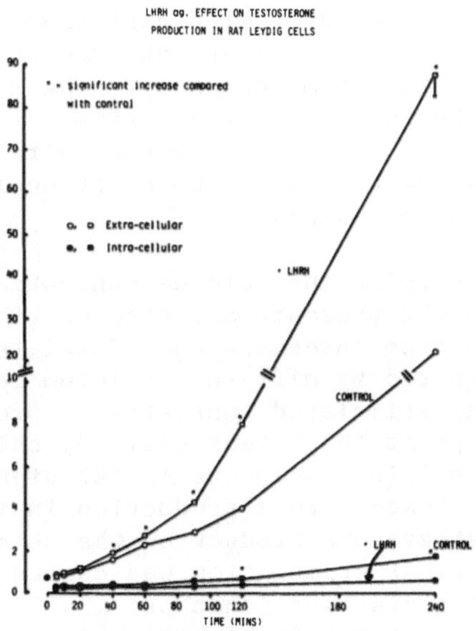

Figure 2

(Data from Sullivan & Cooke 1984 a)

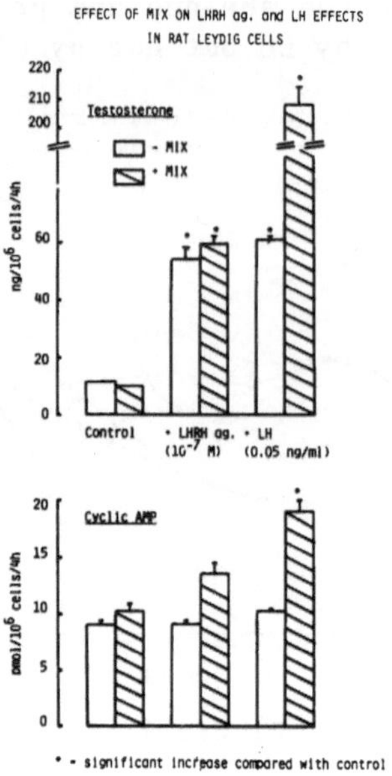

Figure 3

(Data from Sullivan and Cooke 1984 a).
(ii) Calcium: To determine the effect of the calcium ionophore A23187 on LHRH agonist-stimulated testosterone production, cells were incubated with different concentrations of the ionophore in the presence (●) and absence (0) of the agonist (10^{-7} M) for 4 hours (in 2.5 mM calcium). The results obtained (Fig. 4) show that the ionophore itself stimulated testosterone production and that this occurred in a concentration-dependent manner. LHRH agonist had little or no additional effect in the presence of 0.2 - 1.0 μM A23187.

The effect of changing the calcium concentration in the incubation medium in the presence and absence of the ionophore and LHRH agonist was also investigated. Basal testosterone production was unaffected by different calcium concentrations. LHRH agonist (10^{-7} M) stimulated testosterone production 2 - 3 fold ($p < 0.05$) except at the lowest (1.1 μM) calcium concentration. The calcium ionophore A23187 significantly increased ($p < 0.01$) testosterone production in 1 - 10 mM calcium; maximum testosterone production was obtained with 2.5 mM calcium. A small further stimulation was caused by the combination of LHRH agonist and ionophore A23187 at 1.1 μM and 1 mM calcium ($p < 0.05$) but not at higher calcium levels compared with the ionophore alone. With 10 mM calcium, the ionophore effect (in the presence or absence of LHRH agonist) was the same as the effect of LHRH agonist alone.

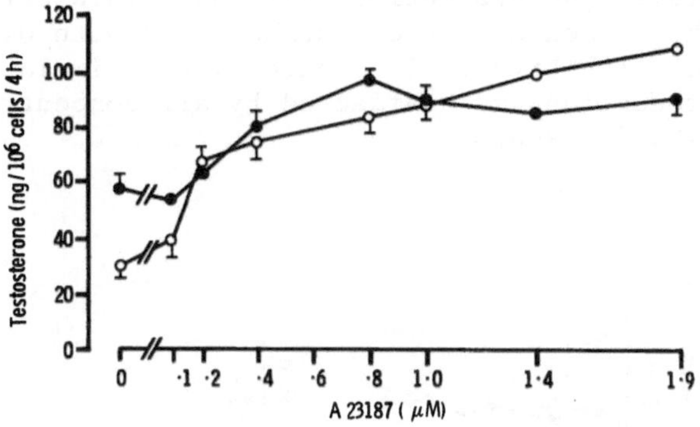

Figure 4

(Data from Sullivan and Cooke 1984 a).

Effects of LHRH agonist and LH

(i) Cyclic AMP and Testosterone production: LHRH agonist potentiated testosterone production at all concentrations of LH ($p < 0.05$). At submaximal levels of LH (0 -0.1 ng/ml), cyclic AMP levels were undetectable (no MIX was added) but were measurable at higher LH concentrations (1.0 - 1000 ng/ml). LHRH agonist decreased LH-induced cyclic AMP production ($p < 0.05$) with 10 ng/ml LH, but not significantly with 100 - 1000 ng/ml LH. However, accumulated data from 5 experiments with 100 ng/ml LH gave a mean significant decrease of $24.5 \pm 6.1\%$ (S.E.M. in cyclic AMP levels below LH-stimulated levels ($p < 0.01$).

(ii) Effects of A23187 and Calcium: In the presence of low calcium levels (1.1 μM and 1.0 mM) LH-stimulated testosterone production was less than 50% of the production with 2.5 mM calcium. Concentrations of calcium higher than 2.5 mM had little further effect. The LHRH agonist potentiated LH-stimulated testosterone production at all calcium concentrations, and was highest at the highest calcium concentration used (10 mM) ($p < 0.05$, with 1.1 μM and 1 mM calcium; $p < 0.01$, with 2.5 - 10 mM calcium).

To examine the effect of the ionophore A23187 on the potentiating effects of LHRH agonist on LH-induced steroidogenesis, cells were incubated with different concentrations of the ionophore with and without LHRH agonist, for 4 hours; LH was added after 2 hours of incubation. Again, in the absence of the calcium ionophore, LHRH agonist potentiated LH-induced testosterone production (Fig. 5). This effects was decreased in the presence of the ionophore and with 0.5 μM A23187 it was completely inhibited. In contrast, LH-stimulated testosterone production was unaffected by all concentrations of the ionophore A23187 used.

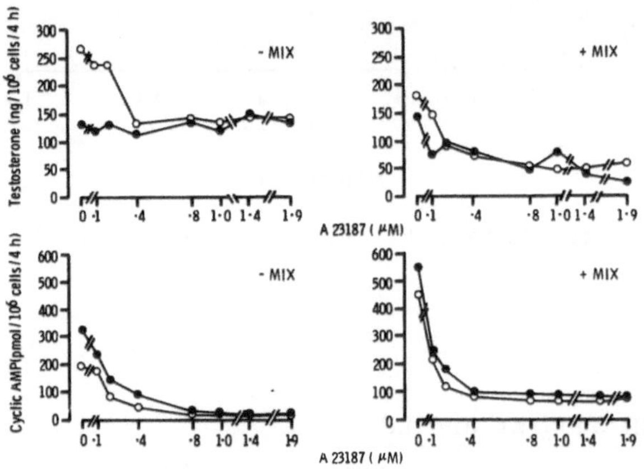

Figure 5

(Data from Sullivan and Cooke 1984 a).

In the presence of the phosphodiesterase inhibitor MIX, the effect of LHRH was negated with lower concentrations of A23187 (0.2 μM) and the LH-stimulated steroidogenesis was decreased; with 1.4 - 1.9 μM A23187 it was decreased to basal levels. In the presence of MIX, higher levels of cyclic AMP were obtained than in the absence of this phosphodiesterase inhibitor (lower graphs, Fig. 5) but when the ionophore was added a marked concentration-dependent decrease in the cyclic AMP levels was found in both cases.

Effects of LHRH agonist and LH on Cholesterol Side Chain Cleavage

In initial experiments it was found that addition of 25-hydroxycholesterol or 22(R) hydroxycholesterol to the rat Leydig cells increased the amounts of testosterone formed above those obtained with maximally stimulatory amounts of LH. The amounts of the hydroxycholesterol metabolized to testosterone were not increased by LH. In fact, with concentrations greater than 0.37 μM 25-hydroxycholesterol the LH-stimulated testosterone production in the presence of the hydroxycholesterol decreased compared with 25-hydroxycholesterol alone; the LH-induced stimulation of testosterone production above basal decreased from 69.5 ± 3.8 ng/10^6 cells/4 h over a range 0 - 0.37 µM 25-hydroxycholesterol to 38.4 ± 6.2 ng with 3.7 µM hydroxycholesterol and to 13.2 ± 5.4 ng with 37 µM hydroxycholesterol. In contrast, LHRH agonist markedly stimulated more 25-hydroxycholesterol metabolism to testosterone with concentrations of the former greater than 0.37 µM; the increase due to LHRH agonist was 16.6 ± 1.2 ng testosterone/10^6 cells/4 h with no hydroxycholesterol present, and increased to 83.5 ± 7.9 testosterone/10^6 cells/4 h in the presence of 37 µM 25-hydroxycholesterol.

Because more testosterone is formed from 22(R)-hydroxycholesterol than the 25-hydroxy compound the metabolism of the former was also investigated. In the above experiments the Leydig cells were incubated with the LHRH agonist for a total of 4 h and the hydroxycholesterol and LH were present during the last 2 h of incubation. An additional experiment was carried out in which LH and/or LHRH agonist was present for 4 h. The 22(R)-hydroxycholesterol (0.1, 1.0 and 10.0 µM) was added after 1 h. LHRH agonist increased the production of testosterone as the concentration of 22(R)-hydroxycholesterol was increased (from 23.4 ng testosterone/10^6 cells/4 h with no hydroxysteroid to 101.2 ng testosterone/10^6 cells/4 h with 10 µM hydroxysteroid) ($p < 0.05$) (Fig. 6). In contrast, the stimulation by LH compared with the hydroxysteroid alone remained constant (61.9 ± 5.2 ng/10^6 cells/4 h over the whole concentration range). LH plus LHRH agonist potentiated steroidogenesis further ($p < 0.05$) compared with the effects of LH and LHRH agonist when present separately, e.g. with 10 µM 22(R)-hydroxycholesterol the testosterone production due to LH + LHRH agonist was 326.4 compared with 101.2 and 52.5 ng/10^6 cells/4 h for LHRH agonist and LH respectively (Fig. 6).

EFFECTS OF LH AND LHRH AGONIST ON 22(R) - HYDROXYCHOLESTEROL METABOLISM

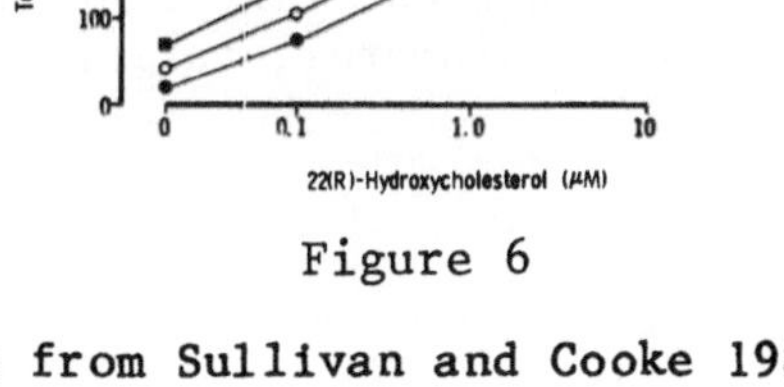

Figure 6

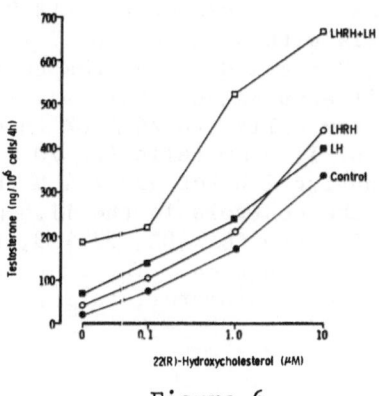

(Data from Sullivan and Cooke 1984 c).

Substitution of 1.6 μM pregnenolone (added in 10 μl ethanol) for 22(R)-hydroxysteroid in the incubations with the Leydig cells also resulted in high testosterone production (562 ± 24 ng/10^6 cells/4 h), but the addition of LHRH agonist had no additional effect on testosterone production (pregnenolone + LHRH agonist: 558 ± 16 ng/10^6 cells)/4 h).

Effects of LHRH agonist and A23187 on Leydig Cell Size

The cells isolated from rat testes were found to vary in size with a mean diameter of 11.8 ± 1.9 μm (means ± S.D. from 8 separate experiments, 2 - 4 rats per experiment) and with a range of 7 to 15 μm. For convenience of counting they were grouped into 3 sizes: 7.7, 11.5 and 15.4 μm. In freshly isolated cells the percentage of cells in these 3 groups was 15.7 ± 5.0, 73.3 ± 6.7 and 11.0 ± 10.7% respectively, (means ± S.D., n=5).

In control experiments (Fig. 7,8 & 9 upper graph) it was found that no changes in cell size occurred within 2 h but after 2 - 4 h there was a decrease in the number of cells of the smallest diameter (7.7 μm) and an increase in the cells of the largest diameter (15.4 μm). When LHRH agonist was added to cells there was a rapid marked increase in the percentage of cells with an average diameter of 15.4 μm and there were corresponding decreases in the percentages of 7.7 μm and 11.5 μm diameter cells (fig. 8). In contrast LH only caused small changes compared with the control during 1 h and after this time no significant changes could be detected (Fig. 9). The calcium ionophore A23187 had very similar effects to the LHRH agonist (Fig. 10) i.e. a rapid increase from 20 to 40% of the largest cells occurred and remained at 30 - 40% throughout the incubation period. These studies were carried out on the cells in culture. Similar results were obtained with the cells were kept in suspension.

The mouse cells had a mean diameter of 13.9 ± 3.3 μm (n=5). The distribution of cells with diameters of 7.7, 11.5, 15.4 and 19.2 was 4 ± 6, 34 ± 7,57 ± 8 and 5 ± 4% respectively. During 4 h incubation of the cell suspensions there was a decrease in the number of 15.4 μm diameter cells (to 26 ± 6% in 4 h) and an increase in the number of 11.5 μm cells (to 70 ± 7%). LHRH agonist had no effect during 2 h but after 4 h there was a small decrease compared with the controls in the 11.5 μm cells (to $p < 0.05$) and the 15.4μm cells (to 40 ± 8%, 57 ± 9, $p < 0.02$). LH had no effect during 2 h incubation. The presence of A23187 prevented any changes in cell diameter, taking place during 2 h incubation.

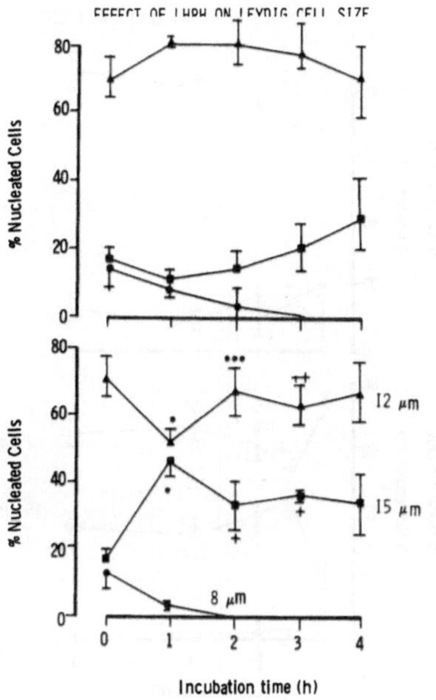

Figure 7

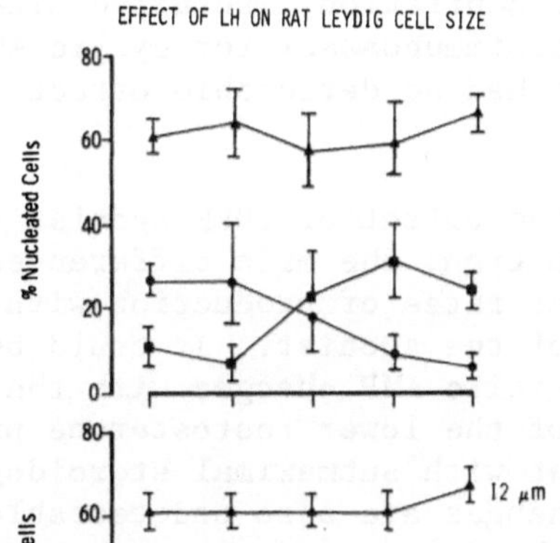

Figure 8

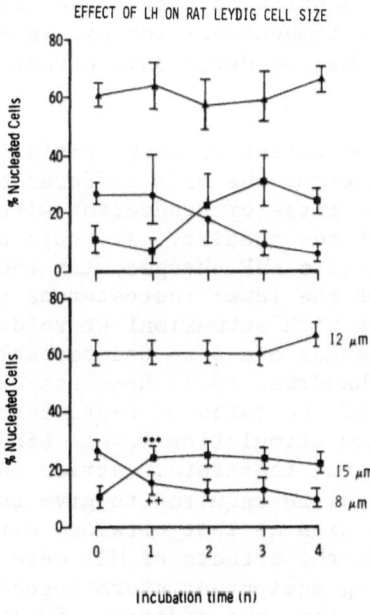

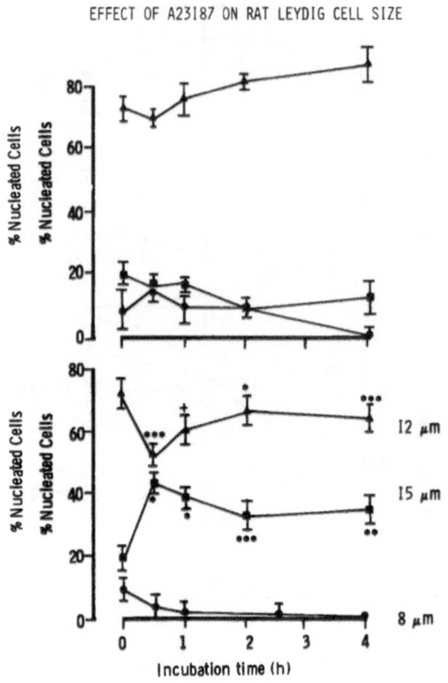

Figure 9

DISCUSSION

The results obtained in this study show that the LHRH agonist required at least 1 mM Ca^{2+} to exert its effects on steroidogenesis, and it has no detectable effect on cyclic AMP levels at any Ca^{2+} concentration. Detailed kinetic studies using a sensitive radioimmunoassay for cyclic AMP also showed that the LHRH agonist had no detectable effect on cyclic AMP levels.

With regard to the effect of LHRH agonist compared with LH on testosterone production, the main differences are the lower maximum production and rates of production with maximum stimulating amounts of the agonist. It could be argued that the inability to detect cyclic AMP changes with the LHRH agonist is simply a reflection of the lower testosterone production levels; it is established that with submaximal steroidogenic amounts of hCG/LH, cyclic AMP changes are also undetectable (Catt and Dufau, 1973; Moyle and Ramachandran, 1973; Rommerts et al.,1973). Also with low amounts of hCG the rates of testosterone production are lower than with maximum stimulating levels (Sharpe and Harmer, 1983). Experiments were, therefore, carried out in the to determine the amounts of LH required to give the same stimulation of testosterone production as that obtained with LHRH agonist; cyclic AMP changes and the effects of MIX were then determined. It was found that using equipotent steroidogenic concentrations of LH and LHRH agonist that the addition of MIX had a marked potentiating effect on LH-induced steroidogenesis, but no effect on LHRH agonist stimulated steroidogenesis during 4 hour incubations. Higher levels of cyclic AMP were found in the presence of MIX in all the incubations. In the absence of MIX using equipotent steroidogenic concentrations of the hormones, a very small but significant ($p < 0.05$) increase in cyclic AMP was induced by LH, but not by LHRH agonist. These data again emphasise the different mechanisms of action of LH and LHRH agonist on steroidogenesis. These results are consistent with a primary role of Ca^{2+} in the action of the LHRH agonist.

The effects of LH and LH plus LHRH agonist on testosterone production were found to be dependent on the concentration of Ca^{2+}. It was anticipated, therefore, that the Ca^{2+} ionophore in the presence of 2.5 mM Ca^{2+} would further stimulate LH and LH plus LHRH agonists effects; however, this was not found; 0.1 - 0.2 μM A23187 had no effect and higher amounts completely negated the effect of LHRH agonist, whereas the LH stimulation was unaltered. Although this effect of the ionophore may have been non-specific this is unlikely because the cell viability was not affected and the LH-stimulated testosterone production remained constant (in the absence of MIX).

In both the absence and presence of MIX a marked decrease (approx. 90%) in cyclic AMP levels was obtained in the presence of increasing concentrations of the ionophore. Similar results were obtained in the presence of A23187 when the Ca^{2+} concentration was increased. Although very low levels of cyclic AMP were attained, they were apparently sufficient for maximal LH-stimulated steroidogenesis; this is in accordance with previous studies (Cooke et al., 1981 [review]). These results indicate that A23187 either inhibited LH stimulation of cyclic AMP production and/or that activation of a phosphodiesterase occurred. Both of these effects may be mediated by Ca^{2+}. The A23187-induced decrease in cyclic AMP levels even in the presence of MIX would seem to argue against an activation of phosphodiesterase. However, MIX does not completely inhibit the latter and the cyclic AMP levels were measured after 4 h of incubation so considerable metabolism could have taken place. The addition of LHRH agonist to LH further decreased the cyclic AMP levels, both in the presence and absence of the ionophore. The inhibitory effects of LHRH agonists on ovarian steroidogenesis have been reported to lower cyclic AMP levels by activation of a phosphodiesterase (Ranta et al., 1983).

It was demonstrated that the LHRH agonist increases 22(R)- and 25-hydroxycholesterol metabolism to testosterone. At high concentrations of 22(R)-hydroxycholesterol, LHRH agonist plus LH also increased testosterone production more than that obtained with the hydroxysteroid alone. In contrast LH did not increase metabolism of the hydroxysteroids; this is in agreement with the results of Taoff et al., (1982), who found that the metabolism of

25-hydroxycholesterol by dispersed rat luteal cells was not influenced by addition of LH. The present results, therefore, indicate a specific action of the LHRH agonist on steroidogenesis which is different from that of LH.

In conclusion, the results of the present study indicate that the LHRH agonist, in contrast to LH, increases the metabolism of 22(R)- and 25- hydroxycholesterol in rat testis Leydig cells to testosterone. This may well result from an increased synthesis of the mitochondrial cytochrome P_{450} enzyme. The results obtained in this study also demonstrate that rat and mouse Leydig cells are heterogenous with respect to their cell sizes and that changes in cell size can be induced in vitro.

To conclude, the results obtained in this in vitro study and those obtained after in vivo exposure of the Leydig cells to various stimulants and inhibitors are consistent with a mechanism for the paracrine control of Leydig cell function. They also provide an explanation for the heterogeneity of Leydig cells with respect to density and size (Cooke et al., 1981), especially if these variations vary according to the stage of spermatogenesis (Bergh 1982). The present observations on effects of LHRH agonist on cell size in vitro will facilitate the investigations of the effects of seminiferous tubular factors on Leydig cell morphology. The significance of the increases in cell size are unknown but they may reflect an increase in Leydig cell activity perhaps as a prelude to cell division.

REFERENCES

Aldred, L.F. & Cooke, B.A. (1982). Int. J. Andrology, 5, 191-195.

Bergh (1982). Int. J. Andrology 5, 325.

Catt, K.J. and Dufau, M.L. (1973). Nature New Biology 224,219-221.

Cooke, B.A., Dix, C.J., Magee-Brown, R. Janszen, F.H.A. and van der Molen, H.J. (1981). Adv. Cyc. Nucl. Res. 14, 593-609.

Harper, J.F. & Brooker, G. (1975). J. Cyclic Nucleotide Res. 1, 207-218.

Hunter, M.G., Sullivan M.H.F., Dix, C.J., Aldred, L.R. & Cooke, B.A. (1982). Mol. Cell. Endocrinol. 27, 31-44.

Massicotte, J., Veilleux, R. Lavoie, M. and Labrie, F. (1980). Biochem. Biophys. Res. Comm. 94, 1362-1366.

Moyle,W.R. and Ramachandran, J. (1973). Endocrinology 93, 127-134.

Ranta, R., Baukal, A., Knecht, M., Korhonen, M. and Catt, K.J. (1983). Endocrinology, 112, 956-964.

Rommerts, F.F.G., Cooke, B.A. & van der Kemp, J.W.C.M. and van der Molen, H.J. (1973). FEBS Letters 33, 114-118.

Sharpe, R.M. and Cooper, I. (1982). Mol. Cell. Endocrinol. 26, 141-150.

Sharpe, R.M. and Harmer, T.J. (1983). In: Hormones and Cell Regulation 7, (Eds. J.E. Dumont, J. Nunez and R.M. Denton). pp217-210.

Sharpe, R.M., Doogan, D.G. and Cooper, I. (1982). Biochem. Biophys. Res. Comm. 196, 1210-1217.

Sullivan, M.H.F. and Cooke, B.A. (1984a). Biochem. J. 216, (in press).

Sullivan, M.H.F. and Cooke, B.A. (1984b). Molec. Cell. Endocr. 34, (in press).

Sullivan, M.H.F. and Cooke, B.A. (1984c). Biochem. J. (submitted for publication).

Steiner, A.L., Parker, C.W. and Kipnis, D.M. (1972). J. Biol. Chem. 247, 1106-1113.

Taoff, M.E., Schleyer, H. and Strauss, J.F. (1982). Endocrinology, 111, 1785-1790.

Verjans, H.L., Cooke, B.A., de Jong, F.H, de Jong, C.M.M. & van der Molen, H.J. J. Steroid Biochem. 4, 665-676.

PHOSPHOLIPID TURNOVER IN GONADOTROPIN-RELEASING HORMONE TARGET CELLS: COMPARATIVE STUDIES

Zvi Naor, Jacob Molcho, Moshe Zilberstein and Haim Zakut

Department of Hormone Research
The Weizmann Institute of Science
Rehovot, 76100, Israel

INTRODUCTION

Gonadotropin releasing hormone (GnRH) stimulates pituitary luteinizing hormone (LH) and follicle stimulating hormone (FSH) biosynthesis and release. Paradoxical antifertility effects of GnRH and its potent agonistic analogs *in vivo* have led to the findings that GnRH and its agonists also exert direct stimulatory and inhibitory gonadal effects (Hsueh and Jones, 1981; Hillensjö and Lemaire, 1980; Clark et al., 1980; Knecht and Catt, 1981; Ekholm et al., 1981; Hunter et al., 1982; Jones and Hsueh, 1982; Dekel et al., 1983; Hsueh et al., 1983; Knecht et al., 1983). The direct inhibitory effects are mainly observed after several hours of coculture of GnRH agonists and gonadotropins. The inhibitory effects might be explained by reversal of the inhibitory effect of FSH on ovarian phosphodiesterase activity and a progressive inhibition of adenylate cyclase (Knecht and Catt, 1981); and/or by inhibition of the side-chain cleavage enzyme and increase in 20-α hydroxysteroid dehydrogenase activity in the ovary (Jones and Hsueh, 1982). The testicular inhibitory effects might be explained by inhibition of 17α-hydroxylase and/or inhibition of 17-20 desmolase (Hsueh et al., 1983). The gonadal stimulatory effects of GnRH, which include stimulation of prostaglandin E (PGE) and steroid production, oocyte maturation and induction of ovulation are not clear at the present time. We have recently demonstrated that cyclic AMP (cAMP) is not involved in GnRH action in the pituitary and the gonads (Naor et al., 1978; and submitted). Therefore, we investigated the possible involvement of phosphatidylinositol (PI) turnover and PGE production in the mediation of GnRH action in both the pituitary and gonads.

PHOSPHATIDYLINOSITOL TURNOVER

The relevance of PI turnover to ligand-receptor interaction was first suggested by Hokin and Hokin (1953) and later proposed as a general mechanism for ligands operating via calcium and cyclic GMP production (Michell, 1975; Fig. 1). It is regarded as one of the earliest biochemical effects that follow the binding to the specific receptor. Multiple phosphorylation of PI will result in the formation of di- and triphosphoinositides (DPI and TPI) that were implicated in nervous conduction, in nicotinic cholinergic receptor activation and in mediating hormone action in steroid producing target cells (Michell, 1975; Farese and Sabir, 1980). More recently, it was observed that a decrease in the ^{32}P content of labeled TPI and DPI after hormonal challenge precedes PI turnover (Kirk et al., 1981; Thomas et al., 1983). It was suggested that the early decrease in polyphosphoinositides might be associated with the release of calcium (at a micromolar range) needed to activate the recently described PI-specific phospholipase C in certain target organs. Thereafter the formation of phosphatidic acid (PA) during the PI cycle will facilitate further calcium entry serving as an endogenous calcium ionophore (Salmon and Honeyman, 1980). The elevated cytosolic calcium can activate phospholipase A_2 leading to the formation of prostaglandins (PG), thromboxanes and leukotrienes.

The arachidonic acid (AA) needed for PG production can be derived from several sources (Fig. 1). The diglyceride formed during the PI cycle can be acted upon by a diglyceride lipase to liberate AA. The second potential source is a PA-specific phospholipase A_2 that acts on PA and results in the formation of lysophosphatidic acid (lyso-PA) and AA. Third, the lyso-PA can also serve as a calcium ionophore and can activate other phospholipases A_2 that act on other phospholipids such as phosphatidylcholine and phosphatidylethanolamine to liberate more AA (Lapetina et al., 1981). Arachidonic acid can also be liberated from cellular phospholipids by phospholipase A_2 independently to the PI cycle. It is interesting to note that although PI is a minor constituent of the phospholipids in the cell, it is the main source of AA needed for PG synthesis at least in platelets (Fain, 1982).

The diglyceride formed during PI-turnover can also activate a recently described cAMP-independent, calcium- and phospholipid-dependent protein kinase C (Kishimoto et al., 1980). This kinase might initiate calcium-activated phosphorylation of key proteins and enzymes. Such a mechanism will link a receptor mediated event at the plasma membrane level, and biochemical reactions within the cell machinery that are dependent on phosphorylation-dephosphorylation.

It is interesting to note that PI turnover and calcium mobilization may be considered a major alternative pathway for peptide hormones which do not act via cyclic nucleotide production. For example, the hormones which activate hepatocyte glycogen phosphorylase can be divided between cAMP-dependent and cAMP-independent activators. Among the first group are glucagon and β-catecholamines and among the second group vasopressin, angiotensin and α-catecholamines. Those which do not increase cAMP levels are thought to activate PI turnover and elevate cytosolic calcium (Fain, 1982).

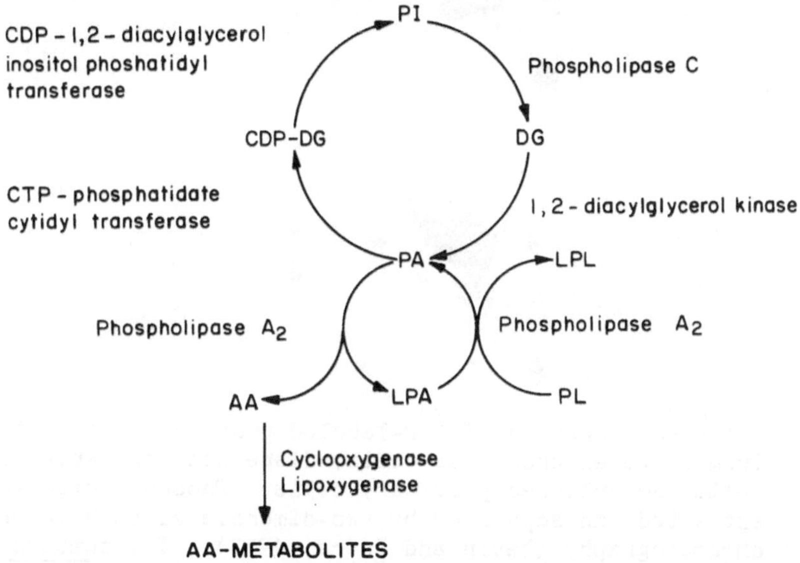

Fig. 1. Phosphatidylinositol (PI) cycle and potential sources of arachidonic acid (AA). Receptor activation results in breakdown of PI to 1,2-diacylglycerol (DG) by a PI-specific phospholipase C. Phosphorylation by ATP and activation by diacylglycerol (DG) kinase forms phosphatidic acid (PA). Conjugation with CTP by phosphatidic acid: CTP cytidyltransferase forms CDP-diacylglycerol (CDP-DG). The final reaction is an exchange of the activated CDP with free inositol by CDP-diacylglycerol inositol phosphatidyltransferase to form PI. PA can be acted upon by a PA-specific phospholipase A_2 to form lysophosphatidic acid (LPA) and AA. LPA can facilitate the activation of other phospholipase A_2 acting on general phospholipids (PL) resulting in the formation of AA and lysophospholipids (LPL).

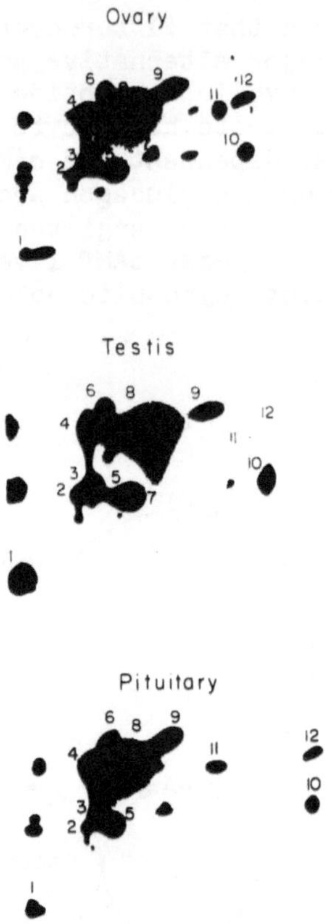

Fig. 2. Relative migration of ^{32}P-labeled phospholipids isolated from cultured granulosa cells, dispersed interstitial cells and cultured pituitary cells. Phospholipids were extracted and separated by two-dimensional thin layer chromatography (Yavin and Zutra, 1977). The numbers in the autoradiographs denote the relative migration of the phospholipids: 1) origin; 2) unidentified, possibly phosphatidylinositol plasmalogen; 3) lysophosphatidylcholine; 4) phosphatidylcholine plasmalogen; 5) PI; 6) phosphatidylethanolamine plasmalogen; 7) phosphatidylserine; 8) phosphatidylcholine; 9) phosphatidylethanolamine; 10) PA; 11) phosphaditylglycerol; 12) cardiolipin.

PHOSPHOLIPID LABELING IN THE PITUITARY AND GONADS

Several methods of phospholipid separation were examined, and the two-dimensional separation used in our studies (Yavin and

Table 1. Rate of phospholipid labeling in GnRH target organs.

Phospholipid	Relative phosphorylation %		
	Pituitary	Ovary	Testis
Phosphatidylglycerol	N.D.	2.0	0.50
Cardiolipin	3.4	2.0	N.D.
Phosphatidylserine (PS)	1.8	2.0	U.D.
Phosphatidic acid (PA)	2.5	1.75	6.6
Phosphatidylethanolamine	4.2	3.5	3.3
Lysolecitin	N.D.	4.0	10
Phosphatidylinositol (PI)	45	6.5	9.6
Cholineplasmalogen	N.D.	8.5	8.5
Phosphatidylcholine (PC)	32	64	62

N.D. not determined
U.D. undetectable

Zutra, 1977) was found to be the most appropriate to ensure a complete separation of PI and PA from other labeled phospholipids. As shown in Fig. 2, at least 20 phospholipids were separated from pituitary and gonadal cells. In the gonads the majority of the radioactivity was incorporated into PC (> 60%) (Table 1), while PI represents only 5-10% of total radioactivity incorporated into the phospholipid fraction. The opposite was observed in pituitary cells, while PI labeling amounted to 45%, that of PC reached only about 30% of total radioactivity of phospholipids.

PHOSPHATIDYLINOSITOL TURNOVER AND ICOSANOID PRODUCTION IN THE PITUITARY

Preliminary reports have appeared recently indicating that GnRH stimulates PI turnover in the pituitary (Snyder et al., 1980; Raymond et al., 1982; Kiesel et al., 1983). We found stimulation of pituitary PA and PI labeling by GnRH after 1 and 5 min of incubation, respectively (Fig. 3.). GnRH-stimulated PI turnover exhibited a lag time of about 5 min before a significant increase could be demonstrated. This is in agreement with the assumption that the PI cycle is initiated by a rapid hydrolysis of the PI head-group via a PI-specific phospholipase C followed by resynthesis from PA. In

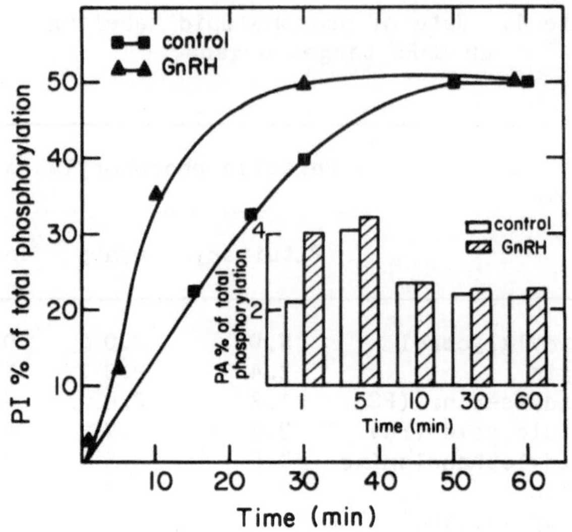

Fig. 3. Time-response study of the effect of GnRH on PA and PI labeling in cultured pituitary cells. The cells were prelabeled for 10 min with [^{32}P]Pi and later incubated with GnRH (10^{-7}M) for the time indicated.

support of this assumption is the finding that PA labeling preceeded that of PI. It is interesting to note that GnRH-stimulation of PA labeling could be detected only up to 1 min of incubation and that of PI only when the prelabeling period was 10 min but not 60 min (Fig. 3, and data not shown). It is possible therefore that pituitary gonadotrophs contain a minor fraction of GnRH-sensitive PA and PI with a very high turnover rate and a larger pool of hormone-insensitive PA and PI pool with lower turnover rate. In short incubation periods the hormone-sensitive pool is labeled and the increased labeling can be detected. On the other hand, the longer incubation periods also label the hormone-insensitive pool and thereby masking the stimulatory effect of GnRH. Additional studies are needed to further substantiate this compartmentalization of PI and PA.

PI turnover in the pituitary apparently results in the formation of PA and is believed to precede the opening of calcium channels (Michell, 1975). Indeed PA was implicated as an endogenous calcium ionophore (Salmon and Honeyman, 1980). It is also well recognized by now that GnRH-stimulated gonadotropin release is calcium depen-

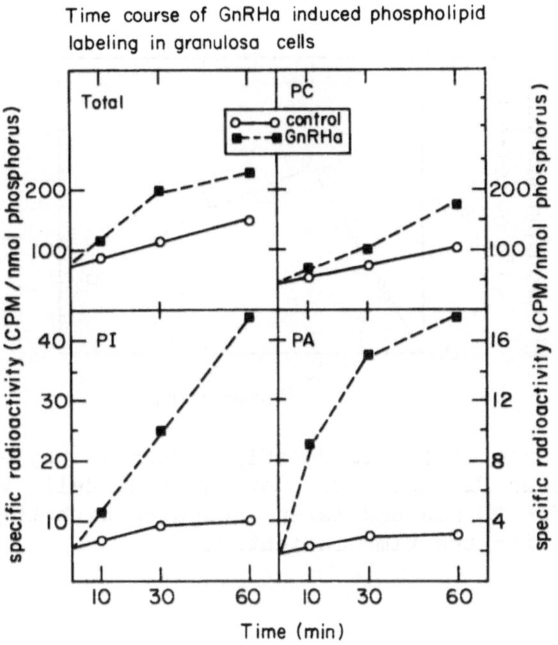

Fig. 4. Time course of [D-Ala^6]GnRH (GnRHa)-induced labeling of phospholipids in granulosa cells from preantral follicles. Prelabeling was conducted for 60 min before the addition of GnRHa (10^{-7}M). (PC-phosphatidylcholine).

dent (Conn et al., 1981a; Naor et al., 1980). The increased levels of cytosolic calcium can interact with calmodulin (Conn et al., 1981b) and activate phospholipase A_2, leading to the formation of free AA (Naor and Catt, 1981). We previously demonstrated that prostaglandins are not involved in GnRH action (Naor et al., 1975; Ojeda et al., 1979). On the other hand, we and others have recently suggested that lipoxygenase or epoxygenase derivatives of AA might mediate GnRH action on gonadotropin release (Naor et al., 1983; Snyder et al., 1983). This was based on findings that lipoxygenase inhibitors blocked GnRH-induced gonadotropin release from cultured pituitary cells (Naor et al., 1983). On the other hand, the prostaglandin synthesis inhibitor, indomethacin, potentiated GnRH action. Moreover, studies in progress reveal the presence of lipoxygenase activity in purified gonadotrophs.

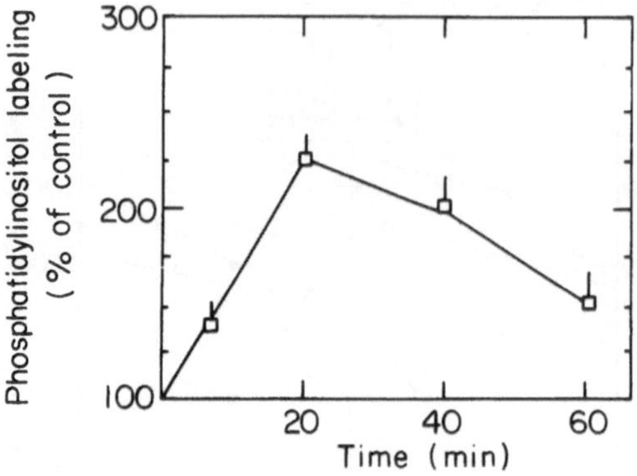

Fig. 5. Time course of [D-Ala^6]desGly^{10}-GnRH N ethylamide-induced testicular PI labeling. Interstitial cells were prelabeled for 20 min and later incubated with the GnRH analog (10^{-7}M) for the time indicated.

We therefore suggest that following the binding of GnRH to its specific receptors in pituitary gonadotrophs, GnRH activates the PI cycle, which in turn results in altered calcium fluxes. Whether an early event in this proposed cascade of events includes TPI and DPI degradation and the release of endogenous bound-calcium is not clear at the present time, and needs further investigation. The elevated calcium apparently initiates a series of biochemical reactions leading to the formation of active metabolites of AA which are not prostaglandins. The lipoxygenase and/or epoxygenase products of AA then mediate the process of exocytosis (Naor et al., 1983; Snyder et al., 1983).

PHOSPHATIDYLINOSITOL TURNOVER AND ICOSANOID PRODUCTION IN THE GONADS

A rapid stimulation of PI and PA labeling by a GnRH-agonist was observed in cultured granulosa cells (Fig. 4 and Naor and Yavin, 1982). The effect could be demonstrated as early as 5 min after the addition of the agonist (Fig. 4). In testicular interstitial

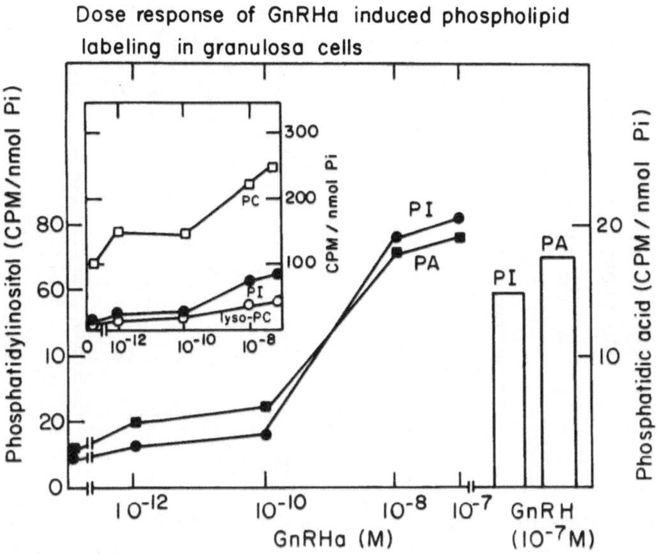

Fig. 6. Dose-response of [D-Ala[6]]GnRH induced phospholipid labeling in the ovary. Granulosa cells were prepared from preantral follicles and prelabeled for 60 min before the addition of GnRH or its potent analog for another 60 min.

cells, addition of a GnRH agonist caused stimulation of PI but not PA labeling which reached a peak at 20 min and declined thereafter (Fig. 5).

The dose-response curves for PI and PA labeling by GnRH agonist in granulosa cells is shown in Fig. 6. A maximal stimulation of PI and PA labeling (8-fold) was obtained after 60 min of incubation with a GnRH analog in cultured granulosa cells. A much smaller effect (30%, $p<0.02$) was obtained with testicular interstitial cells after the addition of a GnRH analog (10^{-8} M) for 60 min (Fig. 7). No consistent effect of GnRH on PA labeling in testicular cells was observed.

GnRH agonists had no effect on gonadal (granulosa and interstitial cell) cyclic AMP (cAMP) production (submitted for publication). On the other hand, it is well documented that LH initiates its stimulatory action on gonadal steroidogenesis by increased cAMP formation. Therefore, in the gonads, LH and GnRH agonists differ in the way in which their early stimulatory action is mediated. GnRH agonists mimic the gonadal effects of LH and stimulate prostaglandin, progesterone and testosterone production (Clark et al., 1980; Hunter et al., 1982). However, while cAMP mediates LH in-

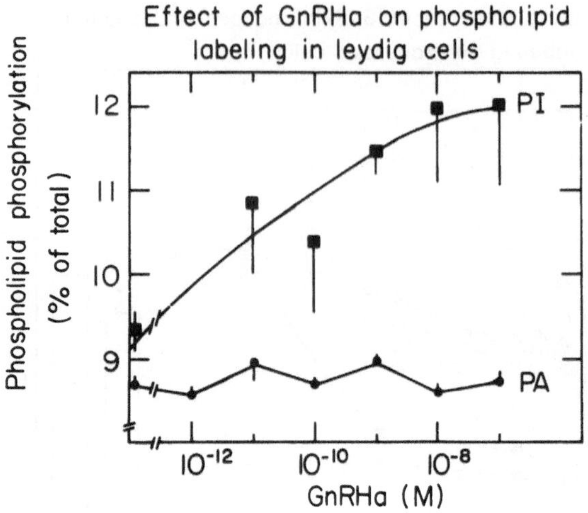

Fig. 7. Dose response of [D-Ala^6]des-Gly^{10}-GnRH N ethylamide-induced phospholipid labeling in interstitial cells. Prelabeled cells (20 min) were incubated with a GnRH analog for 60 min.

duced PGE, progesterone and testosterone formation (Mendelson et al., 1975; Zor and Lamprecht, 1977), we suggest that GnRH-stimulated PGE production is derived from increased PI turnover as is the case with angiotensin II action in the kidney (Benabe et al., 1982) and caerulein action in the exocrine pancreas (Marshall et al., 1981).

It is possible that GnRHa-stimulated PI turnover is also involved in progesterone and testosterone formation via the production of 1,2 diacylglycerol coupled with the activation of the recently discovered calcium-dependent, phospholipid-activated protein kinase C (Kishimoto et al., 1980). Nevertheless, we have excluded the possibility that PGE mediates GnRH-induced progesterone and testosterone formation by demonstrating that indomethacin had no inhibitory action on the peptide induced steroid formation in cultured granulosa and interstitial cells (submitted).

Since GnRH mimics several actions of LH (PGE and progesterone formation; oocyte maturation and induction of ovulation) a mediatory role for ovarian GnRH-like material in LH actions was considered. However, while a potent GnRH antagonist was capable of blocking stimulation of gonadal functions by GnRH, no inhibitory effect was noticed on LH stimulation of oocyte maturation and induction of ovulation (Fig. 8 and Dekel et al., 1983).

Administration of indomethacin blocked the stimulatory effect of both LH and GnRHa on induction of ovulation but had no inhibitory effect on the peptide-induced oocyte maturation in vitro (Fig. 8). On the other hand, we have recently shown that the stimulatory effect of LH and GnRHa on resumption of meiosis in follicle-enclosed rat oocytes in vitro was blocked by dibutyryl cAMP (DBC) and by MIX (Fig. 8 and Dekel et al., 1983). Prostaglandins of the E type (PGE) are involved in mediating the effect of LH on the induction of ovulation but the exact mechanisms involved in oocyte maturation are not yet understood. We suggest here that the direct stimulatory effect of GnRH on oocyte maturation and induction of ovulation are most likely mediated by a rapid PI turnover followed by PGE and progesterone formation. The initially independent pathways of LH and GnRH converge at a step proximal to PGE production and thereafter share similar pathways leading to oocyte maturation and independently to induction of ovulation.

In dispersed interstitial cells, we found that LH and GnRH agonists increase PGE production and that GnRH agonists mimic LH stimulation of testosterone production (submitted). It is possible that GnRH-stimulated PGE production mediates the inhibitory effects of GnRH on testicular functions since it has been demonstrated that administration of PG's decreases the level of spermatogenesis (Isidori et al., 1980). More studies are needed not only to clarify this possibility, but also to examine the diverse effects of PGs in relation to LH and GnRH actions in the testis. Our studies thus far have excluded the possibility that PGE mediates a GnRH effect on testosterone production in dispersed interstitial cells since we have demonstrated that indomethacin has no effect on GnRH-induced testosterone production under conditions where nearly 80% of the cellular content of PGE was depleted (submitted).

The stimulatory actions of GnRH agonists upon gonadal functions are most likely calcium-dependent since PG synthesis is dependent on the presence of elevated calcium. Moreover, it was recently demonstrated that the inhibitory effect of a GnRH agonist upon LH-induced cAMP formation is completely dependent on extracellular calcium (Knecht et al., 1983; Ranta et al., 1983). Since GnRH-induced PI turnover precedes the previously described inhibitory and stimulatory actions of GnRH agonists on gonadal function, it is possible that the PI turnover is responsible for calcium gating which mediates both inhibitory and stimulatory actions of GnRH at the gonadal level.

The inhibitory effects of GnRH agonists upon gonadal functions can be detected only after several hours of exposure to the hormone and are not observed during the initial 4 h of incubation. Thus, binding of GnRH to its specific gonadal receptors is followed by activated PI turnover and increased calcium fluxes. The increased cytosolic calcium modulates adenylate cyclase and phosphodiesterase

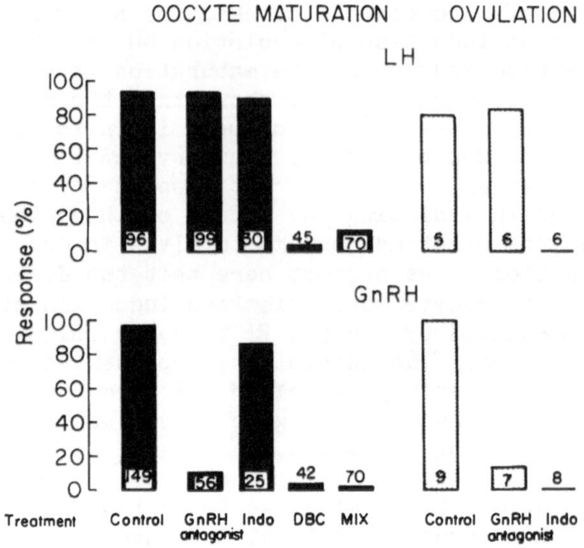

Fig. 8. Comparative studies of GnRH and LH stimulation of ovarian functions. To study oocyte maturation, follicles were isolated from the ovaries of immature rats 48 h after PMSG (15 IU/rat) priming and incubated in the presence of either oLH (0.1 μg/ml) or GnRHa (10^{-7} M) with or without either GnRH antagonist [D-pGlu^1, pclPhe^2,D-Trp^{3,6}]-GnRH, (10^{-5}M), dibutyryl cyclic AMP (DBC, 5 mM), MIX (0.2 mM) or indomethacin (Indo 20 μg/ml). The incidence of maturation was indicated by the breakdown of the germinal vesicles. Ovulation was studied in mature rats hypophysectomized and treated with PMSG (15 IU) on the morning of proestrus and 24 h later injected with hCG (4 IU/rat) or GnRHa (500 ng/rat) with or without a combined treatment with either GnRH antagonist (5 ug/rat) or indomethacin (2 mg/rat). The presence of ovulated oocytes was examined 20 h after hormonal treatment.

activities. Moreover, the inhibition of GnRH on FSH-induced progesterone formation might result from the inhibition of the side chain cleavage enzyme and an increase in 20α-hydroxysteroid dehydrogenase activity (Jones and Hsueh, 1982). Collectively, the inhibitory effects are slow and can commence only after several hours of exposure to a GnRH challenge. On the other hand, we suggest that elevated calcium induced by GnRH via the phospholipid effect can stimulate phospholipase A_2 which leads to increased formation of AA and PGs. The early responses to GnRH agonists might therefore be involved in initiating a series of biochemical events that culminate in stimulatory and inhibitory actions of GnRH upon diverse gonadal functions.

Recently, we have suggested that lipoxygenase products of AA but not PGs might be involved in GnRH action on pituitary gonadotropin release (Naor et al., 1983). In the gonads however, PGs seem to be the pathway of choice for GnRH action. Therefore, GnRH might be an example of a peptide hormone that is capable of activating the different pathways of AA metabolism (cyclooxygenase vs. lipoxygeanse) in different target cells. Nevertheless, it is possible that the lipoxygenase pathway is also involved in mediating GnRH action on gonadal functions by a mechanism that has yet to be elucidated.

Since it is unlikely that hypothalamic GnRH reaches the gonads in sufficient concentrations, it is possible that the data provided here represent insight into the mechanism of action of putative GnRH-like substances that are produced by the gonads of some species (Sharpe et al., 1981; Ying et al., 1981). Until these GnRH-like substances are found and purified, the use of GnRH and its agonists provides an excellent tool for studying the biochemical events involved in oocyte maturation, induction of ovulation, testicular steroidogenesis and spermatogenesis, all of which are fundamental physiological processes that are not yet fully understood.

ACKNOWLEDGEMENTS

The technical assistance of Mrs. Yona Eli and Mrs. Ester Bercovici is greatly appreciated. We also thank Mrs. M. Kopelowitz for typing and editing the review, and Dr. G. Childs for helpful comments. The active collaboration of Drs. Jack Vanderhoek, Ephraim Yavin, Nave Dekel and Kevin Catt made this work possible. Supported in part by NIH grant HD-]6279. Z.N. is the incumbent of the Charles H. Revson Career Development Chair. J.M. and M.Z. were supported by grants in aid from the Office of the Chief Scientist of the Ministry of Health. The permanent address of J.M., M.Z. and H.Z. is The Sackler Faculty of Medicine, Tel-Aviv University, the Wolfson Hospital, Holon, Israel.

REFERENCES

Benabe, J.E., Spry, L.A., and Morrison, A.R., 1982, Effect of angiotensin II on phosphatidylinositol and polyphosphoinositide turnover in rat kidney, mechanism of prostaglandin release. J. Biol. Chem., 257:7430.

Clark, M.R., Thibier, C., Marsh, J.M., and Lemaire, W.J., 1980, Stimulation of prostaglandins accumulation by luteinizing hormone releasing hormone (LHRH) and LHRH analogs in rat granulosa cells in vitro, Endocrinology, 107:17.

Conn, P.M., Marian, J., McMillian, M., Stern, J., Rogers, D., Hamby, M., Penna, A., and Grant, E., 1981a, Gonadotropin releasing hormone action in the pituitary: A three step mechanism, Endocrin. Reviews, 2:174.

Conn, P.M., Chafouleas, J.G., Rogers, D., and Means, A.R., 1981b, Gonadotropin releasing hormone stimulates calmodulin redistribution in rat pituitary, Nature, 292:264.

Dekel, N., Sherizly, I., Tsafriri, A., and Naor, Z., 1983, A comparative study on the mechanism of action of luteinizing hormone and gonadotropin releasing hormone analogs on the ovary. Biol. Reprod., 28:161.

Ekholm, C., Hillensjo, T., and Isaksson, O., 1981, Gonadotropin releasing hormone agonists stimulate meiosis and ovulation in hypophysectomized rats, Endocrinology, 108:2022.

Fain, J.N., 1982, Involvement of phosphatidylinositol breakdown in elevation of cytosol Ca^{2+} by hormones and relationship to prostaglandin formation, in: "Hormone Receptors", L.D. Kohn, ed., John Wiley and Sons, Ltd., p. 237.

Farese, R.V., and Sabir, A.M., 1980, Polyphosphoinositides: Stimulator of mitochondrial cholesterol side chain cleavage and possibile identification as an adrenocorticotropin induced cyclohemimide sensitive, cytostolic, steroidogenic factor, Endocrinology, 106:1869.

Hillensjo, T., and Lemaire, W.J., 1980, Gonadotropin releasing hormone agonists stimulate meiotic maturation of follicle enclosed rat oocyte in vitro, Nature, 287:145.

Hokin, M.R., and Hokin, L.E., 1953, Enzyme secretion and the incorporation of ^{32}P into phospholipids of pancreas slices, J. Biol. Chem., 203:967.

Hsueh, A.J.W., and Jones, P.B.C., 1981, Extrapituitary actions of gonadotropin-releasing hormone, Endocrine Reviews, 2:437.

Hsueh, A.J.W., Bambino, T.H., Zhuang, I.Z., Welsh, T.H., and Ling, N.C., 1983, Mechanism of the direct action of gonadotropin releassng hormone and its antagonist on androgen biosynthesis by cultured rat testicular cells, Endocrinology, 112:1653.

Hunter, M.G., Sullivan, M.H.F., Dix, C.J., Aldred, L.F., and Cooke, B.A., 1982, Stimulation and inhibition by LHRH analogues of cultured rat Leydig cell function and lack of effect on mouse Leydig cells, Mol. Cell. Endocr., 27:31.

Isidori, A., Conte, D., Laguzzi, G., Giovneco, P., and Dondero, F., 1980, Role of seminal prostaglandins in male fertility. I. Relationship of prostaglandin E and 19-OH prostaglandin E with seminal parameters, J. Endocrinol. Invest., 3:1.

Jones, P.B.C., and Hsueh, A.J.W., 1982, Pregnenolone biosynthesis by cultured rat granulosa cells: Modulation by follicle stimulating hormone and gonadotropin releasing hormone, Endocrinology, 111:713.

Kiesel, L., Naor, Z., and Catt, K.J., 1983, Mechanisms of GnRH action: Role of arachidonate metabolites and phosphatidic acid in the stimulation of cyclic GMP production and LH release in pituitary gonadotrophs, Proc. of the 65th Annual Meeting of the Endocrine Society, San Antonio, Abst. 561.

Kirk, C.J., Creba, J.A., Downes, C.P., and Michell, R.H., 1981, Hormone-stimulated metabolism of inositol lipids and its relationship to hepatic receptor function, Biochem. Soc. Trans., 7:377.

Kishimoto, A., Takai, Y., Mori, T., Kikkawa, U., and Nishizuka, Y., 1980, Activation of calcium and phospholipid-dependent protein kinase by diacylglycerol, its possible relation to phosphatidylinositol, J. Biol. Chem., 255:2273.

Knecht, M., and Catt, K.J., 1981, Gonadotropin releasing hormone: Regulation of adenosine 3',5'-monophosphate in ovarian granulosa cells, Science, 214:1346.

Knecht, M., Ranta, T., Naor, Z., and Catt, K.J., 1983, Direct effect of GnRH on the ovary, in: "Factors Regulating Ovarian Function", G.S. Greenwold and P.F. Terranova, eds., Raven Press, p. 225.

Lapetina, E.G., Billah, M.M., and Cuatrecasas, P., 1981, The phosphatidylinositol cycle and the regualtion of arachidonic acid production, Nature, 292:367.

Marshall, P.J., Boatman, D.E., and Hokin, L.E., 1981, Direct demonstration of the formation of prostaglandin E_2 due to phosphatidylinositol breakdown associated with stimulation of enzyme secretion in the pancreas, J. Biol. Chem., 256:844.

Mendelson, C., Dufau, M.L., and Catt, K.J., 1975, Gonadotropin binding and stimulation of cyclic adenosine 3'5' monophosphate and testosterone production in isolated Leydig cells. J. Biol. Chem., 250:8818.

Michell, R.H., 1975, Inositol phospholipids and cell surface receptor function, Biochim. Biophys. Acta, 415:81.

Naor, Z., Koch, Y., Chobsieng, P., and Zor, U., 1975, Pituitary cyclic AMP production and mechanism of luteinizing hormone release, FEBS Lett., 58:318.

Naor, Z., Zor, U., Meidan, R., and Koch, Y., 1978, Sex difference in pituitary cyclic AMP response to gonadotropin releasing hormone, Am. J. Physiol., 235:E37.

Naor, Z., Leifer, A.M., and Catt, K.J., 1980, Calcium dependent actions of gonadotropin releasing hormone on pituitary cGMP production and gonadotropin release, Endocrinology, 107:1438.

Naor, Z., and Catt, K.J. 1981, Mechanism of action of gonadotropin releasing hormone, involvement of phospholipid turnover in luteinizing hormone release, J. Biol. Chem., 256:2226.

Naor, Z. and Yavin, E., 1982, Gonadotropin releasing hormone stimulates phospholipid labeling in cultured granulosa cells, Endocrinology, 111:1615.

Naor, Z., Vanderhoek, J.Y., Lindner, H.R., and Catt, K.J., 1983, Arachidonic acid products as possible mediators of the action of gonadotropin releasing hormone, in: "Advances in Prostaglandin Thromboxane and Leukotriene Research" B. Samuelsson, R. Paoletti and P. Ramwell, eds., Raven Press, Vol. 12, p. 259.

Ojeda, S.R., Naor, Z., and Negro-Vilar, A., 1979, The role of prostaglandins in the control of gonadotropin and prolactin secretion, Prostaglandins Med., 2:249.

Ranta, T., Knecht, M., Darbon, J.M., Baukal, A.J., and Catt, K.J., 1983, Calcium dependence of the inhibitory effect of gonadotropin releasing hormone on luteinizing hormone induced cyclic AMP production in rat granulosa cells. Endocrinology, 113:427.

Raymond, V., Veilleux, R., and Leung, P.C.K., 1982, Early stimulation of the phosphatidylinositol response by LHRH in an enriched population of gonadotrophs in primary culture, Proc. of the 64th Annual Meeting of the Endocrine Society, San Franciso, 821 (Abst.).

Salmon, D.M., and Honeyman, T.W., 1980, Proposed mechanism of cholinergic action in smooth muscle, Nature, 284:344.

Sharp, R.M., Fraser, H.M., Cooper, I., and Rommerts, F.F.G., 1981, Sertoli-leydig cell communication via an LHRH-like factor, Nature, 290:785.

Snyder, G.D., and Bleasdale, J.E., 1982, Effect of LHRH on incorporation of [^{32}P]-orthophosphate into phosphatidylinositol by dispersed anterior pituitary cells, Mol. Cell. Endocrinol. 28:55.

Snyder, G.D., Capdevila, J., Chacos, N., Manna, S., and Falck, J.R., 1983, Action of luteinizing hormone releasing hormone: Involvement of novel arachidonic acid metabolites, Proc. Nat. Acad. Sci., U.S.A., 80:3504.

Thomas, A.P., Marks, J.S., Coll. K.E., and Williamson, J.R., 1983, Quantitation and early kinetics of inositol lipid changes induced by vasopressin in isolated and cultured hepatocytes. J. Biol. Chem., 258:5716.

Yavin, E., and Zutra, A., 1977, Separation and analysis of ^{32}P-labeled phospholipids by a simple and rapid thin-layer chromatographic procedure and its application to cultured neuroblastoma cells. Anal. Biochem., 80:430.

Ying, S.Y., Ling, N., Bohlen, P., and Guillemin, R., 1981, Gonadocrinins: peptides in ovarian follicular fluid stimulating the secretion of pituitary gonadotropins, Endocrinology, 108:1206.

Zor, U., and Lamprecht, S.A., 1977, Mechanism of prostaglandin action in endocrine glands. in: "Biochemical Actions of Hormones", G. Litwack, ed., Academic Press, Vol. 4, pp. 85.

RELATION OF ENDOGENOUS OPIATES TO SECRETION OF GONADOTROPINS

Joseph Meites* and Karen Briski

Department of Physiology
Neuroendocrine Research Laboratory
Michigan State University, East Lansing, MI 48824

INTRODUCTION

In recent years considerable evidence has been reported indicating that the endogenous opioid peptides (EOP) have an important role in regulating secretion of pituitary hormones. B-endorphin, the enkephalins, and dynorphin appear to be the major EOPs and all may participate in control of pituitary hormone secretion. Each of these opiates has different receptors, but can be displaced from their receptors to variable degrees by morphine (MOR) or by the specific opiate antagonists, naloxone (NAL) or naltrexone (NALT). The EOP in the hypothalamus have been shown to be strongly localized in areas that contain GnRH neurons and neurons that secrete neurotransmitters which modulate GnRH release. Their inhibitory effects on gonadotropin release appear to be exerted via hypothalamic neurotransmitters and GnRH, and not directly on the pituitary. Evidence will be presented showing that the EOP are involved in regulating both basal and altered gonadotropin secretion during different endocrine states.

RELATION OF EOP TO BASAL LH SECRETION IN MATURE RATS

Shortly after isolation and characterization of the first opioid peptides in the brain in 1975,[1] we compared the effects of MOR and methionine (Met)-enkephalin on basal secretion of LH and FSH in mature male rats.[2] Twenty minutes after intraperitoneal injection of the two opiates, both depressed serum concentrations of LH, but not FSH. No

*Aided by NIH research grants AM04784 and AG00416.

Table 1. Effects of Morphine, Met-Enkephalin and Naloxone on Serum LH and FSH in Male Rats

n = 10/group	LH	FSH
Controls 0.87% NaCl	19 ± 1	341 ± 33
Morphine 2.0 mg/kg	8 ± 1[b]	340 ± 12
Morphine 10.0 mg/kg	9 ± 2[b]	387 ± 23
Morphine 15.0 mg/kg	13 ± 2	333 ± 13
MET-ENK 5.0 mg/kg	11 ± 2[b]	314 ± 20
NAL & MOR 0.2 + 2.0 mg/kg	17 ± 3	384 ± 9
NAL & MOR 0.2 + 10.0 mg/kg	14 ± 4	369 ± 16
NAL & MET-ENK 0.2 + 5.0 mg/kg	17 ± 3	350 ± 18
Naloxone 0.2 mg/kg	44 ± 5[b]	361 ± 15
Naloxone 2.0 mg/kg	52 ± 8[b]	490 ± 36[b]
Naloxone 5.0 mg/kg	45 ± 8[b]	446 ± 29[b]

[a]X ± SEM; all data are expressed in ng/ml serum
[b]P < 0.05 compared with controls. MET-ENK = met-enkephalin
NAL = naloxone. MOR = morphine
(from ref. 2)

explanation is available at present for the apparent lack of action of opiates on FSH secretion, although there may be differences in opioid receptors for these two hormones. When the specific opioid antagonist, NAL, was injected together with the opiates, their inhibitory effects on LH release were either abolished or diminished. Of greatest interest were the effects of administering NAL alone. All three doses of NAL significantly elevated basal serum levels of LH, and the two highest doses of NAL used also significantly increased basal serum FSH levels (Table 1). On the basis of these initial observations, we suggested that the EOP tonically depressed basal secretion of LH and possibly FSH in male rats. The effects of NAL on basal secretion of gonadotropins have been widely confirmed in the rat, monkey, and man.[3-6] Morley et al.[6] reported that iv injection of 10 mg naloxone to eight normal human subjects (seven males and one female) produced a significant increase in serum LH and FSH levels, whereas saline injection had no effect. Two laboratories have reported that intraventricular injection of opiates raised circulating levels of LH in rats,[7,8] but the significance of this observation is not clear.

Other evidence that the EOP tonically depress basal secretion of LH in rats has been reported recently. Our laboratory observed that injection of a specific antiserum to B-endorphin (kindly provided by H. Friesen, U. of Manitoba, Winnipeg, Canada) into mature male rats elevated plasma LH concentrations approximately 3-fold at 20 and 50 minutes after injection, and LH levels declined by 90 minutes but still remained above pre-injection values[9] (Fig.1). Control rats injected with normal rabbit serum showed no significant change in plasma LH levels. Similar results were reported by Schulz et al.[10] who injected anti-sera to B-endorphin and dynorphin intraventricularly to 12-day old female rats, and found that B-endorphin antiserum was much more potent in elevating basal LH values than dynorphin. It can be concluded, therefore, that B-endorphin tonically depresses basal LH secretion in rats, and may be the major EOP responsible for this action.

RELATON OF EOP TO LH SECRETION IN PREPUBERTAL RATS

The effects of a single sc injection of MOR or NAL on serum LH concentrations were investigated in sexually immature male and female rats at 10, 15, 20, 25 and 30 days of age. MOR depressed the initially low basal levels of LH in both sexes only at 15 days of age. However, NAL significantly raised serum LH values two to 16-fold in female rats during the different ages studied. By contrast, the prepubertal male rats failed to show an LH increase in response to NAL administration except for a small rise on day 30.[4] Blank et al.[3] found a similar sex difference in the LH response of sexually immature female and male rats to NAL.

Recently we determined that the sex difference in the LH response

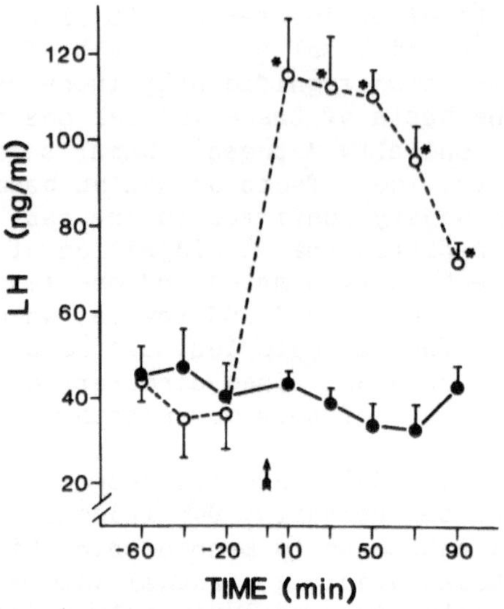

Fig. 1. Effects of B-endorphin antiserum (dashed line) and normal rabbit serum (solid line, controls) on plasma LH levels in adult male rats. Vertical bars indicate standard errors of mean, and stars indicate significant differences from control and pre-injection values. Each solid point is the average of assays from six rats. Each open circle is the average value from seven rats. (from ref. 9)

of prepubertal rats to NAL depends on the early gonadal steroid environment after birth (Sylvester, Sarkar, and Meites, unpublished). Castration of male rats on the day of birth resulted in NAL-induced LH increases when tested on 15, 25, and 35 days of age, as in female rats. These effects were not seen in male rats given testosterone on day three of life. Female rats given testosterone on the day of birth failed to show an LH response to NAL at 15, 25, and 35 days of age, similar to results observed in prepubertal male rats. Thus the presence or absence of testosterone early after birth determines whether prepubertal rats can exhibit increased LH release in response to NAL administration. When estradiol was injected together with NAL into castrate rats of either sex at 15 or 25 days of age, it blocked any LH rise. However, at 35 days of age the same dose of estrogen was no longer able to block the LH rise produced by NAL in either sex. These latter observations indicate that the LH response mechanism is much more sensitive to the negative feedback action of estrogen in the early rather than the later stages of prepuberty, in agreement with the gonadostat theory of puberty onset.

RELATION OF EOP TO ACTIONS OF GONADAL STEROIDS ON LH SECRETION IN MATURE RATS

During the estrous cyle of rats, administration of morphine on the day of proestrus has been shown to block LH release and ovulation.[11,12] Administration of NAL alone (0.2 mg/kg BW) at 1400 hours on the day of proestrus did not alter the peak of the LH surge, but maintained higher levels of LH during the declining phase[13] (Fig. 2). NAL had no effect on the proestrous FSH surge in these animals. In a rat model system which simulated the LH and FSH surges during proestrous afternoon, induced by first administering estrogen to ovariectomized rats followed three days later by progesterone administration, MOR prevented whereas NAL enhanced the LH and FSH surges.[14] In women[15] and in rhesus monkeys[16] during the menstrual cycle, NAL was effective in elevating circulating LH values only during the luteal phase of the cycle. This suggests that inhibition of LH release by gonadal steroids during the luteal phase of the menstrual cycle is mediated, in part at least, via an increase in EOP activity in the hypothalamus. An increase in B-endorphin content in the portal circulation during the luteal phase of the menstrual cycle in monkeys has been observed,[16] and may represent increased B-endorphin release from the pituitary during the luteal phase of the cycle.

It is well known that castration in male rats leads to a rapid and sustained elevation in circulating LH levels. Beginning two hours after castration, and every six hours thereafter, male rats were injected with either MOR or NAL for a period of 170 hours. MOR significantly reduced the LH rise whereas NAL significantly elevated the LH rise after castration.[17] These results suggest that even after castration of male rats, the EOP prevent a maximum increase in LH release, and hence NAL can produce a further increase in LH release.

The negative feedback action of gonadal steroids on LH secretion is at least partially mediated via the EOP, since administration of NAL can partially or completely counteract this inhibitory effect of the gonadal steroids. This was first demonstrated by the ability of NAL to counteract testosterone in castrated male rats.[18] NAL also was

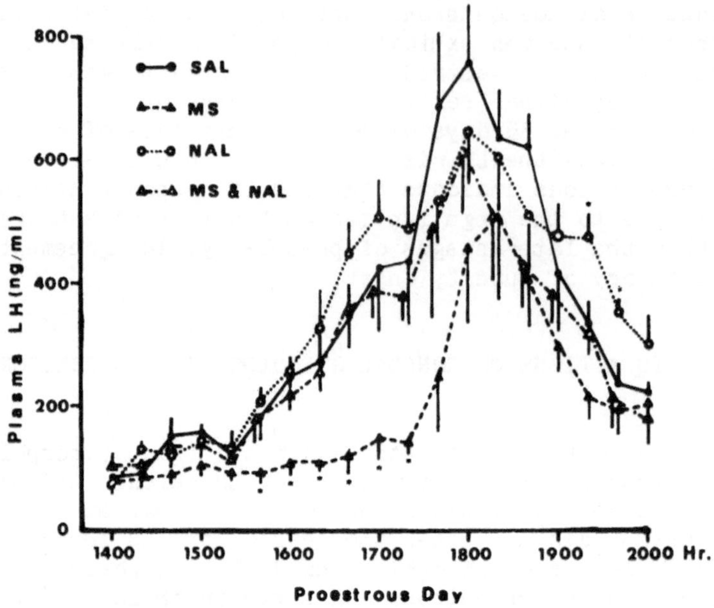

Fig. 2. Effects of 0.9% NACl (SAL), morphine sulfate (MS) (10 mg/kg), naloxone hydrochloride (NAL; 0.2 mg/kg), and combination of both MS and NAL, injected iv at 1400 h, on the LH surge on the afternoon of proestrus. Each point represents mean ± SE of six animals. Asterisk shows significant difference from SAL controls at $P < 0.05$. (from ref. 9)

shown to be able to overcome the inhibitory action of estradiol benzoate or testosterone proprionate on LH release in ovariectomized rats[19] (Fig. 3). Pulsatile release of LH in ovariectomized rats was suppressed by injection of estrogen or estrogen in combination with progesterone. MOR had no effect on this action of the ovarian steroids, but NAL counteracted their inhibitory action on pulsatile LH release.[20] The combination of estrogen and progesterone has been shown to increase β-endorphin content in the hypophysial portal vessels of the monkeys,[21] although the significance of this observation is not clear. There is no convincing evidence that the EOP act directly on the pituitary to inhibit LH secretion.

RELATION OF EOP TO INHIBITION OF LH RELEASE BY STRESS OR STARVATION

Acute stress is known to rapidly elevate LH release, whereas

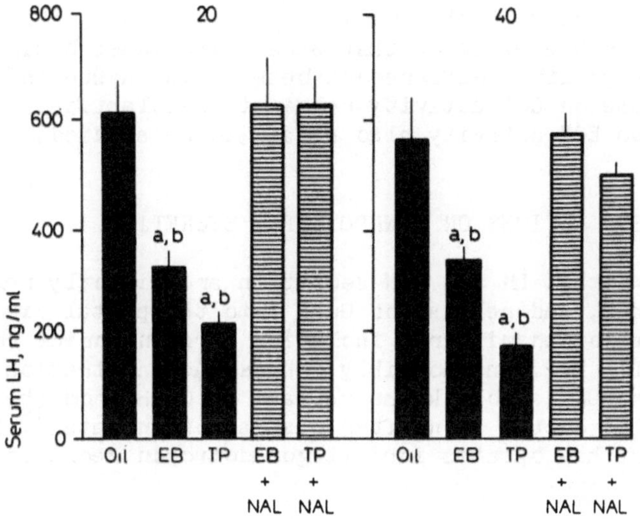

Fig. 3. Effects of NAL on EP or TP inhibition of LH release in ovariectomized rats. EP or TP were injected twice at 24-hour intervals. NAL was injected 3 h after the second steroid injection. Blood samples were collected 20 and 40 min after injection of NAL. Doses were EB = 20 ug; TP = 2 mg; NAL = 2 mg/kg, a = $p < 0.05$ vs. ovariectomized controls; b = $p < 0.05$ vs. EP + NAL or TP + NAL. (from ref. 19)

chronic stress depresses LH release; reduced caloric intake also decreases LH release. Recently, Briski in our laboratory (unpublished) tested the effects of acute and chronic stress as well as complete food removal on LH release in intact male rats injected with NAL or naltrexone (NALT), a longer opiate antagonist. Continuous immobilization of mature male rats resulted in increased plasma LH concentrations during the first hour of restraint, and these were further elevated by administering NALT. Immobilization for eight hours depressed plasma LH levels, and this was prevented by injection of NALT. More prolonged stress was induced by implanting a piece of gauze pad sc for three days. Three daily injections of NALT counteracted the effect of the chronic stress on LH release.

When food, but not water, was completely removed from mature male rats for five days, plasma LH values were significantly lowered. NALT injected three times daily completely overcame the effect of starvation on LH release during the first four days, but by the fifth day plasma LH levels fell to those in the control starved rats. These results suggest that the chronic effects of stress and of starvation on LH release may be partially mediated by increasing EOP activity. There is considerable evidence that stress increases brain EOP activity,[22] but possible differences between the acute and chronic effects of stress on EOP activity remain to be clarified. The effects of starvation on EOP activity also remain to be studied.

MECHANISMS OF EOP ACTIONS ON GONADOTROPIN SECRETION

It is known that LH and FSH secretion are directly regulated by hypothalamic GnRH, and release of GnRH into the portal circulation is modulated by neurotransmitters, including norepinephrine (NE), serotonin (5-HT), EOP, and possibly others. Administration of either testosterone or MOR can block the release of GnRH from the hypothalamus that occurs soon after castration in rats.[19] This explains in part how opiates inhibit gonadotropin secretion. The

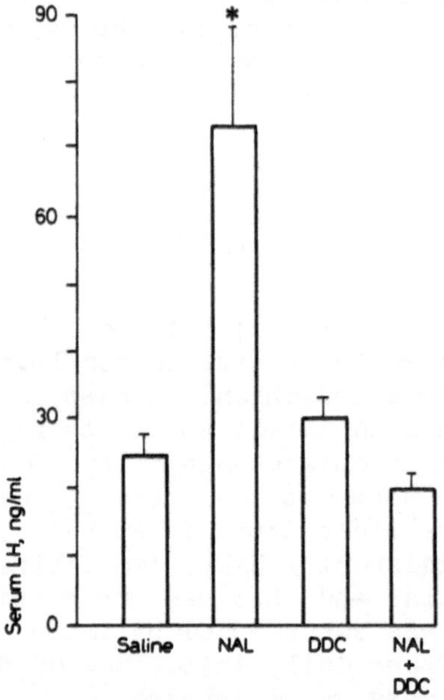

Fig. 4. Effect of DDC on NAL-induced release of LH. * = $p < 0.05$ as compared to controls. Doses used were: DDC = 500 mg/kg BW; NAL = 2 mg/kg BW; n = 8 rats per group. (from ref. 23)

neurotransmitters NE and 5-HT also are influenced by opiates. We have recently reported that when each of three anti-noradrenergic drugs, α-methyl-p-tyrosine, phenoxybenzamine, or diethyldithiocarbamate, were given together with NAL to mature male rats, each completely prevented any increase in release by NAL in release of LH[23] (Fig. 4). Control animals injected only with NAL showed a 2-4 fold increase in LH release. MOR had earlier been shown to reduce NE activity in the brain of rats.[24] Thus, the EOPs help to mediate both the positive and negative feedback effects of gonadal steroids on LH release. Chronic administration of 17 B-estradiol was shown to increase met-enkephalin concentrations in the lateral and medial preoptic nuclei of the hypothalamus, areas which contain GnRH cell bodies.[25] It appears, therefore, that at least part of the mechanism by which opiates inhibit and NAL promotes LH release is via their action on NE activity.

Serotonin also appears to be involved in mediating the effects of opiates on LH release.[4] When male rats were first injected with 5-hydroxytryptophan, the precursor of 5-HT, NAL failed to increase LH release. On the other hand, when parachlorophenylalanine (an anti-serotonergic drug) was first given to reduce 5-HT activity, the action of NAL on LH release was significantly enhanced. Earlier reports had indicated that MOR could increase 5-HT activity in the brain.[24] It appears therefore that the effects of opiates and NAL on LH release are mediated both via NE and 5-HT. Opiates may also operate via other hypothalamic neurotransmitters to alter LH release. There also is the possibility that the EOP may act directly on the hypothalamic neurons secreting GnRH.

CONCLUSIONS

The observations presented here are believed to constitute strong evidence that the EOP are importantly involved in regulating basal and physiologically altered changes in gonadotropin release in animals and man. There is evidence that the EOP participate in mediating secretion of gonadotropins during the prepubertal period, the estrous and menstrual cycles, negative and positive feedback exerted by gonadal steroids in both sexes, and following stressful stimuli or starvation. B-endorphin may be the major EOP involved in regulating gonadotropin secretion, although others may participate as well. The effects of the EOP on gonadotropin secretion have been shown to be mediated via GnRH and hypothalamic neurotransmitters that regulate GnRH release into the pituitary portal vessels.

DEDICATION

I (J.M.) was very saddened to learn last year of the illness and death of Hans Lindner, a friend whom I very much admired both as a scientist and man. I am honored to contribute to this memorial to Hans Lindner. He contributed a great deal to the reputation and high standards of the Department of Hormone Research here at the Weizmann Institute of Science. I shall always treasure the moments I had with him and his family.

REFERENCES

1. J. T. Hughes, W. Smith, H. W. Kosterlitz, L. A. Fothergill, B. A. Morgan, and H. R. Morris, Identification of two related pentapeptides from the brain with potent opiate agonist activity, Nature 258:577 (1975).
2. J. F. Bruni, D. Van Vugt, S. Marshall, and J. Meites, Effects of naloxone, morphine and methionine enkephalin on serum prolactin, luteinizing hormone, follicle stimulating hormone, thyroid stimulating hormone and growth hormone, Life Sci. 21:461 (1977).
3. M. S. Blank, A. E. Paneri, and H. G. Friesen, Opioid peptides modulate luteinizing hormone secretion during sexual maturation, Science 203:1129 (1979).
4. T. Ieiri, H. T. Chen, and J. Meites, Naloxone stimulation of luteinizing hormone release in prepubertal female rats; role of serotonergic system, Life Sci. 26:1269 (1980).
5. D. A. Van Vugt, A. G. Bakst, I, Dryenfurth, and M. Ferin, Naloxone stimulation of luteinizing hormone secretion in the female monkey: influence of endocrine and experimental conditions, Endocrinology 113:1858 (1983).
6. J. E. Morley, N. G. Baranetsky, T. D. Wingert, H. E. Carlson, J. M. Hershman, S. Melmed, S. R. Levin, K. R. Jamison, R. Weitzman, R. J. Chang, and A. A. Varner, Endocrine effects of naloxone-induced opiate receptor blockade, J. Clin. Endocrinol. Metab. 50:251 (1980).
7. J. Takahara, J. Kageyama, S. Yunoki, W. Yakushiji, W. Yamanuchi, N. Kageyama, and T. Ofuji, Effects of 2-bromo-α-ergocryptine on B-endorphin-induced growth hormone, prolactin and luteinizing hormone release in urethane anesthetized rats, Life Sci. 22:2205 (1978).
8. M. Motta and L. Martini, Effect of opioid peptides on gonadotrophin secretion, Acta Endocrinologica 99:321 (1982).
9. L. J. Forman, W. E. Sonntag, and J. Meites, Elevation of plasma LH in response to systemic injection of B-endorphin antiserum in adult male rats, Proc. Soc. Exp. Biol. Med. 173:14 (1983).
10. R. Schulz, A. Wilhelm, K. N. Pirke, C. Gramsch, and A. Herz, B-endorphin and dynorphin control serum luteinizing hormone levels in immature female rats, Nature 294:757 (1981).
11. C. A. Barraclough and C. H. Sawyer, Inhibition of the release of pituitary ovulatory hormone in the rat by morphine, Endocrinology 57:329 (1955).
12. C. N. Pang, E. Zimmerman, and C. H. Sawyer, Morphine inhibition of

the pre-ovulatory surges of plasma luteinizing hormone and follicle stimulating hormone in the rat, *Endocrinology* 101:1726 (1977).

13. T. Ieiri, H. T. Chen, G. A. Campbell, and J. Meites, Effects of naloxone and morphine on the proestrous surge of prolactin and gonadotropins in the rat, *Endocrinology* 106:1568 (1980).
14. P. W. Sylvester, H. T. Chen, and J. Meites, Effects of morphine and naloxone on phasic release of luteinizing hormone and follicle stimulating hormone, *Proc. Soc. Exp. Biol. Med.* 164:207 (1980).
15. J. F. Ropert, M. E. Quigley, and S. S. C. Yen, Endogenous opiates modulate pulsatile luteinizing hormone release in humans, *J. Clin. Endocrinol. Metab.* 52:583 (1981).
16. W. B. Wehrenberg, S. L. Wardlaw, A. G. Frantz, M. Ferin, B-endorphin in hypophyseal portal blood: variations throughout the menstrual cycle, *Endocrinology* 111:879 (1982).
17. D. A. Van Vugt, J. F. Bruni, and J. Meites, Effects of morphine and naloxone on the post-castration rise of luteinizing hormone, *IRCS Med. Sci: Endocrinol.* 7:56 (1978).
18. T. J. Cicero, B. A. Schainker, and E. R. Meyer, Endogenous opioids participate in the regulation of the hypothalamic-pituitary-luteinizing hormone axis and testosterone's negative feedback control of luteinizing hormone, *Endocrinology* 104:1286 (1979).
19. D. A. Van Vugt, P. W. Sylvester, C. F. Aylsworth, and J. Meites, Counteraction of gonadal-steroid inhibition of luteinizing hormone release by naloxone, *Neuroendocrinology* 34:274 (1982).
20. P. W. Sylvester, D. A. Van Vugt, C. F. Aylsworth, E. A. Hanson, and J. Meites, Effects of morphine and naloxone on inhibition by ovarian hormones of pulsatile release of LH in ovariectomized rats, *Neuroendocrinology* 34:269 (1982).
21. L. S. Wardlow, W. B. Wehrenberg, M. Ferin, J. L. Antunes, and A. G. Frantz, Effects of sex steroids on B-endorphin in hypophyseal portal blood, *J. Clin. Endocrinol. Metab.* 55:877 (1982).
22. H. Akil, J. Madden, R. L. Patrick, and J. D. Barchas. Stress-induced increase in endogenous opiate-peptides: concurrent analgesia and its partial reversal by naloxone, *in*: "Opiates and Endogenous Opioid Peptides," H. W. Kosterlitz, ed., North Holland Publishing (1976).
23. D. A. Van Vugt, C. F. Aylsworth, P. W. Sylvester, F. C. Leung, and J. Meites, Evidence for hypothalamic noradrenergic involvement in naloxone-induced stimulation of luteinizing hormone release, *Neuroendocrinology* 33:261 (1981).
24. D. de Wied, J. M. van Ree, and W. de Jong, Narcotic analgesics and the neuroendocrine control of anterior pituitary function, *in*: Narcotics and the Hypothalamus," E. Zimmerman and R. George, eds., Raven Press, New York (1974).
25. P. Savard, N. Barden, Y. Mirand, D. Rouleau, and A. Dupont, Effect of estrogen and haloperidol treatment on brain met-enkephalin levels and receptors in rats, *Endocrine Soc. Absts.*, no. 586, p. 221 (1980).

STRUCTURE - FUNCTION OF LH-RH ANALOGS AND DESIGN APPLICATIONS TO OTHER PEPTIDE SYSTEMS

David H. Coy and Mary V. Nekola

Department of Medicine
Tulane University School of Medicine
New Orleans, Louisiana 70112, USA

INTRODUCTION

It is probable that more synthetic analogs of LH-RH have been made than any other peptide. This considerable research effort, carried out by many groups over a 12 year period since the initial sequencing of the LH-RH decapeptide by Matsuo et al. (1971), has been aimed at the development of increasingly more active competitive antagonists. In the process, the research has provided a tremendous stimulus for improvement of rapid peptide synthesis techniques and general strategies for the speedy development of improved analogs of other peptides. Events leading to the discovery of weak LH-RH antagonists followed by their steady improvement have been frequently reviewed (see for instance, Coy et al. (1981) and Schally et al. (1981). Of tremendous importance to this process was the discovery of the LH-RH superagonist series which was based on the presence of D-amino acids, particularly those with large, aromatic side-chains in place of glycine in position 6 (Monahan et al., 1976; Coy et al., 1976). The increased rigidity and stabilization of the preferred receptor binding conformation produced by D-amino acids has been further utilized in many other positions of the antagonist sequences. The D-amino acid substitution strategy has also become perhaps the prime design approach in many other peptide systems and has yielded many impressive results of late.

OVERVIEW OF LH-RH ANTAGONIST STUDIES

So many varied alterations have been made to the LH-RH decapeptide (pGlu-His-Trp-Ser-Tyr-Gly-Leu-Arg-Pro-Gly-NH_2) that it is quite difficult to devize a generic formula which accurately reflects the most important changes. However, in figure 1 we have attempted to define some of the most beneficial modifications which can be made at certain positions.

Several early alterations to the chain can be considered critical to the steady improvement in antagonist potency. These include the use (de la Cruz et al., 1976) of D-aromatic amino acids in position 6 to boost general levels of antagonism. This was, of course, a direct utilization of the primary superagonist modification. The substitution of D-Trp in position 3 (Coy et al., 1977) and particularly D-p-Cl-Phe in position 2 (Coy et al., 1979) resulted in a two-fold and 10-fold increase in antiovulatory activity, respectively. More recently, N-acetyl-D-aromatic amio acids (Channabasavaiah and Stewart, 1979) in position 1 or, better still, D-p-Cl-Phe incorporated at the N-terminus together with D-Ala at the C-teminus (Erchegyi et al., 1981) resulted in dramatic increases in activity. At this stage of their development, analogs were giving full blockade of ovulation in the cycling, female rat (body weight ca. 250 g) at minimum effective doses in the 15-7.5 ug per animal range.

Needless to say, so many hydrophobic amino acids in the peptide chain resulted in extremely poor solubility in aqueous solvent systems. It was in an effort to improve solubility that we investigated the effects of D-Lys and D-Arg rather than the usual D-aromatic amino acids in position 6 (Coy et al., 1982). Solubility was indeed improved and, furthermore, no loss of antiovulatory activities was experienced with Ac-[D-p-Cl-Phe^{1,2},D-Trp^{3},D-Lys^{6},D-Ala^{10}]-LH-RH. The more basic D-Arg^{6} analog was about twice as active as it D-Lys^{6} and D-Phe^{6} counterparts, producing antiovulatory effects at a 3 ug dose level.

CURRENT APPROACHES TO ANTAGONIST IMPROVEMENT

Since the discovery of the D-Arg^{6} analog, much effort has gone into the re-examination of other positions relative to the new position 6 substitution. In a large part, this work has centered around the N-terminal region of the peptide. The synthesis of a large number of D-Arg^{6} analogs containing various acylated D-amino acids in position 1 (Table 1) clearly demonstrates that increased hydrophobicity can be tolerated as long as D-Arg is present. Indeed, less hydrophobic rJsidues such as dehydro-Pro, Gly and D-Ala which are quite effective in the D-Phe^{6} series now give inferior results in the D-Arg^{6} series. One of the most potent analogs to be found in our laboratory thus far is Ac-[D-B-Nal^{1},D-p-Cl-Phe^{2},D-Trp^{3},D-Arg^{6},D-Ala^{10}]-LH-RH which gives 100% blockade of ovulation at 3 ug per rat and 50% at 1 ug. Another important feature of this particular analog is its

Ac–A–B–C–Ser–Tyr–E–Leu–F–Pro–G–amide

A: D-4-halophenylalanines, D-B-naphthylalanine

B: D-4-Cl-Phe, certain other D-4-halo-Phe's, D-B-Nal

C: D-Trp, certain other D-amino acids resembling Trp

E: D-Arg, D-Lys, certain other basic amino acids

F: Arg or Lys

G: Gly or, better, D-Ala

Figure 1. Some of the main amino acid replacements used in recent LH-RH antagonist design.

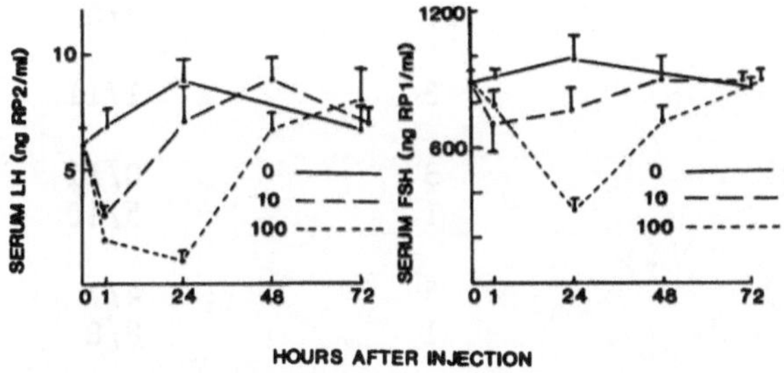

Figure 2. Prolonged suppresion of both LH and FSH release in ovariectomized rats by [Ac-D-B-Nal-1, D-p-Cl-Phe-2, D-Trp-3,D-Arg-6,D-Ala-10]-LH-RH.

prolonged (up to 48h) suppressive effects on both LH and FSH release (figure 2). As far as we are aware, such prolonged activity is unprecedented for a peptide and appears to be the result of prolonged pituitary receptor occupancy with these analogs in general (Dr. K.J. Catt, personal communication). This analog is, for instance, considerably longer acting than Ac-[D-p-Cl-Phe^{1,2},D-Trp^{3},D-Arg^{6},D-Ala^{10}]-LH-RH so that this appears to be another desirable result of increased lipophilicity at the N-terminus. Another analog with slightly higher antiovulatory activity (Table 1) and also prolonged effects (not shown) is [Ac-D-p-Br-Phe^{1},D-p-Cl-Phe^{2},D-Trp^{3},D-Arg^{6},D-Ala^{10}]-LH-RH which again has a bulky, lipophilic amino acid in the first position.

Table I. Position 1 Modifications in the Standard Ac-[D-p-Cl-Phe^{2}, D-Trp^{3},D-Arg^{6},D-Ala^{10}]-Format

RESIDUE IN POSITION 1	ANTIOVULATORY ACTIVITY	
	DOSE (ug)	ANIMALS OVULATING
Ac-Dehydro-Pro	3	9/9
Ac-D-Leu	15	6/8
Ac-Gly	7.5	10/10
Ac-D-Arg	7.5	9/10
Ac-D-Glu	15	8/8
Ac-D-Trp	3	1/11
Ac-D-B-Nal(2)	3	0/11
	1	5/10
Ac-D-B-Nal(1)	5	4/7
	1	8/8
Ac-D-p-Br-Phe	3	0/10
	1	7/9
Ac-D-p-F-Phe	5	0/6
Ac-D-F_5-Phe	3	4/5
Ac-D-His	5	8/9

This much increased tolerance for high lipophilicity at the N-terminus of D-Arg^{6} analogs is further illustrated by the high activity of Ac-[D-B-Nal^{1,2},D-Trp^{3},D-Arg^{6},D-Ala^{10}]-LH-RH (Table 2). If, however, the D-Trp^{3} residue is also replaced by the D-B-Nal residue then an extremely insoluble and far less active analog results. This suggests that there is a sharp cut-off in the degree of hydrophobicity that can be tolerated.

Table II. Additional D-B-Nal Substitutions in the Standard Ac-[D-p-Cl-Phe^{2},D-Trp^{3},D-Arg^{6},D-Ala^{10}]-Format

RESIDUE	ANTIOVULATORY ACTIVITY	
	DOSE (ug)	ANIMALS OVULATING
D-B-Nal^{1}	1	5/10
D-B-Nal^{1,2}	3	0/12
	1	11/11
D-B-Nal^{1,2,3}	7.5	9/9

Present analog studies seem to be taking into account overall considerations of lipophilicity to an increasing extent. A useful model is proving to be one proposed by Dr. Marvin Karten at NIH in which the generally accepted looped structure, stabilized by the position 6 D-amino acid, might lead to the creation of lipophilic and hydrophilic surfaces in roughly equal proportions (figure 3).

Interestingly, this model bears some resemblance to that proposed by Veber (1981) for the conformationally analyzed, short-ring somatostatin analog, cyclo(Phe-D-Trp-Lys-Thr-Pro-Phe), in which the hydrophilic, charged Lys side-chain protrudes on the opposite side of an otherwise highly lipophilic surface, with the Pro residue serving as a conformationally-restricting linking residue. The hydrophilic surface of an LH-RH antagonist would, of course, be considerably more complex thus offering considerably more flexibility in analog design.

With LH-RH analogs, it is evident that modifications to the hydrophilic part of the chain must often be accompanied by suitable changes to the complimentary hydrophobic region in order for antagonist activity to be maintained or increased. In this way, it is possible to alter global properties in an extremely subtle

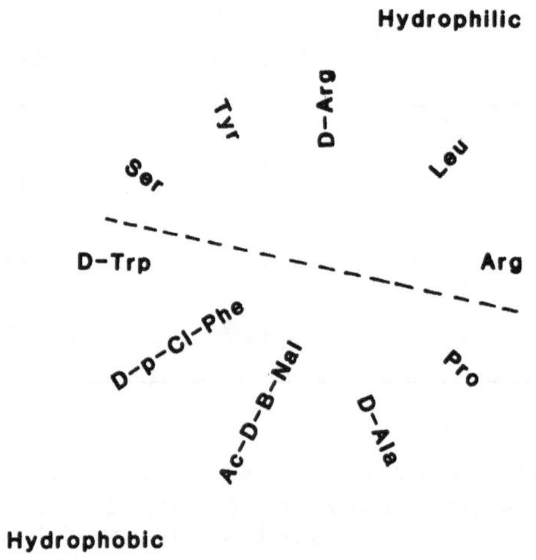

Figure 3. Hydrophilic-hydrophobic surface model for LH-RH antagonists.

manner and this has recently made it possible to decrease antiovulatory doses to the 500 ug region with new compounds.

CONCLUSIONS

The steady progress towards LH-RH antagonists of increasing potency and duration of bction continues unabated. In fact, opportunities for successful analog design appear higher now than at some previous stages of research in the field. The increases in effectiveness of the antagonists have considerable implications for the possible medicinal uses of these compounds both from the viewpoint of cost and more practical routes of administration. We have, for instance, already shown (Nekola et al., 1982) that Ac-[D-p-Cl-Phe^{1,2},D-Trp^{3},D-Arg^{6},D-Ala^{10}]-LH-RH produces complete blockade of ovulation in the rat at an injection dose of 5 ug and an oral dose of 2 mg per animal - a dose ratio of 1:400. If this ratio holds true for analogs active in the ng region after injection, then the oral route of administration may become practical.

It would be hard to overemphasize the value of analog design strategies which were initially developed with LH-RH analogs and which have now been extended to many other important peptides including somatostatin and the enkephalin. Recently, we have used the D-amino acid replacement strategy for some much larger and complex neuro-GI peptides. Replacement of a Gly residue in position 4 of glucagon (Coy et al., 1983) by D-Phe produced an analog with 6 times the glycogenolytic activity of glucagon in the rat. This observation is very analogous to the situation with respect to position 6 of LH-RH which has been referred to throughout this report, and appears to be another example of B-bend stabilization.

Alanine in position 2 of hpGRF(1-29)-NH_2 (Rivier et al., 1983) can be replaced by D-Ala to give a superagonist with 60 times the GH releasing activity of the parent sequence in the anesthetized rat (Lance et al., 1983) . Results such as these should enormously increase the probality of the peptides becoming a major class of therapeutic agents.

ACKNOWLEDGEMENTS

LH-RH antagonist research was supported by NIH NICHD Contract HD-2-2809. We would like to thank Dr. Marvin Karten of NIH for his continuing advice and encouragement on this project.

REFERENCES

Channabasavaiah, K., and Stewart, J.M., 1979, New analogs of luliberin which inhibit ovulation in the rat, Biochem Biophys. Res. Commun. 86: 1266.

Coy, D.H., Horvath, A.., Nekola, M.V., Coy, E.J., Erchegyi, J., and Schally, A.V., 1982, Peptide antagonist of LH-RH: Large increases in antiovulatory activities produced by basic D-amino acids in the six position, Endocrinology, 110: 1445.

Coy, D.H., Mezo, I., Pedroza, E., Nekola, M.V., Vilchez-Martinez, J.A., Piyachaturawat, P., Schally, A.V., Seprodi, J., and Teplan, I., 1979, LH-RH antagonists with potent antiovulatory activity, in "Peptides: Proceedings of the Sixth American Peptide Symposium", E. Gross and J. Meienhofer, eds., p. 775, Pierce, Rockford, Illinois.

Coy, D.H., Nekola, M.V., Erchegyi, J., Coy, E.J., and Schally, A.V., 1981, Contraceptive effects of recent potent LH-RH antagonist analogs, in: "LH-RH Peptides as Female and Male Contraceptives", G.I. Zatuchni, J.D. Shelton, and J.J. Sciarra, eds., p. 37, Harper and Row, NY..

Coy, D.H., Sueiras-Diaz, J., Murphy, W.A., and Lance, V., 1983, Structure-activity studies on glucagon - a position 4 analog with superagonist properties, in "Peptides. Proceedings of the Eighth American Peptide Symposium", V. Hruby and J. Meienhofer, eds., in press, Pierce, Rockford, Illinois.

Coy, D.H., Vilchez-Martinez, J.A., Coy, E.J., and Schally, A.V., 1976, Analogs of LH-RH with increased biological activity produced by D-amino acid substitutions in position 6. J. Med. Chem. 19: 423.

Coy, D.H., Vilchez-Martinez, J.A., and Schally, A.V., 1977, Structure function studies on LH-RH , in "Peptides 1976. Proceeding of the Fourteenth European Peptide Symposium", A. Loffet, ed., p. 463, Editions de l´ Universite de Brusselles, Brussells.

de la Cruz, A., Coy, D.H., Vilchez-Martinez, J.A. Arimura, A. and Schally, A.V., 1976, Blockade of ovulation in rats by inhibitory analogs of LH-RH, Science 191: 195.

Erchegyi, J., Coy, D.H., Nekola, M.V., Coy, E.J., Schally, A.V., Mezo, I., and Teplan I., 1981, LH-RH analogs with increased antiovulatory activity Biochem. Biophys. Res. Commun. 100: 915.

Lance, V.A., Murphy, W.A., Sueiras-Diaz, J.A., and Coy, D.H., 1983, Super-active analogues of growth hormone-releasing factor containing N-terminal D-amino acids, Nature, submitted.

Monahan, M.W., Amoss, M.S., Anderson, H.A. and Vale, W., 1976, Synthetic analogs of the hypothalamic luteinizing hormone releasing factor with increased agonist or antagonist properties, Biochemistry 12: 4616.

Matsuo, H., Baba, Y., Nair, R.M.G., Arımura, A., and Schally, A.V. 1971, Structure of the porcine LH and FSH-releasing hormone. I Proposed amino acid sequence, Biochem.Biophys Res. Commun. 43: 1334.

Nekola, M.V., Horvath, A., Ge, L-J., Coy, D.H. and Schally, A.V., 1982, Suppression of ovulation in the rat by an orally active antagonist of LH-RH, Science 218: 160.

Rivier, J., Spiess, J., Thorner, M., and Vale, W., 1982, Characterization of a growth hormon-releasing factor from a human pancreatic islet tumor, Nature 300: 276

Schally, A.V., Arimura, A., and Coy, D.H., 1980, Recent approaches to fertility control based on derivatives of LH-RH, in "Vitamins and Hormones", P.L. Munson, J. Diczfalusy, J. Glover, and R.E. Olson, eds., p. 257, Academic Press, NY.

Veber, D.F., 1981, Design of a highly active cyclic hexapeptide analog of somatostatin, in "Peptides: Proceedings of the Seventh American Peptide Symposium", D.H. Rich and E. Gross, eds., p. 685, Pierce, Rockford, Illinois

MEDICAL CASTRATION WITH LHRH AGONISTS AND THE NEED FOR COMBINED TREATMENT WITH AN ANTIANDROGEN IN PROSTATE CANCER

F. Labrie, A. Dupont, A. Bélanger,
R. St-Arnaud, C. Labrie and Members of the
Laval University Prostate Cancer Program*

Departments of Medicine and Molecular Endocrinology, CHUL, Québec G1V 4G2, Canada

INTRODUCTION

Cancer of the prostate is the second cause of death due to cancer in man, its annual incidence being approximately 40,000 new cases per 100 millions of population in North America. A major change in the treatment of this disease has been introduced by the pioneering studies of Huggins and collaborators who have recognized the role of androgens of testicular origin in the evolution of this cancer (Huggins and Hodges, 1941; Huggins et al., 1941). Following these observations, during the last forty years, neutralization of testicular androgens has been achieved by surgical castration or treatment with estrogens, two approaches which lead to subjective and/or objective improvement in 60 to 70% of cases for various time intervals (Bailar et al., 1970; Barnes and Ninan, 1972; Byar, 1973; Grayhack and Kozlowski, 1980; Murphy and Slack, 1980; Nesbit and Plumb, 1946; Nesbit and Baum, 1950; Staubiz et al., 1954; Whitmore, 1956). However, surgical castration presents psychological limitations for many patients while high doses of estrogens frequently cause lethal cardiovascular complications (Byar, 1973). There was thus the need for a more ac-

*C. Bossé, R. Delisle, J. Emond, J.G. Girard, J.G. Houle, Y. Lacoursière, G. Monfette, J.P. Paquet and A. Vallières

ceptable way of neutralizing testicular androgens.

INHIBITION OF TESTICULAR STEROIDOGENESIS

Experimental animals

Stimulated by the lack of success of LHRH and its agonists in the treatment of infertility in men (Schwartzstein, 1976; Krabbe and Shakkeback, 1977), we have investigated in detail the effect of acute and chronic administration of these peptides on testicular functions in experimental animals. Somewhat unexpectedly, we then made the observation that short-term administration of the LHRH agonist [D-Leu^6, des-Gly-NH_2^{10}]-LHRH ethylamide, ([D-Leu^6]LHRH-EA), to adult male rats led to a loss of testicular LH and prolactin receptors, as well as decreased serum testosterone levels accompanied by inhibition of ventral prostate, seminal vesicle and testis weight (Auclair et al., 1977a, b; Labrie et al., 1978, 1980).

Man

It is of great interest that inhibitory effects on testosterone secretion similar to those first described in the rat are exerted in the male hamster (Sandow and Hahn, 1978), rabbit and dog. The only exception so far reported is the monkey where androgen biosynthesis is exceptionally resistant to treatment with LHRH agonists (Resko et al., 1982).

Fortunately, among all species studied, man is the most sensitive to the inhibitory effect of LHRH agonist treatment on testicular androgen formation (Labrie et al., 1980; Bélanger et al., 1980; Faure et al., 1982; Santen et al., 1984) and medical castration can be easily achieved (Labrie et al., 1980, 1982, 1983a, 1983b, 1983c, 1983d, 1984a, 1984b; Santen et al., 1984; Tolis et al., 1982).

Despite the initial improvement of symptoms after neutralization of androgens of testicular origin in a large proportion of patients, relapse of the disease usually occurs within one or two years (Resnick and Grayhack, 1975). Moreover, within 6 months after relapse of the disease, the survival is only approximately 50% (Johnson et al., 1975). Since man is unique among species in having a high secretion of precursor adrenal steroids which can be converted into active steroids in the prostate as well as at the periphery, (Geller et al., 1978; Harper et al., 1974; Pike et al., 1970), it is quite possible that reactivation of the cancer and the lack of response in 30 to 40% of patients following orchiectomy or DES treatment are due to the androgens of adrenal origin (Bhanalaph et al., 1974; Cowley et al., 1976; Sanford et al., 1977). We thus felt important to include neutralization of adrenal androgens in our antihormonal treatment regime.

Knowing that chemical castration can be easily achieved with LHRH agonists (Labrie et al., 1980), neutralization of the action of adrenal androgens on the cancer was the next problem to be investigated. Following our preliminary studies using an LHRH agonist and a pure antiandrogen in experimental animals (Lefebvre et al., 1982; Séguin et al., 1981), we have used the same combined therapy in men with advanced prostatic cancer (Labrie et al., 1980, 1982, 1983a, 1983b, 1983c, 1983d, 1984a, 1984b). The present report is a continuation of this study in 97 patients at stage D2 of the disease. The combination therapy was used in 44 previously untreated patients as well as in 24 patients previously treated with DES (diethylstilbestrol) and in 29 patients previously castrated. In support of our previous suggestion (Labrie et al., 1980, 1982, 1983a, 1983b, 1983c, 1983d), the present study clearly indicates drastic changes in our approach to the treatment of prostatic cancer.

SERUM PROSTATIC ACID PHOSPHATASE

Serum prostatic acid phosphatase (PAP) measured by radioimmunoassay was elevated in 70 out of 97 patients at initiation of treatment. It can be seen in Fig. 1 that serum PAP was rapidly reduced to 45% of pretreatment values as early as 5 days after starting the combined antihormonal therapy using the LHRH agonist and the antiandrogen in previously untreated patients. The serum PAP values progressively decreased and normal values were reached within two months in all except 5 patients who all showed normal serum PAP levels at 4 months. A comparable pattern was seen in 9 previously untreated patients who were orchiectomized and received the same dose of the antiandrogen (data not shown).

It can be seen in Fig. 2 that a striking difference is observed when the same treatment is applied to pa-

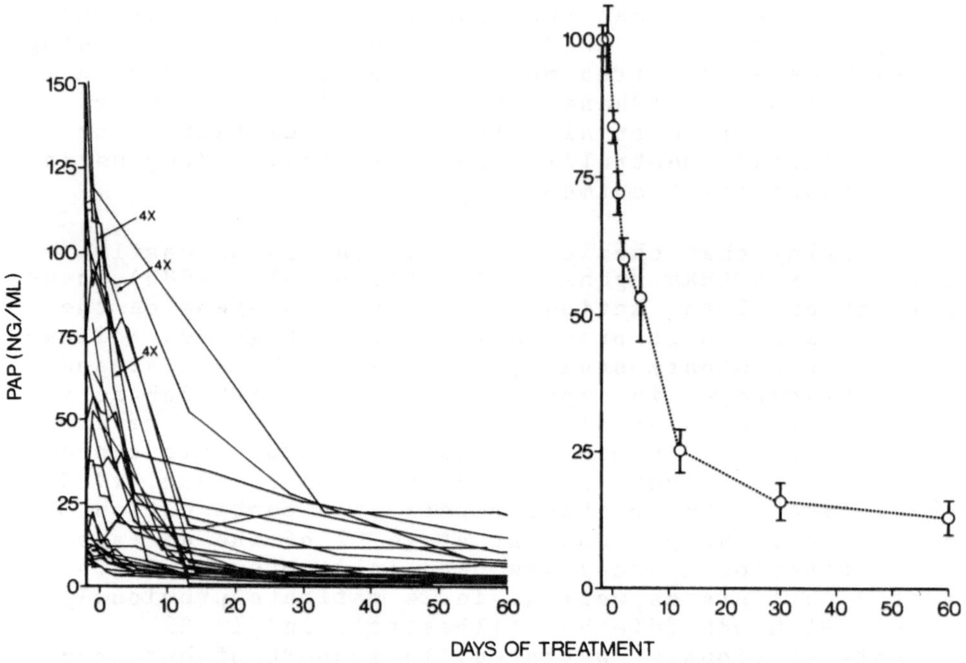

Fig. 1. Effect of combined treatment with an LHRH agonist (HOE-766) and a pure antiandrogen (RU23908) on serum PAP levels in previously untreated patients with advanced (stage D2) prostatic cancer. Individual values are shown on the left panel while means ± SEM are illustrated on the right panel (25 patients).

tients previously treated with DES. In fact, although serum PAP levels decreased to normal values in some patients, the levels of serum PAP continued to increase in 11 out of 24 patients. Similarly, in patients previously castrated, stabilization or an increase of serum PAP levels was seen in 75% of patients (data not shown).

As already seen in the first adult men treated with a high dose of an LHRH agonist (Labrie et al., 1980), treatment with LHRH agonists alone is always accompanied by a rise in serum T and DHT concentration

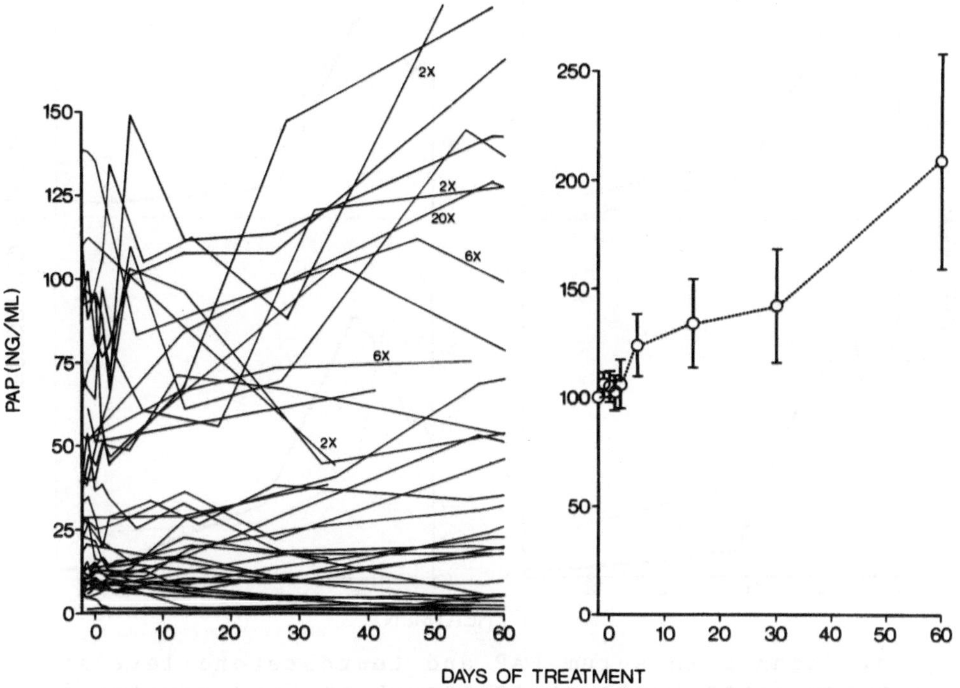

Fig. 2. Effect of combined treatment with an LHRH agonist (HOE-766) and a pure antiandrogen (RU23908) on serum PAP levels in patients with advanced (stage D2) prostatic cancer previously treated with diethylstilbestrol. Individual values are shown on the left panel while means ± SEM are illustrated on the right panel (9 patients).

which lasts for 5 to 15 days (Glode, 1982; Labrie et al., 1982; 1983a, 1983b; Santen et al., 1984; Trachtenberg, 1983) and is accompanied in a significant proportion of cases by a flare of the cancer (Glode, 1982; Santen et al., 1984; Trachtenberg, 1983). It is thus of great interest to see in Fig. 1 and 3 that a 55% decrease in serum PAP is already observed during the first 5 days of treatment with the LHRH agonist at a time when serum androgens are increased by 100 to 200% ($p < 0.01$, Fig. 3).

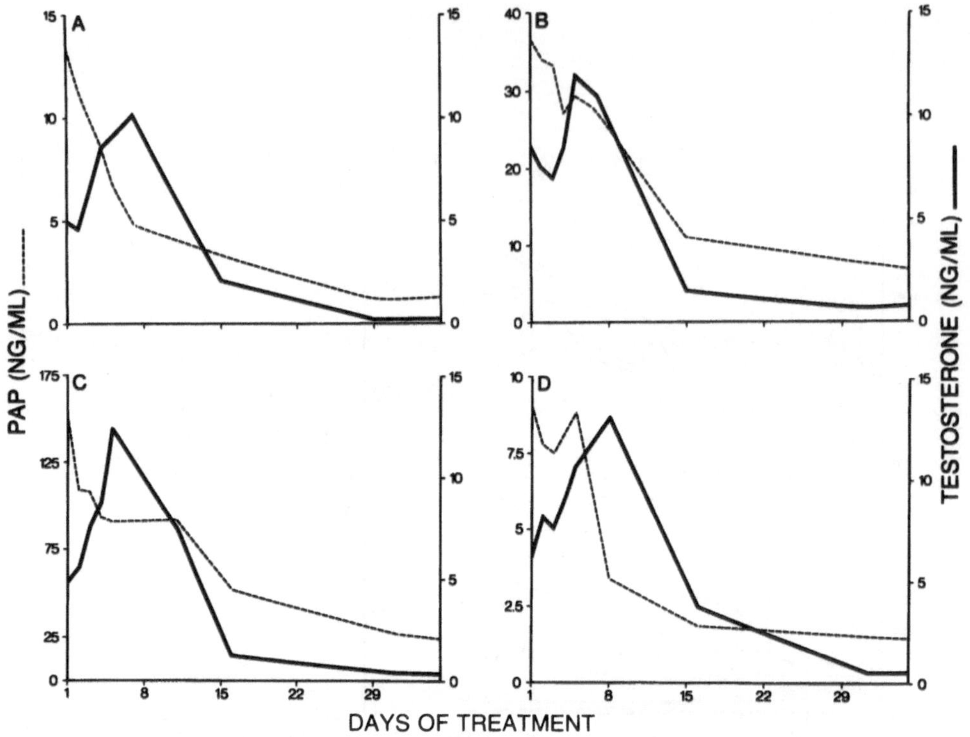

Fig. 3. Changes in serum PAP and testosterone levels during the first month of treatment in four previously untreated patients having advanced prostatic cancer and receiving the combined administration of an LHRH agonist and a pure antiandrogen. Note the rapid and marked decrease in serum PAP concentration in the presence of elevated serum T levels, thus indicating the efficiency of the antiandrogen at the dose used.

Hormonal

The changes in plasma cortisol, dehydroepiandrosterone sulfate and dehydroepiandrosterone levels in 20 patients treated with the LHRH agonist [D-Ser(TBU)^{6}, des-Gly-NH_2^{10}]LHRH ethylamide (LHRH-A) and the pure antiandrogen RU23908 are illustrated in Fig. 4. While the plasma levels of cortisol are unchanged after 60 days of combined treatment with the LHRH agonist and the antiandrogen, the plasma concentrations of DHEA-S and DHEA are reduced to 45 ± 7 ($p < 0.01$) and 64 ± 4% ($p < 0.01$) of control, respectively. After 60 days of combined treatment with the LHRH agonist and the antiandrogen, the plasma levels of testosterone are reduced from 5.44 ± 0.45 to 0.450 ± 0.052 ng/ml (2.5% of control).

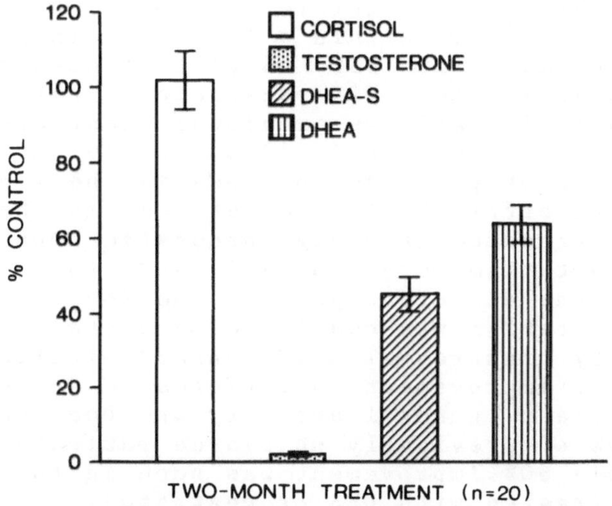

Fig. 4. Effect of combined treatment with the LHRH agonist [D-Ser(TBU)^6, des-Gly-NH$_2$^{10}]LHRH ethylamide and the antiandrogen RU23908 or surgical castration and RU23908 on the basal serum levels of cortisol, dehydroepiandrosterone (DHEA) and dehydroepiandrosterone sulfate (DHEA-S) in patients with prostate cancer. Serum steroid levels were measured before and after 2 months of treatment. Control levels of cortisol, dehydroepiandrosterone sulfate and dehydroepiandrosterone were respectively 156 ± 6, 834 ± 147 and 1.9 ± 0.3 ng/ml in patients (n = 20) treated with the LHRH agonist and respectively 239 ± 26, 738 ± 120 and 1.83 ± 0.27 ng/ml in castrated patients (n = 19).

Bone scanning

In 32 previously untreated patients having metastatic disease, the combined therapy led to at least a 50% decrease in uptake accompanied by a normalization of serum PAP and no appearance of new lesions. A complete disappearance of bone lesions was seen within 5 months in 4 patients, thus indicating complete objective response. In the other 12 patients classified as stable, serum PAP levels are decreasing but have not yet reached normal values. A most important finding is that none of the 44 previously untreated patients receiving the combined therapy showed progression of the disease (Table 1).

Clinical signs and symptoms

In the previously untreated patients, a rapid and compleve relief of pain was observed in all patients presenting this symptom before treatment. Disappearance of bone pain was seen within a few days. In patients previously treated with DES, complete blockade of androgens also led to a disappearance of pain in all patients while in patients previously castrated, disappearance of pain was seen in 12 out of 16 patients. A partial relief of pain was obtained in the 4 others. Although more difficult to evaluate due to the frequent concomitant presence of benign prostatic hyperplasia, signs of prostatism were improved in 80 to 100% of patients in the different groups. The improvement in signs of prostatism was confirmed by rectal examination as well as by transrectal and transabdominal echography in all cases. Improvement in performance and well-being (appetite, sleep, general activity and body weight) was seen in 100% of previously untreated patients while an approximately 60% improvement was seen in the patients previously treated with DES or castrated.

As shown earlier (Labrie et al., 1980, 1982, 1983a, 1983b, 1983c, 1983d), approximately 50% of patients receiving the combined therapy developed, to various degrees, climateric-like vasomotor phenomena consisting of perspiration and hot flushes. These symptoms decreased or disappeared after a few months of treatment. Most patients complained of a decrease in libido and erectile potency after two to three weeks of treatment. However, in a few cases, libido and erectile potency were maintained despite complete androgen neutralization. No other side-effects were observed.

Table 1. Objective response to the complete blockade of androgens

Previous treatment	Months of RX	Current RX	No of pts	% OBJECTIVE RESPONSE Complete	Partial	Stable	Progression	Escape
		LHRH-A		9%	71%	20%	0%	2/35
NIL	9.9	+ANTI-	35	(3)	(25)	(7)	0%	
	(4-18)	ANDR.						4.5%
		CASTR.		11%	33%	56%	0%	2/44
NIL	7.3	+ANTI-	9	(1)	(3)	(5)	0	0/9
	(4-11)	ANDRO.						
		LHRH-A		4%	37%	17%	42%	
DES	8.5	+ANTI-	24	(1)	(9)	(4)	(10)	4/14
	(3-14)	ANDROG.						25%
		LHRH-A		0%	8%	31%	61%	6/24
CASTR.	8.1	+ANTI-	13	0	(1)	(4)	(8)	2/5
	(4-11)	ANDRO.						
CASTR.	6.5	ANTI-	16	0%	19%	12%	69%	0/5
+ DES	(4-10)	ANDR.		0	(3)	(2)	(11)	

Objective response according to the NPCP criteria to the combined treatment with an LHRH agonist (or surgical castration) and a pure antiandrogen in previously un- treated patients with prostate cancer at stage D2 or previously treated with DES as well as to treatment with the antiandrogen in stage D2 patients previously castrated.

As revealed by a series of standard biochemical and hematological tests, treatment with the LHRH agonist and the antiandrogen has no detectable effect on any of the following parameters: complete (WBC, RBC, hemoglobin, hematocrit and platelets) and differential blood count, γ-glutamyl transaminase, glutamic oxaloacetic transaminase, glutamic pyruvic transferase, lactic dehydrogenase, creatinine, total biliburin and other parameters of blood biochemistry (SMA-12).

A most consequent conclusion of this study is that prostate cancer, even at the metastatic stage, is exquisitely sensitive to androgens. In fact, when complete androgen neutralization is achieved in patients previously untreated, a positive objective response assessed according to the criteria of the National Prostatic Cancer Project has so far been observed in all patients. In fact, in the 44 patients who received the combined therapy with the LHRH agonist or surgical castration in association with the antiandrogen, no progression of the disease has been observed in any patient.

Since patients at stage D2 have an average of at least ten metastases each, for a total of approximately 450 metastases, and only two tumors showed relapse, the present data indicate that even at the late metastatic stage, more than 99% of prostatic tumors are androgen-sensitive. This finding has major implications for therapy. In a large study, including 600 patients who could be followed up to five years, Nesbit and Baum (1950) concluded that 30% of patients with metastases showed no response whatever to castration and/or estrogen therapy, an indication, according to the authors, of a high incidence of androgen independence. The same percentage of patients with advanced prostatic cancer who responded to standard hormonal therapy has been reported by Menon and Walsh (1979), Whitmore (1956) and Fowler and Whitmore (1980). The most likely explanation for this major difference between our results and those of previous studies is that previous hormonal therapy was limited to the neutralization of androgens of testicular origin by surgical castration and/or high doses of estrogens while the present approach achieves complete neutralization of all androgens of both testicular and adrenal origin (Fig. 5).

After neutralization of testicular androgens by surgical castration, high doses of estrogens or LHRH agonists alone, the adrenals continue to secrete a large amount of weak androgens and also low amounts of testosterone. These weak adrenal androgens are converted into strong androgens in prostatic tissue (Acevedo and Goldziecker, 1965; Geller et al., 1978) as well as at the peripheral level. The skin does in fact convert DHEAS and DHEA into androstenedione and DHT (Gallegos and Berliner, 1967; Schubert, 1975; Sommerville et al., 1971). Even blood cells can transform androstenedione into T (Blaquier et al., 1967; Van der Molen and Groen, 1968) while the brain can transform DHEA into T and DHT (Knapstein et al., 1968).

That androgens of adrenal origin play a role in prostatic cancer after removal of testicular androgens is clearly demonstrated by the finding that relatively high levels of DHT have been found to accumulate in

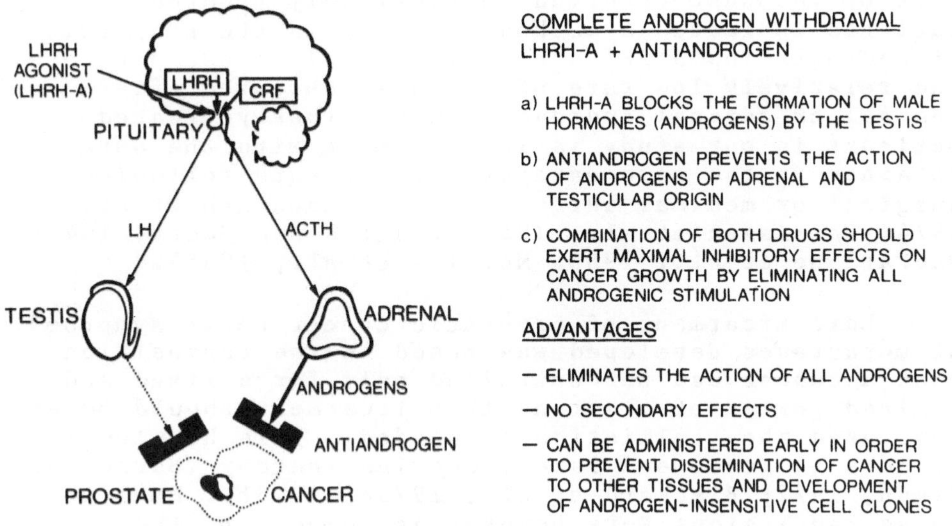

LHRH AGONIST (LHRH-A)
LHRH
CRF
PITUITARY
LH
ACTH
TESTIS
ADRENAL
ANDROGENS
ANTIANDROGEN
PROSTATE
CANCER
COMPLETE ANDROGEN WITHDRAWAL
LHRH-A + ANTIANDROGEN
a) LHRH-A BLOCKS THE FORMATION OF MALE HORMONES (ANDROGENS) BY THE TESTIS
b) ANTIANDROGEN PREVENTS THE ACTION OF ANDROGENS OF ADRENAL AND TESTICULAR ORIGIN
c) COMBINATION OF BOTH DRUGS SHOULD EXERT MAXIMAL INHIBITORY EFFECTS ON CANCER GROWTH BY ELIMINATING ALL ANDROGENIC STIMULATION
ADVANTAGES
— ELIMINATES THE ACTION OF ALL ANDROGENS
— NO SECONDARY EFFECTS
— CAN BE ADMINISTERED EARLY IN ORDER TO PREVENT DISSEMINATION OF CANCER TO OTHER TISSUES AND DEVELOPMENT OF ANDROGEN-INSENSITIVE CELL CLONES

Fig. 5. Schematic representation of the combined treatment with an LHRH agonist and a pure antiandrogen in prostate cancer.

accumulate in prostatic cancer tissue in patients after surgical castration (Geller et al., 1978). That cancer cells which are androgen-sensitive remain active after surgical castration or high doses of estrogens is also clearly illustrated by the finding that 33 to 39% of patients already castrated or treated with estrogens showed a positive response to the antiandrogen Flutamide (Sogani et al., 1975; Stoliar and Albert, 1974).

Another most important conclusion of the present study is that a large proportion of prostatic cancer cells which continue to grow under the influence of androgens of adrenal origin become insensitive to androgens in this "androgen-poor" milieu. This is clearly demonstrated by the finding that complete androgen neutralization in patients previously treated with estrogens or castrated leads to only 30 to 40%

positive/objective responses as compared to more than 95% in previously untreated patients. The much lower rate of response observed in previously treated patients indicates a marked increase in the proportion of androgen-insensitive cancer cells in these patients. The relatively low rate of response observed after removal of adrenal androgens in previously treated patients in our study is in agreement with the data obtained in the same category of patients following surgical or medical adrenalectomy (Bhanalaph et al., 1974; Harrisson et al., 1953; Huggins and Scott, 1945; MacFarlane et al., 1960; Morales et al., 1955).

Late treatment of prostatic cancer until symptoms of metastases developed was based on the supposition that a cancer can be controlled only for a fixed and limited period of time and that treatment should be at best used when palliation is needed. This has led most authors to recommend late endocrine therapy (Barnes and Ninan, 1972; Blackard et al., 1975a; 1975b). Much of these conclusions were however influenced by the serious cardiovascular side-effects related to the use of estrogens. In addition, the suggestion of late endocrine therapy was based on the supposition that hormone-insensitive cells are present early in the tumors and are those responsible for the ultimate failure of hormonal therapy (Markland et al., 1978; Murphy and Slack, 1980). However, complete removal of androgens of both testicular and adrenal origins shows that more than 99% of prostatic tumors, even at the stage of metastases, are still androgen-sensitive (Scott, 1983). Instead of being present at the beginning of treatment, our data clearly indicate that most of the androgen-insensitive cells appear when the tumor cells are exposed to the "low androgen" milieu provided by the adrenal androgens.

Hormone dependence of prostatic cancer cells is a characteristic of the tissue of origin. This property of cancer cells can be progressively lost during cell division (De Grouchy, 1973; Schubert, 1975). It is logical that as the disease advances, a greater chance of appearance of androgen-resistant cell clones develops. In animal models, survival is related to the size of the tumor at the time treatment is administered (Fowler and Whitmore, 1980). Our present data strongly support the suggestion that antihormonal therapy should be started as early as possible after diagnosis, at least in advanced prostatic cancer.

Another important finding in the present study is that concomitant treatment with the pure antiandrogen completely prevents disease flare, a complication unfortunately observed in a significant proportion of patients treated with LHRH agonists alone (Glode, 1982; Santen et al., 1984; Trachtenberg, 1983). With the present knowledge, there remains no rationale for the use of LHRH agonists alone since the adverse effects of the initial rise in serum androgens can be so easily prevented, thus eliminating any unnecessary risk to the patient.

Due to its excellent tolerance and lack of secondary effects other than those related to hypoandrogenecity, the present findings strongly suggest that complete androgen blockade achieved by the present approach should be initiated as early as possible after diagnosis (at least at stages C and D) in order to obtain remission in a greater proportion of patients and to minimize the appearance of androgen-insensitive cell clones, thus improving the quality of life and faciliting the possible application of other treatments such as radiotherapy and/or chemotherapy in the cases developing androgen-independent tumors.

REFERENCES

Acevedo, H.F., and Goldziecker, J.W., 1965, Further studies on the metabolism of 4-[4-^{14}C]androstene-3,17-dione by normal and pathological human prostate tissue. Biochim. Biophys. Acta., 97:564.

Auclair, C., Kelly, P.A., Coy, D.H., Schally, A.V., and Labrie, F., 1977a, Potent inhibitory activity of [D-Leu^{6}, des-Gly-NH$_2$^{10}]LHRH ethylamide on LH/hCG and PRL testicular receptor levels in the rat. Endocrinology, 101:1890.

Auclair, C., Kelly, P.A., Labrie, F., Coy, D.H. and Schally, A.V., 1977b, Inhibition of testicular luteinizing hormone receptor levels by treatment with a potent luteinizing hormone-releasing hormone agonist or human chorionic gonadotropin. Biochem. Biophys. Res. Commun., 76:855.

Bailar, J.C., Byar, D.P., and Vet. Adm. Coop. Urol. Res. Group, 1970, Estrogen treatment for cancer of the prostate. Cancer, 26:257.

Barnes, R.W., and Ninan, C.A., 1972, Carcinoma of the prostate: biopsy and conservative therapy. J. Urol., 108:897.

Bélanger, A., Labrie, F., Lemay, A., Caron, S. and Raynaud, J.P., 1980, Inhibitory effects of a single intranasal administration of [D-Ser(TBU)^6, des-Gly- NH_2^{10}]LHRH ethylamide, a potent LHRH agonist, on serum steroid levels in normal adult men. J. Steroid Biochem., 13:123.

Bhanalaph, T., Varkarakis, M.J., and Murphy, G.P., 1974, Current status of bilateral adrenalectomy of advanced prostatic carcinoma. Ann. Surg. 179:17.

Blackard, C.E. and The Veteran's Administration Cooperative Urology Research Group, 1975a, Studies of carcinoma of the prostate: a review. Cancer Chemother. Rep., 59:225.

Blackard, C.E., Byar, D.P., Seal, U.S., Doe, R.P. and VACURG, 1975b, Correlation of pretreatment serum nonprotein-bound cortisol and total 17-hydroxycorticosteroid values with survival in patients with prostatic cancer. New Engl. J. Med., 291:751.

Blaquier, J., Forchielli, E. and Dorfman, R.I., 1967, In vitro metabolism of androgens in whole human blood. Acta Endocrinol., 55:697.

Byar, D.P., 1973, The Veterans Administration Cooperative Urological Research Group's studies of cancer of the prostate. Cancer, 32:1126.

Cowley, T.H., Brownsey, B.G., Harper, M.E., Peeling, W.B., and Griffiths, K., 1976, The effect of ACTH on plasma testosterone and androstenedione concentrations in patients with prostatic carcinoma. Acta Endocrinol., 81:310.

De Grouchy, J., 1973, Cancer and the evolution of species: a ransom. Biomedicine, 18: 6.

Faure, N., Labrie, F., Lemay, A., Bélanger, A., Gourdeau, Y., Laroche, B., and Robert, G., 1982, Inhibition of serum androgen levels by chronic intranasal administration of a potent LHRH agonist in adult men. Fertil. Steril., 37:416.

Fowler, J.E. Jr., and Whitmore, W.F. Jr., 1980, The response of metastatic adenocarcinoma of the prostate to exogenous testosterone. J. Urol., 126:372.

Gallegos, A.J., and Berliner, D.L., 1967, Transformation and conjugation of dehydroepiandrosterone by human skin. J. Clin. Endocrinol. Metab., 27:1214.

Geller, J., Albert, J., Loza, D., Geller, S., Stoeltzing, W., and De La Vega, D., 1978, DHT concentrations in human prostate cancer tissue. J. Clin. Endocrinol. Metab., 46: 440.

Glode, L.M. (Abbott Prostatic Cancer Study), 1982, Leuprolide therapy of advanced prostatic cancer. : LASCO Proc., Abst., p. 110.

Grayhack, J.T. and Kozlowski, J.M., 1980, Endocrine therapy in the management of advanced prostatic cancer: the case for early initiation of treatment. Urol. Clin. North Amer., 7: 639.

Harper, M.E., Peeling, W.B., Cowley, T., Bronsey, B.G., Phillips, M.E.Z., Groom, G., Fahmy, D.R., and Griffiths, K., 1974, Plasma steroid and protein hormone concentration in patients with prostatic carcinoma before and during estrogen therapy. Acta Endocrinol., 81: 409.

Harrisson, J.H., Thorn, G.W., and Jenkins, D., 1953, Total adrenalectomy for reactivated carcinoma of the prostate. N. Engl. J. Med., 248:86.

Huggins, C., and Hodges, C.V., 1941, Studies of prostatic cancer. I. Effect of castration, estrogen and androgen injections on serum phosphatases in metastatic carcinoma of the prostate. Cancer Res., 1:293.

Huggins, C., Stevens, R.E., and Hodges, C.W., 1941, Studies on prostatic cancer. II. The effects of castration of advanced carcinoma of the prostate gland. Arch. Surg., 43:209.

Huggins, C., and Scott, W.W., 1945, Bilateral adrenalectomy in prostatic cancer. Ann. Surg., 122:1031.

Johnson, D.E., Kaesler, K.E., and Ayala, A.G., 1975, Megestrol acetate for treatment of advanced carcinoma of the prostate. J. Surg. Oncol. 7:9.

Knapstein, P., David, A., Wu, C.H., Archer, D.F., Flickinger, G.L., and Touchstone, J.C., 1968, Metabolism of free and sulfoconjugated DHEA in brain tissue in vivo and in vitro. Steroids 11:885.

Krabbe, S. and Shakkeback, N.E., 1977, Gonadotropin-releasing hormone (LHRH) and human chorionic gonadotropin in the treatment of two boys with hypogonadotrophic hypogonadism. Acta Paediatr. Scand., 66:361.

Labrie, F., Auclair, C., Cusan, L., Kelly, P.A., Pelletier, G. and Ferland, L., 1978, Inhibitory effects of LHRH and its agonists on testicular gonadotropin receptors and spermatogenesis in the rat. In Hansson, V. (ed.), Endocrine Approach to Male Contraception, Int. J. Androl. (Suppl. 2), pp. 303.

Labrie, F., Bélanger, A., Cusan, L., Séguin, C., Pelletier, G., Kelly, P.A., Lefebvre, F.A., Lemay, A., and Raynaud, J.P., 1980, Antifertility effects of LHRH agonists in the male. J. Androl., 1:209.

Labrie, F., Dupont, A., Bélanger, A., Cusan, L., Lacourcière, Y., Monfette, G., Laberge, J.G., Emond, J.P., Fazekas, A.T.A., Raynaud, J.P. and Husson, J.M., 1982, New hormonal therapy in prostatic carcinoma: combined treatment with an LHRH agonist and an antiandrogen. J. Clin. Invest. Med., 5:267.

Labrie, F., Dupont, A., Bélanger, A., Lacourcière, Y., Raynaud, J.P., Husson, J.M., Gareau, J., Fazekas, A.T.A., Sandow, J., Monfette, G., Girard, J.G., Emond, J. and Houle, J.G., 1983a, New approach in the treatment of prostate cancer: complete instead of only partial withdrawal of androgens. The Prostate, 4:579.

Labrie, F., Dupont, A., Bélanger, A., Lefebvre, F.A., Cusan, L., Raynaud, J.P., Husson, J.M. and Fazekas, A.T.A., 1983b, New Hormonal therapy in prostate cancer: combined use of a pure antiandrogen and an LHRH agonist. Hormone Res., 18:18.

Labrie, F., Dupont, A., Bélanger, A., Lefebvre, F.A., Cusan, L., Monfette, G., Laberge, J.G., Emond, J.P., Raynaud, J.P., Husson, J.M. and Fazekas, A.T.A., 1983c, New hormonal treatment in cancer of the prostate: combined administration of an LHRH agonist and an antiandrogen. J Steroid Biochem., 19:999.

Labrie, F., Bélanger, A., Carmichael, R., Séguin, C., Lefebvre, F.A., Faure, N., and Dupont, A., 1983d, Inhibition of the testicular steroidogenic pathway in experimental animals and men, in: "Recent Advances in Male Reproduction: Molecular Basis and Clinical Implications", R. D'Agata, M.B. Lipsett and H.J. Van der Molen (eds), Raven Press, New York, p. 239.

Labrie, F., Dupont, A., Bélanger, A., Labrie, C., Lacourcière, Y., Raynaud, J.P., Husson, J.M., Emond, J., Houle, J.G., Girard, J.G., Monfette, G., Paquet, J.P., Vallières, A., Bossé, C., and Delisle, R., 1984a, Combined antihormonal treatment in prostate cancer, a new approach using an LHRH agonist or castration and an antiandrogen, in: Hormones and Cancer, Raven Press, New York, in press.

Labrie, F., Dupont, A., Bélanger, A., Emond, J., and Monfette, G., 1984b, Pure antiandrogens permit to take advantage of the well-tolerated LHRH agonists for the treatment of prostate cancer. Proc. Natl. Acad. Sci. USA, in press.

Lefebvre, F.A., Séguin, C., Bélanger, A., Caron, S., Sairam, M.R., Raynaud, J.P., and Labrie, F., 1982, Combined long-term treatment with an LHRH agonist and a pure antiandrogen blocks androgenic influence in the rat. The Prostate, 3:569.

MacFarlane, D.A., Thomas, L.P., and Harrison, J.H., 1960, A survey of total adrenalectomy in cancer of the prostate. Amer. J. Surg. 99:562.

Markland, F.S., Chiopp, R.T., Cosgrove, M.D., and Howard, E.B., 1978, Characterization of steroid hormone receptors in the Dunning R-3327 rat prostatic adenocarcinoma. Cancer Res., 38:2818.

Menon, M. and Walsh, P.C., 1979, Hormone therapy for prostatic cancer. in: "Prostatic Cancer", G.P. Murphy, ed., Littleton, Massachusetts, PSG Publishing Co., p. 175.

Morales, P.A., Brendler, H., and Hotchkiss, R.S., 1955, The role of the adrenal cortex in prostatic cancer. J. Urol., 73: 399.

Murphy, G.P. and Slack, N.H., 1980, Response criteria for the prostate of the USA National Prostatic Cancer Project. Urol. Clin. North Amer., 7:631.

Nesbit, R.M. and Plumb, R.T., 1946, A follow-up on 795 patients treated prior to the endocrine era and a comparison of survival rates between these and patients treated by endocrine therapy. Surgery, 20:263.

Nesbit, R.M. and Baum, W.C., 1950, Endocrine control of prostatic carcinoma. Clinical and statistical survey of 1818 cases. J. Amer. Med. Assoc. 143:1317.

Pike, A., Peeling, W.B., Haerper, M.E., Pierrepoint, C.G., and Griffiths, K., 1970, Testosterone metabolism in vivo by human prostatic tissue. Biochem. J., 120:443.

Resko, J., Bélanger, A., and Labrie, F., 1982, Effects of chronic treatment with a potent LHRH agonist on serum LH and steroid levels in the male rhesus monkey. Biol. Reprod., 26:378.

Resnick, M.I., and Grayhack, J.T., 1975, Treatment of stage IV carcinoma of the prostate. Urol. Clin. North Amer., 2:141.

Sandow, J. and Hahn, M., 1978, Chronic treatment with LHRH in golder hamsters. Acta Endocrinol. 88:601.

Sanford, E.J., Paulson, D.F., Rohner, T.J., Drago, J.R., Santen, R.J. and Bardin, C.W., 1977, The effects of castration on adrenal testosterone secretion in men with prostatic carcinoma. J. Urol., 118:1019.

Santen, R.J., Warner, B., Demers, L.M., Dufau, M., and Smith, J., 1984, Use of GnRH hormone agonists analogues. in: " LHRH and its analogs -a new class of contraceptive and therapeutic agents", B. Vickery, J.J. Nestor, Jr. and E.S.E. Hafez (eds), MTP Press, Lancaster-Boston, in press.

Schubert, G.E., 1975, Hormone dependency and histological types of tumors, in: "Hormone Therapy of Prostate Cancer", U. Bracci and F. Di Silverio, (eds), Cofese Edizione, Rome, Palermo, p. 43.

Schwartzstein, L., 1976, Diagnostic and therapeutic use of LHRH in the infertile man, in: "Hypothalamus and endocrine functions", F. Labrie, J. Meites and G. Pelletier, eds, Plenum Press, New York, p. 73.

Scott, W.W., 1983, Historical overview of the treatment of prostatic cancer. The Prostate 4:435.

Séguin, C., Cusan, L., Bélanger, A., Kelly, P.A., Labrie, F., and Raynaud, J.P., 1981, Additive inhibitory effects of treatment with an LHRH agonist and an antiandrogen on adrogen-dependent tissues in the rat. Mol. Cell. Endocrinol., 21:37.

Sogani, P.C., Ray, B., and Whitmore, W.F. Jr., 1975, Advanced prostatic carcinoma: flutamide therapy after conventional endocrine treatment. Urology, 6:164.

Sommerville, I.F., Flamigni, C., Collins, W.P., Koullapis, E.N., and Dewhurst, C.J., 1971, Androgen metabolism in human skin. Proc. Roy Soc. Med., 64:845.

Staubiz, W.J., Oberlkircher, O.J. and Lent, M.H., 1954, Clinical results of the treatment of prostatic carcinoma over a ten-year period. J. Urol., 72:939.

Stoliar, B., and Albert, D.J., 1974, SCH 13521 in the treatment of advanced carcinoma of the prostate. J. Urol., 111: 803.

Tolis, G., Ackman, D., Stellos, A., Mehta, A., Labrie, F., Fazekas, A.T.A., Comaru-Schally, A.M. and Schally, A.V., 1982, Tumor growth inhibition in patients with prostatic carcinoma treated with agonists of LHRH. Proc. Natl. Acad. Sci. USA, 79:1658.

Trachtenberg, J., 1983, The treatment of metastatic prostatic cancer with a potent luteinizing hormone-releasing hormone analogue. J. Urol., 129:1149.

Van der Molen, H.J., and Groen, D., 1968, Interconversion of progesterone and 20α-dihydroprogesterone and of androstenedione and testosterone in vitro by blood and erythrocytes. Acta Endocrinol., 58:419.

Whitmore, W.F. Jr., 1956, Hormone therapy in prostatic cancer. Amer. J. Med., 21:697.

POTENTIAL USE OF LHRH AND ANALOGUES: CLINICAL IMPLICATIONS

J. Sandow, K. Engelbart and W. von Rechenberg

Hoechst AG
Pharmacology H821
D-623 Frankfurt 80, Germany, F.R.

INTRODUCTION

The development of LHRH-related peptides has been very rapid since the elucidation in 1971 of the structure of LHRH (see reviews by Schally et al., 1981, Yen, 1983, Swerdloff and Heber, 1983, Sandow, 1983). Today, the established clinical role for synthetic LHRH is in stimulation of gonadal function by pulsatile activation of gonadotrophin secretion (Knobil, 1980, Leyendecker et al., 1980, Hoffman and Crowley, 1982). LHRH analogues are predominantly used for reversible suppression of gonadal steroid secretion. The therapeutic potential of agonists and antagonists of LHRH is exerted through different mechanisms of action. Agonists stimulate gonadotrophin release at low doses, when given at suitable intervals so that pituitary sensitivity can recover between stimulations. At higher doses, they suppress pituitary function when given repeatedly. Several important clinical indications are now studied based on reversible suppression of pituitary and gonadal function by agonists. The LHRH antagonists block the action of endogenous and exogenous LHRH for extended time periods, and cause reversible pituitary-gonadal involution without a stimulation phase. Antagonists are now studied in preclinical animal models, and the inhibitory activity has been confirmed in humans. The future clinical application of agonists and antagonists will depend on suitable ways of self-administration, to facilitate long-term use and patient convenience, but also on the development of sustained release formulations, to improve patient compliance and increase the efficacy of peptide absorption. Future progress in the therapeutic use of LHRH related peptides requires development of convenient biomedical devices for pulsatile administration and sustained drug delivery. In the past, studies on the physiology, pharmacology and clinical use of LHRH have revealed many surprising facts, and a better understanding of the therapeutic potential has been achieved. The major advantage of LHRH related peptides is their highly specific hormonal action, and favourable biological tolerance with absence of systemic side effects. The reversibility of pituitary-gonadal inhibition has facilitated their clinical acceptance. New pathophysiological insights have resulted from the diagnostic and therapeutic use of agonists, with a close exchange of information between experimental endocrinology, biochemical endocrinology and clinical investigation. Many new mechanisms discovered in preclinical studies, in particular the direct gonadal effects of LHRH agonists (Sharpe, 1982), still await clinical investigation of their relevance. The highly specialized requirements for hypothalamic activation of pituitary gonadotrophin secretion are now well established. The subtle interactions of ovarian and testicular functional units remain to be investigated.

PITUITARY STIMULATION

This is the clinical domaine of LHRH given by pulsatile infusion pumps. Under physiological conditions, pituitary function is sequentially activated by LHRH, at low frequency to initiate FSH secretion during puberty, and at higher frequency for subsequent LH secretion. Apparently, gonadotrophin secretion is frequency modulated by LHRH, with an additional amplitude modulation by gonadal steroids, in particular by progesterone. There are marked species differences in the role of steroids during the preovulatory LH surge. In the monkey, the variable frequency and amplitude of FSH and LH pulses observed during the menstrual cycle appears to be due to steroid conditioning in the presence of an unvarying LHRH pulsatility. Similarly, in women with secondary amenorrhoea, pulsatile infusion of LHRH with constant frequency is sufficient to support follicular development, induce ovulation and subsequently maintain luteal function. Our understanding of pulsatile pituitary activation has been greatly advanced by studies on dispersed pituitary cells suspended in suitable columns for superfusion experiments. Regular LH pulses are elicited by short-lasting LHRH exposure, and desensitization is observed after changing to a continuous LHRH infusion (Badger et al., 1983). In intact animals, desensitization is elicited by frequent LHRH stimulation (5 pulses per hour), or by continuous exposure to an infusion (Knobil, 1980). There is a threshold dose for pituitary stimulation as well as a critical frequency for consistent pituitary activation, which has been defined in women with secondary amenorrhoea, and in men with idiopathic hypogonadotropic hypogonadism (Hoffman and Crowley, 1982). The shape of the LHRH stimulus is of relevance. In some patients, subcutaneous pulsatile stimulation is less effective than intravenous stimulation with the same dose. It is likely that such differences are related to the higher peak concentrations reached immediately after an intravenous pulse.

Pituitary stimulation by pulsatile LHRH will be the method of choice in a variety of clinical conditions, where the cause for pituitary involution or transient dysfunction is related to a hypothalamic deficiency. The use of pulsatile infusion pumps is mandatory to ensure consistent stimulation over weeks and months.

PITUITARY DESENSITIZATION

In the presence of LHRH antagonists, the pituitary LHRH receptors are unresponsive to endogenous LHRH pulses, or to test injections of LHRH. This is due to receptor occupancy, and the receptors regain responsiveness once the antagonist is degraded, or dissociates from the receptor. The process initiated by LHRH agonists is more complex. The LH release after a single physiological LHRH pulse is short-lived, whereas an agonist pulse elicits a similar LH increase but with more prolonged duration (Yeo et al., 1981). Repeated agonist pulses result in diminishing LH release with transient unresponsiveness to LHRH stimulation. Desensitization is a post-receptor event not associated with an immediate change of LHRH receptors. When supraphysiological doses of LHRH or an agonist, eliciting a near-maximal LH stimulation are injected once daily or repeatedly in rats, there is a gradual decrease in basal LH release, reduced responsiveness to test injections of LHRH, and a depletion of pituitary gonadotrophin content. Continuous exposure to a stimulatory concentration of LHRH also reduces pituitary responsiveness, by a direct inhibitory effect on the pituitary in the absence of gonadal steroids. This inhibition of responsiveness is maintained for extended time periods by infusion of LHRH or agonists. It is associated with gradual decrease in LHRH receptors to low levels, and with a marked depletion of gonadotrophins (Clayton, 1982, Sandow, 1982). The therapeutic implications are obvious. LHRH agonists rapidly induce pituitary refractoriness when administered subcutaneously from suitable pumps, or by sustained release from implant materials (Clayton, 1982, Vickery, 1981, Bint Akhtar et al., 1983). Agonists act via an initial stimulation phase, which is absent with antagonists. During the second phase of desensitization, agonists and antagonists have similar effects although operating through entirely different mechanisms. LH and FSH secretion decline to a basal rate, and profound gonadotrophin depletion of the pituitary confirms inhibition of de novo synthesis. This inhibition may be a consequence of neutralizing the trophic effect of endogenous LHRH stimulation. Pituitary inhibition by continuous agonist stimulation has been compared to a "chemical hypophysectomy". The important difference to hypophysectomy is reversibility, and preservation of a basal secretion rate of FSH and LH, even though the pituitary becomes refractory to endogenous LHRH stimulation.

INHIBITION OF GONADAL FUNCTION

The pituitary process initiated by supraphysiological agonist stimulation is enhanced by a marked effect of near-maximal LH release on gonadotrophin receptors. The regulatory event is due to excessive LH stimulation, and can be mimicked by injections of LH or hCG. The decrease in gonadotrophin receptors is associated with a deficiency in biosynthesis of gonadal steroids (steroidogenic lesion). There are characteristic qualitative changes in androgen biosynthesis, the secretion of active androgen is reduced and C-21 androgen precursors of low androgenic activity are secreted in increased amounts. The net effect of reduced gonadotrophin receptors plus deficient biosynthesis is a decrease in the secretion of androgenic gonadal steroids, which has been compared to a "chemical castration", characterized by post-gonadectomy levels. The two combined processes, pituitary gonadotrophin inhibition and gonadal steroid decrease depend on the dose of agonist administered, on the type of the stimulus (daily injections or continuous infusion), and on the duration of treatment. There are marked species differences in the extent of gonadal steroid suppression, as well as sex differences. In the following sections, the preclinical basis for the contraceptive use of LHRH agonists, and clinical conditions requiring a block of gonadal steroid secretion will be discussed, with particular reference to parameters which can be derived from the preclinical analysis in animal species.

CLINICAL USE OF LHRH AGONISTS

In general, there are two groups of indications which require different regimens. A low dose range is effective for incomplete suppression of pituitary function (as in female contraception), and high doses are necessary for maximal suppression (as in precocious puberty, endometriosis and hormone-dependent tumours). Our own studies have been performed with the highly active agonist, 6-D-Ser(But)-LHRH(1-9)-nonapeptide-ethylamide (buserelin, Hoe 766). The effective doses found in clinical studies are similar to the effective doses for other LHRH(1-9)-nonapeptide-ethylamide agonists of related structure, and for LHRH(1-10)-decapeptide agonists substituted in 6-glycin with particular D-aminoacids.

FEMALE CONTRACEPTION

Many different protocols have been tested, based on preclinical observations of inhibition of fertility (Sandow et al., 1982). Attempts to modify follicular function by inducing an FSH deficit during the early follicular phase, resulting in luteal insufficiency (Skarin et al., 1982) were not successful. This approach depends on FSH suppression at a critical early stage of follicular development, and requires close monitoring of the menstrual cycle. If an agonist is administered throughout the follicular phase of the menstrual cycle, follicular maturation and ovulation are suspended. However, immediately after treatment, a normal menstrual cycle will start with ovulation at an appropriate time, and a normal luteal phase. This indicates that pituitary suppression requires daily agonist administration throughout the entire cycle. Once treatment is stopped, pituitary function recovers within 3-4 days. The luteolytic approach, as indicated by the marked post-coital contraceptive effects of agonists in rats and rabbits has been investigated extensively in the human. After high dose treatment, there is a slight reduction in luteal progesterone secretion, but the luteolytic activity is not of practical importance, because the corpus luteum is protected by hCG, as soon as pregnancy is established. High doses of agonists can terminate pregnancy in animals, but there is no abortifacient effect in the human during early pregnancy. Attempts to disrupt the menstrual cycle at an arbitrary time have failed. Primate studies have confirmed the efficacy, reversibility, and safety of a long-term contraceptive approach based on daily treatment (Fraser et al., 1981, Fraser, 1983). In women, a reliable contraceptive effect is achieved by an agonist administered daily from the first day of the follicular phase on. This method relies on menstrual bleeding as the starting point for the contraceptive regimen. Daily administration is facilitated by the use of a nasal spray delivering 400-600 ug buserelin/day (Bergquist et al., 1982a, Schmidt-Gollwitzer et al., 1981), but daily injections are equally effective (Baumann et al., 1980). There is a wide range of individual reactions in oestradiol secretion and endometrial proliferation to the continuous contraceptive regimen (one or two daily administrations). All endometrial changes are within the range found during a normal menstrual cycle, they may range from involution to incipient hyperplasia (Schmidt-Gollwitzer et al., 1981). There is no diagnostic procedure to predict the individual response.

In view of the absence of luteal progesterone increases, a discontinuous contraceptive regimen has been investigated (Hardt et al., 1982). During the first and second week, ovulation is inhibited by daily administration of a peptide nasal spray for 21 days. During the third week, an orally active progestagene is added for 3-7 days to obtain secretory transformation of the endometrium. This regimen with sequential progestagen administration results in a predictable bleeding pattern. Absence of bleeding after the progestagen may be a symptom of oestrogen suppression, or of contraceptive failure, and a pregnancy test should be performed to re-assure the patient.

MALE CONTRACEPTION

Prospects for a male contraceptive method based on agonist suppression plus androgen substitution are difficult to evaluate. Testosterone secretion is reduced in normal men (Bergquist et al., 1979), and also in prostate carcinoma (Borgmann et al., 1982) by daily agonist injections. The androgen deficit leads to reduced libido, and inhibition of spermatogenesis. In a male contraceptive method, the primary target would be to suppress FSH secretion, and disrupt spermatogenesis. In rhesus monkeys, a regimen based on sequential induction of azoospermia followed by testosterone substitution was found to be highly effective (Bint Akhtar et al., 1983). Constant infusion of buserelin 48 µg/day for 20 weeks induced azoospermia within 10 weeks, associated with a decrease in testicular volume. After testosterone substitution from silastic implants, the ejaculatory behaviour was re-established, while azoospermia persisted. Inhibition of spermatogenesis was reversible within 6 weeks after treatment. The crucial question remains, whether testosterone substitution will reinitiate spermatogenesis in men even in the presence of low FSH levels (Bremner et al., 1981).

PRECOCIOUS PUBERTY

In experimental animals, sexual maturation is reversibly inhibited by LHRH agonists. The physiological role of endogenous hypothalamic activity has been firmly established by induction of puberty by LHRH in sexually immature monkeys, by the increase in urinary LHRH excretion found in children at puberty, and by spontaneous onset of FSH and LH secretion in children with gonadal dysgenesis at the appropriate age for puberty. Precocious puberty is an indication for high dose treatment with agonists. Clinical experience with daily injections of 6-Trp-LHRH(1-9)nonapeptide-ethylamide 4-8 µg/kg s.c. is encouraging. More frequent administration of smaller doses, e.g. by nasal spray 3 x 400 µg buserelin may be effective as a maintenance therapy. The long-term effects on fertility of children with precocious puberty treated with agonists are not known. Preclinical safety studies indicate no impairment of fertility in prepubertal animals suppressed with agonist injection for extended time periods. In precocious puberty, agonists may be of significant advantage because of good biological tolerance and absence of biological side effects. Sexual maturation is inhibited reversibly (Comite et al., 1981). The secretion of gonadal steroids is blocked to prevent premature closure of the epiphyses, and the growth velocity is decelerated. Treatment also improves psychosocial adjustment of these children to their age group. Uninterrupted treatment is required until the appropriate age for puberty.

ENDOMETRIOSIS

The characteristic symptoms of endometriosis are related to bleeding from dystopic endometrium, and can be controlled by pituitary suppression with progestagenic or androgenic synthetic steroids (cyproterone acetate, danazol). The treatment is effective, if it causes amenorrhoea, and the therapeutic effect is always associated with symptoms of a pseudomenopause state (hot flushes), and symptoms of oestrogen deficiency. Agonists have to be injected at high doses to suppress oestradiol secretion sufficiently to prevent endometrial proliferation. It is desirable to shorten the initial phase of pituitary stimulation (associated with an oestradiol increase) by high dose therapy (e.g. by injections of 3 x 1 mg s.c. daily for 3-7 days), followed by maintenance injections or nasal spray administered in 4-5 divided daily doses. Frequent pituitary stimulation is more effective to maintain desensitization, and sustained release formulations or constant rate infusions by suitable small infusion pumps should be investigated. The clinical efficacy of agonist suppression in endometriosis has been confirmed (Lemay and Quesnel, 1982, Meldrum et al., 1982). Injection of 100 µg 6-D-Trp-LH-RH-ethylamide once daily s.c. for 28 days lowered plasma oestradiol to an extent causing endometrial involution. Implants releasing the peptide over prolonged periods of time are suitable, but their pharmaceutical development is not sufficiently advanced for clinical studies. In polycystic ovarian disease (PCO), the elevated secretion of serum androgens of ovarian origin can be suppressed selectively by daily injection of 6-D-Trp-LHRH-ethylamide 100 µg s.c. for 28 days. This treatment does not alter the secretion of adrenal steroids either in normal women or in women with polycystic ovarian disease (Chang et al., 1983).

The increased secretion of gonadotrophins during the menopause is not causally related to the hot flushes, and agonist suppression is ineffective in this indication (Casper and Yen, 1981). Hot flushes are reported after hypophysectomy, after agonist suppression of oestradiol secretion in endometriosis, and in premature ovarian failure. Normal men and prostate cancer patients also experience hot flushes after androgen suppression by agonist treatment.

HORMONE-DEPENDENT TUMOURS

Agonist treatment is effective to suppress androgen or oestrogen secretion in experimental tumour models in animals (Redding and Schally, 1981, Corbin, 1982), provided that sufficiently high doses are administered. In clinical oncology, the beneficial effect of castration in hormone-sensitive prostate cancer is well documented. A pharmacological block of testosterone production can be achieved by high dose agonist injections, followed by lower maintenance doses given by nasal spray administration, or by sustained release formulations. This treatment is effective in metastatic prostate cancer (Tolis et al., 1982, Borgmann et al., 1982, Waxman et al., 1983). The stimulatory effect of the residual non-suppressible adrenal androgens on the primary tumour, and metastases of hormone-sensitive prostate cancer can further be reduced by androgen receptor blockers (antiandrogens) like cyproterone acetate, flutamide or RU 23,908 (Labrie et al., 1982).

A similar protocol for pituitary-ovarian suppression may be useful in the treatment of hormone-dependent breast cancer. The therapeutic aim is to reduce oestradiol secretion to levels found after ovariectomy. Preliminary clinical experience (Klijn et al., 1982) confirms the therapeutic principle, and dual suppression by combining LHRH agonists and antioestrogens may be most effective (Furr and Nicholson, 1982).

CONCLUSIONS

LHRH and its agonist analogues have a stimulatory and/or inhibitory action on gonadotrophin release and gonadal steroid secretion which can be adjusted by appropriate selection of the pharmacological stimulus. Pulsatile stimulation with LHRH is the therapy of choice in the presence of a functional pituitary gland, and hypothalamic deficiency. The suppression of gonadal steroid secretion by daily supraphysiological stimulation or continuous infusion/sustained release is effective with highly active LHRH agonists, and has been successfully explored in several clinical indications requiring transient or permanent reduction of gonadal steroid levels. In female contraception, ovulation is inhibited by daily administration of an agonist nasal spray, either alone or together with a progestagen to obtain a regular bleeding pattern. In male contraception, inhibition of spermatogenesis with simultaneous androgen substitution is difficult to achieve, but may be reached if a transitory phase of androgen deficiency is accepted. It depends on the selection of the stimulus (continuous infusion vs. daily injection), whether a state of "chemical hypophysectomy" or "chemical gonadectomy" is attained. During continuous stimulation, a basal rate of gonadotrophin secretion remains intact, in contrast to surgical hypophysectomy. Protocols of daily agonist injection have been investigated successfully in precocious puberty, endometriosis, and hormone-dependent tumours (prostate and mammary carcinoma). The clinical investigation of sustained release preparations for peptides opens new fields of research. Future physiological and pharmacological studies with LHRH agonists and antagonists will significantly enlarge our therapeutic options for clinical conditions requiring reversible or permanent suppression of gonadal steroid secretion.

REFERENCES

Badger, T.M., Loughlin, J.S. & Naddaff, P.G. (1983): The luteinizing hormone-releasing hormone (LHRH)-desensitized rat pituitary: luteinizing hormone responsiveness to LHRH in vitro. Endocrinology 112:793-799

Baumann, R., Kuhl, H., Taubert, H.D. & Sandow, J. (1980): Ovulation inhibition by daily i.m. administration of a highly active LHRH analog (D-Ser(TBU)^6-LHRH(1-9)nonapeptide-ethylamide). Contraception 21:191-197

Bergquist, C., Nillius, S.J., Bergh, T., Skarin, G. & Wide, L. (1979): Inhibitory effects on gonadotropin secretion and gonadal function in men during chronic treatment with a potent stimulatory luteinizing hormone-releasing hormone analogue. Acta Endocrinol. (Kbh.) 91:601-608

Bergquist, C., Nillius, S.J. & Wide, L. (1982): Intranasal LHRH agonist treatment for inhibition of ovulation in women: clinical aspects. Clin. Endocrinol. 17:91-98

Bint Akhtar, F., Marshall, G.R., Wickings, E.J. & Nieschlag, E. (1983): Reversible induction of azoospermia in rhesus monkeys by constant infusion of a gonadotropin-releasing hormone agonist using osmotic minipumps. J. Clin. Endocrinol. Metab. 56:534-540

Borgmann, V., Hardt, W., Schmidt-Gollwitzer, M., Adenauer, H. & Nagel, R. (1982): Sustained suppression of testosterone production by the luteinizing-hormone releasing-hormone agonist buserelin in patients with advanced prostate carcinoma. A new therapeutic approach? Lancet (May 82):1097- 1099

Bremner, W.J., Matsumoto, A.M., Sussman, A.M. & Paulsen, C.A. (1981): Follicle-stimulating hormone and human spermatogenesis. J. Clin. Invest. 68:1044-1052

Casper, R.F. & Yen, S.S.C. (1981): Menopausal flushes: effect of pituitary gonadotropin desensitization by a potent luteinizing hormone-releasing factor agonist. J. Clin. Endocrinol. Metab. 53:1056-1058

Chang, R.J., Laufer, L.R., Meldrum, D.R., DeFazio, J., Lu, J.K.H., Vale, W.W., Rivier, J.E. & Judd, H.L. (1983): Steroid secretion in polycystic ovarian disease after ovarian suppression by a long-acting gonadotropin-releasing hormone agonist. J. Clin. Endocrinol. Metab. 56:897-903

Clayton, R.N. (1982): GnRH modulation of its own pituitary receptors: evidence for biphasic regulation. Endocrinology 111: 152-161

Comite, F., Cutler Jr., G.B., Rivier, J., Vale, W.W., Loriaux, D.L. & Crowley Jr., W.F. (1981): Short-term treatment of idiopathic precocious puberty with a long-acting analogue of LHRH. New Engl. J. Med. 305:1546-1550

Corbin, A. (1982): From contraception to cancer: a review of the therapeutic applications of LHRH analogues as antitumor agents. Yale J. Biol. Med. 55:27-47

Fraser, H.M. (1983): Effect of treatment for one year with a luteinizing hormone-releasing hormone agonist on ovarian, thyroidal, and adrenal function and menstruation in the stumptailed monkey (macaca arctoides). Endocrinology 112: 245-253

Fraser, H.M., Laird, N.C. & Blakely, D.M. (1980): Decreased pituitary responsiveness and inhibition of the luteinizing hormone surge and ovulation in the stumptailed monkey (macaca arctoides) by chronic treatment with an agonist of luteinizing hormone-releasing hormone. Endocrinology 106: 452-457

Furr, B.J.A. & Nicholson, R.I. (1982): Use of analogues of LHRH for the treatment of cancer. J. Reprod. Fertil. 64:529-539

Hardt, W., Schmidt-Gollwitzer, K., Nevinny-Stickel, J. & Schmidt-Gollwitzer, M. (1982): Fortschritte in der kontrazeptiven Anwendung des LHRH-Agonisten Buserelin: diskontinuierliche Medikation mit gestageninduzierter Abbruchblutung. Geburtshilfe Frauenheilkd. 42:874-877

Hoffman, A.R. & Crowley, W.F. (1982): Induction of puberty in men by long-term pulsatile administration of low-dose gonadotropin-releasing hormone. New Engl. J. Med. 307:1237-1241

Klijn, J.G.M. & de Jong, F.H. (1982): Treatment with a luteinizing-hormone-releasing-hormone analogue (buserelin) in premenopausal patients with metastatic breast cancer. Lancet (May 1982):1213-1216

Knobil, E. (1980): The neuroendocrine control of the menstrual cycle. Recent Prog. Horm. Res. 36:53-88

Labrie, F., Dupont, A., Bélanger, A., Cusan, L., Lacourcière, Y., Monfette, G., Laberge, J.G., Emond, J.P., Fazekas, A.T.A., Raynaud, J.P. & Husson, J.M. (1982): New hormonal therapy in prostatic carcinoma: combined treatment with an LHRH agonist and an antiandrogen. J. Clin. Invest. Med. 5:267-275

Lemay, A. & Quesnel, G. (1982): Potential new treatment of endometriosis - reversible inhibition of pituitary-ovarian function by chronic intranasal administration of a LHRH agonist. Fertil. Steril. 38:376-377

Leyendecker, G., Wildt, L. & Hansmann, M. (1980): Pregnancies following chronic intermittent (pulsatile) administration of GnRH by means of a portable pump (Zyklomat). A new approach in the treatment of infertility in hypothalamic amenorrhea. J. Clin. Endocrinol. Metab. 51:1214-1216

Meldrum, D.R., Chang, R.J., Lu, J., Vale, W., Rivier, J. & Judd, H.L. (1982): "Medical oophorectomy" using a long-acting GnRH agonist - a possible new approach to the treatment of endometriosis. J. Clin. Endocrinol. Metab. 54:1081-1083

Redding, T.W. & Schally, A.V. (1981): Inhibition of prostate tumor growth in two rat models by chronic administration of $D-Trp^6$ analogue of luteinizing hormone-releasing hormone. Proc. Natl. Acad. Sci. USA 78:6509-6512

Sandow, J. (1982): Inhibition of pituitary and testicular function by LHRH analogues. In: Progress towards a male contraceptive (eds. S.L. Jeffcoate & M. Sandler), John Wiley & Sons Ltd., London, pp. 19-39

Sandow, J. (1983): Clinical applications of LHRH and its analogues. Clin. Endocrinol. 18:571-592

Sandow, J., Kuhl, H., Jerzabek, G., Kille, S. & Rechenberg, W.v. (1982): The reproductive pharmacology and contraceptive application of LHRH and its analogues. In: The Gonadotropins: Basic Science and Clinical Aspects in Females (eds. C. Flamigni & J.R. Givens), Academic Press, London, pp. 77-105

Schally, A.V., Arimura, A. & Coy, D.H. (1981): Recent approaches to fertility control based on derivates of LHRH. Vitam. Horm. 38:257-310

Schmidt-Gollwitzer, M., Hardt, W., Schmidt-Gollwitzer, K. & Nevinny-Stickel, J. (1981): Influence of the LHRH analogue buserelin on cyclic ovarian function and on endometrium. A new approach to fertility control? Contraception 23:187-196

Sharpe, R.M. (1982): Cellular aspects of the inhibitory actions of LHRH on the ovary and testis. J. Reprod. Fertil. 64:517-527

Skarin, G., Nillius, S.J. & Wide, L. (1982): Early follicular phase luteinizing hormone-releasing hormone agonist administration - effects on follicular maturation and corpus luteum function in women. Contraception 25:31-39

Swerdloff, R.S. & Heber, D. (1983): Superactive gondotropin-releasing hormone agonists. Ann. Rev. Med. 34:491-500

Tolis, G., Ackman, D., Apostolos, S., Metha, A., Labrie, F., Fazekas, A.T.A., Comaru-Schally, A.M. & Schally, A.V. (1982): Tumor growth inhibition in patients with prostatic carcinoma treated with luteinizing hormone-releasing hormone agonist. Proc. Natl. Acad. Sci. USA 79:1658-1662

Vickery, B.H. (1981): Physiology and antifertility effects of LHRH and agonistic analogs in male animals. In: LHRH peptides as female and male contraceptives (eds. G.I. Zatuchni,

J.D. Shelton & J.J. Sciarra), Harper & Row, Philadelphia, pp. 275-290

Waxman, J.H., Wass, J.A.H., Hendry, W.F., Whitfield, H.N., Besser, G.M., Malpas, J.S. & Oliver, R.T.D. (1983): Treatment with gonadotrophin releasing hormone analogue in advanced prostatic cancer. Br. Med. J. 286:1309-1312

Yeo, T., Grossman, A., Belchetz, P. & Besser, G.M. (1981): Response of LH from colums of dispersed rat pituitary cells to a highly potent analogue of LHRH. J. Endocrinol. 91:33-41

Yen, S.S.C. (1983): Clinical applications of gonadotropin-releasing hormone and gonadotropin-releasing hormone analogs. Fertil. Steril. 39:257-266

APPLICATION OF GnRH FOR INDUCTION OF OVULATION IN ANOVULATORY MENSTRUATING WOMEN

Vaclav Insler, Gershon Hochberg, Joseph Levy,
Gad Potashnik and David Goldstein

Division of Obstetrics and Gynecology
Soroka Medical Center and
Ben-Gurion University of the Negev
Beer-Sheba, Israel

The presence of LH-releasing activity in hypothalamic extracts was reported by McCann and co-workers in 1960. Shortly afterwards Campbell et al.(1964) showed that similar extracts, when injected into the pituitary gland were capable of inducing ovulation. In less than 10 years Luteinizing Hormone Releasing Hormon (LHRH or GnRH) was purified, its amino-acid sequence was identified and confirmed by synthesis (Matsuo et al., 1971).This opened new exciting avenues for important physiological studies and for the development of antisera which could be used as a basis for devising radioimmunoassays of GnRH and for precise localization of the peptide by immunocytochemistry. Synthesis of large quantities of GnRH enabled large-scale clinical studies which, in turn, produced important information on the role of this hormone in the reproductive process. Synthesis of new GnRH analogs, both agonistic and antagonistic (Schally et al.,1981) further expanded the application of this hormone for clinical and research purposes.

Three characteristics of the mode of action of GnRH were soon discovered and shown to be of utmost importance for further studies and developments:

a) For stimulating gonadotropin secretion capable of inducing full follicular maturation and ovulation, GnRH must be applied in a pulsatile manner (Knobil, 1980; Leyendecker et al., 1980).
b) GnRH action upon the pituitary gland is mediated and/or modified by natural and synthetic sex steroids (Insler and Lunenfeld, 1983; Genazzani et al., 1978).
c) Continuous administration of GnRH or its analogs causes "down regulation" of gonadotropin secretion eventually leading to a reversible medical castration (Rivier et.al.,1978; Berquist

et al., 1979;Meldrum et al., 1982).
The first two characteristics are the cornerstones of ovulation inducing therapy using GnRH. Recently, the intermittent(pulsatile) therapy has become the prevailing form of GnRH application for stimulation of the pituitary_gonadal axis. The mediating role of sex steroids is of importance in planning prolonged GnRH therapy designed to induce several consecutive ovulations,in avoiding ovarian hyperstimulation and in combined therapy using clomiphene, epimestrol or other steroid-like compounds together with GnRH (Maia et al., 1980).
The "down regulation" of pituitary-gonadal response following prolonged application of GnRH or its analogs serves as a basis for designing treatments aimed at reduction of undesirable gonadal activity in precocious puberty (Growley et al., 1980), endometriosis (Meldrum et al., 1982) or hormone-dependent cancer (Faure et al., 1982; Borgmann et al., 1982) as well as for developing contraception agents (Nillius et al., 1978; Sheehan et al., 1982).
The main clinical applications of GnRH and its analogs are listed in Table 1.

Table 1. Clinical Application of GnRH and its Analogs

Diagnosis and classification of infertility	
	Anovulatory females
	Azoospermic males
Stimulation of Pituitary-Gonadal Function	
	Induction of ovulation
	Induction of spermatogenesis
	Delayed puberty
	Cryptorchidism
Inhibition of Pituitary-Gonadal Function	
	Precocious puberty
	Endometriosis
	Hormone dependent tumors (breast, prostatic)
Contraception	
	Inhibition of ovulation
	Interference with corpus luteum function
	Inhibition of spermatogenesis
	Interference with development of early pregnancy.

This article is going to discuss only the application of GnRH in diagnosis and treatment of infertility.

The GnRH Test

The idea that a short-term GnRH stimulation test may help to diagnose and classify anovulatory and/or amenorrheic women and azoospermic men into different functional cathegories was put forward shortly after the synthetic hormone has become available. It has been sized upon by numerous investigators and generated a great number of publications (Table 2).

Table 2. Clinical Value of GnRH Test

Author & year	No. of patients	Dose (μg) & route	Diagnost. value	Prognost. value
Bergh et al. (1978)	287	100 i.v.	no	no
Keller (1973)	31	12.5 i.v.	?	yes
Aono et al. (1974)	80	100 i.v.	yes	not examined
Insler et al. (1974)	10	500 i.v.	?	no
Shaw (1979)	134	100 i.v.	?	no
Feore & Taymor (1976)	31	10 i.v.	not exam.	yes
Soules et al. (1979)	130	100 s.c.	?	not examined

The initial enthusiasm for the GnRH test faded when it became clear that the majority of amenorrheic women and azoospermic men did respond to GnRH stimulation regardless of the type of functional disturbance leading to amenorrhea (or azoospermia) and infertility. Moreover, it has also been pointed out that in some patients the short-term GnRH stimulation may not result in an appreciable pituitary response while repeated application of the hormone may do so (Insler & Lunenfeld, 1983). Also, as shown by Meidan et al., (1982) on isolated pituitary cells of the rat, lack of estrogen results in a significantly reduced response to GnRH stimulation probably due to the decrease in the number of GnRH binding sites. Thus, the endogenous estrogen production (or lack of it) may influence the results of the GnRH test and mask the true responsive capability of the pituitary. It seems, at present, that the GnRH stimulation test is of some clinical value in ascertaining the completeness of hypophysectomy (Insler & Lunenfeld, 1983), in pinpointing a very specific group of normogonadotropic azoospermic men that are likely to respond to gonadotropin therapy (Lunenfeld & Glezerman, 1981) and possibly in predicting the dose requirement of GnRH in amenorrheic women about to receive this therapy (Leyendecker et al.,1981).

Induction of Ovulation

Anovulation is the main cause of infertility in up to 49% of infertile couples (Insler et al., 1981). During the last 25 years a whole series of ovulation inducting agents such as clomiphene citrate, tamoxifen, epimestrol, ergoline derivatives and gonadotropin preparations have been made available for clinical use. Because their target organs and mode of action are different, each of these agents is particularly effective in a specific group of patients. For this reason a treatment - oriented classification of anovulatory states was proposed in 1968 (Insler et al., 1968) and later modified and adopted by the WHO Scientific Group (1973). Development of proper dosage schemes and monitoring protocols made the ovulation inducing therapy reasonably efficient and safe. However, wide scale clinical use of the above fertility promoting drugs soon revealed that, even with the best planned and executed therapy, the conception rates rarely exceed 75% and in some groups of patients remain dismally low (11-25%) leaving a sizable proportion of anovulatory women uncured (Insler & Lunenfeld, 1983).Thus, the commercial availability of GnRH raised new hopes for patients with treatment resistant anovulation. At first, GnRH has been used, alone or in combination with other agents in the traditional manner of 1-3 injections per-day (Kastin et al., 1971; Keller, 1972; Nillius et al.,1981; Henderson et al., 1976; London, 1973; Phansey et al., 1980). It has soon become evident that conception rates achieved with this type of treatment were unacceptably low. Indeed, Hammond and his co-workers(1979) in a well controlled study using placebo and 2 or 3 daily doses of GnRH in treatment cycles of 28 days duration, showed that GnRH therapy resulted in 2 conceptions out of 33 cycles as compared to one pregnancy out of 30 placebo cycles. It is of interest to note that 3 additional women conceived during the 6 months post-treatment observation period. The introduction of intermittent(pulsatile) mode of treatment resulted in a significant improvement of conception rates(Table 3). It was initially postulated that, due to ovarian control of the pituitary response, induction of ovulation with GnRH should be free of complications such as ovarian hyperstimulation and multiple pregnancies. These high hopes were not entirely fulfilled and the occurence of both complications has already been reported(Bogchelman et al.,1982; Yen, 1983). It seems, nevertheless, that in comparison to hMG/hCG therapy, induction of ovulation with GnRH may indeed be safer although not yet as efficient as gonadotropin therapy.

Table 3. Induction of Ovulation with Pulsatile Application of GnRH

Author & Year	Dose µg/pulse	Pulse frequency (min)	Route	No.of cycles	No.of ovulat.	No.of pregn.
Bogchelman et al.(1982)	15 - 20	90	i.v.	1	1	1
Crowley & McArthur (1980)	1.75	120	s.c.	1	1	0*
Keogh et al. (1981)	3.41	62	s.c.	1	1	1
Leyendecker et al.(1980)	2.5-20	90	i.v.	26	26	6
Miller et al. (1983)	1 - 5	96 -120	i.v.	23	20	7
Reid et al. (1981)	0.5- 5	90 -120	s.c.	2	2	2
Schoemaker et al.(1981)	10- 20	90 - 120	i.v.	3	3	1
Seibel et al. (1983)	12- 20	120	s.c.	3	3	1
Skarin et al. (1982)	20	90	s.c.	12	12	1**
Valk et al. (1981)	1.75	120	i.v.	1	0	0
Insler et al. (1983)	20	90	i.v.	8	5	1

* Kallman's Syndrome ; ** Only 4 of 7 women treated were infertile

Up till now GnRH therapy has been applied for induction of ovulation mainly in amenorrheic women with low endogenous estrogens and low-normal gonadotropin levels (Group I according to the WHO classification). In these patients hMG/hCG therapy is also very efficient resulting in conception rates of 50-80%. However, the bulk of infertile patients requiring induction of ovulation consists of spontaneo bleeders rather than amenorrheic women(Bettendorf et al., 1981; Lunenfeld et al., 1981)(WHO Group IIa)and in this group ovulation inducing therapy has proven to be less successful with pregnancy rates in the range of 20-40%. Thus, special effort should be invested to device new efficient means of treatment for this group of anovulatory women. That was the main reason why our group decided to try pulsatile GnRH treatment in this particular cathegory of infertile women.
8 patients gave informed consent to participate in this study. Their relevant clinical characteristics are listed in Table 4.

Table 4. Clinical Characteristics of Patients

Patient	Age (Years)	Type and duration of infert.	Clinical diagnosis	Additional fertility disturbances
B.R.	27	I - 2 y.	LPD	none
E.Z.	29	II - 6 y.	LPD	OTA
N.M.	34	II - 6 y.	LPD	OTA
G.I.	35	II - 7 y.	LPD	none
P.S.	29	I - 3 y.	LPD	none
L.Z.	31	I - 6 y.	Oligomen. Anovulat.	none
A.M.	30	II - 3 y.	Oligomen. Anovulat.	none
C.Sh.	25	I - 7 y.	Oligomen. Anovulat.	OTA

LPD = luteal phase deficiency

OTA = oligo-terato-astheno-spermia

The diagnosis of anovulation or luteal phase deficiency was established on the basis of basal body temperature (BBT) records, cervical mucus examinations and 2 plasma progesterone assays. In some patients

premenstrual endometrial biopsy was also carried out. The diagnosis was accepted when 2 consecutive cycles or the majority of several cycles showed the same disturbance. Within 3 months prior to this study the women did not receive any hormonal therapy.
GnRH was administered through an indwelling i.v. catheter using a computerized pump (generously supplied by Ferring, West Germany) that delivered pulses of 20 µg of the hormone every 90 min. The application of GnRH started on the 4th or 5th menstrual day and continued for 3 days after presumed ovulation, when 10,000 IU of hCG were injected daily for 3 consecutive days in order to sustain the corpus luteum. If ovulation failed to occur within 21 days of GnRH therapy, the treatment was discontinued. Patients were examined every 2 to 3 days throughout the treatment cycles. On each examination the ovaries were palpated, the cervical mucus was evaluated and the evaluation was expressed as a cervical score using a scale of 0 to 12 points (Insler et al.,1972), blood was drawn for FSH,LH, prolactin, 17β - estradiol and progesterone assays and the women were questioned about any possible side effects. Plasma FSH, LH and prolactin were assayed using commercial radioimmunoassay kits supplied by Diagnostic Product Corporation of California, U.S.A. For radioimmunoassay of progesterone and 17β - estradiol antibodies from Radioassay Systems Laboratory (California, U.S.A) and radioactive steroids from Amersham (England) were used. Plasma was extracted prior to the steroid assays. In all hormone measurements the intra-assay and inter-assay coefficient of variation did not exceed 4.1% and 9.2% respectively.The results of treatment are summarized in Table 5 and the course of therapy in the patient that conceived is presented in Fig.1.

The duration of GnRH therapy was 6 to 14 days. No side-effects were observed. One patient conceived. In the remaining 7 women; the duration of cycle was between 26 and 31 days in 5 patients, one woman had a long cycle of 35 days and in one the bleeding appeared after 25 days. Three patients had a short thermal shift (8, 8 and 9 days respectively). An unequivocal FSH rise was observed in 4 cycles and in 4 others it was either questionable or absent. An LH peak could be detected in 7 of the 8 cycles. A distinct estradiol peak, however, was seen in only 3 cycles. In the remaining 5 women the estradiol peak was either absent or missed. Progesterone levels were compatible with ovulation in 5 cycles and low (less than 10ng/ml) in 3 others. The clinical results of treatment of anovulation in these 8 anovulatory patients could thus be summarized as follows: one patient conceived, 3 had a probably normal ovulatory cycle, one had an ovulatory cycle with luteal phase deficiency and in three women GnRH therapy failed to induce ovulation. An ovulation rate of 50% is rather low, as compared to that obtained in amenorrheic patients (see Table 3).

Table 5. Results of GnRH Therapy in Infertile Spontaneously Menstruating Women

Pat- ient	Duration of GnRH therapy (days)	Cycle length (days)	Sust- ained high temper. (days)	FSH rise	LH peak*	E_2 peak*	Prog- ester- one
B.R.	14	31	15	yes	yes	?	high**
A.Z.	10	28	12	yes	yes	?	high**
N.M.	9	25	8	yes	yes	?	high**
G.I.	12	27	13	?	yes	yes	high**
P.S.	10	PREGNANCY		?	yes	yes	high**
L.Z.	6	35	9	no	yes	?	low
A.M.	14	26	14	no	no	yes	low
C.SH	12	28	8	yes	yes	yes	low

* one value exceeding by 100% the mean of all othe examinations

** at least 2 values exceeding 10 ng/ml

The significant difference of the efficacy of ovulation inducing therapy in patients of Group I as compared to women of Group II (WHO classification) may be explained as follows:

In women with negligible endogenous gonadotropin activity(Group I), at the beginning of each treatment cycle the ovaries are at a quiescent state with all follicles atat early stage of development as evidenced by the very low endogenous estrogen production. Pulsatile application of GnRH or administration of hMG supply gonadotropin stimulation of a magnitude and duration adequate for the recruitment of a population of follicles and sufficient for the maturation of some of them as well as the progession of at least one follicle until the preovulatory stage. In these cases, ovulation inducing treatment is essentially a straightforward replacement therapy providing the specific hormone which the patient is unable to produce.

In contrast, women of Group II although not ovulating, do have some endogenous gonadotropic activity albeit inadequate or ill-timed. Their ovaries are capable of spontaneous follicular maturation although rarely, if ever, reaching the ovulation stage. It has been postulated that in a spontaneously menstruating woman, the recruitment of follicles destined to mature and possibly ovulate during a particular cycle begins in the luteal phase of the preceding cycle.

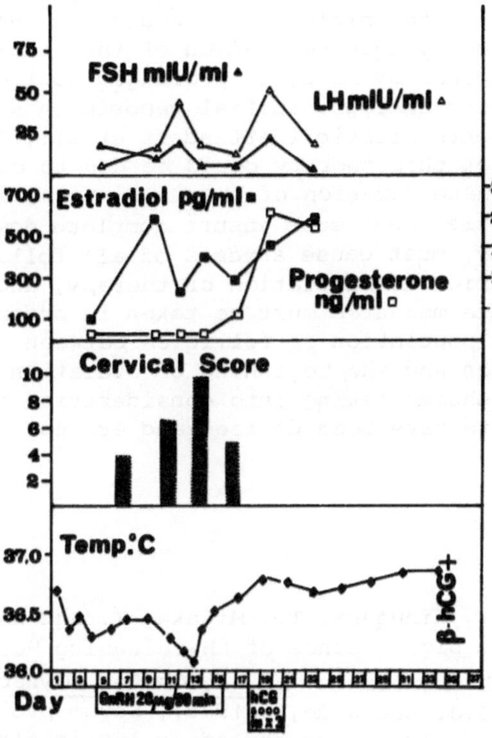

Fig. 1

The course of GnRH therapy in a patient P.S. with luteal phase deficiency.

Ovulation inducing therapy initiated a few days following menstruation acts upon ovaries containing a number of follicles that have already begun their maturation process, but the precise stage of their development is not known. Thus, in these women, the course of treatment is difficult to predict, the control of therapy is complicated and the results are unrewarding.

Another element possibly hindering the ovulation inducing therapy in patients of Group II may be due to the hypersensitivity of the pituitary gland to estrogen. In such cases, even a relatively low level of estrogen may provoke an untimely release of LH interferring with full maturation of follicles and/or with ovulation. Indeed, in three out of the eight treatment cycles presented here, the elevated LH levels were spread over 4 to 6 days. Theoretically it might be possible to overcome the above undesirable effects by suppressing the endogenous pituitary activity and consequently rendering the ovaries quiescent prior to initiation of ovulation inducing therapy. This could be achieved by down regulation of the pituitary and possibly ovarian response by means of prolonged application of GnRH or its long-acting analogs. Initial reports on such trials have been rather un-enthusiastic (Bettendorf et al.,1981). The rather low efficacy of this therapy could be due to either insufficient dose of inadequate duration of the GnRH analog administration. To be effective the treatment must ensure complete down-regulation of pituitary activity, must cause atresia of all follicles that started to develop prior to initiation of therapy, and last but not least, appropriate measures must be taken in order to prevent recruitment of a new population of follicles between the completion of the down-regulation and the beginning of ovulation inducing therapy. Treatment schemes taking into consideration the above mentioned requirements have been devised and are now applied in clinical trials.

REFERENCES

Aono,T., Minagawa, J., Kinugasa, T., Miyake, A. and Kurachi,K.(1974), The diagnostic significance of LH-releasing Hormone test in patients with amenorrhea. Am. J. Obstet. Gynecol. 119:740.

Bergh, T., Nillius, S.J. and Wide,L.(1978), Serum prolactin and gonadotropin levels before and after luteinizing hormone-releasing hormone in the investigation of amenorrhea. Brit. J. Obstet. Gynec. 85:945.

Berquist, C., Nillius, S.J. and Wide, L.(1979), Reduced gonadotropin secretion in postmenopausal women during treatment with a stimulatory LRH analogue. J. Clin. Endocrinol. Metab.49:472.

Bettendorf, G., Braendle, W., Sprotte, Ch., Weise, Ch.and Zimmermann. R.(1981), Overall results of gonadotropin therapy ,in Advances in Diagnosis and Treatment of Infertility, Edts. V. Insler, G. Bettendorf and K-H. Geissler, Elsevier/North Holland, New York, p. 21.

Bettendorf, G., Braendle W., Weise C. and Poels W.(1981 b). Effect of gonadotropin treatment during inhibited pituitary function,in Advances in Diagnosis and Treatment of Infertility, Edts. V. Insler,G.Bettendorf and K-H. Geissler, Elsevier/North Holland, New York, p. 43.

Bogchelman, D., Lappohn, R.E. and Janssens, J.(1982), Triplet pregnancy after pulsatile administration of gonadotropin releasing hormone. Lancet 2:45.

Borgmann, V., Hardt, W., Schmidt-Gollwitzer, M., Adenauer, H. and Nagel, R.(1982), Sustained suppression of testosterone production by the luteinizing hormone-releasing hormone agonist Buserelin in patients with advanced prostate carcinoma : a new therapeutic approach? Lancet 1:1097.

Campbell , H.J., Feure, G. and Harris, G.W. (1964), The effect of intrapituitary infusion of median eminence and other brain extracts on anterior pituitary gonadotropin secretion. J. Physiol. (London) 170:474.

Crowley, W.F. and McArthur, J. (1980), Simulation of thé normal menstrual cycle in Kallman's Syndrome by pulsatile administration of luteinizing hormone-releasing hormone (LHRH). J. Clin. Endocrinol. Metab. 51:173.

Crowley, W.F., Comite, F., Vale, W., Rivier, J., Loriaux, D.L. and Cutler, G.B. (1980), Therapeutic use of pituitary desensitization with a long-acting LH-RH agonist : a potential new treatment for idiopathic precocious puberty. J. Clin. Endocrinol. Metab. 52:370.

Faure, N., Labrie, F., Lamey, A., Gourdeau, Y., Larche,B.and Belanger,A. Robert, G. (1982), Inhibition of serum androgen levels by chronic intranasal and subcutaneous administration of a potent luteinizing hormone-releasing hormone (LH-RH) agonist in adult men. Fertil. Steril. 37:416.

Feore, J.C. and Taymor, M.L. (1976), The relationship between the pituitary response to luteinizing hormone-releasing hormone and the ovulatory response to clomiphene citrate. Fertil. Steril. 27:1240.

Genazzani, A., Facchinetta, F., Vicenzo, L., Piccioieni, E., Franchi, F., Penini, D. and Kicovic, P. (1978), Effect of epimestrol on gonadotropin and prolactin plasma levels and response to luteinizing hormone-releasing hormone in secondary amenorrhea and oligomenorrhea. Fertil. Steril. 30:654.

Hammond, Ch.B., Weibe, R.H., Haney, A.F. and Yancy, S.C. (1979), Ovulation induction with luteinizing hormone-releasing hormone in amenorrheic, infertile women. Am. J. Obstet. Gynecol. 135:924.

Henderson, S.R., Bonnar, J., Moore, A. and McKinnon, P.C.B.(1976), Luteinizing hormone-releasing hormone for induction of follicular maturation and ovulation in women with infertility and amenorrhea. Fertil. Steril.27:621.

Insler, V., Lunenfeld, B., Serr, D.M. and Eshkol, A. (1974), Differential diagnosis of hypogonadotropic amenorrheic patients using GnRH. Israel J. Med. Sci.10:796.

Insler, V. and Lunenfeld, B. (1983), Diagnose und therapie Endokriner Fertilitaetsstoerungen der Frau, Grosse, Berlin.

Insler, V., Melmed, H., Mashiah, S., Monselise, M., Lunenfeld, B. and Rabau, E . (1968), Functional classification of patients selected for gonadotropin therapy. Obstet. Gynec. 32:620.

Insler, V., Melmed, H., Eichenbrenner, I., Serr, D.M. and Lunenfeld, B. (1972), The cervical score - a simple semiquantitative method for monitoring of the menstrual cycle. Internat. J. Gynecol. Obstet. 10:223.

Insler, V., Potashnik, G. and Glassner M.(1981), Some epidemiological aspects of fertility evaluation, in Advances in Diagnosis and Treatment of Infertility, Edts. V. Insler, G. Bettendorf and K-H. Geissler, Elsevier/ North Holland, New York, p. 165.

Kastin, A.J., Zarate, A., Midgley, A.R., Canales, E. and Schally, A.V. (1971), Ovulation confirmed by pregnancy after infusion of porcine LHRH. J. Clin. Endocrinol. Metab. 33:980.

Keller, P. (1972), Induction of Ovulation by synthetic luteinizing hormone-releasing factor in infertile women. Lancet 2:570.

Keller, P.J. (1973), A pituitary function test with synthetic LH-releasing hormone. J. Obstet.Gynecol. Brit. Commonw. 80:72

Keogh, E.J., Mallal, S.A., Giles, P.F.H. and Evans, D.V. (1981), Ovulation induction with intermittent subcutaneous LHRH. Lancet 1:147.

Knobil, E. (1980), The neuroendocrine control of the menstrual cycle. Recent Prog. Horm. Res. 36:53.

Leyendecker, G., Wildt, L. and Hansmann, M. (1980), Pregnancies following chronic intermittent (pulsatile) administration of GnRH by means of portable pump (Zyklomat) : a new approach in the treatment of infertility in hypothalamic amenorrhea. J. Clin. Endocrinol. Metab. 52:882.

Leyendecker, G., Wildt, L. and Plotz, E.J. (1981) Die Hypothalamische ovarialinsuffizienz. Gynaekologe 14:84.

London, D.R. (1973) Effects of luetinizinghormone releasing hormone given intranasally. J. Endocrinol. 33:153.

Lunenfeld, B. and Glezerman, M. (1981), Diagnose und therapie maennlicher fertilitaetsstorungen, Grosse, Berlin, p. 100.

Lunenfeld, B., Serr, D.M., Mashiah, S., Oelsner, G., Blankstein, J., Frenkel, Y., Ben-Raphael, Z., Tokotzky, D. and Snyder, M. (1981), Therapy with gonadotropins: where are we today, in Advances in Diagnosis and Treatment of Infertility, Edts. V. Insler, G. Bettendorf and K-H Geissler, Elsevier/North Holland, New York, p. 27.

Maia, H., Barbosa, I., Maia, H., Nascimento, A.J. and Bonfin de Souza, M. (1980), Induction of ovulation with epimestrol and luteinizing hormone-releasing hormone. Int. J. Gynecol. Obstet. 17:431.

Matsuo, H., Baba, Y., Nair, R.M., Arimura, A. and Schally, A.V. (1971), Structure of the porcine LH and FSH - releasing hormone. I. The proposed amino acid sequence. Biochem. Biophys. Res. Communw. 43:134.

McCann, S.M., Taleisnik, S. and Friedman, H.M. (1960), LH-releasing activity in Hypothalamic extracts. Proc. Soc. Exp. Biol. Med. 104:432.

Meidan, R., Ben Aroya, N. and Koch, Y. (1981), Variations in the number of pituitary LHRH receptors correlated with altered responsivenese to LHRH. Life Sci. 30:535

Meldrum, D.R., Chang, R.J., LU, J., Val , W., Rivier, J. and Judd, H.L. (1982) "Medical Oophorectomy" using a long-acting GnRH agonist - a possible new approach to the treatment of endometriosis. J. Clin. Endocrinol. Metab. 54:1081.

Miller, D.S., Reid R., Catel, N. and Yen, S.S.C. (1983), Cited in: Yen S.S.C. Clinical Applications of gonadotropin-releasing hormone and gonadotropin- releasing hormone analogs. Fertil. Steril. 39:257.

Nillius,S.J., Berquist, C. and Wide L. (1978), Inhibition of ovulation by chronic treatment with stimulatory LRH analogue-a new approach to birth control ? Contraception 17:537.

Nillius, S.J., Skarin, G. and Wide, L. (1981), Gonadotropin releasing hormone and its agonists for induction of follicular maturation and ovulation, in: Advances in Diagnosis and Treatment of Infertility. Edts. V. Insler, G. Bettendorf and K-H. Geissler, Elsevier/ North Holland, New York, p. 5.

Phansey, S.A., Barnes, M.A., Williamson, H.O., Sagel, J. and Nair, R.M.G. (1980), Combined use of clomiphene and intranasal luteinizing hormone-releasing hormone for induction of ovulation in chronically anovulatory women. Fertil. Steril. 34:448.

Reid, R.L., Leopold, G.R. and Yen, S.S.C. (1981), Induction of ovulation and pregnancy with pulsatile luteinizing hormone releasing factor: dosage and mode of delivery. Fertil. Steril. 36:553.

Rivier, C., Rivier, J. and Vale, W. (1978), Chronic effects of D-Trp^6-Pro^9-NEt-luteinizing hormone-releasing factor on reproductive processes in the female rat. Endocrinol. 103:2299.

Schally, A.V., Arimura, A. and Coy, D.H. (1981), Recent approaches to fertility control based on derivatives of LH-RH. Vitam. Horm. 38:257.

Seibel, M.M. Kamrava, M., McArdie, C. and Taymor, M.L. (1983), Ovulation induction and conception using subcutaneous pulsatile luteinizing hormone-releasing hormone. Obstet. Gynecol. 61:292.

Schoemaker, J., Simons, A.H.M., Van Osnabrugge, G.J.C.,Lugtenburg, C. and Van Kessel, H. (1981), Pregnancy after prolonged pulsatile administration of luteinizing hormone-releasing hormone in a patient with clomiphene-resistant secondary amenorrhea. J. Clin. Endocrinol. Metab. 52:882.

Shaw, R., (1979), differential response to LHRH following oestrogen therapy in women with amenorrhea. Brit. J. Obstet. Gynec. 86:69.

Sheehan, K.L., Casper, R.F. and Yen, S.S.C. (1982), Luteal phase defects induced by and agonists of luteinizing hormone-releasing factor: a model for fertility control. Science 215!170.

Soules, M.R. Jelovsek, F.R., Wiebe, R.H., Tyrey, L., Paulson, D.F. and Hammond, Ch.B. (1979), Amenorrhea : Observations based on the analysis of luteinizing hormone-releasing hormone testing. Am. J. Obstet. Gynecol. 13 :651.

Skarin G., Nillius, S.J. and Wide, L. (1982),pulsatile low dose luteinizing hormone-releasing hormone treatment for induction of follicular maturation and ovulation in women with amenorrhea. Acta Endocr. 101:78

Valk, T.W., Marshall, J.C. and Kelch, R.P. (1981),stimulation of the follicular phase of the menstrual cycle by intravenous administration of low-dose pulsatile gonadotropin releasing hormone. Am. J. Obstet. Gynecol. 141:842.

WHO Scientific Group Report on Agents stimulating gonadal function in the Human. Technical Report Series No. 514.

Yen, S.S.C. (1983), Clinical applications of gonadotropin-releasing hormone and gonadotropin-releasing hormone analogs. Fertil. Steril. 39:257.

PULSATILE ADMINISTRATION OF Gn-RH IN HYPOTHALAMIC AMENORRHEA

G. Leyendecker and L. Wildt

Department of Obstetrics and Gynecology
University of Bonn
53 Bonn, Federal Republic of Germany

INTRODUCTION

Gonadotropin releasing-hormone (Gn-RH) was the second of the neurohumoral agents postulated by Harris more than three decades ago to mediate hypothalamic control of anterior pituitary function that has been isolated, identified in its structure and synthesized. Since this was achieved by the groups of Schally and Guillemin in 1971 and the synthetic hormone became available, Gn-RH has been used extensively as a tool in neuroendocine research. Early attempts to use this decapeptide clinically for the treatment of reproductive disorders supposed to be due to an inadequate secretion of endogenous Gn-RH, however, were of only limited sucess. Effective therapeutic use had to await further progress in the understanding of the physiologic significance of pulsatile gonadotropin secretion and gonadal function. The demonstration that the pattern of the hypophysiotropic stimulation is of critical importance in this respect and the elucidation of the physiologic significance of pulsatile Gn-RH-secretion have provided the rational basis for the efficient use of synthetic Gn-RH in the treatment of Gn-RH deficiency. These findings have also furthered the understanding of the seemingly paradoxical antifertility effects of long acting Gn-RH analogues initially designed to compensate for the short action of the parent decapeptide and thus to simplify treatment of infertility. In this communication, following a short review on physiologic and pathophysiologic aspects of hypothalamic control of gonadotropin secretion in the human female, clinical data obtained with chronic-intermittent (pulsatile) administration of Gn-RH in hypothalamic amenorrhea (HA) will be presented.

THE PULSATILE PATTERN OF GONADOTROPIN SECRETION DURING THE NORMAL MENSTRUAL CYCLE

The pattern of gonadotropin secretion during the normal menstrual cycle is characterized by low serum levels of LH and FSH during the follicular and luteal phases of the cycle interrupted by a sharp increase of LH and FSH during midcycle which causes ovulation. It has been shown by numerous investigators that this cyclic pattern of pituitary gonadotropin secretion can be ragarded as a result of negative and positive feedback effects of ovarian steroids on pituitary function (Knobil, 1980; Leyendecker and Wildt, 1983a).

As first demonstrated in the castrated rhesus monkey, the pituitary release of LH is pulsatile in nature reflecting a pulsatile stimulation of the pituitary gonadotrophs by hypothalamic Gn-RH (Dierschke et al., 1970). By measurement of immunoreactive Gn-RH in the portal stalk effluent (Carmel et al., 1976) and in the cerebrospinal fluid of the third ventricle (Van Vugt et al., 1983) of the rhesus monkey direct evidence for the secretory pattern of hypothalamic Gn-RH could be provided. The pulsatile secretion of Gn-RH is directed by the arcuate nucleus of the mediobasal hypothalamus (Knobil, 1980). Selective destruction of this region in the brain will abolish pituitary secretion of LH and FSH. Moreover, electrophysiological studies have shown that rhythmic increases in multiunit activity in the region of the arcuate nucleus are coincident with the initiation of LH pulse in serum (Knobil, 1981).

In the agonadal female high amplitude LH pulses are observed every 90 minutes on the average (Yen et al., 1982; Santen and Bardin, 1973). The same studied had established that pulses with approximately this frequency, but a lower amplitude occur during the follicular phase of the cycle, while during the luteal phase low-frequency-high-amplitude pulses prevail. A more close analysis of the pulsatile pattern of the LH release revealed that from day 3 - 5 of the follicular phase until after the midcycle surge pulse frequency does not change and is maintained at one pulse every 90 minutes (Leyendecker and Wildt, 1983a; Wildt et al., 1983). During the luteal phase there is a progressive decline in LH pulse frequency, which is lowest immediately before menstruation and increases again during the first few days of early follicular phase. There is no direct relationship between progesterone concentrations and the reduction in LH pulse frequency. The reduction, however, appears to be correlated with the duration of the progesterone elevation. The physiologic significance of the changing frequency of gonadotrpin secretion during the menstrual cycle, particularly during the luteal phase, remains to be elucidated. The observation that normal menstrual cycles can be induced women (leyendecker et al., 1980a, 1981) and in rhesus monkeys (Knobil, 1980) with essentially abolished endogenous Gn-RH secretion by the pulsatile administration of Gn-RH at an unvarying frequency, however, argues strongly against any major physiologic importance of this phenomenon for the regulation of luteal function and of follicular development.

PATTERN OF GONADOTROPIN SECRETION IN PATIENTS WITH HYPOTHALAMIC AMENORRHEA

Complete absence or severe reduction of pulsatile gonadotropin release results in impairment of follicular maturation, anovulation and amenorrhea (Leyendecker, 1979; Leyendecker et al., 1981). While this obtains physiologically before puberty or during pregnancy and lactation, it is pathological in other periods of reproductive life. Since there is substantial indirect evidence that cause of this kind of amenorrhea is a reduced stimulation of the anterior pituitary gland by Gn-RH and since Gn-RH is secreted from the hypothalamus, it is referred to as hypothalamic amenorrhea (Leyendecker, 1979; Leyendecker and Wildt, 1983b).

The term "hypothalamic amenorrhea" was coined by Klinefelter and associates in 1943 to describe amenorrhea of suprapituitary origin. Due to some cases described in the original publication, however, it was later on confined to psychogenic amenorrhea. In this communication, hypothalamic amnorrhea is used in its broader original sense and consequently applies for patients with lesions of the pituitary stalk or hypothalamus, anorexia nervosa, Kallmann's syndrome as well as for idiopathic or psychogenic amenorrhea.

Since endogenous Gn-Rh cannot be measured reliably in peripheral blood direct evaluation of hypothalamic function is presently not possible. Therefore, the diagnosis of hypthalamic amenorrhea is essentially based on the exclusion of other causes of amenorrhea, such a hyperprolactinemia, hyperandrogenemia, primary ovarian failure, genital tract defects as well as internal and neurological diseases. Primary pituitary failure is exluded by the ability to stimulate pituitary gonadotropic function by pulsatile administration of Gn-RH.

Based on studies in amenorrhoic patients, prepubertal subjects and experimental animals the view has been advanced that hypothalamic amenorrhea forms a pathophysiological continuum, reflecting a gliding scale of imapirment of hypothalamic Gn-RH secretion and consequently gonadotropin production and follicular development and it was furthermore proposed that the extent of this impairment can be assessed by the response to Gn-RH-, gestagen-, and clomiphene-administration (Leyendecker, 1979; Leyendecker and Wildt, 1983b). The reactions in those simple tests have therefor been used as criteria for grading of amenorrhoic patients according to the severity of hypothalamic impairment and for selection of the appropriate therapy (table 1).

Table 1. Grading of hypothalamic amenorrhea on the basis of clomiphene-, gestagen- and Gn-RH-tests, respectively

Grade	Result of test
1	Clomiphene positive (bleeding)
2	Gestagen positive (bleeding) Clomiphene negative (no bleeding)
3	Gestagen negative (no bleeding) with pituitary response to 100 μg of Gn-RH i.v.
3a	"adult" response
3b	"prepubertal" response"
3c	no response

Recent studies on the pulsatile pattern of LH in serum (figure 1), the frequency of LH pulses, overall LH and FSH levels during a 24 hour steroid as well as on ultrasonographic visualization of ovarian follicles in 20 patients suffering from hypothalamic amenorrhea supported this view (figure 2) (Wildt et al., 1983). The number of LH pulses was lowest in grade 3c patients and increased gradually until a value comparable of that of the normal menstrual cycle was reached in grade 2 patients. Only in grade 3b patients an increase in pulse frequency during sleep became apparent, while in all other grades pulses were found to be evenly distributed between sleep and awake periods. Amplitude of some LH pulses however, was considerably larger during sleep than during awake periods in grade 3b, 3a and grade 2 subjects. Overall LH and FSH levels increased parallel to the number of LH pulses up to grade 3a and 2, respectively, but failed to reach values typical for the early follicular phase of the cycle. In clomiphene positive patients, LH and particularly FSH levels declined again and this may be attributed to negative feedback inhibition by the elevated levels of estradiol found in those patients.

Considerable follicular development up to large antral stage has been found in ovarian biopsies of amenorrhoic patients (Nakano et al., 1982). This was reflected by the number of follicles indentified by ultrasound, which increased parallel to the number of LH pulses from essentially undetectable in grade 3c patients to a hight comparable to that found during the phase of maximal follicular development during the early follicular phase of the cycle in clomiphene positive patients. Thus, hypothalamic amenorrhea is characterized by a reduced frequency and amplitude of gonadotropin secretion which is reflected by the concomitant reduction of ovarian follicular growth. In this context, a reduction of frequency of pulsatile gonadotropin secretion is distinctive for the most severe grades of hypothalamic amenorrhea, while a reduction in amplitude characterizes less pronounced grades of this disorder.

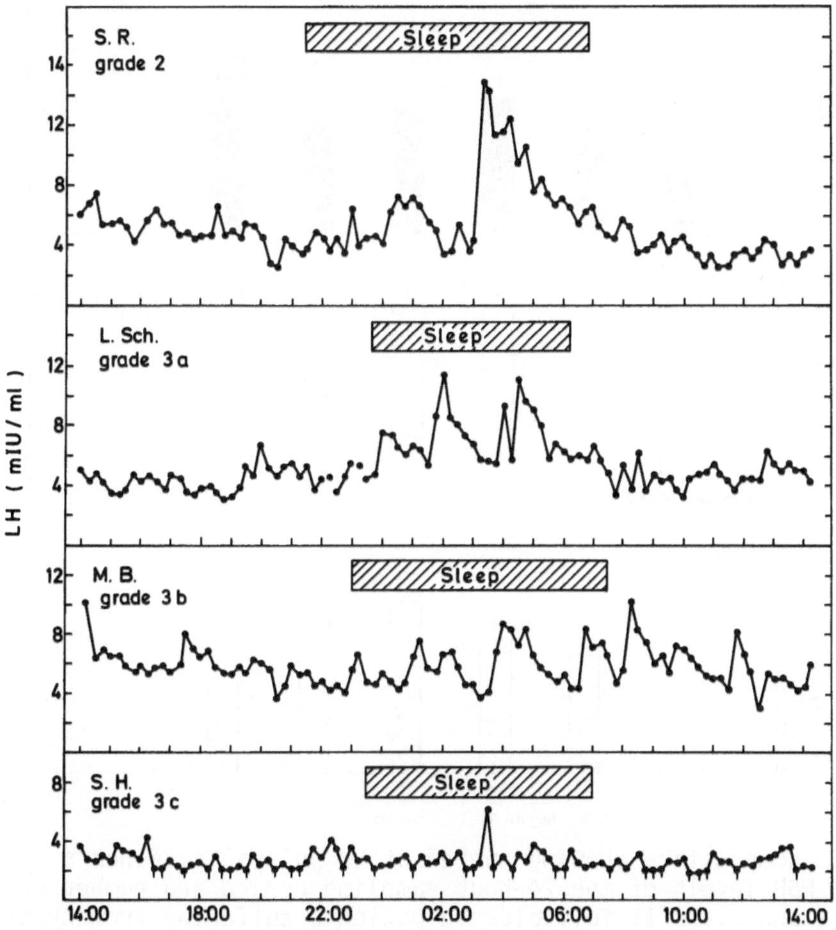

Fig. 1. Composite of the 24-hour secretory pattern of LH in representative patients suffering from different grades of hypothalamic amenorrhea, grading from virtually absent pulses in grade 3c to frequent pulsations with sleep-related increase in amplitude in grade 2. Vertical lines underneath data points indicate levels below assay sensitivity. From Leyendecker G, Wildt L (1983b), with permission.

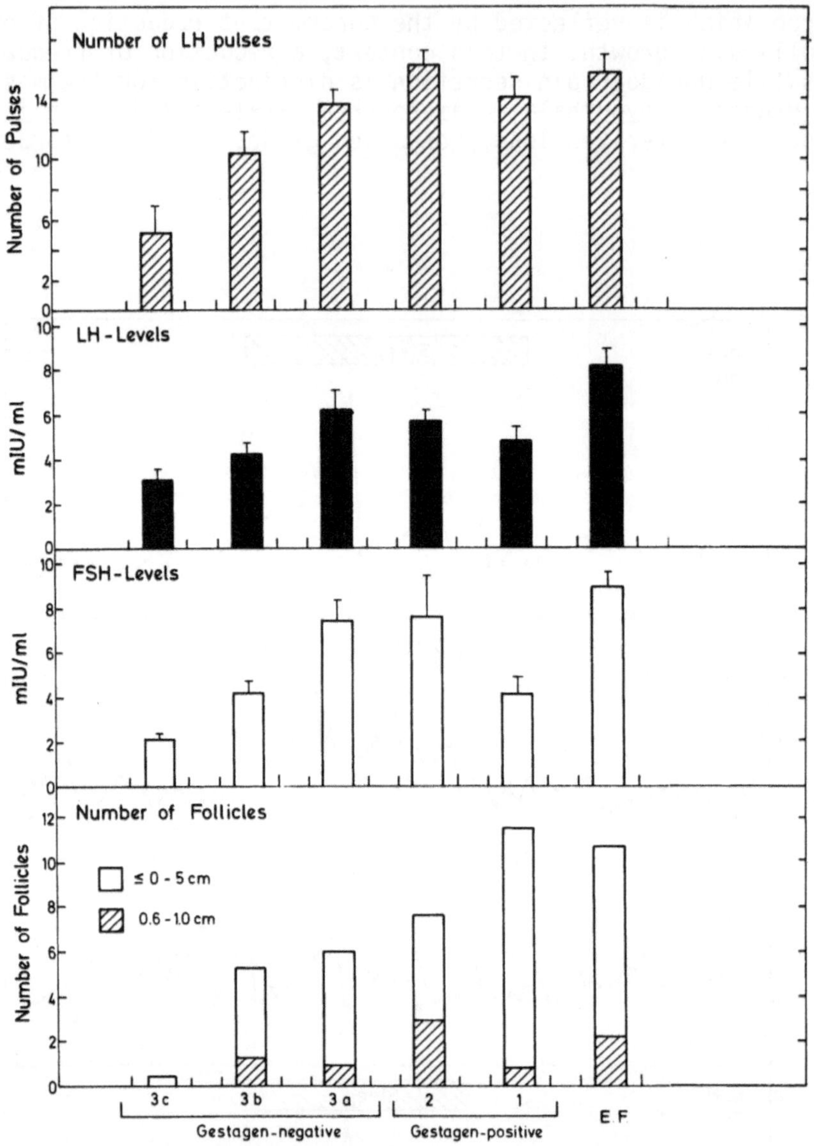

Fig. 2. Compositive showing number of LH pulses in 24 hours, mean LH and FSH levels of the 24-hour sampling period and number of class I and class II follicles in patients suffering from hypothalamic amenorrhea grades according to response to Gn-RH-,gestagen- and clomiphene-administration. Bars indicate mean ± SEM. The corresponding values for the early follicular phase (day 3 - 7) of 13 normal menstrual cycles (EF) are given for comparison and represent values of 8-hour sampling periods. The number of follicles given under EF represents the maximum number observed for each class of follicles. From Wildt et al. (1983), with permission.

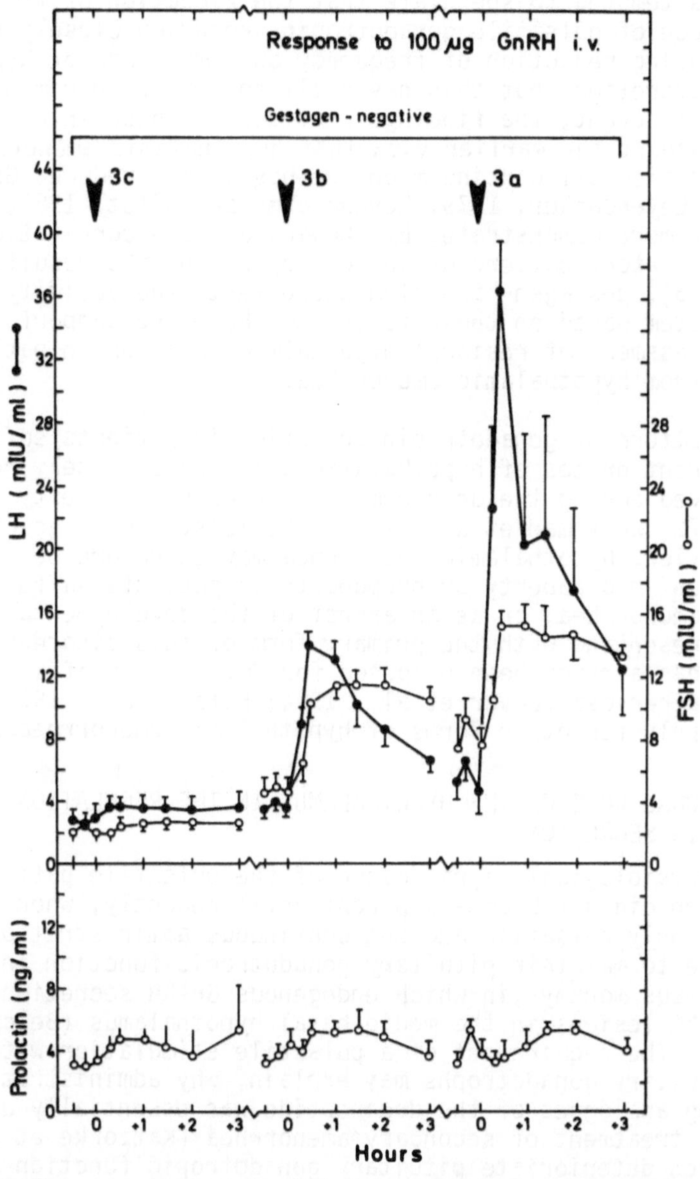

Fig. 3. Pituitary response to the i.v. injection of 100 µg Gn-RH in 13 gestagen negative patients with hypothalamic amenorrhea. Note the three clearly distinguishable response patterns: no response (grade 3c), prepubertal (grade 3b) and adult (grade 3a) response of LH and FSH. Each point represents mean ± SEM of 4 (3a), 6 (3b) and 3 (3a) observations, respectively. From Leyendecker and Wildt (1983b) with permission.

One is tempted to speculate that the reduction of frequency and amplitude of pulsatile gonadotropin secretion closely reflects a corresponding reduction of frequency and amplitude of hypothalamic Gn-RH secretion, but this has still to await experimental proof. In any event, the findings provided by these investigations strongly support the earlier view that hypothalamic amenorrhea forms a pathophysiological continuum on the basis of a reduced Gn-RH secretion (Leyendecker, 1979; Leyendecker and Wildt, 1981, 1983b). They furthermore demonstrate, by showing a close correlation between the secretory pattern of gonadotropins and the results of Gn-RH (figure 3), gestagen- and clomiphene tests the validity of the grading system based on these tests and therefore support its use for the assessment of residual hypothalmic function in patients suffering from hypothalamic amenorrhea.

The pattern of gonadotropin secretion in patients suffering from different grades of hypothalamic amenorrhea closely resembles that observed during the developmental process ob puberty (Boyar et al., 1972; Weitzman et al., 1975). At least from a descriptive points of view, hypothalamic amenorrhea may therefore be viewed as a regression into puberty or prepuberty in patients suffering from secondary amenorrhea, or as an arrest of the developmental process in those presenting with the primary form of this disorder. Such a mechanism has already been proposed for development of amenorrhea in anorexia nervosa (Boyar et al., 1974; Katz et al., 1977) but seems to apply for other forms of hypothalamic amenorrhea also.

THE FUNCTIONAL ROLE OF THE HYPOTHALAMUS IN THE REGULATION OF GONADOTROPIN SECRETION

The physiological significance of the pulsatile pattern of Gn-RH secretion did not become apparent until recently, when it was shown that only pulsatile and not continuous administration of Gn-RH was able to maintain pituitary gonadotropic function in ovariectomized rhesus monkeys,in which endogenous Gn-RH secretion had been abolished by lesions in the medio-basal hypothalamus (Belchetz et al., 1980). The requirement of a pulsatile stimulation with Gn-RH by the pituitary gonadotrophs may explain, why administration of long acting analogues of the decapeptide was essentially unsuccessful in the treatment of secondary amenorrhea (Katzorke et al.,1980) and did even deterioriate pituitary gonadotropic function in normal women (Derick-Tan et al., 1977; Bergquist et al., 1979). Moreover, it could be demonstrated with the model of the hypothalamus lesioned rhesus monkey that the site of action of estradiol in exhibiting negative and positive feedback effects on the pituitary secretion of LH and FSH is localized on the level of the pituitary rather than on the level of the brain (Nakai et al., 1978). In hypothalamus lesioned but otherwise intact female rhesus monkeys the pulsatile administration of an unvarying amount of Gn-RH at a physiologic frequency induced menstrual cycles which were not different from spontaneous ones (Knobil et al., 1980). Thus, the endocrine regulation of the menstrual cycle of primates appears to be fundamentally different from that of the estrous cycle of the rat. While in the rat the rostral part of the hypothalamus seems to be essential in the mediation of chrono-biological signals and positive feedback reactions, the assumption of such a "cyclic center" appears no longer to be justified for the primate. In the primate the function of the hypothalamus in the regulation of the menstrual cycle is only a "permissive" one (Knobil et al., 1980).

In women with severe hypothalamic amenorrhea, a condition functionally comparable with that of the hypothalamus lesioned female rhesus monkey, chronic intermittent (pulsatile) administration of Gn-RH with an unvarying dose and at an unchanged frequency of one pulse every 90 minutes resulted in follicular maturation, ovulation and corpus luteum formation (Leyendecker, 1979; Leyendecker et al., 1980a). The endocrine pattern of the normal menstrual cycle could be completely replicated.

Thus, it could be shown that the concept of the permissive function of the hypothalamus developed in the rhesus monkey could be extended to the human female. These results have been confirmed by other investigators (Crowley and McArthur, 1980; Keogh et al., 1981; Schoemaker et al., 1982; Skarin et al., 1982) and with the development of chronic-intermittent (pulsatile) administration of Gn-RH by means of a small computerized pump ("Zyklomat", Ferring GmbH, Kiel, FRG) as a new and practical mode of treatment of infertility in hypothalamic amenorrhea clinical advantage has been taken of these new insights into the physiology of the human menstrual cycle (Leyendecker et al., 1980b; Leyendecker and Wildt, 1981, 1983b).

CLINICAL RESULTS OF PULSATILE ADMINISTRATION OF GN-RH IN HYPOTHALAMIC AMENORRHEA

Since the first introduction of pulsatile administration of Gn-RH to women with hypothalamic amenorrhea 130 experimental and treatment cycles made so far been performed in our institution. The patients were selected for pulsatile treatment on the basis of the criteria described above. Only patients with hypothalamic amenorhhea of grades 2 - 3c were considered suitable for Gn-RH substitution.

Dose of Gn-RH

Intravenous administration of Gn-RH with a dose of 10 µg per pulse did not result in full follicular maturation over a tretment period of 17 days in a patient with primary hypothalamic amenorrhea grade 3c (Leyendecker et al., 1980a). The same patient did however ovulate and exhibit normal luteal phases repeatedly when i.v. doses of 15-20 μg/pulse were used. Dose of 2.5 and 5 μg/pulse again resulted only in ovulatory bleeding (Leyendecker et al., 1981). However, another patient with grade 3c hypothalamic amenorrhea ovulated with a dose of 5 μg of Gn-RH per pulse. Presently, the different dosage requirement of some patients of the same degree of hypothalamic impairment as determined with our grading system is not fully understood. It indicates that pulsatile administration of Gn-RH in hypothalamic amenorrhea may provide information which may lead to a better understanding of the pathophysiology of different forms of hypothalamic amneorrhea. All women with hypothalamic amenorrhea grades 3b, 3a and 2, respectively, ovulated with i.v. doses ranging from 2.5 - 20 μg/pulse, indicating that in less severe cases than grade 3c a smaller dose of Gn-RH might be sufficient to induce menstrual cycles reliably. However, in these patients a dose of 1 - 2,5 μg/pulse might constitute a critical dose range for induction of ovulation. In a patient with secondary hypothalamic amenorrhea grade 2 with a dose of 1 μg/Pulse ovulation could not be induced over a treatment period of 41 days. When the dose was increased to 5 μg/pulse ovulation was obtained and the patient conceived during that treatment course (figure 4). As a consequence

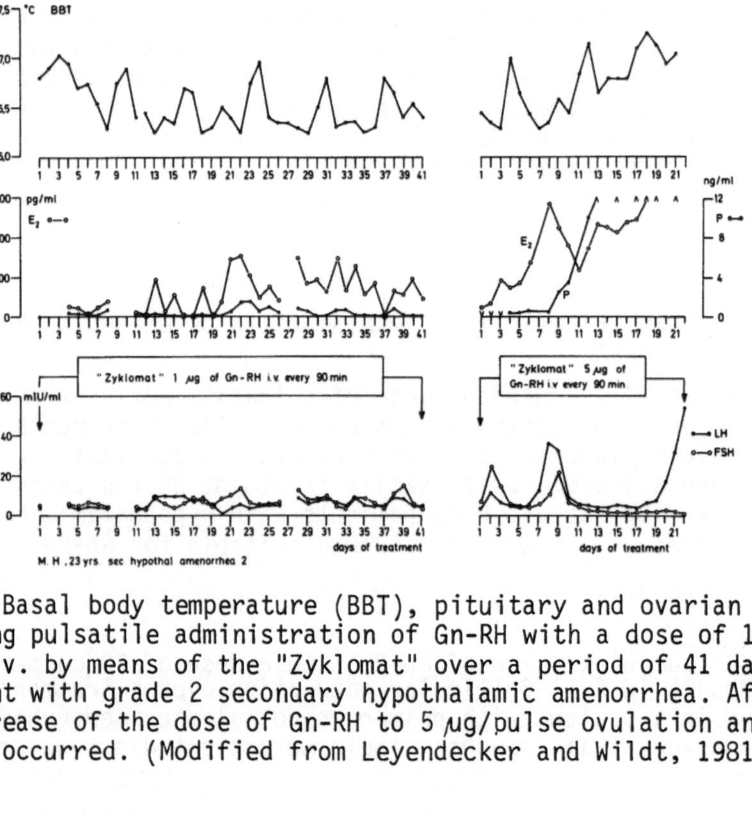

Fig. 4. Basal body temperature (BBT), pituitary and ovarian response during pulsatile administration of Gn-RH with a dose of 1 μg/pulse i.v. by means of the "Zyklomat" over a period of 41 days in a patient with grade 2 secondary hypothalamic amenorrhea. After the increase of the dose of Gn-RH to 5 μg/pulse ovulation and conception occurred. (Modified from Leyendecker and Wildt, 1981).

of these findings, patients with hypothalamic amenorrhea grade 3c (usually patients with primary amenorrhea or pituitary stalk and hypothalamic lesions exhibit this degree of severity) are now routinely treated with 15-20 μg/pulse and the less serious cases with 5 μg/pulse when the i.v. route is used. With this dose regimen of Gn-RH all i.v. treatment cycles performed so far resulted in ovulation.

There is a dose response relationship between the dose of Gn-RH administered per pulse and the ovarian response, as reflected by estradiol and progesterone levels in serum (figure 5). The mean estradiol and progesterone levels of the cycles induced with 15-20 μg/pulse were all above those obtained in cycles with 2.5 - 5 μg/pulse. The results depicted in figure 5 were all obtained in patients suffering from hypothalamic amenorrhea grade 3b.

Duration of the follicular phase

The duration of the follicular phase after pulsatile administration of Gn-RH is a reflection of the ovarian functional status at the beginning of the Gn-RH substitution. As indicated by ovarian biopsies (Nakano et al., 1982) and ultrasonography of the ovaries, there is an increased chance of developed or even dominant follicles being present in grades 3a and 2 of hypothalamic amenorrhea. Ultrasonographic follow-up demonstrates that there is a "cyclic" growth of these follicles ("occult anovulatory cycles"), which can reach a size of 14-18 mm in diameter before they become atretic (G. Leyendecker and L. Wildt, unpublished observations). This also resembles the prepubertal state, in which the ovaries contain a population of "cyclically" growing large antral follicles which become atretic (Peters, 1979). Proliferative phases of short duration, ovulations and conceptions show that these follicles can be further stimulated and bear a competent egg. The first child born after induction of ovulation with Gn-RH resulted from such a large antral follicle which was present before initiation of treatment (Leyendecker et al., 1980b). The presence of large antral follicles explains the observation that there is an immediate dramatic rise in serum oestradiol levels in some patients with the onset of Gn-RH substitution (Leyendecker et al., 1980a).

Substitution during the Luteal Phase

The normal luteotrophic hormone in the human is pituitary LH (Van de Wiele et al., 1970). In severe hypothalamic amenorrhea corpus luteum function immediately caeses following termination of pulsatile Gn-RH substitution a few days after ovulation (Leyendecker and Wildt, 1981). Continuation of pulsatile administration of Gn-RH during the whole luteal phase resulted in normal luteal function as indicated by the length of the luteal phase, the progesterone levels in serum and conceptions. Previously, it was suggested to support the luteal function by one to three injections of 2500 IU of HCG once ovulation had been obtained by Gn-RH (Leyendecker et al., 1980). There is, however, no indication on the basis of our data (Leyendecker and Wildt, 1983b) that one method of luteal substitution is superior over the other in terms of pregnancy rate obtained.

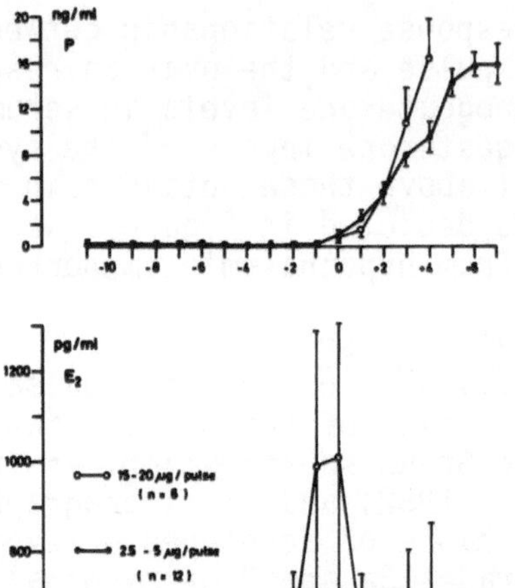

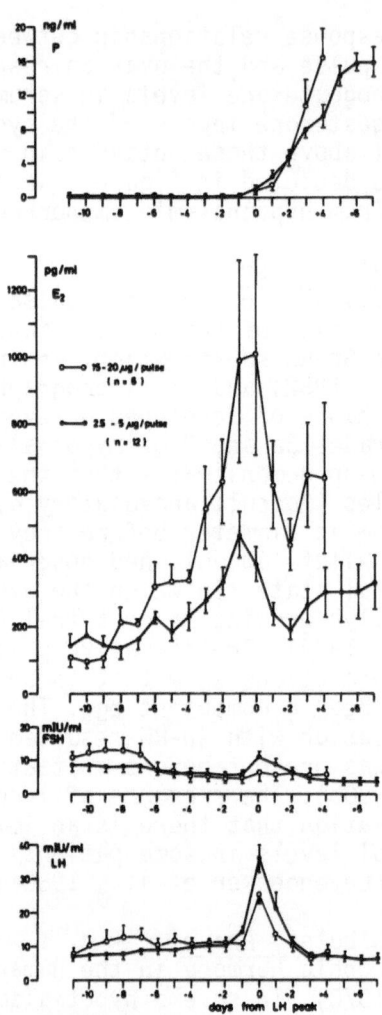

Fig. 5. The serum concentrations of FSH, LH, estradiol and progesterone in patients with hypothalamic amenorrhea grade 3b treated with 15 - 20 µg/pulse or with 2.5 - 5 µg/pulse of Gn-RH intravenously.

Intravenous Versus Subcutaneous Application of Gn-RH

The same catheter used for the i.v. application of Gn-RH was also used for the subcutaneous route, however without the addition of heparin to the hormone containing solution. The catheter was placed into the fat tissue of the lower abdominal wall. Ovulations could be induced with doses of 5-20 µg/pulse in patients with hypothalamic amenorrhea of grades 2 - 3b and with 20 µg/pulse in a patient with hypothalamic amenorrhea grade 3c following the removal of a craniopharyngeoma (Leyendecker and Wildt, 1981). Four pregnancies were obtained with the s.c. route. However, in contrast to the i.v. application with a 100% ovulation rate, the adequate dose per pulse provided, there was an incidence of only 13 ovulatory cycles in 21 s.c. applications of Gn-RH. However, all these patients who did not ovulate during s.c. application, had ovulatory cycles when Gn-RH was intravenously applied at the same dose level. Delayed resorption of Gn-RH from the subcutaneous fat tissue might result in insufficient serum levels on Gn-RH for adequate stimulation of the pituitary gonadotrophs.

Ovulation- and Pregnancy-Rate

The adequate dose of Gn-RH provided (15 - 20 µg/pulse i.v. in hypothalamic amenorrhea grade 3c and 2.5 - 5 µg/pulse in grades 3b - 2) ovulation and normal luteal function can be excepted in every treatment cycle. The ovulation rate is reduced, when the s.c. route is chosen. Definitive treatment failure (no ovulation) was only observed when the diagnosis of hypothalamic amenorrhea was not correct. In the beginning of our studies, mild hyperandrogenemia was not taken into account carefully.In these patients pulsatile administration of Gn-RH could not induce ovulatory cycles. PCO and related pathological entities are, on the basis of our experiencies, not considered to be suitable for pulsatile Gn-RH administration. Recent studies indicate, however, that pulsatile Gn-RH treatment might be successfully applied in polycystic ovarian disease (Coelingh Bennink, 1983).

The pregnancy rate isremarkably high. Of 30 patients 26 became pregnant. One patient had two successful pregnancies two years apart. Twenty four pregnancies are completed with 29 children born, among them 3 sets of heterozygous twins and one set of triplets. Five patients aborted of whom one patient had two sequential abortions probably due to active cytomegaly. Four of these patients conceived thereafter again and had uneventful pregnacies so far. Totally 32 conceptions were obtained in 30 patients.

The pregnancy rate, however, is critically dependent upon whether or not additional factors causing infertility of the couple are present (i.e. tubal or andrological factors). 64 treatment cycles were applied in 27 "favourable couples", in whom the hypothalamic amenorrhea constitutes the only cause of infertility of the couple, and 29 pregnancies were obtained (2.2 cycle per pregnancy). Totally, the pregnancy rate is comparable to the normal population. In 97 ovulatory treatment cycles 32 conceptions occurred (3.0 cycles per pregnancy).

Ovarian Overstimulation and Multiple Pregnancies

The feedback mechanisms of ovarian steroids on the pituitary secretion of the gonadotropic hormones are operative during pulsatile adminstration of Gn-RH. Clinical signs of ovarian overstimulation have therefore not been observed during 130 experimental and treatment cycles. As shown in figure 4, there is, however, a dose response relationship between the dose of Gn-RH and the ovarian response, which is mediated by adose related pituitary secretion of gonadotropins. If it is taken into consideration that the mechanisms of recruitment of follicles, the selection of the dominant follicle and the suppression of the other accompanying follicles are dependent to a certain degree upon the gonadotropic stimulation, it has to be expected that a gonadotropic stimulation of the ovaries resulting in discrete chemical overstimulation must cause an increased incidence of multiple pregnancies as compared to the normal population. In our study 4 multiple pregnancies were obtained out of 30 conceptions. One of these multiple pregnancies was obtained by too high a dose for the respective grade (20 µg/pulse in grade 3b of hypothalamic amenorrhea).

CONCLUSIONS

Pulsatile administration of Gn-RH by means of a portable pump ("Zyklomat") has proven to be an efficient and practical method for the induction of ovulation as a treatment of infertility in hypothalamic amenorrhea. The results obtained with this method of treatment are critically dependent upon the correct selection of patients as far as the diagnosis of hypothalamic amenorrhea is concerned. Patients with hypothalamic amenorrhea, previously treated with human gonadotropins are suitable for this mode of treatment. Further intensive studies have to demonstrate whether other anovulatory conditions, such as polycystic ovarian disease and hyperprolactinemia (Leyendecker et al., 1980a), are also suitable for pulsatile Gn-RH administration.

In our study 30 conceptions were obtained in 28 patients. These favourable results are obtained due to a rather physiological stimulation of the ovaries during chronic intermittent (pulsatile) administration of Gn-RH. On the basis of operating negative and positive feedback mechanisms of the ovarian steroids on the pituitary secretion of the gonadotropins during treatment, the follicle itself regulates the required amount of gonadotropin stimulation. However, since there is a relationship between the [3]Gn-RH dose per pulse applied and the reaction of the pituitary-ovarian axis, the lowest efficient dose of Gn-RH in reliably inducing ovulatory cycles should be chosen.

ACKNOWLEDGEMENT

The skillful technical assistance of Miss Roswitha Klasen is gratefully acknowledged.

REFERENCES

Belchetz PE, Plant TM, Nakai Y, Keogh EJ, Knobil E,1978, Hypophyseal responses to continous and intermittent delivery of hypothalamic gonadotropin releasing hormone (Gn-RH).Science 202: 631

Bergquist C, Nillius SJ, Wide L.,1979, Reduced gonadotropin secretion in postmenopausal women during treatment with a stimulatory LRH analogue. J Clin Endocrinol Metab 49:472

Boyar RM, Finkelstein J, Roffwarg H, Kapen S, Weitzman ED, Hellman L, 1972, Synchronization of augmented luteinizing hormone secretion with sleep during puberty. N Eng J Med 287:582

Boyar RM, Katz J, Finkelstein J, Kapen S, Weiner H, Weitzman ED, Hellman L, 1974, Anorexia nervosa: Immaturity of the 24-hour luteinizing hormone secretion pattern. N Eng J Med 291:861

Carmel PW, Araki S, Ferin M, 1976, Pituitary stalk portal blood collection in rhesus monkeys: Evidence for pulsatile release of gonadotropin releasing hormone (Gn-RH). Endocrinology 99: 243

Coelingh-Bennink HJT, 1983, Induction of ovulation by pulsatile intravenous administration of LHRH in polycystic ovarian disease. Present at the Sixty-Fifth Annual Meeting of The Endocrine Society, San Antonio, Texas, 1983. Published by The Endocrine Society, in Programs and Abstracts, p 81

Crowley jr WF, McArthur JW, 1980, Stimulation of the normal menstrual cycle in Kallmann's syndrome by pulsatile administration of luteinizing hormone -releasing hormone (LH-RH). J Clin Endocrinol Metab 51:173

Dericks-Tan JSE, Hammer E, Taubert HD, 1977, The effect of D-Ser (TBU)^{6}-LH-RH-EA^{10} upon gonadotropin release in normally cyclic women. J Clin Endocrinol Metab 45:597

Dierschke DJ, Bhattacharya AN, Atkinson LE, Knobil E, 1970, Circhoral oscillations of plasma LH levels in the ovariectomized rhesus monkey. Endocrinology 87:850

Katz JL, Boyar RM, Roffwarg H, Hellman L, Weiner H, 1977, LHRH reponsiveness in anorexia nervosa: Intactness despite prepubertal circadian LH pattern. Psychosom Med 39:241

Katzorke T, Popping D, Ohe von der M, Tauber PF, 1980, Clinical evaluation of the effects of a new long acting superactive luteinizing-release hormone (LH-RH analog. D-Ser (TBU)^{6}-des Gly-10-Ethylamide-LH-RH, in women with secondary amenorrhea. Fertil Steril 33:35

Keogh EJ, Mallal SA, Giles PFH, Evans DV, 1981, Ovulation induction with intermittent subcutaneous LH-RH. Lancet I, 147

Klinefelter jr HF, Albright F, Griswold G, 1943, Experience with a quantitative test for normal or decreased amounts of follicle stimulating hormone in the uterus in endocrinological diagnosis. J Clin Endocrinol Metab 3:529

Knobil E, 1980, The neuroendocrine control of the menstrual cycle. Recent Prog Hormone Res 36:53

Knobil E, 1981, Patterns of hypophysiotropic signals and gonadotropin secretion in the rhesus monkey. Biol Reprod 24:44

Knobil E, Plant TM, Wildt L, Belchetz DE, Marshall G, 1980, Control of the rhesus monkey menstrual cycle: permissive role of hypothalamic gonadotropin releasing (Gn-RH). Science 207:1371

Leyendecker G, 1979, The pathophysiology of hypothalamic ovarian failure - diagnostic and therapeutical considerations. Eur J Obstet Gynec Reprod Biol 9:175

Leyendecker G, Struve T, Plotz EJ, 1980a, Induction of ovulation with chronic-intermittent (pulsatile) administration of LH-RH in women with hypothalamic and hyperprolactinemic amenorrhea. Arch Gynecol 229:117

Leyendecker G, Wildt L, Hansmann M, 1980b, Pregnancies following chronic-intermittent (pulsatile) administration of Gn-RH by means of a portable pump ("Zyklomat") - a new approach to the treatment of infertility in hypothalamic amenorrhea. J Clin Endocrinol Metab 51:1214

Leyendecker G, Wildt L, Plotz EJ, 1981, Die hypothalamische Ovarialinsuffizienz. Gynäkologe 14:84

Leyendecker G, Wildt L, 1981, Chronisch intermittierende Gabe von Gn-RH. Ein Beitrag zur Physiologie und Pathophysiologie der endokrinen Regulation des menstruellen Zyklus sowie ein neues Verfahren zur Ovulationsauslösung bei hypothalamischer Amenorrhoe. Therapiewoche 31:6711

Leyendecker G, Wildt L, 1983a, Control of gonadotropin secretion in the human female In: Brenner RM, Phoenix CH, Norma L (eds) Neuroendocrine aspects of Reproduction. Academic Press, New York

Leyendecker G, Wildt L, 1983b, Induction of ovulation with chronic-intermittent (pulsatile) administration of Gn-RH in women with hypothalamic amenorrhea. J Reprod Fertil 69:397

Nakai Y, Plant TM, Hess DL, Keogh EJ, Knobil E. 1978, On the sites of the negative and positive feedback actions of estradiol in the control of gonadotropin secretion in the rhesus monkey. Endocrinology 102:1008

Nakano R, Washio M, Hashiba N, Tojo S, 1982, Ovarian morphologic features and endocrine profile in amenorrhoic patients. Gynecol Obstet Invest 14:19

Peters H, 1979, The human ovary in childhood and early maturity. Eur J Obstet Gynec Reprod Biol 9:137

ON THE MODE OF ACTION OF AN LHRH AGONIST IN MAN AND ITS POTENTIAL USE AS CONTRACEPTIVE

David Rabin, Robert M. Evans, and Gregory C. Doelle

Vanderbilt University School of Medicine
Division of Endocrinology
Nashville, Tennessee 37232

1. INTRODUCTION

The isolation of LHRH (Schally et al., 1971; Burgus et al., 1971) was followed by the development of a large number of analogs (Vale et al., 1977). The compound D-Trp^6-Pro^9-N-Ethylamide LHRH ($LHRH_A$) has a potency 144 times that of native LHRH in causing LH release in *in vitro* systems (Vale et al., 1977). However, when administered *in vivo* to the rat, "paradoxical" gonadal atrophy was observed (Tcholakian et al., 1978; Sandow et al., 1980).

We have reported similar findings in a group of normal male volunteers - reversible inhibition of steroidogenesis and spermatogenesis after 50 μg $LHRH_A$ daily for ten weeks. Figure 1 shows results in a typical subject (Linde et al., 1981). Other laboratories have reported very similar data (Berquist et al., 1979; Swerdloff et al., 1983).

2. MODE OF ACTION OF $LHRH_A$ IN MAN

At least three loci of action of $LHRH_A$ have been identified in the rat. First, there is the desensitization of the gonadotroph, that is reduced responses to repeated stimulation with the agonist (Rivier and Vale, 1979). Second, there is loss of testicular receptors, particularly for LH, thought to be due to excessive or inappropriate release of LH (Auclair et al., 1977; Hsueh et al., 1976). Third, $LHRH_A$ exerts a direct inhibitory effect on the gonad (Hsueh and Erickson, 1979; Clayton et al., 1980). The position is much less clear in man. We studied hor-

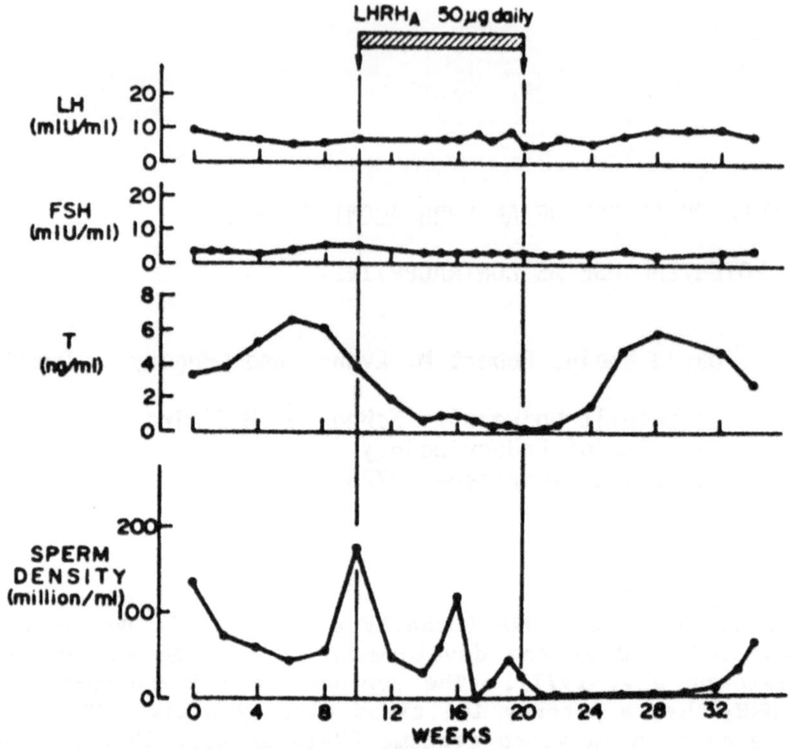

Fig. 1. Levels of luteinizing hormone (LH), follicle stimulating hormone (FSH), and testosterone (T) and sperm density in subject 7 during the basal period, treatment period (LHRH$_A$), and recovery period. Reprinted with permission from N. Engl. J. Med. 305:665, 1981.

Table I. Mean Serum LH Values During Treatment with LHRH$_A$

Subject	0	4 Weeks	8 Weeks
1	11.7 ± 0.5	6.4 ± 0.1	--
2	11.1 ± 0.5	7.3 ± 0.1	5.9 ± 0.7
3	15.5 ± 0.5	5.1 ± 0.2	5.7 ± 0.3
4	8.2 ± 0.5	24.3 ± 1.2	18.3 ± 0.4
5	8.3 ± 0.5	8.4 ± 1.2	--
6	15.6 ± 0.7	15.3 ± 0.4	19.5 ± 0.4
7	7.1 ± 0.4	10.6 ± 0.4	13.8 ± 0.3

Mean serum LH values in 7 subjects before (0) and 4 and 8 weeks after commencement of LHRH$_A$.

Table II. Bioactive and Immunoreactive Serum LH Levels During $LHRH_A$

Subject		Day 0	Day 12
1	B	207	218
	I	37	84
2	B	285	63
	I	48	91
3	B	212	101
	I	14.6	65
4	B	182	88
	I	32	87

B = ng LER 907/ml; I = ng LER 907/ml.

Bio-(B) and immuno-(I) assayable LH values in 4 subjects before (0) and after 12 days of $LHRH_A$ treatment.

monal profiles in seven subjects under basal conditions and after four and eight weeks of drug treatment with $LHRH_A$, 50 μg daily. Samples were taken every 20 minutes between 0700 and 1900 hours. Mean LH values are shown in Table I. Mean serum LH fell modestly in three subjects, remained unchanged in one and rose significantly in the other three (Evans et al., 1984b). Serum testosterone fell in all. The episodic pattern of LH secretion was lost during $LHRH_A$ treatment. We examined the gonadal response to human LH in four other subjects receiving $LHRH_A$. The rise in serum testosterone after infusion of LH for 48 hours was similar in normal controls and in men treated with $LHRH_A$ for up to eight weeks (Evans et al., 1984b). These results suggested that $LHRH_A$ acts primarily at the level of the pituitary in man, possibly by producing a qualitative change in LH.

To explore this notion, we gave four subjects 500 μg $LHRH_A$ daily for two weeks. We measured serum testosterone and bio-(B) and immuno-(I) assayable LH daily (Evans et al., 1984a). Figure 2 shows the time course of serum testosterone and I - LH. Note the fall in testosterone while I - LH remains increased above basal. Table II gives the B to I ratios in each subject before treatment and on the 12th day of $LHRH_A$. A significant fall was observed in all four subjects. When these samples were subjected to G-100 chromatography, a consistent change was noted. The LH eluted later than labeled LH, and this pattern was clearly different from that found in the same individual examined when he was not receiving $LHRH_A$ (Figure 3). The reason for this is not known. The altered LH eluted before LHβ, and the cross-reactivity of the latter is only 4% in our LH assay (Figure 3).

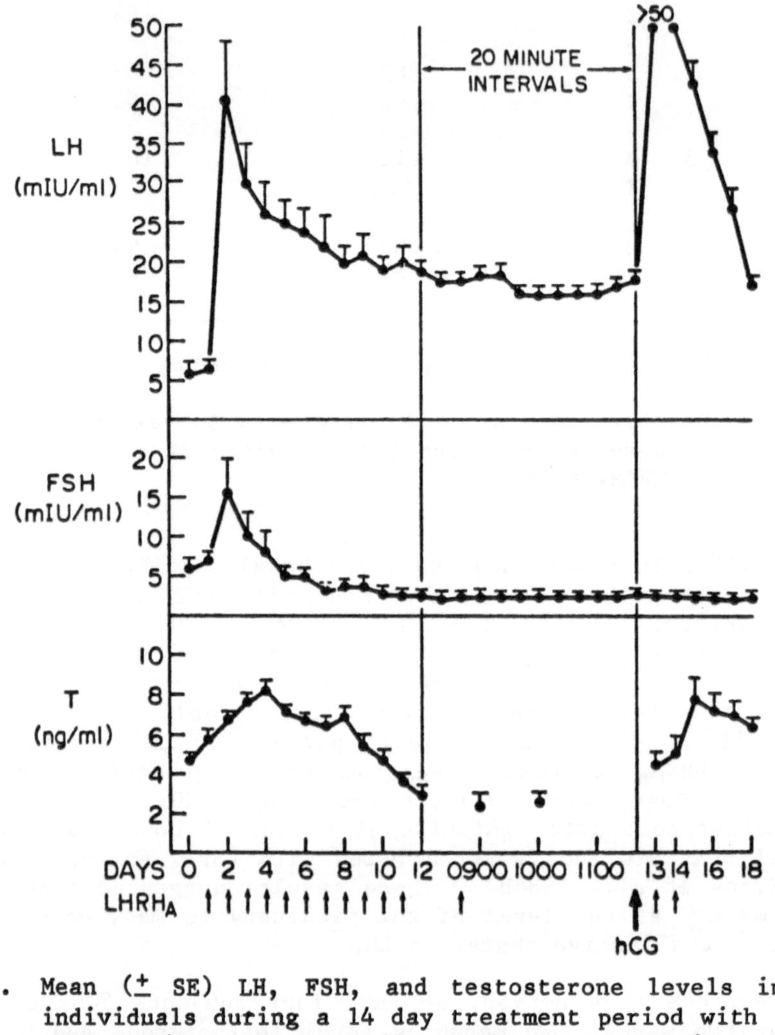

Fig. 2. Mean (± SE) LH, FSH, and testosterone levels in four individuals during a 14 day treatment period with 500 μg $LHRH_A$ daily. On day 12 samples were obtained at 20-minute intervals. Arrows indicate injections of $LHRH_A$. All subjects received a single injection of 4,000 units hCG I.M. on day 12. Reprinted with permission from J. Clin. Invest. 73:262-266, 1984.

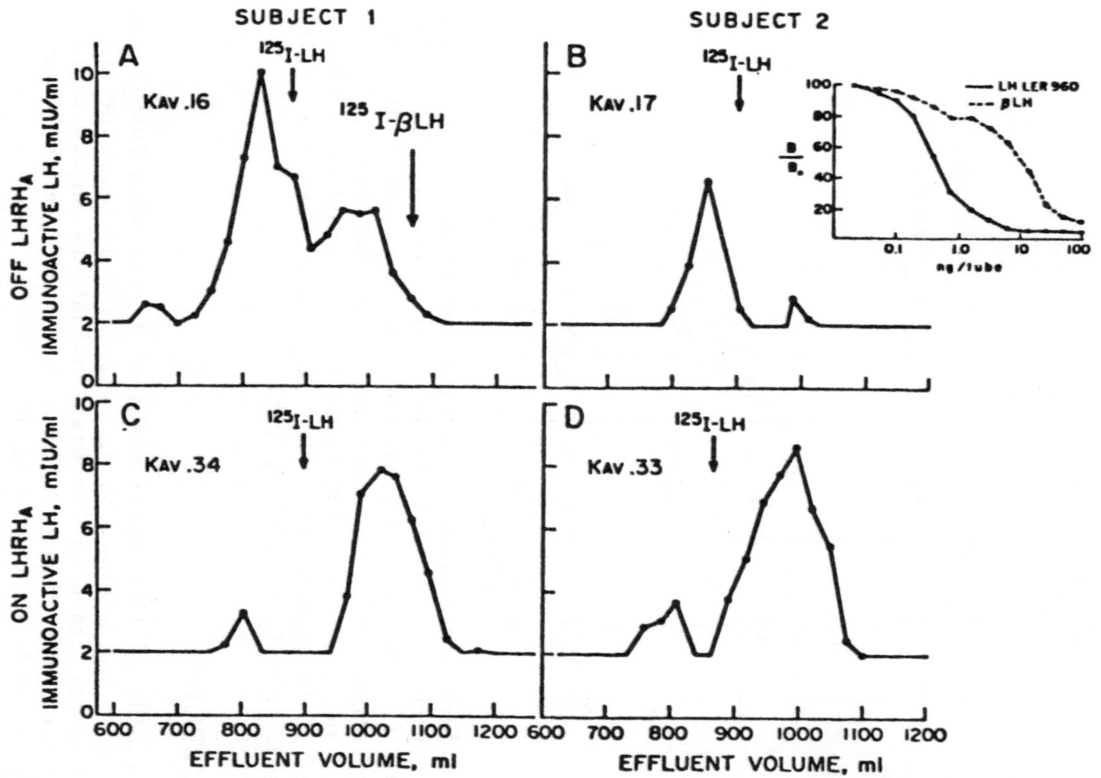

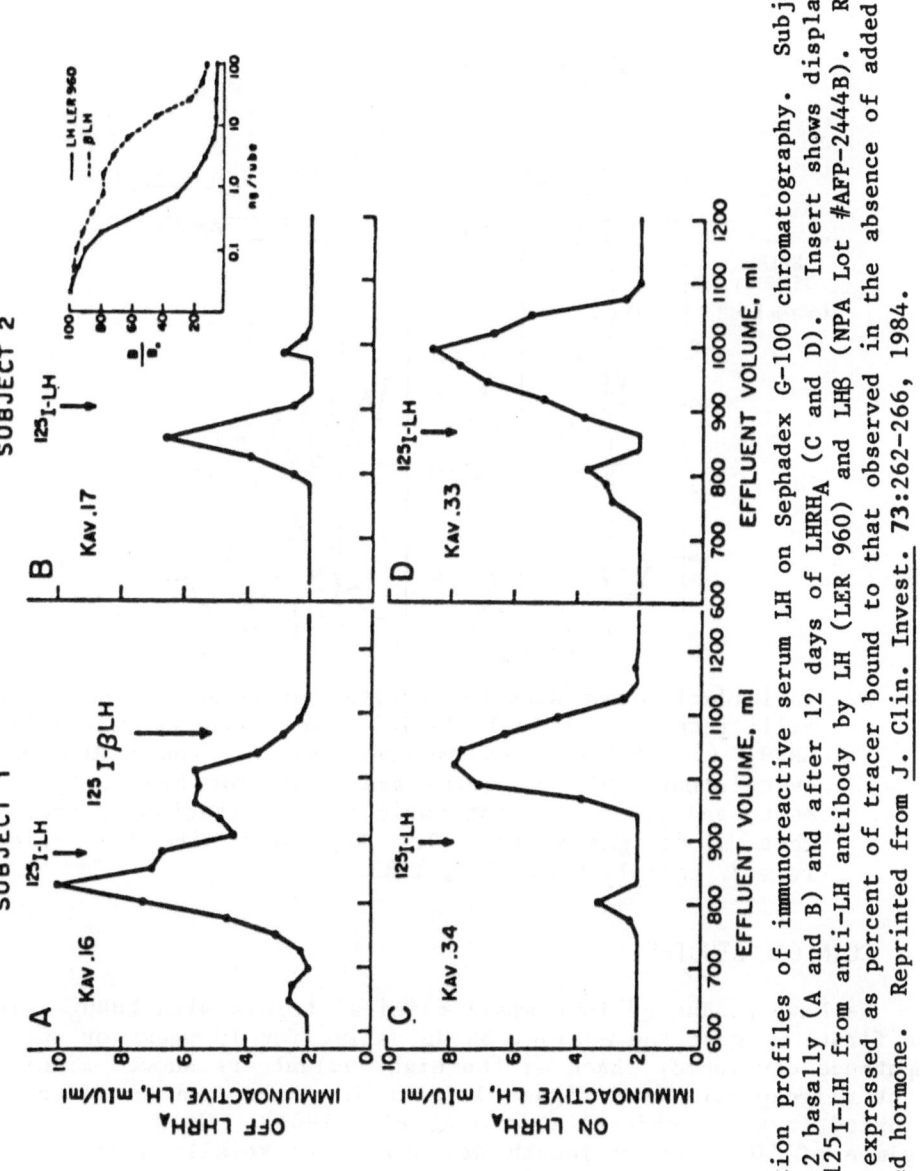

Fig. 3. Elution profiles of immunoreactive serum LH on Sephadex G-100 chromatography. Subjects 1 and 2 basally (A and B) and after 12 days of LHRH$_A$ (C and D). Insert shows displacement of ^{125}I-LH from anti-LH antibody by LH (LER 960) and LHβ (NPA Lot #AFP-2444B). Results are expressed as percent of tracer bound to that observed in the absence of added unlabeled hormone. Reprinted from J. Clin. Invest. 73:262-266, 1984.

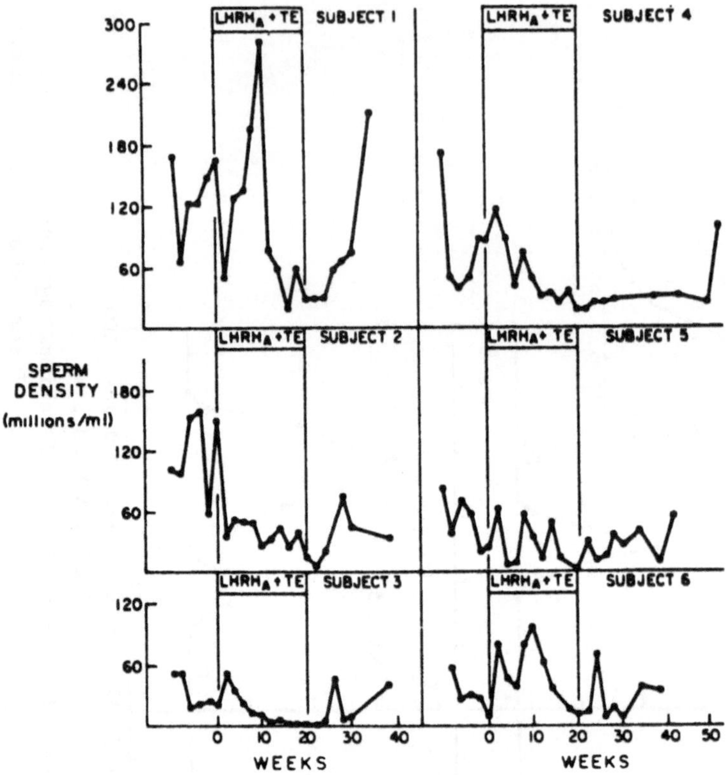

Fig. 4. Individual sperm density results (millions of sperm per milliliter of seminal fluid) for subjects receiving $LHRH_A$ (50 μg/day) and testosterone enanthate 100 mg/ every other week. Results are shown for basal, treatment, and post-treatment periods. Institution of treatment is designated week 0. Reprinted with permission from J. Androl. 4:298-301, 1983.

3. CLINICAL STUDIES

We have conducted four small clinical trials with $LHRH_A$. In the first, we gave the analog, 50 μg daily, for 10 weeks or until impotence developed. Each of the eight volunteers showed significant oligospermia (see Figure 1), but impotence and hot flashes occurred in most subjects (Linde et al., 1981). We next tried a regimen of 50 μg every fourth day which was totally ineffective (Doelle et al., 1982).

In the third study, we administered $LHRH_A$, 50 μg daily, plus a dosage schedule of testosterone enanthate (TE), 100 mg IM every two weeks, which we had shown did not influence sperm density (Doelle et al., 1983). Results appear in Figure 4. A fall in sperm density was noted in all six subjects, but the degree was quite variable, and while the addition of TE had eliminated the side effects of impotence and hot flashes, the regimen was not satisfactory as a contraceptive (Doelle et al., 1983). We wondered whether we could improve results by increasing the amount of $LHRH_A$ to 100 or 500 μg daily. The dosage of TE remained 100 mg every other week. Figure 5 shows that heterogeneity in sperm density profiles persisted even with the higher $LHRH_A$ dosages.

4. CONCLUSIONS

It appears from our data that the mode of action of $LHRH_A$ differs in the rat and in man. The pituitary is the principal locus in man. We concur with those who caution against extrap-

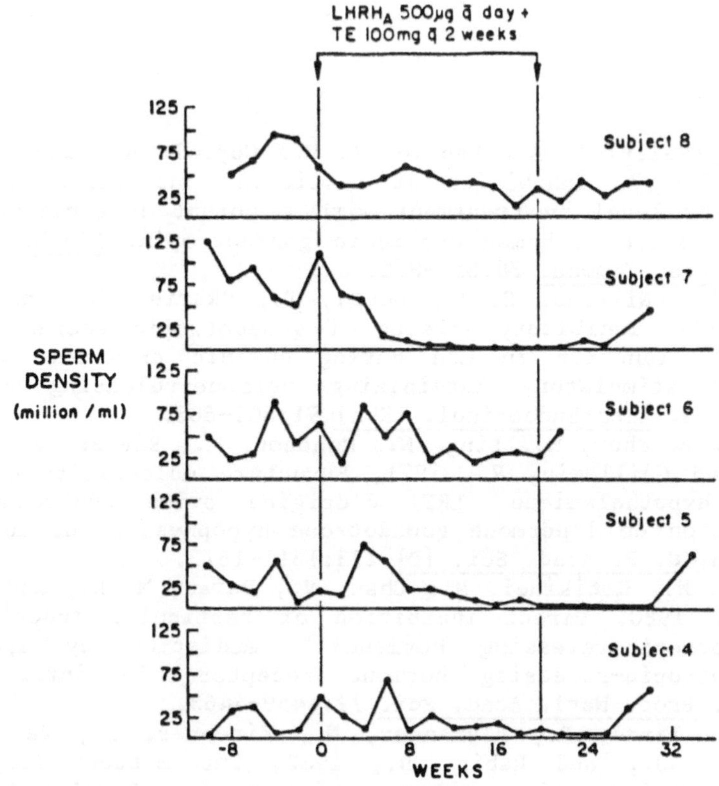

Fig. 5. Values of sperm density in five subjects before, during, and after treatment with $LHRH_A$, 500 μg daily for 20 weeks, and testosterone enanthate, 100 mg intramuscularly every two weeks.

olating findings in the rat - the most frequently used experimental model for LHRH analogs - to humans. We have explored various clinical regimens using $LHRH_A$ with TE, but none has yielded results sufficiently consistent to warrant large-scale testing as a male contraceptive. Other studies are in progress.

ACKNOWLEDGEMENTS

D.R. wishes to pay tribute to Dr. Hans Lindner, scientist, academic leader, and generous colleague who inspired a generation of endocrinologists.

We thank Dr. Wylie Vale and Dr. Jean Rivier of the Salk Institute for provision of $LHRH_A$ and cordial cooperation. Ms. A. N. Alexander, Mr. D. P. Island, and Ms. Jill Lindner made valuable contributions to our studies. We thank Ms. Bettye Rid ley for expert secretarial assistance. This work was supported by the following grants and grants-in-aid: Ford Foundation #810-0297, NIH #R01-HD16453, and Clinical Research Center #5-M01 RR-95.

REFERENCES

Auclair C., Kelly, P. A., Labrie, A. V., Coy, D. H., and Scally, A. V., 1977, Inhibition of testicular luteinizing hormone receptor level by treatment with a potent luteinizing hormone agonist or human chorionic gonadotropin, Biochem. Biophys. Res. Commun. **76**:855-862.

Berquist, D., Nillius, S. J., Bergh, T., Skarin, G., and Wide, L., 1979, Inhibitory effects of gonadotropin secretion and gonadal function in men during chronic treatment with a potent stimulatory luteinizing hormone-releasing hormone analogue, Acta Endocrinol. (Kbh) **91**:601-608.

Burgus, R., Butcher, M., Ling, N., Monahon, M., Rivier, J., Vale, W., and Guillemin, R., 1971, Structure moleculaire du facteur hypothalamique (LRF) d'origine ovine controlant la secretion de l'hormone gonadotrope hypophysaire de luteinisation, C. R. Acad. Sci. [D] **273**:1611-1613.

Clayton, R. N., Katikinei, M., Chan, V., Dufau, M. L., and Catt, K. J., 1980, Direct inhibition of testicular function by gonadotropin-releasing hormone: mediation by specific gonadotropin-releasing hormone receptors in interstitial cells, Proc. Natl. Acad. Sci. **77**:4459-4463.

Doelle, G., Linde, R., Alexander, N., Kirchner, F., Vale, W., Rivier, J., and Rabin, D., 1982, Intermittent long-term administration of a potent gonadotropin-releasing hormone agonist in normal men, Int. J. Fertil. **27**:234-237.

Doelle, G. C., Alexander, A. N., Evans, R. M., Linde, R., Rivier, J., Vale, W., and Rabin, D., 1983, Combined treatment with an LHRH agonist and testosterone in man, J. Androl. **4**:298-302.

Evans, R. M., Doelle, G. C., Alexander, A. N., Uderman, H. D., and Rabin, D., 1984a, Gonadotropin and steroid secretory patterns during chronic treatment with a luteinizing hormone releasing hormone agonist analog in men, J. Clin. Endocrinol. Metab., in press.

Evans, R. M., Doelle, G. C., Lindner, J., Bradley, V., and Rabin, D., 1984b, A luteinizing hormone agonist analog modifies the biologic activity and chromatographic behavior of luteinizing hormone, J. Clin. Invest. **73**:262-266.

Hsueh, A. J. W., and Erickson, G. F., 1979, Extrapituitary inhibition of testicular function by luteinizing hormone releasing hormone, Nature **281**:66-67.

Hsueh, A. J. W., Dufau, M. L., and Catt, K. J., 1976, Regulation of luteinizing hormone receptors in testicular interstitial cells by gonadotropin, Biochem. Biophys. Res. Commun. **72**:1145-1152.

Linde, R., Doelle, G. C., Alexander, N., Kirchner, F., Vale, W., Rivier, J., and Rabin, D., 1981, Reversible inhibition of testicular steroidogenesis and spermatogenesis by a potent gonadotropin-releasing hormone agonist in normal men: an approach toward the development of a male contraceptive, N. Engl. J. Med. **305**:663-667.

Rivier, C., and Vale, W., Hormonal secretion of rats chronically treated with D-Trp^6,Pro^9-NEt-LRF, Life Sci. **25**:1065-1074.

Sandow, J., v Rechenberg, W., Baeder, C., and Engelbart, K., 1980, Antifertility effects of an LH-RH analogue in male rats and dogs, Int. J. Fertil. **25**:213-221.

Schally, A. V., Animura, A., Kashin, A. J., Matsuo, H., Boba, Y., Redding, T. W., Nair, R. M. G., and Dabeljuk, L., 1971, Gonadotropin-releasing hormone: one polypeptide regulates secretion of luteinizing and follicle-stimulating hormones, Science **173**:1036-1038.

Swerdlow, R. S., Heber, D., Bhasin, S., and Rajfer, J., 1983, Effect of GnRH superactive analogs (alone and combined with androgen) on testicular function in man and experimental animals, J. Steroid Biochem. 19:491-497.

Tcholakian, R. K., De La Cruz, A., Chowdhury, M., Steinberger, A., Coy, D. H., and Schally, A. V., 1978, Unusual antireproductive properties of the analog [D-Leu^6,Des-Gly-NH_2^{10}]-luteinizing hormone-releasing hormone ethylamide in male rats, Fertil. Steril. **30**:600-603.

Vale, W., Rivier, C., Brown, M., and Rivier, J., 1977, Pharmacology of thyrotropin releasing factor (TRF), luteinizing hormone releasing factor (LRF), and somatostatin, Adv. Exp. Med. Biol. **87**:123-156.

HYPOTHALAMIC-PITUITARY-GONADAL AXIS: CONCLUDING REMARKS

George Fink

MRC Brain Metabolism Unit
Department of Pharmacology
1 George Square
Edinburgh EH8 9JZ, Scotland

During the last five days we have been treated to a feast of sophisticated data on the interactions that occur between the brain, the anterior pituitary gland and the gonads. In the female of most mammals these interactions result in a spontaneous surge of LH which causes ovulation and the formation of corpora lutea (Figs. 1 and 2). Essentially, the hypothalamic-pituitary system and the ovary can be considered as two oscillators which achieve resonance at regular intervals (with a frequency of 4 days to a year) to result in the LH surge and ovulation. In the male the interactions between the hypothalamic-pituitary system and the gonads are less dramatic than in the female, but lead to the equally important production of sperm and androgens. The nature of the interactions within and between components of the hypothalamic-pituitary-gonadal axis was the subject of this meeting, and Hans Lindner would have been delighted with the level of most of the presentations and discussion.

Neural control of the pituitary gland is mediated by the decapeptide LHRH. Most of the LHRH cell bodies are in the rostral diencephalon and send their projections to the primary plexus of the hypophysial portal vessels which convey the peptide (Fig. 3) to the anterior pituitary gland. There are phylogenetic differences in the amino acid sequence of LHRH with changes occurring mainly at the Arg^8 position. The synthesis and release of LHRH is greatly influenced by steroids whose action is mediated and/or modulated by other transmitter systems such as monoaminergic, cholinergic and opioid.

LHRH is synthesized as a component of a 28,000 MW precursor, the mRNA for which is present in the hypothalamus of man, rat and normal mouse. The decapeptide is released into hypophysial portal

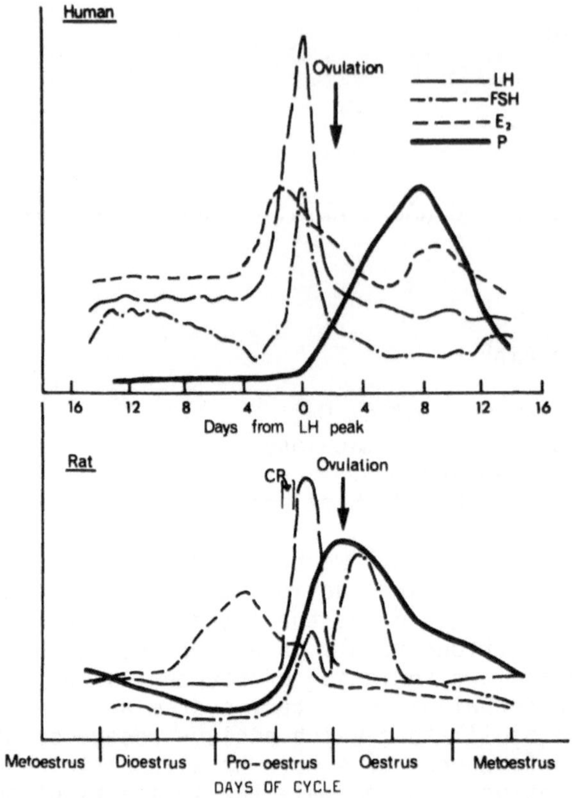

Fig. 1 Schematic diagram of the key hormonal changes during the menstrual cycle of the human and estrous cycle of the rat. The critical period (CP) in the rat is the time before which administration of neural blocking agents will block the LH surge and ovulation. Reproduced with permission of Churchill Livingstone from ref. 2.

blood in amounts consistent with its role in releasing LH under most physiological and experimental conditions. Many studies, including those on the hypogonadal mouse, a mutant totally deficient in LHRH (and the LHRH precursor mRNA), have shown that LHRH is a potent stimulus for the synthesis and release of FSH as well as LH. Processing of the LHRH precursor and degradation of LHRH itself depends upon peptidases which offer potentially important alternative mechanisms for biological regulation and methods for pharmacological intervention.

At the level of the pituitary gland (Figs. 2 and 3), the

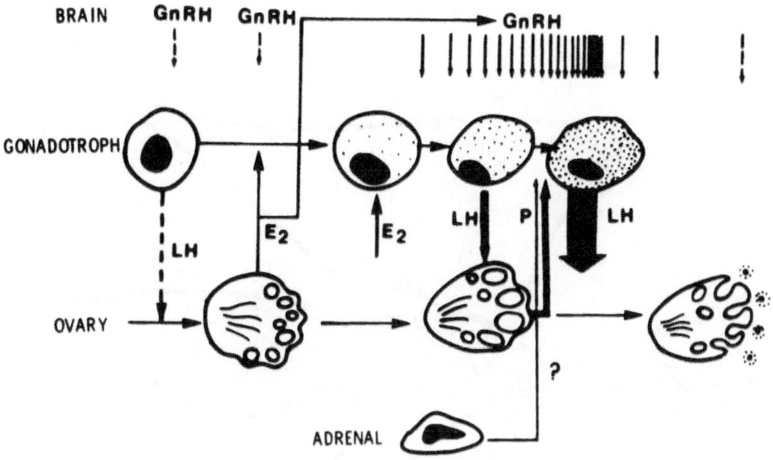

Fig. 2 Schematic diagram illustrating the interactions between the brain, pituitary gonadotrophs and the ovary in producing the spontaneous ovulatory surge of LH and ovulation. 'Basal' secretion of FSH and LH stimulates growth of ovarian follicles and the secretion of estradiol-17β (E_2). This ovarian signal (E_2) increases the responsiveness of the pituitary gonadotrophs (increased stippling) to GnRH (referred to as LHRH elsewhere in this section) and also triggers the surge of LHRH. Pituitary responsiveness to GnRH is further increased by progesterone (P) secreted from the ovary in response to the LH released during the early part of the LH surge and by the priming effect of GnRH. (Adrenal P may also play a role in some mammals.) The priming effect of GnRH coordinates the surge of GnRH with increasing pituitary responsiveness so that the two events reach a peak at the same time. The conditions are thereby made optimal for a massive surge of LH. This cascade, which represents a form of positive feedback, is terminated by the rupture of ovarian follicles (ovulation). Although this scheme is based mainly on studies on the rat, a similar cascade with some variations seems to operate in other spontaneously ovulating mammals including man. The broad descriptive physiology is now well established but the details of the cellular mechanisms at each level are yet to be elucidated. Adapted from ref. 3 and published with permission of the British Council.

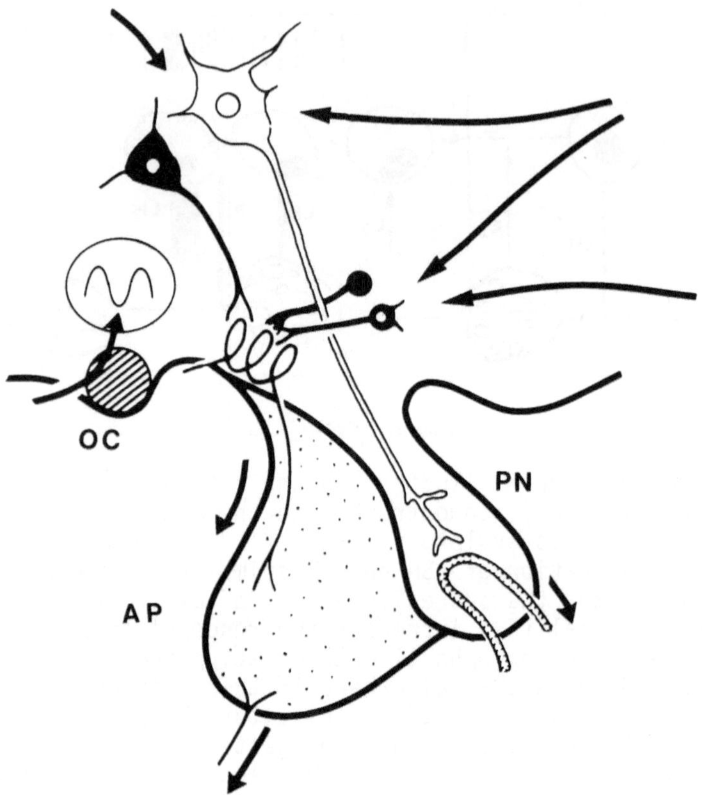

Fig. 3 A schematic diagram showing the main features of the hypothalamic-pituitary system showing the magnocellular (white) projections directly to the systemic vessels in the pars nervosa (PN) and the parvocellular (black) projections to the primary plexus of the hypophysial portal vessels which convey transmitters to the pars distalis of the anterior pituitary gland (AP). Dorsal to the optic chiasm (OC) are the suprachiasmatic nuclei which receive direct projections from the retina and play a key role in the control of circadian and other rhythms. The activity of the intrinsic neurons of the hypothalamus is greatly influenced by projections (arrows) from numerous areas of the forebrain and hindbrain, particularly the limbic system, as well as by hormones.

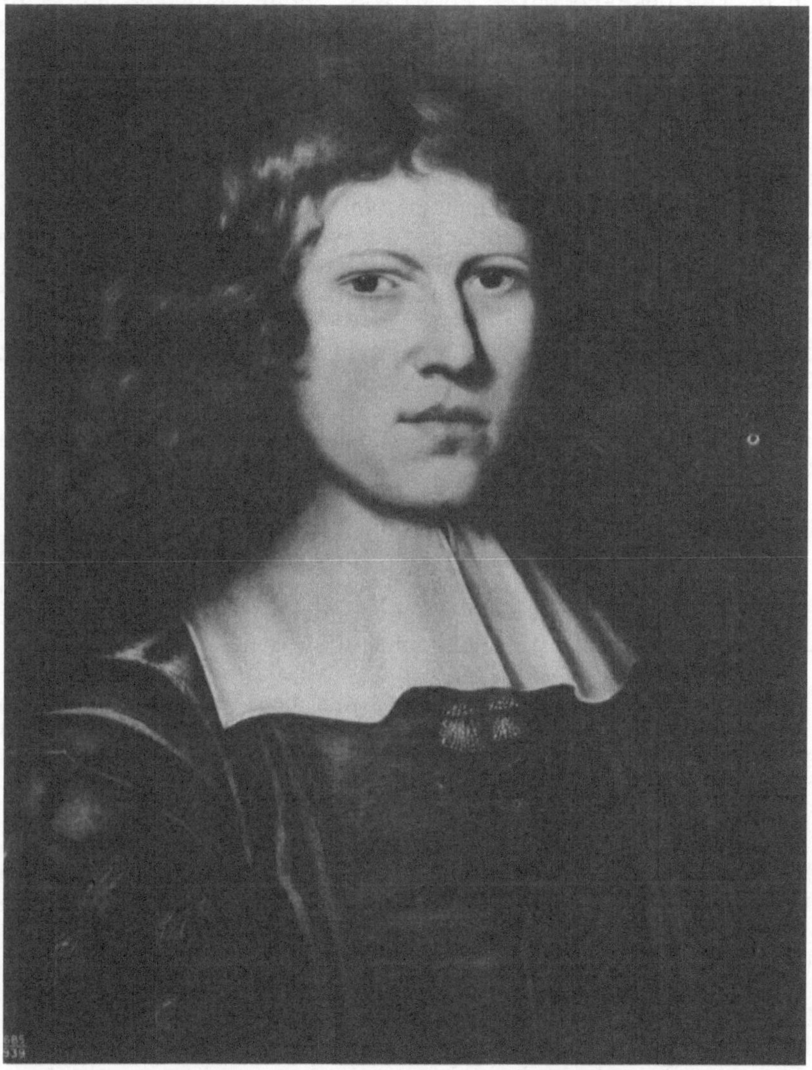

Fig. 4 Richard Lower (1631-1691), the Oxford physician and physiologist who overturned Galen's hypothesis regarding the fate of 'vital' and 'animal spirits' in the brain, and provided a template for the modern neurohumoral hypothesis of the control of the anterior pituitary gland. Reproduced with the kind permission of The Wellcome Institute Library, London.

abundance of LHRH receptors is increased ('up-regulation') by exposure to low concentrations of LHRH, or by intermittent exposure to LHRH, and reduced ('down-regulation') by continuous exposure to relatively high concentrations of LHRH. Aggregation and internalization of the LHRH-receptor complexes occur, but are not a prerequisite for LHRH-induced LH release and in this respect LHRH differs from some other biologically active peptides whose action appears to be dependent upon aggregation and internalization.

Photoaffinity labelling studies showed that LHRH binds to a single 60,000 MW protein in the pituitary gland while in the ovary two protein bands of 54,000 and 60,000 bind LHRH. The acute LH-releasing action of LHRH appears to involve mainly the Ca^{2+} generating system. The action of LHRH on Ca^{2+} generation may be mediated by phospholipids, especially, phosphatidic acid which, derived from phosphatidylinositol, may serve as a Ca^{2+} ionophore. The turnover of phosphatidylinositol is increased significantly by LHRH both in pituitary as well as gonadal cells.

Recent ultrastructural studies of gonadotrophs challenged the accepted view that all secretory products are packaged in the Golgi, while Erlich's dictum, 'Alles ist die Methode', was exemplified by recent immunohistochemical studies of thin ($\sim$ 1 μm) pituitary sections which showed that a relatively large proportion of gonadotrophs, in fact, contained only LH or FSH, but not both. That is, in contrast to earlier findings which were based on the results of using thicker (4-8 μm) sections, many gonadotrophs are 'monohormonal'.

A most important recent finding was that deglycosylated gonadotropins are potent and specific antagonists which can be used as probes to investigate the action of gonadotropins on the gonads, and may in addition provide another alternative method for fertility control.

A series of elegant papers reviewed in detail the data on the mechanism of action of the gonadotropins on the gonads and the way these interact with intricate intrinsic mechanisms to control gametogenesis and steroidogenesis.

In addition to the gonadotropins and endogenous steroids, peptides might be produced by the gonads which may have local effects. Thus, for example, there is evidence for a peptide ovum maturation inhibiting factor, and for an action of LHRH agonists on both the ovary and the testis. Whether a LHRH-like substance with physiological actions is actually produced by the gonads is yet to be established.

The meeting concluded with the lectures on the clinical applications of data produced mainly by experimental studies. Here, information on the fact that continuous exposure to super-active agonists of LHRH down-regulate LHRH receptors while pulsatile LHRH administration can produce normal, or by way of the priming effect, increased gonadotropin release, has been used to employ LHRH analogues for the treatment of prostatic cancer (in combination with anti-androgens) and infertility, and for the development of alternative methods of contraception.

The meeting showed that there were still large gaps in our understanding of mechanisms at the cellular level. How does E_2 actually modulate LHRH synthesis and release? What is the precise mechanism of action of LHRH - why does its releasing action differ from its priming action? What factors are involved in selecting the ovarian follicle of the month, what factors regulate meiosis, and what determines the precision of the spermatogenic cycle? The answers to these and other questions may require major conceptual leaps as well as in-depth research. An example of a major conceptual leap was the neurohumoral hypothesis of the control of the anterior pituitary gland. There is no doubt that the intelligent and elegant studies of Geoffrey Wingfield Harris proved the hypothesis, but there has been debate as to whether Harris, Hinsey or Friedgood were the first to propose the hypothesis in a form that could be tested by experiment. In fact, broadly speaking it may be argued that Richard Lower (Fig. 4) was the first to propose the neurohumoral hypothesis. In 1670, Lower, an Oxford physician and physiologist who was assistant to Thomas Willis and eventually physician to Charles II, appended to his 'de Corde' a short account 'Dissertate de Origine Catarrhi' (1) in which he overturned Galen's thesis that 'animal spirit' was formed from 'vital spirit' in the brain and that the waste products passed through the ventricles to be distilled in the pituitary gland into the nose as nasal mucus ('pituita'). Lower showed by experiment that there was no connection between the pituitary gland and the nose and therefore concluded; 'whatever fluid is secreted into the ventricles of the brain and goes from there to the infundibulum to the glandular pituitaria distils not upon the palate but is passed again into the blood and mixed with it'. Thus, Lower not only provided the template for the modern neurohumoral hypothesis, but also, by way of a conceptually difficult but technically simple experiment, overturned Galen's view that had been held firmly for more than a millenium. There is a direct link between Lower and Lindner in that the renaissance in Biology led by men such as William Harvey and Richard Lower led directly to the development of the great schools of Zoology and Physiology at Edinburgh, Cambridge and Oxford in whose furnaces was tempered the steel of men such as W. Heape, F.H.A. Marshall, E.B. Verney, G.W. Harris and Hans Lindner.

REFERENCES

1. R. Lower (1670) Dissertation de origine catarrhi (an addendum to the second edition of De Corde). At the press of J. Redmayne, at the expense of Jacobi Allestry, at the sign of the Rose and Crown, St. Paul's Churchyard, London.

2. G. Fink, in: Recent Advances in Obstetrics and Gynaecology, J. Stallworthy and G. Bourne, eds., pp. 4-54, Churchill Livingstone, Edinburgh (1977).
3. G. Fink, Brit. Med. Bull. 35:155 (1979).

INDEX